Pediatric and Adult Hand Fractures

Joshua M. Abzug · R. Glenn Gaston
A. Lee Osterman · Richard J. Tosti
Editors

Pediatric and Adult Hand Fractures

A Clinical Guide to Management

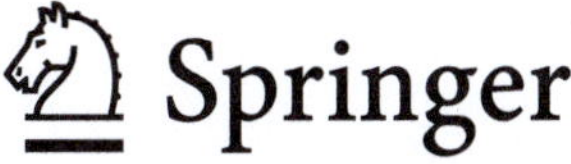
Springer

Editors
Joshua M. Abzug
Department of Orthopedic Surgery
University of Maryland School of Medicine
Baltimore, MD, USA

A. Lee Osterman
Philadelphia Hand to Shoulder Center
Thomas Jefferson University Hospital
Philadelphia, PA, USA

R. Glenn Gaston
Atrium Health Carolinas Medical Center
Charlotte, NC, USA

Richard J. Tosti
Rothman Orthopaedic Institute
Department of Orthopaedic Surgery
Thomas Jefferson University
Philadelphia, PA, USA

ISBN 978-3-031-32074-3   ISBN 978-3-031-32072-9   (eBook)
https://doi.org/10.1007/978-3-031-32072-9

This Springer imprint is published by the registered company Springer Nature Switzerland AG
The registered company address is: Gewerbestrasse 11, 6330 Cham, Switzerland

Contents

Anatomy and Osseous and Functional Development of the Hand

Catherine C. May, Haley A. Jacobs, and Joshua M. Abzug

Introduction

Hand fractures are one of the most common injuries in pediatric patients. Around 50% of all fractures in children and adolescents occur in the distal radius, metacarpals, and phalanges [1]. These injuries, which often take place during sports-related activities, are a leading cause of emergency room visits in this population [2]. Proper diagnosis of hand fractures in pediatric patients may be challenging due to the presence of the physes and incomplete ossification of the bony structures [3]. Currently, there is a misdiagnosis rate of 8% associated with pediatric hand fractures [3]. Therefore, it is crucial to establish a thorough understanding of the anatomy and development of the pediatric hand to ensure timely and appropriate treatment of an injury. With proper management, pediatric hand fractures may heal quickly with minimal complications [3, 4].

Anatomy

The hand is one of the most intricate structures in the human body, designed to accomplish complex tasks unique to humans [5, 6]. Due to the delicate nature of its movements, both sensory and mechanical features must be intact for normal

---

Disclaimers: The views expressed in the submitted article are our own and not an official position of the institution.

C. C. May · H. A. Jacobs · J. M. Abzug (✉)
Department of Orthopedic Surgery, University of Maryland School of Medicine, Baltimore, MD, USA
e-mail: catherine.may@som.umaryland.edu; haley.jacobs@som.umaryland.edu; jabzug@som.umaryland.edu

functioning and development of the hand to be possible [5, 6]. Injuries to this region may interfere with the interdependent structures of the hand [6]. In order to understand pediatric hand fractures and their management, this chapter will outline the anatomy of the hand as well as its osseous and functional development [5].

Bones

The bones of the hand and wrist region may be divided into three categories: carpals, metacarpals, and phalanges [5]. The carpals are the most proximal and are often referred to as the "wrist" of the hand due to their articulation with the metacarpals and anatomical location at the base of the hand clinically (Fig. 1.1) [5]. The carpus consists of eight small bones arranged in two rows [5]. The more proximal row contains the scaphoid, lunate, triquetrum, and pisiform bones (anatomical position lateral/radial to medial/ulnar), which articulate with the radius and ulna [5]. Intercarpal ligaments restrict movement of this carpal row by tightly connecting the bones to one another [6]. The distal row is made up of the trapezium, trapezoid,

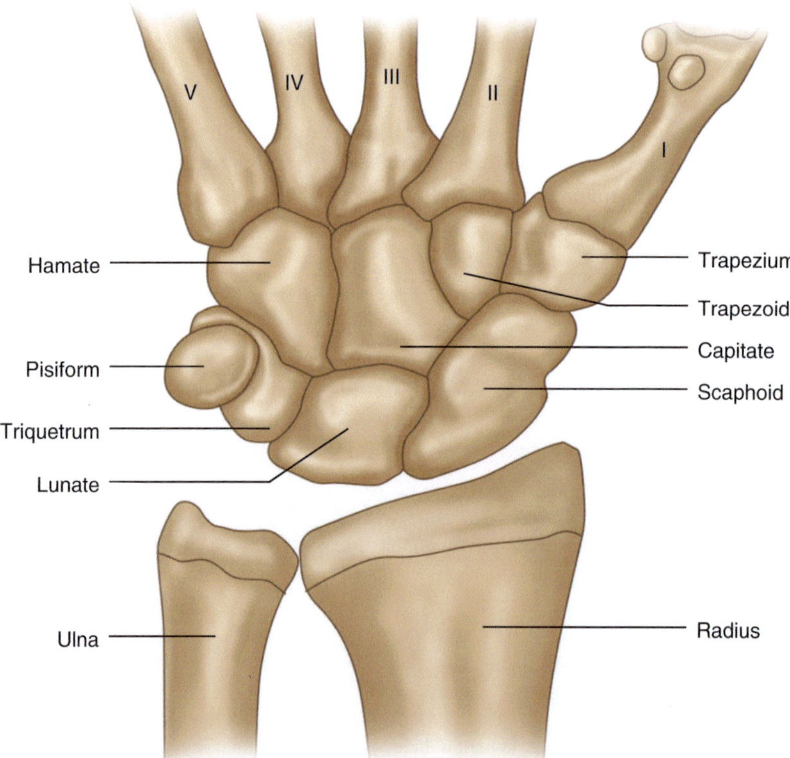

Fig. 1.1 Schematic drawing of the carpal bones (Courtesy of Catherine C. May, BS)

capitate, and hamate bones (anatomical position lateral/radial to medial/ulnar) [5]. The bones in this row are subject to movement based on neighboring articulations [6]. Additionally, there is intercarpal articulation present between the two rows of carpal bones [5].

The metacarpals articulate with the distal extent of the distal row of carpal bones to create the palm of the hand (Fig. 1.2). There are five metacarpal bones that are

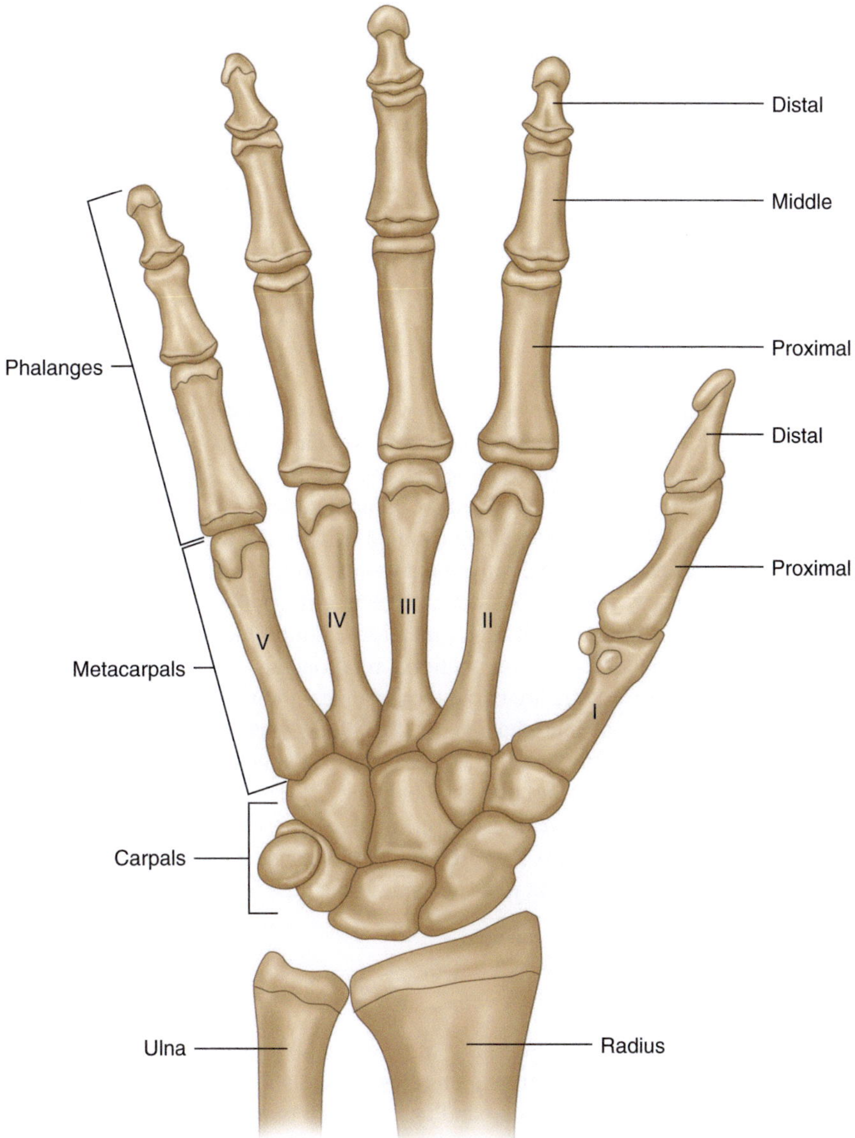

Fig. 1.2 Schematic drawing of the bones of the hand (Courtesy of Catherine C. May, BS)

numbered I through V, with the first metacarpal (I) located at the base of the thumb and the fifth metacarpal (V) located at the base of the small finger [5]. The metacarpals are classified as long bones with a base, diaphysis, and metacarpal head/neck region distally [7]. The proximal aspect of each metacarpal articulates with the carpal bones, while the distal metacarpal head articulates with the phalanges [5]. Due to the close articulation of the metacarpals to the adjacent carpals, the digits are not able to move independently without some movement from the other digits [5]. The thumb is an exception to this as it has increased mobility about the articulation between the carpals and the first metacarpal [5].

The distal aspect of the hand is comprised of the digits, each of which has three phalanges, except for the thumb which has two phalanges. Phalanges are also classified as long bones (Fig. 1.2). Digits II through V have the same anatomical design with three phalanges called the proximal phalanx, middle phalanx, and distal phalanx [5]. The thumb has only two phalanges, called the proximal phalanx and the distal phalanx [5]. Digits II through V may also be termed the index finger, long/middle finger, ring finger, or small/little finger, respectively.

Joints

Between the bones, there are several joints which permit movement of the hand and the digits (Fig. 1.3) [5]. The intercarpal joints are plane joints which rest between the carpal bones and allow them to glide past one another [5]. The junction between the carpals and the metacarpals is called the carpometacarpal (CMC) joint [5]. Most of the CMC joints allow rotation along a single axis [6]. However, IV and V CMC joints may experience additional movement compared to the II and III CMC joints because the fifth CMC joint is considered to be a semi-saddle joint [6]. The thumb contains a saddle CMC joint that offers increased motion including flexion, extension, abduction, adduction, and conjunctional rotation [6].

In digits II through V, there are two interphalangeal joints between the three phalanges [5]. The proximal interphalangeal (PIP) joint rests between the proximal phalanx and middle phalanx, while the distal interphalangeal (DIP) joint is located between the middle phalanx and the distal phalanx [5]. The PIP joints are stabilized by ligaments to prevent hyperextension of the digits [6]. Often, the PIP joint must maintain flexion in order to flex the DIP joint [6]. Because the thumb contains only two phalanges, there is only one joint present, termed the interphalangeal joint [6].

Muscles and Tendons

Each digit is controlled by six muscles: three extrinsic muscles and three intrinsic muscles (Table 1.1) [6]. The extrinsic muscles of the hand originate in the forearm and cross the wrist to insert in the hand and produce movement [5]. Each digit is controlled by two long flexors and one long extensor [6]. Additional extrinsic extensors are present in the small finger and index fingers [6]. The muscles stem from

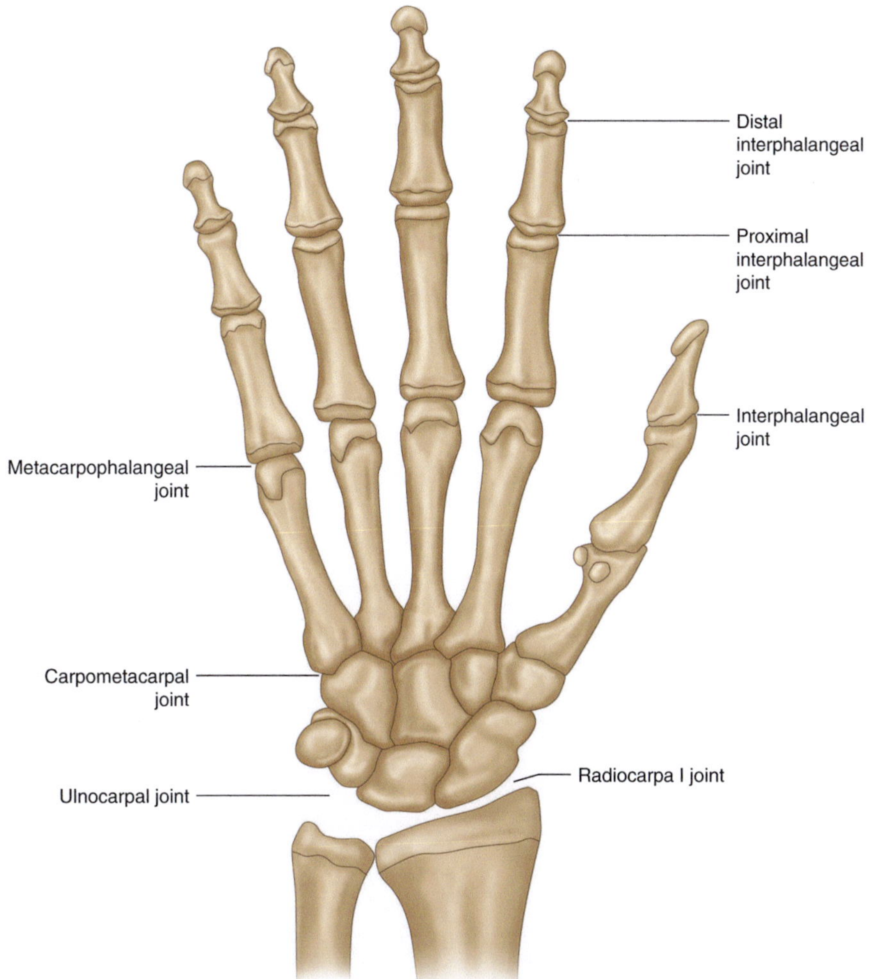

Fig. 1.3 Schematic drawing of the joints of the hand (Courtesy of Catherine C. May, BS)

various locations within the forearm in order to generate specific movements [5]. For example, the muscles responsible for flexion may originate on the medial epicondyle of the humerus, as well as the volar portions of the ulna and radius [5]. Conversely, muscles which generate extension originate on the lateral epicondyle or the ulna and insert across the dorsal portion of the wrist and hand [5].

The intrinsic hand muscles both originate and insert within the hand [5, 6]. The intrinsic muscles may be categorized as thenar, hypothenar, lumbricals, and interosseous muscles [5, 8]. Each digit is controlled by three intrinsic muscles including a dorsal interosseous, palmar interosseous, and lumbrical muscle [6]. The movements produced by these muscles include abduction and adduction of the digits, as well as aid in flexion of the MCP joints and extension of the IP joints [5, 8].

Table 1.1 Muscles of the forearm, hand, and fingers

Muscle		Origin	Insertion	Function
Supinator		Lateral epicondyle of humerus	Proximal end of radius	Supination of wrist
Pronator quadratus		Distal anterior ulna	Anterior distal radius	Pronation of forearm
Pronator teres		Medial epicondyle of humerus	Midshaft of radius	Pronation of wrist
Dorsal interossei	I	Medial side of the proximal end of metacarpal I and lateral side of metacarpal II	Lateral base of proximal phalanx II and extensor expansion	Abduction of fingers: Flexion of the MCP joints: Extension of the IP joints
	II	Medial side of metacarpal II and lateral side of metacarpal III	Lateral base of proximal phalanx III and extensor expansion	
	III	Medial side of metacarpal III and lateral side of metacarpal IV	Medial side of proximal phalanx III and extensor expansion	
	IV	Medial side of metacarpal IV and lateral side of metacarpal V	Medial side of proximal phalanx IV and extensor expansion	
Palmar interossei	I	Lateral side of metacarpal I	Sesamoid bone on proximal phalanx of thumb and extensor expansion	Adduction of fingers: Flexion of MCP joints: Extension of PIP and IP joints
	II	Metacarpal II	Ipsilateral extensor expansion of phalanx II	
	III	Medial side of metacarpal IV	Medial side of proximal phalanx IV and extensor expansion	
	IV	Medial side of metacarpal V	Proximal phalanx V and extensor tendon	
Hypothenar	Abductor digiti minimi	Pisiform bone and dorsal aponeurosis	Lateral side of proximal phalanx V and extensor expansion	Abduction of small finger at MCP joint; flexion of IP joint
	Flexor digiti minimi brevis	Hamate bone and flexor retinaculum	Medial side of proximal phalanx V	Flexion of small finger; lateral rotation and opposition of small finger
	Opponens digiti minimi	Hamate bone and flexor retinaculum	Lateral side of metacarpal V	Flexion of small finger; lateral rotation and opposition of small finger
	Palmaris brevis	Palmar aponeurosis and flexor retinaculum	Dermis of hypothenar skin	Tighten palmar aponeurosis

Table 1.1 (continued)

Muscle		Origin	Insertion	Function
Thenar	Abductor pollicis brevis	Scaphoid and trapezium bones, flexor retinaculum	Lateral side of proximal phalanx I	Abduction of thumb at CMC joint; opposition and flexion of thumb
	Adductor pollicis	Metacarpal II, III, and capitate bone	Medial side of proximal phalanx I	Adduction of thumb at CMC joint; opposition of thumb
	Flexor pollicis brevis	Flexor retinaculum, trapezium, trapezoid, and capitate bones	Proximal phalanx I	Flexion of thumb at MCP and CMC joints; medial rotation of thumb
	Opponens pollicis	Trapezium bone and flexor retinaculum	Lateral side of metacarpal I	Opposition of thumb at CMC joint
Lumbricals	I	Medial side of most radial tendon of flexor digitorum profundus	Extensor expansion near MCP joint of index finger	Flexion of MCP joint; extension of PIP and DIP joints
	II	Medial side of the second most radial tendon of flexor digitorum profundus	Extensor expansion near MCP joint of middle finger	
	III	Radial side of flexor digitorum profundus tendon near ring finger and lateral side of tendon for middle finger	Extensor expansion of ring finger	
	IV	Medial side of flexor digitorum profundus tendon of small finger and lateral side of tendon for ring finger	Extensor expansion of small finger	

The interosseous muscles ensure balance and stability of the digits. When damaged, the interosseous muscles shorten, causing what is referred to as "intrinsic tightness" [6]. Swelling of the muscle tissue results in the development of scar tissue and muscle shortening [6].

The lumbricals originate on the flexor digitorum profundus (FDP) and insert on the lateral portion of the extensor tendon [6]. The lumbrical muscles are involved in MCP joint flexion, and proximal and distal interphalangeal joint extension [6]. Movements produced by the lumbricals allow humans to perform quick alternation of the digits [6].

Flexors

The flexor tendons are housed and protected by flexor tendon sheaths (Table 1.2). These sheaths contain three cruciate and four annular pulleys, which allow the tendons to glide smoothly along the digital bones [6]. When the tendons move, they often change position and shape [6]. Interconnections between the flexor tendons within the carpal tunnel reduce displacement and restrict the fingers from moving independently [6]. In addition, the tendons are moved by the common muscle belly of the FDP, which further limits independent motion [6]. The flexor digitorum superficialis (FDS) is responsible for flexion of the index, middle, ring, and small finger PIP joints. It is also controlled by a common muscle belly, which divides into four tendons. In 38% of individuals, the function of the FDS of the small finger is dependent on the ring finger [6].

Extensors

The twelve extensor tendons are contained by the extensor retinaculum, the thick portion of the antebrachial fascia (Table 1.2). The extensor retinaculum creates six separate compartments for the tendons and serves as a pulley during motion to hold the tendons near the wrist [6]. Lesions of the extensor tendons may result in adhesion formation. However, these adhesions often do not impede extensor function due to the minimal need for tendon gliding and excursion and the largely movable skin in which the adhesions attach. The terminal tendon, which is created by two conjoined lateral bands at the proximal interphalangeal joints, inserts on the dorsal lip of the distal phalanx [6]. The conjoined bands are held in place by the triangular ligament and the transverse retinacular ligaments [6]. The terminal tendon functions to extend the DIP joint.

Nerves

The muscles of the hand are innervated by three nerves: the ulnar nerve, the median nerve, and the radial nerve. The ulnar nerve is derived from the C8 and T1 nerve roots. It travels along the inside of the upper arm to the inside of the forearm where it controls both forearm and hand muscles. In the forearm, the ulnar nerve powers flexion of the wrist, small finger, and ring finger. In the hand, the ulnar nerve powers the hypothenar muscles, the lumbricals of the ring and small finger, the palmar and dorsal interossei muscles, the adductor pollicis, and the flexor pollicis brevis. It is responsible for sensation on the side of the hand closest to the small finger, and to the small finger itself as well as the ulnar aspect of the ring finger. Injuries to the ulnar nerve may result in formation of a claw posture of the small and/or ring finger.

The median nerve is derived from the C5, C6, C7, C8, and T1 nerve roots. The nerve travels near the brachial artery towards the forearm where it innervates the flexor and pronator muscles of the forearm. It helps supply muscles responsible for

Table 1.2 Tendons of the forearm, hand, and fingers

Tendon	Origin	Insertion	Function
Flexor carpi radialis	Medial epicondyle of humerus	Base of metacarpals II, III, and trapezium	Radial deviation and flexion of wrist
Flexor carpi ulnaris	Medial epicondyle of humerus, olecranon, posterior ulna	Base of metacarpal V, hamate, pisiform	Ulnar deviation of wrist; flexion and adduction of wrist
Palmaris longus	Medial epicondyle of humerus	Palmar aponeurosis	Flexion of wrist; abduction of hand
Extensor carpi radialis brevis	Lateral epicondyle of humerus	Posterior base of metacarpal III	Straighten and stabilize wrist; extension of wrist; abduction of wrist
Extensor carpi radialis longus	Lateral epicondyle of humerus	Posterior base of metacarpal II	Straighten and stabilize wrist; extension of wrist; radial deviation
Extensor carpi ulnaris	Lateral epicondyle of humerus; posterior ulna	Dorsal ulnar base of metacarpal V	Extension of wrist; ulnar deviation; stabilize DRUJ
Flexor digitorum profundus	Anteromedial ulna; coronoid process	Distal phalanx of II, III, IV, V	Flexion of MCP and IP joints
Flexor digitorum superficialis	Medial epicondyle, radial head, ulna	Middle phalanx of II, III, IV, V	Flexion of MCP and PIP joints
Extensor digitorum communis	Lateral epicondyle of humerus	Extensor expansion of digits II, III, IV, V	Extension of MCP and IP joints
Extensor digiti minimi	Lateral epicondyle of humerus	Extensor expansion of digit V	Extension of MCP joint
Extensor indicis proprius	Distal third of ulna	Extensor expansion of digit II	Extension of wrist; extension of MCP and IP joints
Abductor pollicis longus	Proximal radius and ulna	Base of metacarpal I, trapezium	Extension of wrist; extension and abduction of CMC joint
Flexor pollicis longus	Anterior radius	Palmar surface of distal phalanx of thumb	Flexion of thumb, MCP, and IP joints
Extensor pollicis longus	Posterior ulna	Posterior base of distal phalanx of thumb	Extension of wrist, thumb, MCP, and IP joints
Extensor pollicis brevis	Posterior ulna	Posterior base of proximal phalanx of thumb	Extension of thumb, CMC, and MCP joints

flexing the wrist and fingers. The median nerve supplies the thenar eminence and the lumbricals of the index and middle finger. It permits sensation on the side of the hand closest to the thumb. Compression of the median nerve near the carpal bones may lead to carpal tunnel syndrome. Although carpal tunnel syndrome is more common in the adult population, pediatric patients may develop carpal tunnel syndrome due to sports participation, trauma, congenital conditions, and/or anatomic anomalies [9].

The radial nerve is derived from the C5, C6, C7, C8, and T1 nerve roots. The radial nerve travels on the lateral side of the elbow and into the forearm to power all extrinsic muscles responsible for extending the wrist and fingers. Damage to the radial nerve may lead to wrist drop, which may be identified as the inability to actively extend the wrist.

Vascular System

The forearm and hand receive blood supply from vessels derived from the radial and ulnar arteries (Fig. 1.4) [10]. The radial artery branches off the brachial artery in the cubital fossa [11]. It runs along the forearm and connects with the superficial branch

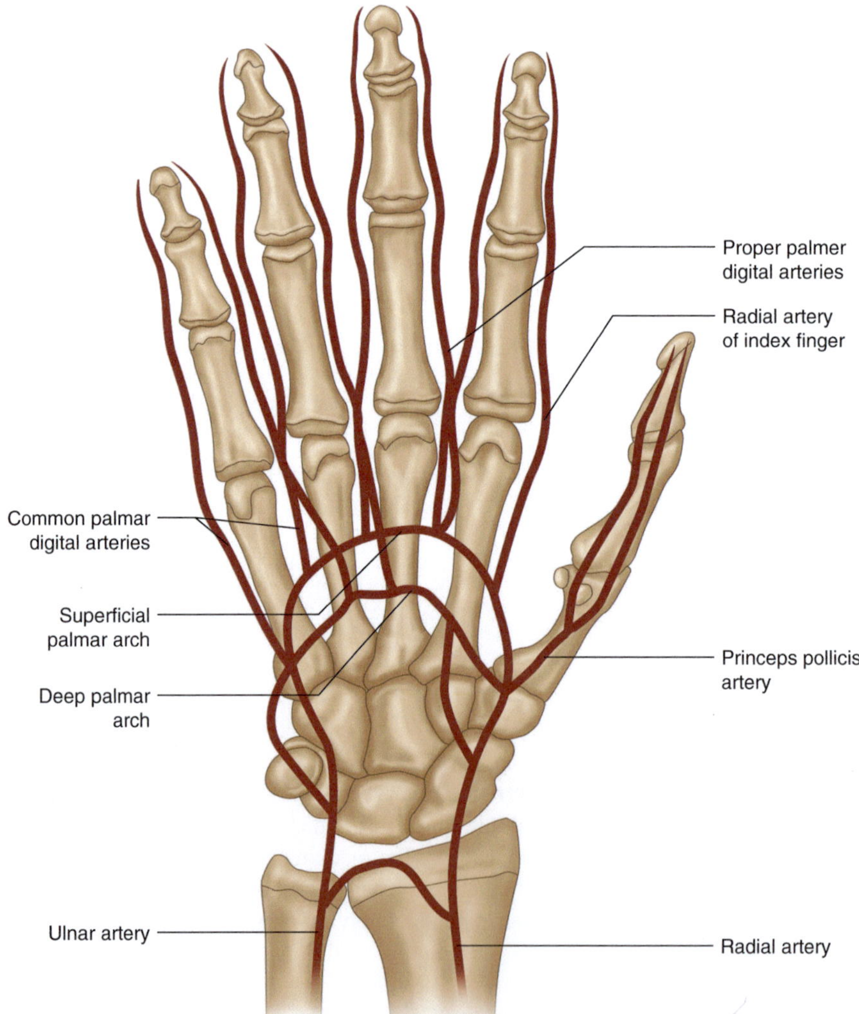

Fig. 1.4 Schematic drawing of the vascular supply of the hand (Courtesy of Catherine C. May, BS)

of the ulnar artery at the radiocarpal joint to form the superficial palmar arch [10]. The dorsal branch of the radial artery enters the palm through the first interosseous space, where it becomes the princeps pollicis, the radialis indicis, and the deep palmar arch [10]. The ulnar artery also branches off the brachial artery in the cubital fossa. The ulnar artery runs along the forearm to the carpus, where the radial and ulnar arteries interact to form three dorsal and three palmar arches. The dorsal arches include the dorsal radiocarpal arch, the dorsal intercarpal arch, and the dorsal proximal metacarpal arch. The palmar arches include the palmar radiocarpal arch, the palmar intercarpal arch, and the distal palmar arch.

The structures of the hand are supplied by the superficial palmar arch, the deep palmar arch, and the dorsal metacarpal arteries, which are derived from the dorsal metacarpal arch. Branches of the digital arteries vascularize the subcutaneous tissue in the palm of the hand and the fingers. The proper digital arteries originate in the center of the palm from the superficial palmer arch, or less commonly, the deep palmar arch [10]. The radial digital arteries are typically larger in the ring and small fingers, while the ulnar digital arteries are larger in the index and middle fingers [10]. The thumb is supplied by two arterial systems, the palmar system and the dorsal system, both of which contain an ulnar digital artery and a radial digital artery [10].

Osseous Development

To understand the functional development of the human hand, it is important to review the process of bone formation. Bone formation begins during the sixth week of embryonic development in a process called osteogenesis [12]. The long and short bones of the hand are developed through a specific type of osteogenesis known as endochondral ossification [12]. The process begins as mesenchymal cells differentiate into chondrocytes [12]. The chondrocytes then proliferate to produce a hyaline cartilage model with a cancellous bone collar, called the periosteum, to serve as a guide for future bone growth [12, 13]. This region is the site of the primary ossification center [12]. Within the center of the cartilage model, chondrocytes experience hypertrophy and produce a matrix of collagen and fibronectin that permits calcification of the tissue [12, 13].

As the extracellular matrix becomes calcified, chondrocytes are unable to reach nutrients needed for their survival [12]. Therefore, the cells are forced to undergo apoptosis [12]. Blood vessels take over the newly created space and carry osteogenic cells into the area to help form the periosteum, a layer of thicker, compact bone located in the diaphysis [12]. The newly created region, called the medullary cavity, helps to supply nutrients to the growing osseous tissues [12]. In each end of the bone, cartilage proliferates resulting in an increase in bone length [12]. These regions, known as the epiphyseal plates, continue to supply growth until they close around age 14.5 for females and 16.5 for males [12, 14]. After birth, the process repeats itself with the secondary ossification centers growing in the epiphysis (Fig. 1.5) [12].

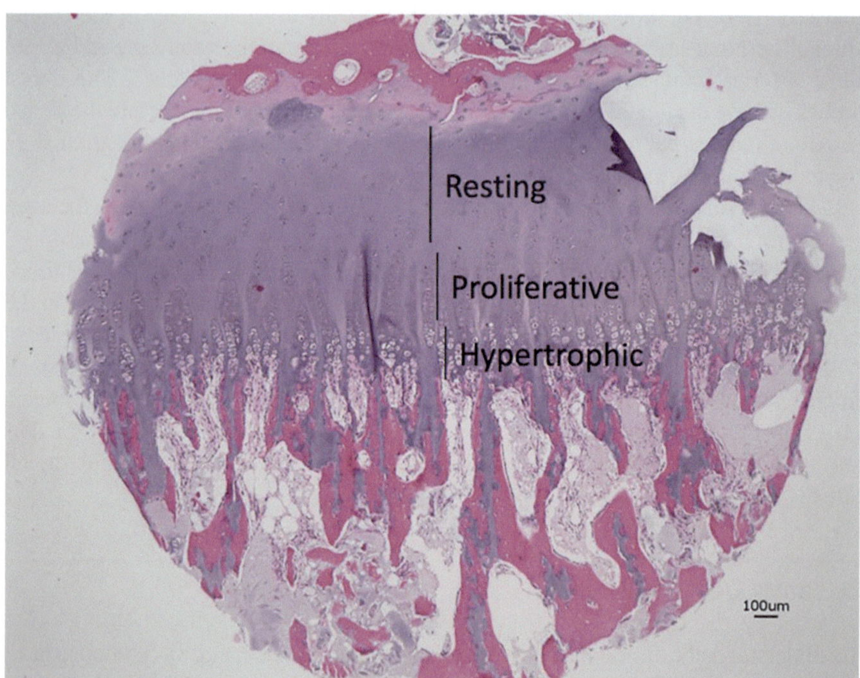

Fig. 1.5 Histology slide of a core of the physis from the distal ulna of a 14-year-old male. (Courtesy of Motomi Iwamoto, Ph.D.)

In younger patients, the physeal plate appears in radiographs as a line separating the epiphysis and the metaphysis of the long bones (Fig. 1.6) [15]. The physes are located distally in metacarpals II-V, and proximally in metacarpal I and all phalanges. The physeal plate, also known as the growth plate, is comprised of cartilage and bony tissue [15]. The bony component protects the cartilage that allows for growth of the young bone [15]. The cartilage region may be divided into three zones: the reserve zone which contains stores of lipids, glycogen, and proteoglycan, the proliferative zone which houses the chondrocytes responsible for longitudinal bone growth, and the hypertrophic zone which is the site of chondrocyte maturation [12, 15].

Ossification timelines will differ between each bone. Secondary ossification center growth will begin in the proximal phalanges within the first 2 years of life beginning in the third finger, followed by the second, fourth, fifth, and thumb [16]. The

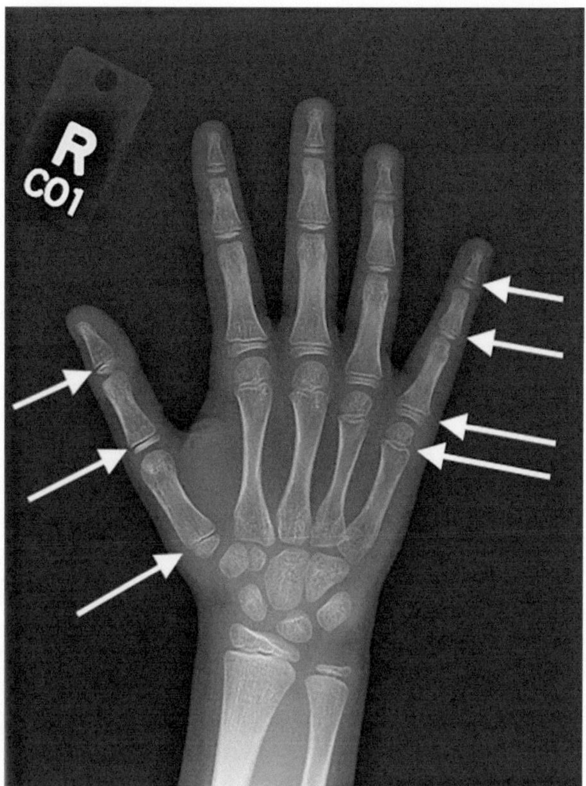

Fig. 1.6 Posteroanterior (PA) hand radiograph of a 9-year-old patient with open physes of the hand. Note the physes are located distally in metacarpals II–V, but proximally in the first metacarpal and all of the phalanges. (Courtesy of Joshua M. Abzug, MD)

middle and distal phalanges will begin the secondary ossification center growth process around ages 2–3 years [16]. Secondary ossification centers form later in the metacarpals. In the II through V metacarpals, the secondary ossification begins at the metacarpal head around ages 5–6 years, while the secondary ossification will begin around ages 7–8 years in the base of the first metacarpal [16]. These bones continue to grow until around age 17, when the growth plate becomes fully ossified [8, 17]. At this point, the adult bone will appear to have cancellous bone surrounded by compact bone (Fig. 1.7) [15].

The carpal bones have a circumferential ossification pattern different than the longitudinal pattern in most long and short bones [18]. The carpal bones will initially appear on radiographs as small ossification centers (Fig. 1.8). The scaphoid and lunate ossific nuclei will not appear until 2–6 years of age. As the patient increases in age, the carpal bones will increase in size, ultimately closing the gap between each bone. By the end of adolescence, the carpal bones will be fully ossified (Fig. 1.9).

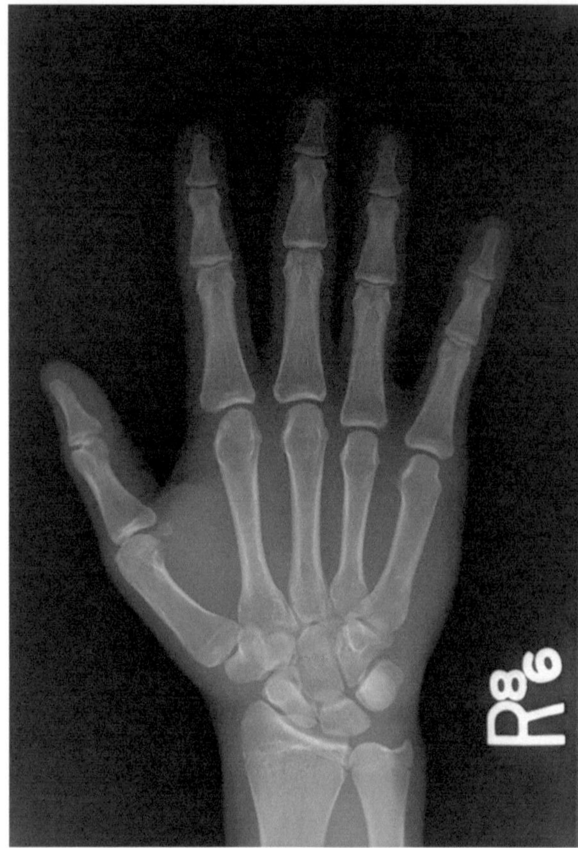

Fig. 1.7 Posteroanterior (PA) hand radiograph of a 16-year-old patient with closed physes of the hand (Courtesy of Joshua M. Abzug, MD)

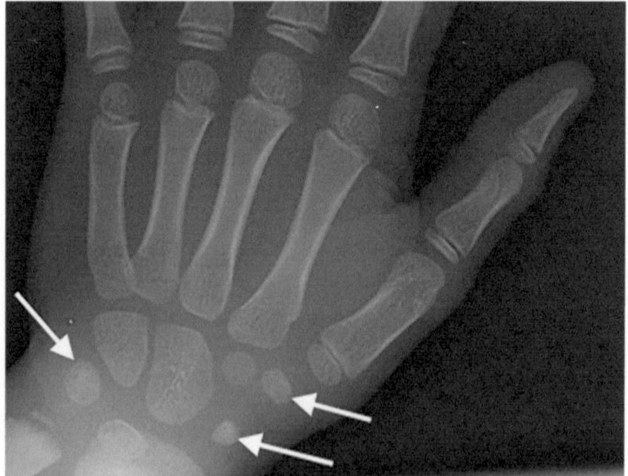

Fig. 1.8 Posteroanterior (PA) wrist radiograph of an 8-year-old male patient with incomplete ossification of the carpals (Courtesy of Joshua M. Abzug, MD)

Fig. 1.9 Posteroanterior (PA) wrist radiograph of a 17-year-old patient with complete ossification of the carpals (Courtesy of Joshua M. Abzug, MD)

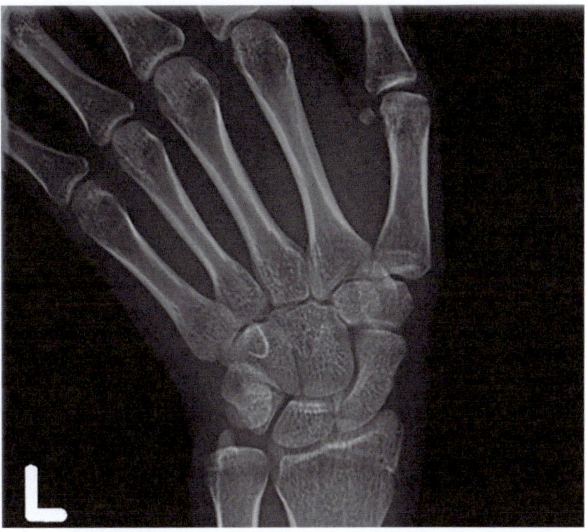

Table 1.3 Salter-Harris Classification System

Type I	Transverse fracture through the physis
Type II	Fracture through the physis and metaphysis
Type III	Fracture through the physis and epiphysis
Type IV	Fracture through the physis, metaphysis, and epiphysis
Type V	Compression fracture of the physis

During the growth process, the physes are particularly susceptible to fracture as the physis is biomechanically weaker compared to the surrounding ligamentous structures and mature bone [19, 20]. Fractures involving the physis comprise approximately 15–18% of all pediatric fractures [11, 20]. Physeal fractures are more common in males and adolescent patients ages 11–14 years [11, 20]. Approximately 30% of all physeal injuries occur in the phalanges [11]. The Salter-Harris classification system describes these injuries based on the fracture pattern (Table 1.3) [17]. Salter-Harris Type II fractures are the most common (75%) followed by Type IV (10%), Type III (8%), Type I (6%), and Type V (1%) [11]. The likelihood of growth arrest increases as the fracture classification in the Salter-Harris classification increases [11].

Successful management of physeal fractures is dependent on the anatomic location of the injury, the age of the patient, and the timing of intervention. Remodeling potential at the fracture site is dependent on the number of years of growth remaining prior to physeal closure, as well as the plane of deformity. Remodeling is increased in planes of motion. For example, there is more remodeling potential in the sagittal plane about the distal radius, due to flexion and extension, compared to the coronal plane, where there is minimal motion in regard to radial and ulnar deviation. Additionally, certain physes have greater remodeling potential than others. It is important to treat physeal injuries within 24 hours of the initial presentation, if possible. Attempts at reduction should be gentle to avoid additional trauma. The risk of causing growth arrest during treatment increases as the fracture begins to heal.

Damage to the physeal region prior to the closure of the physeal plate may result in reduced longitudinal growth, bony deformity, and joint impairment [12]. Complications may occur in approximately 2–14% of patients with physeal injuries [21]. While incidence depends on the location of the physis, the injury characteristics, and treatment, growth arrest may occur in 5–10% of patients [21]. Therefore, it is important to identify and treat these injuries as soon as possible.

Functional Development

Henderson and Pehoski describe the human hand as both an "executive" and "perceptual" organ, meaning that the hand is used to complete tasks and explore the environment by seeking and processing sensory information [22]. Both functions are necessary for proper development and function of the hand. It is important to understand the functional development of the human hand in order to properly diagnose and treat injuries to this region.

Around 8 weeks of gestation, a fetus develops webbed hands and feet. By week 12, the fetus has separate fingers and toes which it is able to open and close [23]. At 14 weeks, the fetus begins manual exploration of the womb with their hands [18]. These initial movements are spontaneous and will continue after birth [23]. Infants have primitive reflexes, such as the grasping reflex, in which they will close their fingers into a fist in response to stroking of the palm. This reflex will last until about 6 months of age.

Infants will wave, rotate, and extend their arms in attempts to reach for objects. As they increase in age, these movements become smoother and subsequently more successful [23]. The action of grasping an object in order to perform action is called prehension. Prehension requires the ability to position the hand and grip the object [24]. Around 4 months, infants will reach for objects in a circuitous motion, accelerating and decelerating the arm in order to reach the object [24]. Movements will become increasingly straight, smooth, and efficient with age [24]. Kinematics of hand reaching improve rapidly until around 7 months of age, after which improvements are more gradual [24]. Differences in spatial layout and velocity control persist in children from age 3 until adulthood [24].

As children age, they will adjust their grip aperture to account for the size and shape of the target object [24]. According to the study conducted by Kuhtz-Buschbeck et al., younger children are more likely to open their hands wider than older children during visually guided reaching [24]. This may be explained by younger children having poorer control over their hand transport [24]. Grip formation improved between ages 4 and 12 with more coordinative organization between the opening and closing of the fist and deceleration in hand transport [24]. Younger children moved largely in response to feedback control, while older children operated under anticipatory control [24].

Younger children have greater dependence on visual control than older children [24]. If the object is not in the visual field, the individual must internally determine distance, location, size, and shape of the object of interest [24]. In the experiment conducted by Kuhtz-Buschbeck et al. which removed the object from the visual field, hand transport velocity remained the same; however, the grip formation varied with wider grip aperture to account for less precise hand transport [24]. Younger children were more likely to miss the target object than older children [24]. Vision of the hand during grasping is not as important as vision of the object, as children were able to reach the target when the hand was removed from the visual field [24].

The process of searching the environment and interpreting sensory information through tactile scanning and hand manipulation is called haptic perception. Haptic perception allows children to identify common objects and inquire about new objects through identification of texture, hardness, size, weight, and shape [22]. A child's ability to identify objects through touch improves with age. Children are able to recognize common objects around ages 2 to 3, match topologic forms around ages 3–5, and recognize geometric figures around age 4 [22]. The complexity and consistency of recognition improves rapidly between ages 4 and 7 [22]. A general consensus suggests that haptic-visual matching of geometric figures develops around age 4 and haptic perception of common objects is reliable around age 5 [22]. The interaction between the hand and the visual senses begins around 4 months of age and continues to progress as the child grows older [22]. Children will develop the ability to explore objects with their hand and recognize objects using their vision within their first year of life [22]. Previous research suggests that haptic perception of size, texture, and weight improves between ages 4 and 9 years old, with rough textures being more easily identified than smooth textures [22]. In addition, haptic abilities are typically similar between males and females [22].

As children continue to explore their environments, they will develop a hand preference for acquiring objects. Around 11 months of age, a child will begin to show preferences for unimanual object manipulation [25]. This hand preference continues to increase until around age 2 [25]. According to a study by Nelson et al., 80% of children with a hand preference at 18 months will have the same preference at 24 months [26]. Hand dominance may be informative in the clinical evaluation; therefore, it is important to understand at what age this preference develops.

Conclusion

The human hand is designed to perform various intricate tasks. In a developing child, the presence of the physes makes various injury patterns unique to children. It is important for clinicians to develop a robust understanding of the anatomy and development of the pediatric hand to properly identify and treat hand fractures. If pediatric hand fractures are managed properly and efficiently, they may heal with minimal complications.

References

1. Arora R, Fichadia U, Hartwig E, Kannikeswaran N. Pediatric upper-extremity fractures. Pediatr Ann. 2014;43(5):196–204. https://doi.org/10.3928/00904481-20140417-12.
2. Nellans KW, Chung KC. Pediatric hand fractures. Hand Clin. 2013;29(4):569–78. https://doi.org/10.1016/j.hcl.2013.08.009.
3. Kreutz-Rodrigues L, Gibreel W, Moran SL, Carlsen BT, Bakri K. Frequency, pattern, and treatment of hand fractures in children and adolescents: a 27-year review of 4356 pediatric hand fractures. Hand (N Y). 2022;17(1):92–7. https://doi.org/10.1177/1558944719900565.
4. Meals C, Meals R. Hand fractures: a review of current treatment strategies. J Hand Surg Am. 2013;38(5):1021–31. https://doi.org/10.1016/j.jhsa.2013.02.017.
5. Taylor CL, Schwarz RJ. The anatomy and mechanics of the human hand. Artif Limbs. 1955;2(2):22–35. https://search.ebscohost.com/login.aspx?direct=true&db=cmedm&AN=13249858&site=eds-live. Accessed 17 Aug 2021.
6. Schreuders TAR, Brandsma JW, Stam HJ. Functional anatomy and biomechanics of the hand. In: Duruöz MT, editor. Hand function. New York: Springer; 2014. p. 3–22. https://doi.org/10.1007/978-1-4614-9449-2_1.
7. Clarke B. Normal bone anatomy and physiology. Clin J Am Soc Nephrol. 2008;3(Suppl 3):S131–9. https://doi.org/10.2215/CJN.04151206.
8. Li Z-M, Tang J. Coordination of thumb joints during opposition. J Biomech. 2007;40(3):502–10. https://doi.org/10.1016/j.jbiomech.2006.02.019.
9. Codd CM, Abzug JM. Upper extremity compressive neuropathies in the pediatric and adolescent populations. Curr Rev Musculoskelet Med. 2020;13(6):696–707. https://doi.org/10.1007/s12178-020-09666-4.
10. Tan RES, Lahiri A. Vascular anatomy of the hand in relation to flaps. Hand Clin. 2020;36(1):1–8. https://doi.org/10.1016/j.hcl.2019.08.001.
11. Mallick A, Prem H. Physeal injuries in children. Surgery (Oxford). 2017;35(1):10–7. https://doi.org/10.1016/j.mpsur.2016.10.008.
12. Breeland G, Sinkler MA, Menezes RG. Embryology, bone ossification. In: StatPearls. StatPearls Publishing; 2021. http://www.ncbi.nlm.nih.gov/books/NBK539718/. Accessed 18 Aug 2021.
13. Rivas R, Shapiro F. Structural stages in the development of the long bones and epiphyses: a study in the New Zealand white rabbit. J Bone Joint Surg Am. 2002;84(1):85–100. https://doi.org/10.2106/00004623-200201000-00013.
14. Case AL, Hosseinzadeh P, Baldwin KD, Abzug JM. Hand fractures in children: when do I need to start thinking about surgery? Instr Course Lect. 2019;68:415–26.
15. Von Pfeil DJF, DeCamp CE. The epiphyseal plate: physiology, anatomy, and trauma. Compend Contin Educ Vet. 2009;31(8):E1–E11. https://search.ebscohost.com/login.aspx?direct=true&db=cmedm&AN=19866441&site=eds-live. Accessed 25 Aug 2021.
16. Limb D, Loughenbury PR. The prevalence of pseudoepiphyses in the metacarpals of the growing hand. J Hand Surg Eur Vol. 2012;37(7):678–81. https://doi.org/10.1177/1753193411436295.
17. Salter RB, Harris WR. Injuries involving the epiphyseal plate. J Bone Joint Surg Am. 1963;45:587–622.
18. Butler P, Mitchell AWM, Ellis H. Applied radiological anatomy. Cambridge: Cambridge University Press; 2012.
19. Abzug JM, Dua K, Bauer AS, Cornwall R, Wyrick TO. Pediatric phalanx fractures. J Am Acad Orthop Surg. 2016;24(11):e174–83. https://doi.org/10.5435/JAAOS-D-16-00199.
20. Meyers AL, Marquart MJ. Pediatric physeal injuries overview. In: StatPearls. StatPearls Publishing; 2022. http://www.ncbi.nlm.nih.gov/books/NBK560546/. Accessed 12 Dec 2022.
21. Dabash S, Prabhakar G, Potter E, Thabet AM, Abdelgawad A, Heinrich S. Management of growth arrest: current practice and future directions. J Clin Orthop Trauma. 2018;9(Suppl 1):S58–66. https://doi.org/10.1016/j.jcot.2018.01.001.

22. Henderson A, Pehoski C. Hand function in the child: foundations for remediation. St. Louis: Elsevier Health Sciences; 2005.
23. Adolph KE, Franchak JM. The development of motor behavior. Wiley Interdiscip Rev Cogn Sci. 2017;8(1-2):10.1002/wcs.1430. https://doi.org/10.1002/wcs.1430.
24. Kuhtz-Buschbeck JP, Stolze H, Jöhnk K, Boczek-Funcke A, Illert M. Development of prehension movements in children: a kinematic study. Exp Brain Res. 1998;122(4):424–32. https://doi.org/10.1007/s002210050530.
25. Nelson EL, Campbell JM, Michel GF. Early handedness in infancy predicts language ability in toddlers. Dev Psychol. 2014;50(3):809–14. https://doi.org/10.1037/a0033803.
26. Nelson EL, Campbell JM, Michel GF. Unimanual to bimanual: tracking the development of handedness from 6 to 24 months. Infant Behav Dev. 2013;36:181–8. https://doi.org/10.1037/a0033803.

Examination of the Pediatric Hand

2

Catherine C. May and Joshua M. Abzug

Introduction

The sophisticated anatomical design of the human hand allows humans to operate with superior fine motor abilities [1, 2]. In the pediatric population, the hand is used to explore and make sense of the surrounding environment, often without fear or ample motor control [3, 4].

Consequently, the hand is susceptible to frequent injury, especially early in life [3]. Although these injuries are not often life threatening, they may significantly impact the overall function of the hand and digits [1, 5].

The age and developmental stage of the patient must be considered to ensure successful fracture management and maintenance of hand function and stability [6]. The ossification centers present at the physes are responsible for longitudinal bone growth in children [7]. In the metacarpals, the physes are present at the distal end of the second through fifth metacarpal bones, and at the proximal extent of the first metacarpal (Fig. 2.1). In the phalanges, the physis is present at the proximal portion of each bone (Fig. 2.1). The physes will appear as a radiolucent line separating the epiphysis and the metaphysis of the metacarpal bones between 12 and 27 months of age and between 10 and 36 months of age for the phalanges [6–8]. The physes may remain open until the bone is completely ossified, which occurs around age 14.5 for females and 16.5 for males (Fig. 2.2) [6, 8]. Due to the biomechanically weak nature

---

Disclaimer: The views expressed in the submitted article are our own and not an official position of the institution.

Supplementary Information The online version contains supplementary material available at https://doi.org/10.1007/978-3-031-32072-9_2.

C. C. May · J. M. Abzug (✉)
Department of Orthopedic Surgery, University of Maryland School of Medicine, Baltimore, MD, USA
e-mail: catherine.may@som.umaryland.edu; jabzug@som.umaryland.edu

© The Author(s), under exclusive license to Springer Nature Switzerland AG 2023
J. M. Abzug et al. (eds.), *Pediatric and Adult Hand Fractures*,
https://doi.org/10.1007/978-3-031-32072-9_2

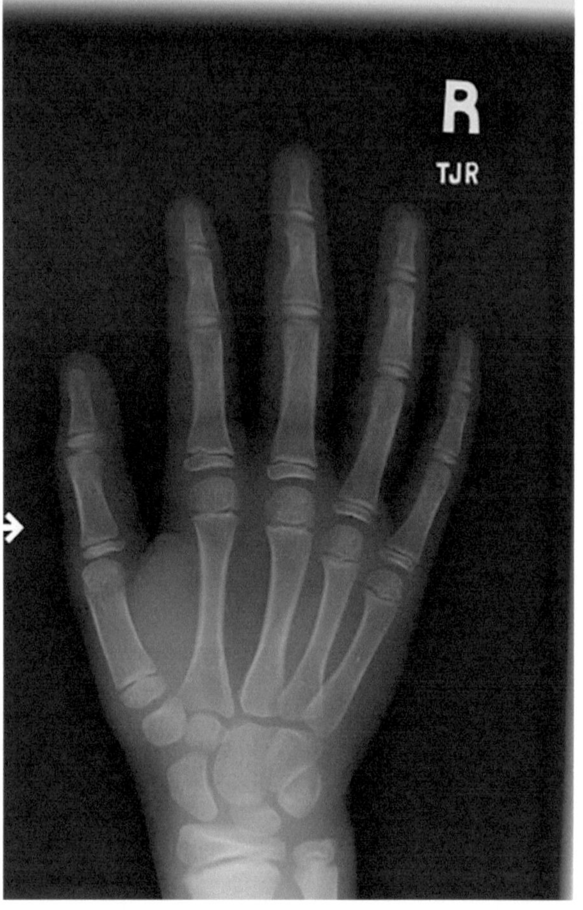

Fig. 2.1 Postero-anterior view of the right hand of a 10-year-old male patient with open physes of the metacarpals and phalanges. Note the presence of the physis distally in the second through fifth metacarpals and proximally in the first metacarpal and all of the phalanges. (Courtesy of Joshua M. Abzug, MD)

of the physis, fractures about the physes are relatively common, accounting for 34–45% of all hand fractures in children [6, 7]. If an injury to this region occurs prior to physeal closure, the hand may suffer permanent growth plate damage [8]. The growth arrest rate following a physeal fracture of the phalanx is approximately 1% [7]. While this rate is relatively low, growth arrest caused by the fracture may lead to growth discrepancies and deformities [8]. In some cases, ongoing pediatric bone growth may be used to promote bone remodeling as a method of deformity correction. Extensive periosteal blood flow allows cell differentiation and tissue regeneration to occur at the fracture site. Therefore, correction of angular displacement via remodeling is possible in young patients, leading to a lower rate of persistent malunion [6].

The prevalence of pediatric hand fractures has risen as participation and intensity of sports has increased. As a result, it is likely that physicians will encounter a greater number of hand fractures in pediatric patients [9]. Proper management of these injuries is crucial as they may disrupt physical function in a developing child.

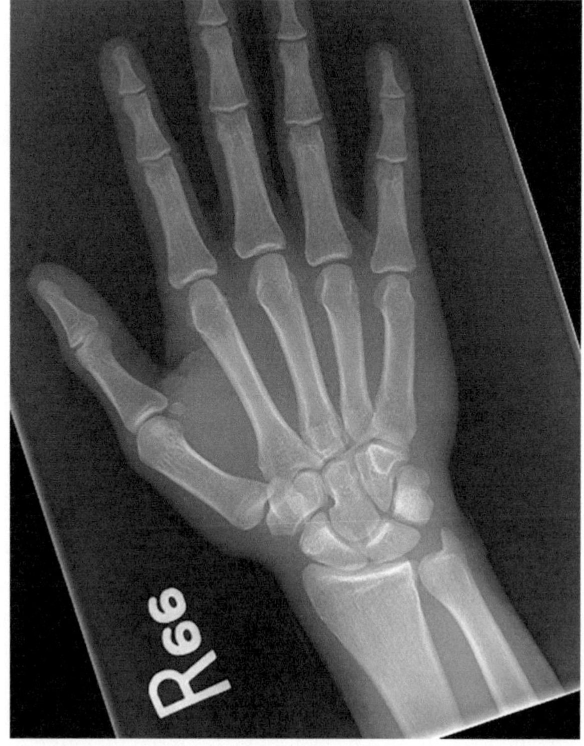

Fig. 2.2 Postero-anterior (PA) view of the right hand of a 16-year-old male patient with closed physes of the metacarpals and phalanges. (Courtesy of Joshua M. Abzug, MD)

Patient history, observation, range of motion assessment, tendinous and neurovascular examination, and radiographic evaluation should be performed to develop the proper clinical diagnosis of the injury [5]. In this chapter, the recommended approach for history, physical and radiographic examination of pediatric hand injuries will be explored. Variations between diagnostic techniques for different presenting injuries will be discussed.

General Examination

Before evaluating the area of injury, the physician should observe the patient as a whole and collect a thorough patient history [5, 6, 10]. According to Dincer and Samut, taking a thorough patient history alone can allow for a diagnosis to be made with 60% accuracy [5]. The patient history should identify demographic information such as the child's age, hand dominance if known, hobbies, sports and positions played, and other activities [5, 6]. Hand dominance emerges around 6 months of age and will become consistent around age 2 years [11]. Any previously existing conditions or illnesses should be assessed for [5]. The child and/or parent should describe the acute trauma responsible for the injury in detail as specific mechanisms may be more characteristic of certain fractures [5, 6]. Any pain experienced by the child should be reported including whether or not the patient experiences relief from the pain, the most prevalent location of the pain, and the relative intensity of the pain [5]. Patients should report any other symptoms they experience after the trauma [5]. The examiner should obtain a history regarding any prior evaluations to determine if there have been attempts at reduction and/or if there is a need for obtaining repeat radiographs. In addition, any treatments provided thus far should be noted including prescription of pain medicine and/or antibiotics. The observer should note the patient's walking pattern, gestures, speech, and habits to identify any abnormalities in the context of the visit [5, 10]. Once the general examination is completed, the physician will develop a clinical suspicion that may inform additional tests that may be needed to confirm the diagnosis [5].

Physical Examination

The next step of the evaluation is to carefully examine the affected region of the patient [5, 10]. The entire upper extremity should be observed to establish any differences in posture, asymmetry, swelling, or congenital differences which may impact the diagnosis. In most cases, it is useful to compare the injured region to the contralateral side to determine any abnormal features that may be present.

To identify any lacerations, ecchymosis, abrasions, and/or edema in the region, the inspection should begin at the skin [6]. Ecchymosis may be indicative of disruptions or changes to the vascular supply of the hand [5]. Changes in skin color/appearance may also be caused by bacterial infection or loss of nerve function, both of which may necessitate immediate treatment [5].

Abrasions and lacerations may pose additional risk for infection; therefore, they must be treated quickly and appropriately [5, 6]. The fight bite, which appears after a patient strikes another individual in the mouth, has one of the highest rates of complications of any closed fist injury or bite wound [12]. The patient will typically present with a laceration about the region of the dorsal metacarpophalangeal (MCP) joint [12]. Due to the high concentration of microbes in the human saliva and the avascular nature of the extensor tendon and joint, the fight bite has a high overall infection rate of around 10% [12]. Fight bites may be treated through irrigation and debridement and a course of antibiotics as well as the repair of any extensor tendon lacerations if present [12].

Bite wounds caused by animals are also fairly common with approximately 2% of the population receiving an animal bite each year [13]. Complications of animal bites may vary depending on the location, the biting animal, and the ferocity of the attack [13, 14]. Individuals with high-risk wounds should be closely monitored and prescribed antibiotics [13].

Additionally, certain mechanisms of injury may result in concomitant skin burns. For example, treadmill injuries are commonly associated with friction and electrical burns [15]. Depending on the extent of the injury, the burns may be managed through dressing changes and/or reconstructive interventions [15]. However, early detection and adequate conservative management is associated with excellent outcomes [15].

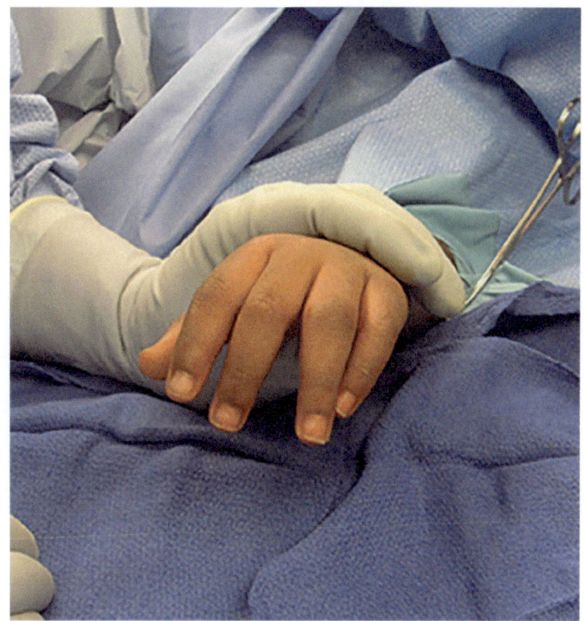

Fig. 2.3 Clinical photograph of a digital cascade assessment in a patient with a phalangeal fracture of the left ring finger. Note the gapping between the long and ring finger fingertips indicating the substantial coronal plane deformity present. (Courtesy of Joshua M. Abzug, MD)

The pattern and amount of edema can be used to inform the diagnosis [5]. Generalized swelling may be caused by circulatory issues, while acute or localized swelling is characteristic of fractures, tumors, cysts, or infections [5]. Additionally, localized swelling may be caused by improper splinting or wound dressings, specifically if these dressings are too tight [16, 17].

Observation of the digital cascade is performed to determine any malrotation and/or deviation of the digits [6]. Comparison to the uninjured hand/digits helps to identify the presence of abnormalities which may be congenital or acquired through previous injury and/or trauma. Gapping of the fingertips in the injured hand may indicate the presence of angular deviation (Fig. 2.3), while malalignment of the nail plates suggests the presence of malrotation. Disruption of the tenodesis effect may indicate possible tendon involvement. If the tendons are intact, the fingers will straighten/extend when the wrist is in flexion and curl up/flex when the wrist is in extension.

Common deformities seen after pediatric hand trauma include mallet finger type presentations and swan neck deformities [18]. A mallet finger is often associated with a sudden blow to an extended finger. The digit presents with a flexed posture of the distal phalanx resulting from an imbalance between the terminal extensor tendon and the flexor digitorum profundus tendon or an avulsion fracture at the site of the extensor tendon insertion [18, 19]. Mallet finger injuries may be confirmed with proper posterior-anterior (PA) and lateral radiographs of the digit (Fig. 2.4) [19]. A Seymour fracture is a juxta-epiphyseal fracture of the distal phalanx that occurs through the physis and has an associated nail bed laceration [20]. The digit will have a similar appearance to a mallet finger due to the deformity that occurs at the level

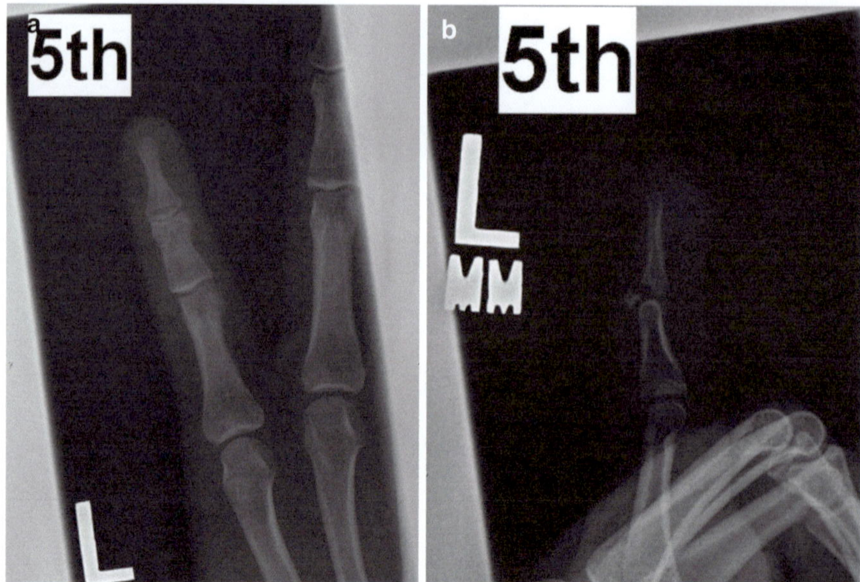

Fig. 2.4 A 15-year-old male with a bony mallet fracture of the left small finger. (**a**) PA view of the digit which appears normal, (**b**) lateral view of the digit demonstrating the fracture fragment. (Courtesy of Joshua M. Abzug, MD)

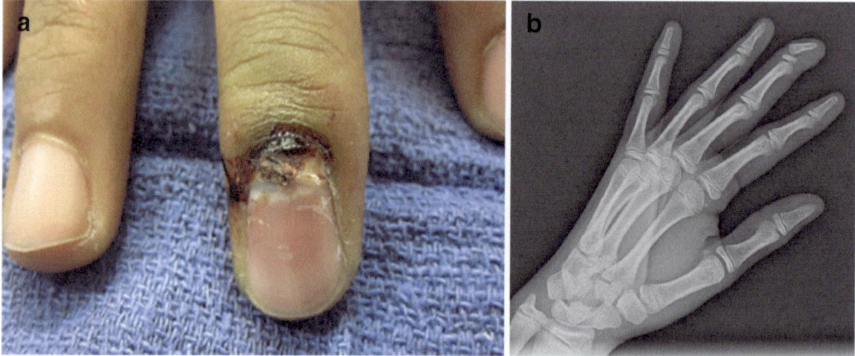

Fig. 2.5 A 12-year-old male with a Seymour fracture and an associated nailbed laceration. (**a**) Clinical photograph of the nail plate lying superficial to the eponychial fold with eschar present. (**b**) Oblique radiograph of the hand demonstrating the displaced physeal fracture of the distal phalanx of the long finger. (Courtesy of Joshua M. Abzug, MD)

of the fracture (Fig. 2.5). However, unlike a mallet fracture, there is no disruption of the extensor mechanism in a Seymour fracture due to the extensor tendon insertion onto the epiphysis [21]. A swan neck deformity occurs due to hyperextension of the proximal interphalangeal (PIP) joint and compensatory flexion of the distal interphalangeal (DIP) joint [18]. It may be present in many conditions including as a complication of a mallet injury [18].

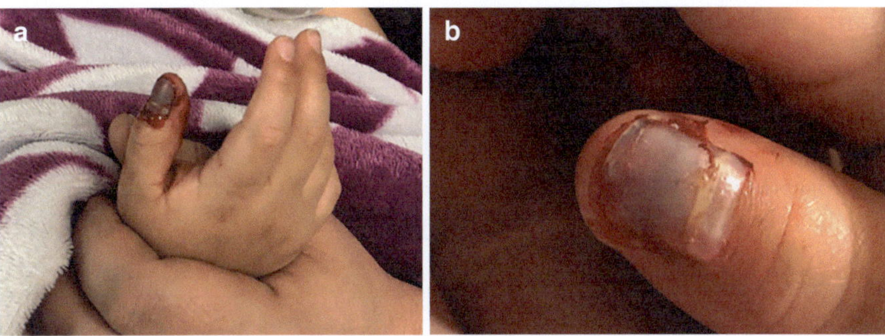

Fig. 2.6 Clinical photographs (**a**) and (**b**) of a thumb with a distal tuft fracture and an associated nail complex injury. (Courtesy of Joshua M. Abzug, MD)

Examination of the patient's nail complex is an important step in the identification of concomitant injuries [6]. Certain injuries to the distal phalanx will often present with a concomitant injury to the nail complex [6]. For example, Seymour fractures are open fractures of the distal phalanx with associated nailbed lacerations [6]. The nailbed injury may not be easily visible, as it often presents with the nail plate lying superficial to the eponychial fold [19]. It is possible that eschar present at the proximal extent of the nail complex will obscure the evaluation (Fig. 2.5); however, clinical suspicion for an associated nailbed injury should remain high when such eschar is present. Assessment of a nail plate abnormality is more easily recognized when comparing the injured distal phalanx/nail complex to an uninjured digit [19]. Distal tuft fractures may also present with an associated injury to the nail complex following a crush injury to the distal phalanx (Fig. 2.6) [6]. This nail complex injury may inhibit the ability to achieve a closed reduction; therefore, open injuries may require additional surgical intervention to remove the nail plate and reduce the fracture [6].

Palpation

Following the visual inspection, the entire upper extremity including the shoulder, arm, elbow, forearm, wrist, and hand should be palpated beginning far away from the site of injury to gain the trust of the child [6]. Palpation is an examination technique in which the examiner uses their hands and/or fingers to feel the body part to identify the texture, tenderness, and temperature of the region [5]. Examination of identifiable regions within the hand and digits may help to make important distinctions in diagnosis [5]. The metacarpal base, located at the proximal extent of the bone, can be felt distal to the carpal bones, whereas the bulbous head of the metacarpal may be identified at the distal end of the bone. Within the phalanges, the observer may palpate the base on the proximal extent of the bone and the head/neck region at the distal end of the bone.

Range of Motion

Assessment of active and passive range of motion is a crucial step in the physical evaluation of any pediatric hand injury [19]. Injury to the wrist, hand, or fingers may limit movement and hand function [5, 19]. Therefore, assessing range of motion is important in diagnosing and treating fractures of the hand [19, 20]. Range of motion may be determined through visual observation and/or measurement using a goniometer [5]. A systematic review conducted by van de Pol et al. examined 21 studies to determine inter-rater reliability of measurements of range of motion in the upper extremity [20]. Measurements using instruments such as a goniometer were found to be more reliable than measurements using vision alone [20]. Therefore, the researchers recommended the use of goniometers and inclinometers when assessing range of motion to increase reliability of decision making [20].

Active range of motion consists of movement performed by the patient without additional assistance [5, 19]. This is dependent on the individual's muscle power, pain, and cooperation level [5]. If an individual has full active range of motion, there is no need to conduct a passive range of motion assessment [5]. Passive range of motion is the movement about a joint with the help of an external force [5]. For example, the examiner may apply pressure with their hand to assess joint mobility [5].

Measurements of active and passive range of motion should be compared to the contralateral hand to identify any deviation from normal. Normal range of motion values may serve as a guideline for comparison. Measuring the range of motion of the second through fifth digits requires the wrist to maintain neutral positioning [5]. The normal range of motion values for these digits can be found in Table 2.1. Due to differences in functional needs, range of motion differs slightly at each digit [23]. Digits closer to the radial aspect of the hand are involved in performing pinching motions. There is greater functional range of motion in the PIP and DIP joints in these digits as compared to the MCP joints [23]. Digits closer to the ulna aspect of the hand are involved in performing power grip; therefore, there is greater functional range of motion of the MCP and DIP joints in these digits as compared to the PIP joints [23]. Due to its anatomically unique design, the thumb has separate values for normal range of motion [5]. These normal range of motion values can be found in Table 2.2.

Digital motion may also be assessed via tendon integrity tests [6]. To evaluate tenodesis, the patient is instructed to move the wrist into extension and flexion

Table 2.1 Normal range of motion of the second through fifth digits[a]

Location	Range of motion
Metacarpophalangeal (MCP) joint	
Flexion	43° - 70°
Extension	0–15°
Hyperextension	0–45°
Proximal interphalangeal (PIP) joints	0–110°
Distal interphalangeal (DIP) joints	0–60/70°

[a]Data adapted from Springer and Journal of Hand Therapy [5, 22]

Table 2.2 Normal range of motion of the thumb[a]

Location	Range of motion
Carpometacarpal (CMC) joint	
Flexion	15°
Palmar abduction	50–71°
Radial abduction	53–71°
Retropulsion	25–38°
Opposition	9–10 grade
Adduction	5–20°
Metacarpophalangeal (MCP) joint	
Flexion	0–80°
Extension	0–10°
Interphalangeal joint	
Flexion	80–90°
Extension	0–45°

[a]Data adapted from Hand and Springer [5, 24]

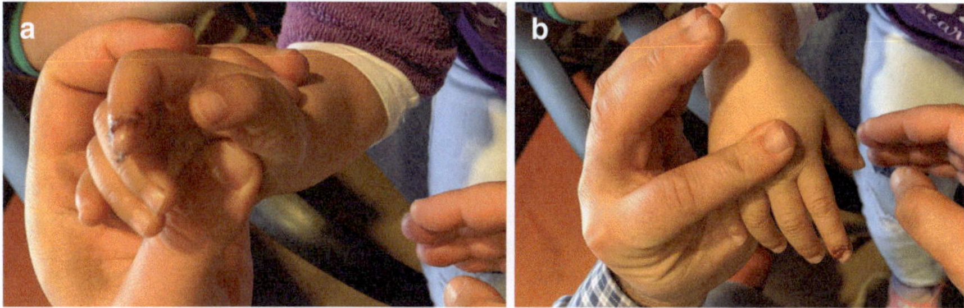

Fig. 2.7 Clinical demonstration of a tenodesis assessment in a 3-year-old female with a right index finger distal tuft fracture and an associated nail complex laceration. Note (**a**) the flexion of the fingers when the wrist is in extension and (**b**) the extension of the fingers when the wrist is in flexion. (Courtesy of Joshua M. Abzug, MD)

(Fig. 2.7) (Video 2.1). If the tendons are intact, the fingers will curl up/flex while the wrist is in extension and straighten/extend when the wrist is in flexion. The results can inform the examiner of possible tendon involvement associated with the injury which will influence the course of management [6]. Alternatively, to determine the presence of tendon congruity, the observer can squeeze the volar musculature in the forearm [6]. If all of the fingers flex together, there is tendon congruity present (Fig. 2.8) (Video 2.2) [6].

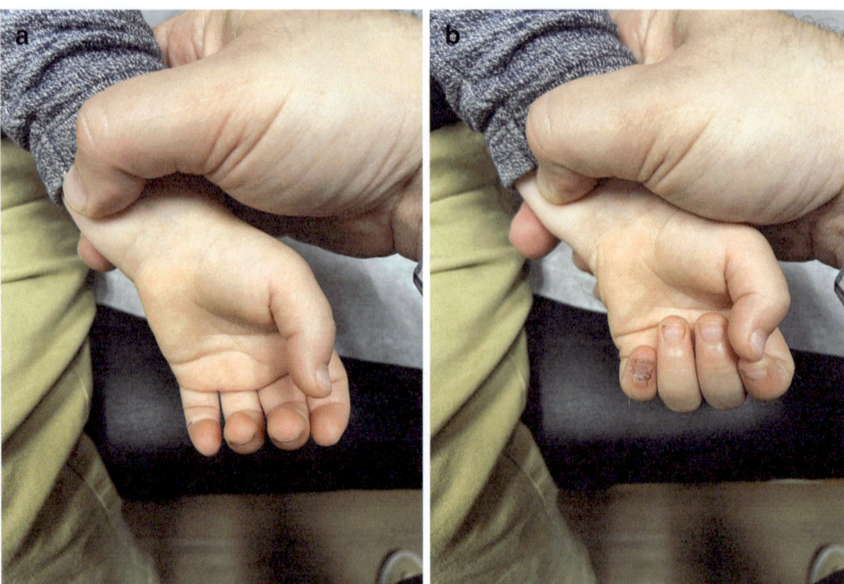

Fig. 2.8 Clinical demonstration of a tendon congruity assessment utilizing volar forearm compression in a 2-year-old male with a left small finger closed, nondisplaced fracture of the distal phalanx. (**a**) Fingers in relaxed state. (**b**) Fingers flex in concert when the volar forearm musculature is squeezed. (Courtesy of Joshua M. Abzug, MD)

Neurovascular Examination

A thorough neurovascular evaluation is used to assess individual finger status, particularly in cases with more severe injury [6, 19]. To evaluate digital sensation, the two-point discrimination test is performed [6]. The two-point discrimination test is a test of digital sensation used in patients ages 6 and above [19]. In this test, patients are evaluated on their ability to identify two points on an area of interest. Observers record their ability to identify the object at varying distances (Fig. 2.9) (Video 2.3).

Younger children under the age of 6 years are unable to commonly have two-point discrimination assessed. Instead, their digital sensation is assessed using the wrinkle and/or the sweat tests [19]. The wrinkle test measures autonomic peripheral nerve function [19]. Patients place their hand in warm water for a 10 min period [19, 25]. If they develop wrinkles on their fingers, sensory function is considered to be intact (Fig. 2.10) [19, 25]. The sweat test is a quicker, easier test which assesses sensory function through identification of the presence or absence of sweat, with intact sweat presence indicating intact sensory nerves [19, 25].

It is important to evaluate the vascular supply of each digit to identify any injury to the radial digital, ulnar digital, and/or common digital arteries. The Allen's test is

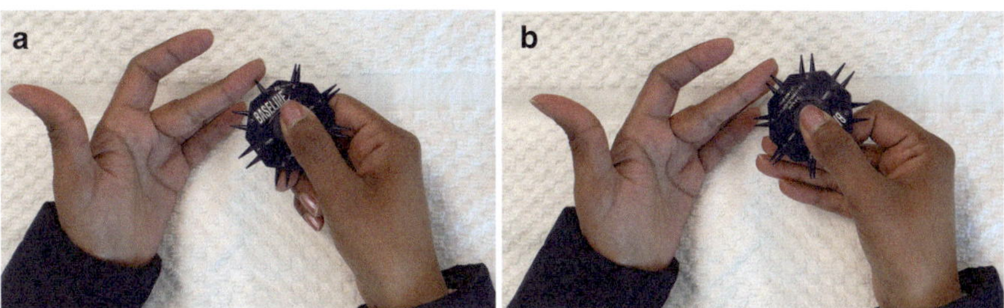

Fig. 2.9 Clinical demonstration of performing the Two-Point discrimination test. (**a**) 1-point of the two-point discriminator wheel, (**b**) 5 mm assessment utilizing the two-point discriminator wheel. (Courtesy of Ritu Goel, MS, OTR/L)

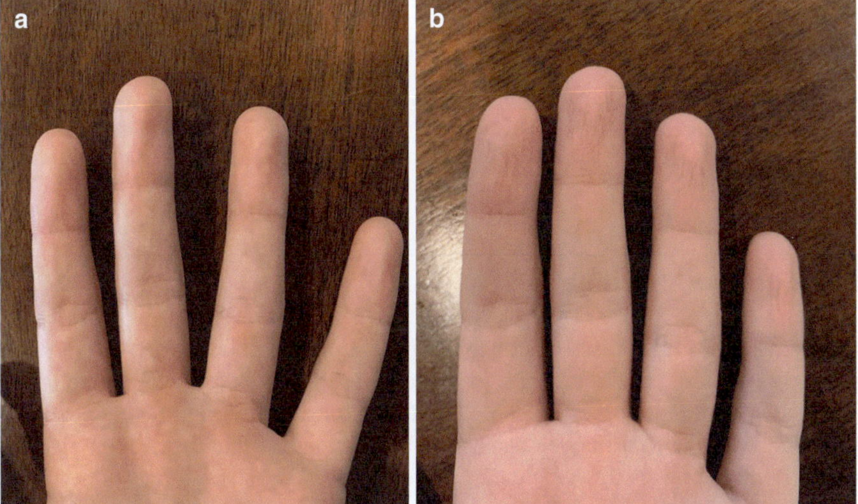

Fig. 2.10 Clinical demonstration of the Wrinkle Test. (**a**) Pre-test with smooth texture of the fingertips. (**b**) Post-test with wrinkles of the fingertips. (Courtesy of Joshua M. Abzug, MD)

a noninvasive test used to assess vascular supply by observing change in color during restriction of arteries [26]. Using two fingers, the observer will apply direct pressure to both of the digital arteries [26, 27]. The observer squeezes the finger in a distal-to-proximal direction to remove blood from the finger. The digit becomes pale in color due to the slowing blood supply [26, 28]. The observer will then remove the pressure over one artery and observe the restoration of the flushed color [26, 28]. The test is repeated to release pressure over the other digital artery [28]. If the color returns within approximately 5 seconds, the artery is considered to be intact (Fig. 2.11) (Video 2.4) [26, 28].

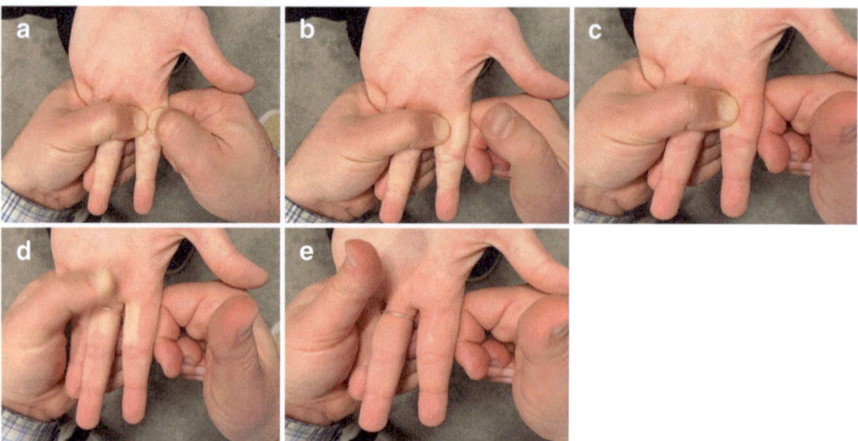

Fig. 2.11 Clinical demonstration of the Digital Allen's test. (**a**) Examiner applies pressure to both of the digital arteries to remove blood from the finger. (**b**) The digit becomes pale in color due to the slowing blood supply. (**c**) The observer removes pressure over one artery to observe restoration of the flushed color. (**d**) Pressure is held over the other digital artery. (**e**) The observer removes pressure over the other artery and observes the restoration of the flushed color. (Courtesy of Joshua M. Abzug, MD)

Radiographic Examination

Following an in-depth history and physical examination, the provider will develop clinical suspicions which may be confirmed through the use of radiographic imaging. Young children may experience difficulty sitting still during the collection of radiographic images. It may be beneficial for someone to hold the digit in place to obtain optimal images. In some cases, posteroanterior (PA) views may appear normal; therefore, both PA and lateral radiographs of the injured digit should be obtained (Fig. 2.4) [6, 19]. If multiple injuries and/or articular phalanx fractures are suspected, oblique radiographs should be obtained in addition to the PA and lateral views [6, 19]. For clear viewing, it is recommended to take isolated images of the injured digit as opposed to the entire hand [6]. However, the interpretation of the radiographic images should begin away from the site of the suspected injury to assess for concomitant injuries.

The impression collected through the history and physical examination may guide more specific imaging techniques. For example, children may not have completely ossified phalangeal condyles, making radiographic assessment more difficult [29]. Abzug et al. proposed a technique using the volar phalangeal line (VPL) as a tool to assess the alignment of phalangeal neck fractures [29]. This technique is analogous to the technique described by Herman et al., which uses the anterior humeral line (AHL) to determine alignment of supracondylar humerus fractures [27, 29]. The VPL predictably intersects the phalangeal condyles based on the age of the patient [29]. The intersection of the VPL and phalangeal condyles will occur

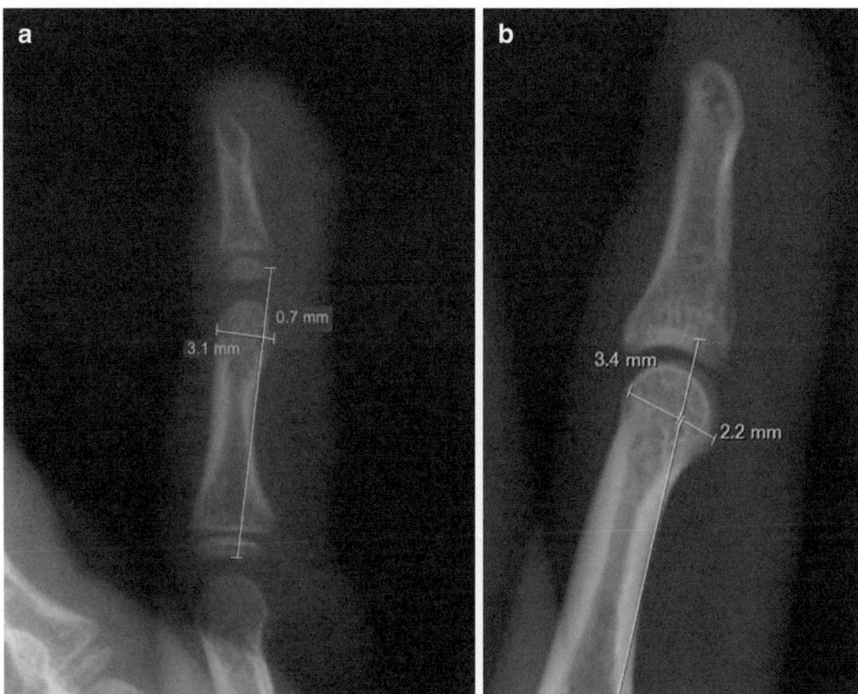

Fig. 2.12 Radiographs demonstrating volar phalangeal line measurements. (**a**) Patient under 9 years of age showing the VPL intersect the volar third of the condyles. (**b**) Patient over 9 years of age showing the VPL intersect the middle third of the condyles. (Courtesy of Joshua M. Abzug, MD)

in the anterior one third of the condyles in patients under the age of 9, and in the middle one third of the condyles in patients older than 9 years of age (Fig. 2.12) [29].

Fractures of the metacarpal may require additional images. To view the second and third metacarpals, a semi-pronated (30 degrees) oblique view should be obtained [30]. To view the fourth and fifth metacarpals, a semi-supinated (30 degrees) view should be obtained [30]. A Brewerton view may be used to specifically assess the metacarpal head [30]. In this view, the dorsal aspect of the hand is placed on the x-ray plate, while the MCP joints are flexed to 65 degrees [30]. In complex fractures and injuries involving the CMC joint, computed tomography (CT) may be useful [30].

In some patients with phalangeal condyle or unicondylar fractures, double density signs are present on a true lateral radiograph. This represents displaced offset of the condyles relative to one another, suggesting a displaced and/or malrotated fracture fragment (Fig. 2.13). In cases of an avulsion fracture, a "two fleck sign" may be present, representing the detached bone fragment [31]. Identification of signs such as this one will help to improve diagnosis and appropriate treatment of the fracture.

The use of fluoroscopy is more effective and efficient than plain radiographs [32, 33]. A study conducted by Ghazala et al. identified several advantages to

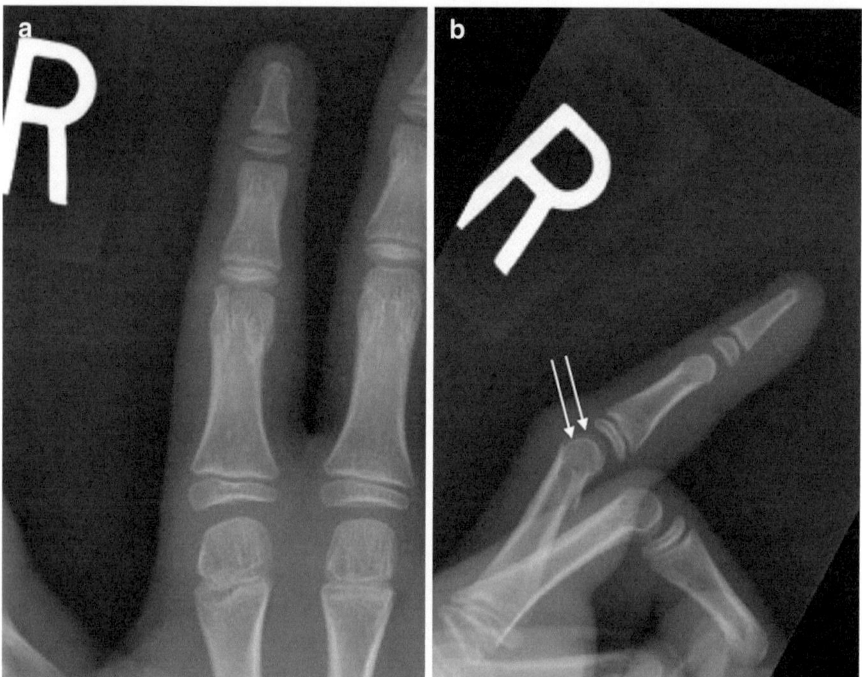

Fig. 2.13 Radiographs of a phalangeal condyle fracture in an 11-year-old male. (**a**) PA and (**b**) lateral views. Note the double density sign which represents displaced offset of the condyles relative to each other. The proximal displacement of the fracture fragment causes a step-off at the articular surface. (Courtesy of Joshua M. Abzug, MD)

utilizing a portable bedside fluoroscopy machine including decreased waiting time, improved accuracy of predicting post-reduction fracture alignment, and decreased radiation exposure [32]. A second study conducted by Fanelli et al. determined that the use of mini C-arm fluoroscopy can improve quality and efficiency of pediatric orthopedic outpatient clinics [33]. Wait times decreased by 23 min; however, there was a slightly higher radiation dose than with standard plain radiographs [33].

While advanced imaging is typically unnecessary in the pediatric population, additional imaging may assist in the diagnosis and treatment in some cases [9, 19]. Magnetic resonance imaging (MRI) can be used to diagnose a stress fracture which cannot be seen through a plain radiograph [9]. CT scans can be used during the assessment of intra-articular fractures to develop plans for operative intervention [9]. It is important to educate providers on the proper imaging techniques in order to limit radiation exposure, the delay to definitive treatment, and the burden of cost on patients and the healthcare system [34].

Conclusion

In the pediatric and adolescent populations, the hand is the most frequently injured region of the body. Careful history, physical and radiographic examinations of the hand are necessary to properly diagnose and treat pediatric hand fractures. It is important to obtain a thorough patient history, range of motion, and tendinous and neurovascular evaluation to identify any behavior or function that is considered abnormal. Following the history and physical examination, physicians may develop a clinical suspicion which can be subsequently confirmed through radiographic imaging. Understanding of proper examination techniques is important to quickly and accurately diagnose pediatric hand fractures.

References

1. Schreuders TAR, Brandsma JW, Stam HJ. Functional anatomy and biomechanics of the hand. In: Duruöz MT, editor. Hand function. New York: Springer; 2014. p. 3–22. https://doi.org/10.1007/978-1-4614-9449-2_1.
2. Taylor CL, Schwarz RJ. The anatomy and mechanics of the human hand. Artif Limbs. 1955;2(2):22–35. https://search.ebscohost.com/login.aspx?direct=true&db=cmedm&AN=13249858&site=eds-live. Accessed 24 Aug 2021.
3. Meals C, Meals R. Hand fractures: a review of current treatment strategies. J Hand Surg Am. 2013;38(5):1021–31. https://doi.org/10.1016/j.jhsa.2013.02.017.
4. Cornwall R, Ricchetti ET. Pediatric phalanx fractures: unique challenges and pitfalls. Clin Orthop Relat Res. 2006;445:146–56. https://doi.org/10.1097/01.blo.0000205890.88952.97.
5. Dincer F, Samut G. Physical examination of the hand. In: Duruöz MT, editor. Hand function: a practical guide to assessment. Springer; 2014. p. 23–40. https://doi.org/10.1007/978-1-4614-9449-2_2.
6. Case AL, Hosseinzadeh P, Baldwin KD, Abzug JM. Hand fractures in children: when do I need to start thinking about surgery? Instr Course Lect. 2019;68:415–26.
7. Peterson HA. Phalanges of the hand. Epiphyseal growth plate fractures. Springer; 2007. p. 201–26.
8. Abzug JM, Little K, Kozin SH. Physeal arrest of the distal radius. J Am Acad Orthop Surg. 2014;22(6):381–9. https://doi.org/10.5435/JAAOS-22-06-381.
9. Arora R, Fichadia U, Hartwig E, Kannikeswaran N. Pediatric upper-extremity fractures. Pediatr Ann. 2014;43(5):196–204. https://doi.org/10.3928/00904481-20140417-12.
10. Campbell EW, Lynn CK. The physical examination. In: Walker HK, Hall WD, Hurst JW, editors. Clinical methods: the history, physical, and laboratory examinations. 3rd ed. Butterworths; 1990. http://www.ncbi.nlm.nih.gov/books/NBK361/. Accessed 31 Aug 2021.
11. Nelson EL, Campbell JM, Michel GF. Early handedness in infancy predicts language ability in toddlers. Dev Psychol. 2014;50(3):809–14. https://doi.org/10.1037/a0033803.
12. Perron AD, Miller MD, Brady WJ. Orthopedic pitfalls in the ED: fight bite. Am J Emerg Med. 2002;20(2):114–7. https://doi.org/10.1053/ajem.2002.31146.
13. Dendle C, Looke D. Review article: animal bites: an update for management with a focus on infections. Emerg Med Australas. 2008;20(6):458–67. https://doi.org/10.1111/j.1742-6723.2008.01130.x.
14. Meyer CL, Abzug JM. Domestic bird bites. J Hand Surg Am. 2012;37(9):1925–7. https://doi.org/10.1016/j.jhsa.2012.02.044.

15. Banever GT, Moriarty KP, Sachs BF, Courtney RA, Konefal BL. Pediatric hand treadmill injuries. J Craniofac Surg. 2003;14(4):487–90.
16. Schwartz BS, Abzug J. Appropriateness and adequacy of splints applied for pediatric upper extremity fractures in an emergency department/urgent care environment: level 2 evidence. J Hand Surg. 2014;39(9):e18. https://doi.org/10.1016/j.jhsa.2014.06.051.
17. Abzug JM, Schwartz BS, Johnson AJ. Assessment of splints applied for pediatric fractures in an emergency department/urgent care environment. J Pediatr Orthop. 2019;39(2):76–84. https://doi.org/10.1097/BPO.0000000000000932.
18. American Society for Surgery of the Hand. The hand, examination and diagnosis. 3rd ed. Churchill Livingstone; 1990. https://search-ebscohost-com.proxy-hs.researchport.umd.edu/login.aspx?direct=true&db=cat01362a&AN=hshs.003015098&site=eds-live. Accessed 30 Nov 2021.
19. Abzug JM, Dua K, Bauer AS, Cornwall R, Wyrick TO. Pediatric phalanx fractures. J Am Acad Orthop Surg. 2016;24(11):e174–83. https://doi.org/10.5435/JAAOS-D-16-00199.
20. van de Pol RJ, van Trijffel E, Lucas C. Inter-rater reliability for measurement of passive physiological range of motion of upper extremity joints is better if instruments are used: a systematic review. J Physiother. 2010;56(1):7–17. https://doi.org/10.1016/s1836-9553(10)70049-7.
21. Abzug JM, Kozin SH. Seymour Fractures. J Hand Surg Am. 2013;38(11):2267–70. https://doi.org/10.1016/j.jhsa.2013.08.104.
22. Hayashi H, Shimizu H. Essential motion of metacarpophalangeal joints during activities of daily living. J Hand Ther. 2013;26(1):69–74. https://doi.org/10.1016/j.jht.2012.10.004.
23. Bain GI, Polites N, Higgs BG, Heptinstall RJ, McGrath AM. The functional range of motion of the finger joints. J Hand Surg Eur Vol. 2015;40(4):406–11. https://doi.org/10.1177/1753193414533754.
24. Barakat MJ, Field J, Taylor J. The range of movement of the thumb. Hand (N Y). 2013;8(2):179–82. https://doi.org/10.1007/s11552-013-9492-y.
25. Feng Y, Schlösser FJ, Sumpio BE. The Semmes Weinstein monofilament examination as a screening tool for diabetic peripheral neuropathy. J Vasc Surg. 2009;50(3):675–82. https://doi.org/10.1016/j.jvs.2009.05.017.
26. Mcconnell EA. Performing Allen's test. Nursing. 1997;27(11):26.
27. Herman MJ, Boardman MJ, Hoover JR, et al. Relationship of the anterior humeral line to the capitellar ossific nucleus: variability with age. J Bone Joint Surg Am. 2009;91:2188–93.
28. Ashbell TS, Kutz JE, Kleinert HE, E LK. The digital Allen test. Plast Reconstr Surg. 1967;39(3):311–2.
29. Dua K, O'Hara NN, Shusterman I, Abzug JM. Ossification of the proximal and middle phalangeal condyles: radiographic aid in phalangeal neck fracture reduction. J Pediatr Orthop. 2019;39(3):e222–6. https://doi.org/10.1097/BPO.0000000000001255.
30. Kollitz KM, Hammert WC, Vedder NB, Huang JI. Metacarpal fractures: treatment and complications. Hand (N Y). 2014;9(1):16–23. https://doi.org/10.1007/s11552-013-9562-1.
31. Thirkannad S, Wolff TW. The "'two fleck sign'" for an occult Stener lesion. J Hand Surg Eur Vol. 2008;33(2):208–11. https://doi.org/10.1177/1753193408087106.
32. Sharieff GQ, Kanegaye J, Wallace CD, McCaslin RI, Harley JR. Can portable bedside fluoroscopy replace standard, postreduction radiographs in the management of pediatric fractures? Pediatr Emerg Care. 1999;15(4):249–51.
33. Fanelli MG, Hennrikus WL, Slough HJM, Armstrong DG, King SH. The mini C-arm adds quality and efficiency to the pediatric orthopedic outpatient clinic. Orthopedics. 2016;39(6):e1097–9. https://doi.org/10.3928/01477447-20160808-01.
34. Hill AD, Catapano JS, Surina JB, Lu M, Althausen PL. Clinical and economic impact of duplicated radiographic studies in trauma patients transferred to a regional trauma center. J Orthop Trauma. 2015;29(7):e214–8. https://doi.org/10.1097/BOT.0000000000000279.

Pediatric Metacarpal Fractures

3

Daniel A. London, Keith T. Aziz, and Kevin J. Little

Epidemiology

Pediatric metacarpal fractures are a relatively common injury. They represent 30–40% of all fractures that occur in the hand [1–3] and have an approximate incidence of 250/100,000 children [4]. Among metacarpal fractures, injury to the fifth metacarpal is most common which accounts for over 40% of all metacarpal fractures [1]. In general, metacarpal fractures are a result of sports injuries, with football being the most common cause [5], followed by physical altercations, accidental closure of a hand in a door, and finally falling [1]. Metacarpal fractures are more commonly seen in males [1, 6–8], and in children older than 14 years of age [8]. Rajesh et al. better delineated the frequency of metacarpal fractures by finger as well as location within the metacarpal, as fractures can occur in the metacarpal base, diaphysis, neck, and/or epiphysis (Fig. 3.1) [2].

D. A. London
Department of Orthopaedic Surgery, University of Missouri, Columbia, MO, USA
e-mail: d.london@health.missouri.edu

K. T. Aziz
Department of Orthopaedic Surgery, Mayo Clinic Jacksonville, Jacksonville, FL, USA
e-mail: Aziz.Keith@mayo.edu

K. J. Little (✉)
Department of Orthopaedic Surgery, Cincinnati Children's Hospital, Cincinnati, OH, USA
e-mail: Kevin.Little@cchmc.org

© The Author(s), under exclusive license to Springer Nature Switzerland AG 2023
J. M. Abzug et al. (eds.), *Pediatric and Adult Hand Fractures*,
https://doi.org/10.1007/978-3-031-32072-9_3

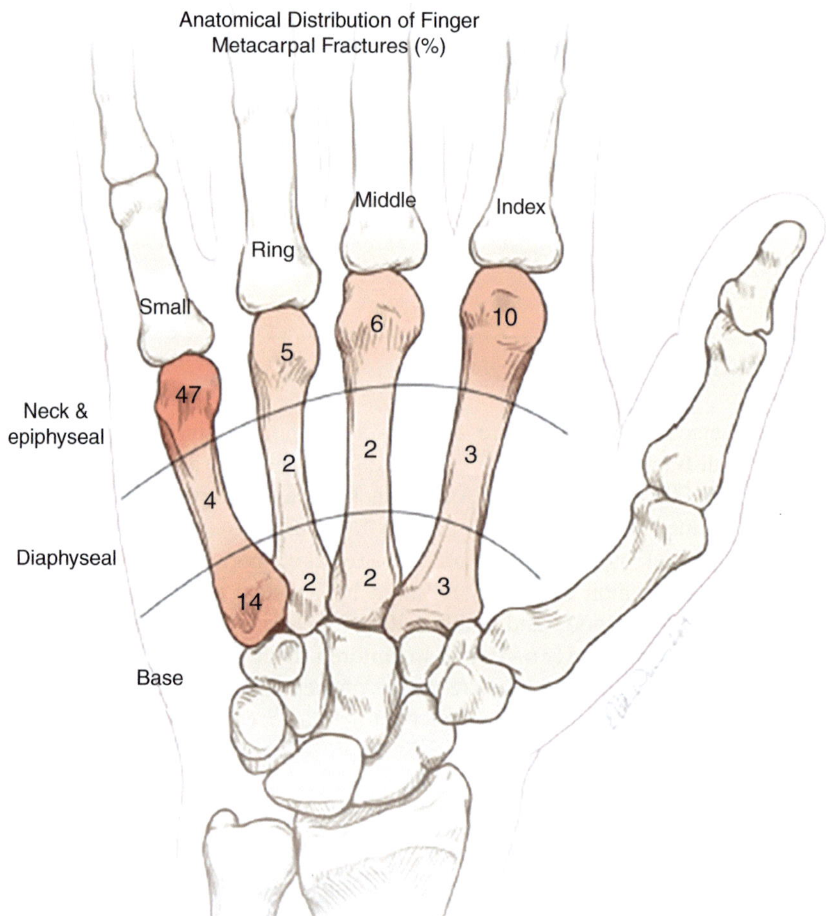

Fig. 3.1 Distribution (in percent) of finger metacarpal injuries according to Rajesh A, Basu AK, Vaidhyanath R, Findlay D. Hand fractures: a study of their site and type in childhood. Clin. Radiol. 2001;56 (8):667–669 [2]. Note that the majority of metacarpal injuries involve the small finger metacarpal

Anatomy

To understand how to treat pediatric metacarpal fractures, it is first helpful to understand the normal anatomy. The metacarpal epiphyses are located distally on the index, middle, ring, and small finger metacarpals, and they first appear between 10 months and 3 years of age after the epiphyses of the proximal phalanges appear

[9]. The physes will close between ages 13 and 16, typically after the distal and proximal phalanges. Frequently by age 15 in females and age 17 in males, the metacarpal epiphyses are completely fused. Whether or not the physes are closed can play an important role in the nonoperative and operative techniques used in the treatment of metacarpal fractures. Additionally, there can also be an accessory epiphysis or pseudoepiphysis at the base of the radial metacarpals which can contribute to some longitudinal growth of that metacarpal. These are relatively common incidental findings and do not represent fractures. Limb and Loughenbury identified that these occur most frequently in the index finger (15.25%), followed by the small finger (7.21%), and finally the middle finger (0.49%) [10].

Anatomically, the metacarpals have a natural arc in the axial plane, and a natural inclination with the index finger metacarpal typically being the longest. This natural arc and inclination results in a slight overlap in the fingers when making a composite fist, typically with the radial digits overlapping the ulnar digits with all fingers pointing towards the scaphoid if alignment is maintained. This overlap is no more than half of the fingernail width, and any overlap of more than 50% is considered to be pathologic. Any divergence of this natural overlap is an indication of malalignment from trauma or disordered growth.

Clinical Assessment

When examining a child with a suspected metacarpal fracture it is important to begin by obtaining the history. While most fractures occur in sports scenarios, it is important to consider other mechanisms of injury. An important mechanism to consider is that of an altercation, which therefore raises the possibility of a "fight bite." If the patient has sustained multiple metacarpal fractures, a crushing mechanism needs to be considered. This is especially important, as such a mechanism of injury can lead to a hand compartment syndrome.

Beyond obtaining an appropriate history, a thorough clinical examination is key. There will often be soft tissue swelling at the level of the fracture, with the potential for ecchymosis. The degree of swelling should be noted, as in some cases it can be so significant that it limits finger flexion and the ability to assess potential malrotation. Additionally, if substantial soft tissue swelling is present, then the patient should be evaluated for compartment syndrome and temporary immobilization with a splint, rather than a cast, should be considered. Furthermore, soft tissues need to be inspected for any lacerations, especially for injuries caused by an altercation and those near the metacarpophalangeal (MCP) joint. It is not uncommon for a tooth to lacerate the skin and potentially introduce oral flora into the MCP joint. Perhaps the most critical aspect of the exam is to assess for any finger malrotation as a result of the injury. The presence of malrotation will be a key determinant of what type of treatment is indicated. This can be assessed by asking the patient to make a composite fist and looking for any finger cross-over. If the patient is unable to make a fist independently, then the tenodesis effect with wrist flexion and extension can be utilized, along with pressure on the volar forearm muscles to aid in digital flexion.

Additionally, shortening and angulation of metacarpals secondary to a displaced fracture can also be assessed clinically, and this can be noted by a less prominent metacarpal head, or first knuckle, dorsally.

The next step in assessing these injuries is obtaining radiographs. An AP and lateral view of the metacarpal is necessary to properly assess the fracture. Due to the collinearity between multiple metacarpals, it may be needed to take multiple oblique radiographs of the hand in order to clearly obtain a lateral view of the injured metacarpal. It must be noted, however, that cadaveric studies have suggested that oblique radiographs may over-estimate the true degree of angulation [11]. When critically reviewing the radiographs you want to measure shortening and fracture angulation. While never studied in pediatric patients, every 2 mm of shortening in adults results in a loss of 7 degrees of extension [12]. Additionally, acceptable angulation in the sagittal plane depends on which metacarpal is injured. The metacarpals corresponding to the index and middle fingers are more rigidly constrained compared to the ring and small fingers, meaning that less angulation is acceptable for these digits. In adults, typically 10–20 degrees of angulation is acceptable for the index and long finger, while 30 degrees is acceptable for the ring finger, and up to 40 degrees is acceptable for the small finger. In pediatrics, it is possible that more angulation can be accepted as these patients have greater remodeling potential with open physes, especially in the planes of motion of the MCP joint, which is predominantly in the sagittal plane but also in the coronal plane (Fig. 3.2). However, there is very little agreement on what level of angulation requires a reduction and what level of angulation is acceptable to be left alone. These values vary by the affected finger as well as the location on the fracture. It must also be remembered that the metacarpal epiphysis is located distally in the second through fifth digits.

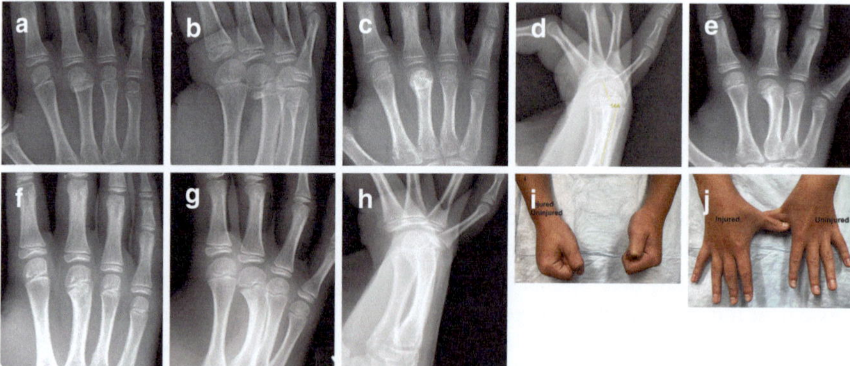

Fig. 3.2 A 9-year-old male sustained a middle finger metacarpal neck fracture. (**a**) AP and (**b**) oblique radiographs demonstrate substantial angulation and slight displacement. (**c**) AP and (**d**) lateral views 4 weeks later show shortening and substantial angulation of the fracture with resultant mild extensor lag. (**e** and **f**) Radiographs at 5 months demonstrate early remodeling which is improved at (**g** and **h**) 11 months post injury. Clinical photographs at 11 months post injury demonstrate full (**i**) flexion and (**j**) extension of the fingers. (Images courtesy of Kevin J. Little, MD)

Treatment

Treatment choices are largely dictated by the location of the metacarpal fracture coupled with the associated deformity in regard to shortening, angulation, and malrotation. In discussing treatment options, we will base our discussion initially on the fracture location. It should be noted in the largest case series, most of these fractures do well, regardless of treatment method [13].

Base

Metacarpal base fractures are relatively uncommon, and most are nondisplaced. These fractures tend to be transverse in pattern and are thought to be due to an axial load [14]. At times these injuries can be associated with crush injuries, and as outlined previously, suspicion for compartment syndrome should be high. For the majority of these injuries, nonoperative treatment with immobilization is indicated, with 3–4 weeks of immobilization required for healing. Intra-articular fractures may be associated with carpometacarpal joint dislocation, and advanced imaging is helpful to determine if operative intervention is warranted.

If the fracture is displaced it can frequently be treated with a closed reduction utilizing longitudinal traction and a volarly directed force at the displaced fracture fragment. In pediatric patients, conscious sedation is frequently needed to successfully accomplish this. Once reduced, immobilization in a cast is required, which should stay in place for 3–4 weeks. If the fracture pattern is unstable, then fixation is required, which is frequently accomplished with placement of Kirschner wires across the fracture site. Wires should be maintained for 4–5 weeks and then can be pulled in the office.

Fracture dislocations of the metacarpal base can also occur, although these are quite rare injuries in children. To best assess this injury pattern a computed tomography (CT) scan is recommended with evaluation of the sagittal cuts. These injuries can also be closed reduced, and if stable, can be treated nonoperatively with immobilization in a cast. If the reduction cannot be maintained, then Kirschner wires placed across the carpometacarpal joint should be utilized and kept for 5–6 weeks. Finally, if a reduction cannot be obtained via closed methods, then a longitudinal, dorsal incision directly over the dislocation can be used to perform an open reduction followed by placement of Kirschner wires as previously described.

There are no case series or larger studies reporting outcomes of these fractures. Most patients do well with appropriate treatment. Potential complications of these injuries can include shortening of the affected ray with subluxation or dislocation of the CMC joint, nonunion, malunion, recurrent instability, and persistent malrotation.

Shaft

Overall, most metacarpal shaft fractures can be treated nonoperatively in pediatric patients. The thick periosteum present in children provides stability and also permits rapid healing times. The mechanism of injury for shaft fractures is frequently torsional, and this results in the subsequent fracture likely having a long spiral or oblique pattern. In these fracture patterns rotation must be closely examined. No amount of malrotation that results in scissoring or finger cross-over is acceptable. As discussed previously, the amount of residual angulation in the sagittal plane that is acceptable is dependent upon the injured metacarpal. Additionally, because these fractures are more proximal than metacarpal neck fractures, the amount of acceptable angulation is reduced. For the second and third metacarpals, typically only 10 degrees of angulation is acceptable, while this increases to 20 degrees for the fourth and fifth metacarpals. Most of these fractures can be treated with cast immobilization for 4–6 weeks, as diaphyseal fractures do not heal as quickly as metaphyseal or epiphyseal fractures. Traditional teaching recommends placing the MCP joints in flexion and the interphalangeal (IP) joints in extension (intrinsic plus positioning) to limit subsequent MCP stiffness. However, when casting the MCP joint in flexion or extension, regardless of how the IP joints are placed, no significant differences have been found in the position the fracture heals or resultant finger range of motion [15].

Surgery is required in fractures that cannot be adequately closed reduced and in multiple metacarpal fractures. Surgical fixation methods can vary with Kirschner wires and intramedullary fixation being common, especially for transverse fracture patterns. Kirschner wires can be placed either intramedullary in a bouquet fashion with entry at the collateral recesses (Fig. 3.3) to avoid the physis or transversely across multiple metacarpals (if the adjacent metacarpals are not injured). For long oblique and spiral fracture patterns, both Kirschner wires and independent lag screws can be considered. Placement of a plate and screws is another option for severely displaced or angulated fractures, as well as in malunions, but these constructs typically require greater dissection, which can result in increased risk for postoperative stiffness secondary to tendon adhesions (Fig. 3.4).

Again, there are no data reporting outcomes of treatment for these fractures specifically. There are also no defined limits to acceptable angulation. Nevertheless, most patients with these injuries recover with full motion and strength, despite some have noticeable deformity. Complications for both operative and nonoperative management include malunion, nonunion, and malrotation. With surgical treatment, additional complications include physeal arrest, hardware failure, stiffness, and tendon adhesions.

Neck

Metacarpal neck fractures are thought to be due to axial loading and bending, which causes a transverse fracture pattern with an apex-dorsal angulation [14]. For most metacarpal neck fractures, nonoperative treatment can be pursued, although treatment algorithms are far from standardized. A recent survey study demonstrated that orthopedic surgeons are more likely to operate with greater than 55 degrees of angulation on the PA x-ray and 47 degrees angulation on the lateral

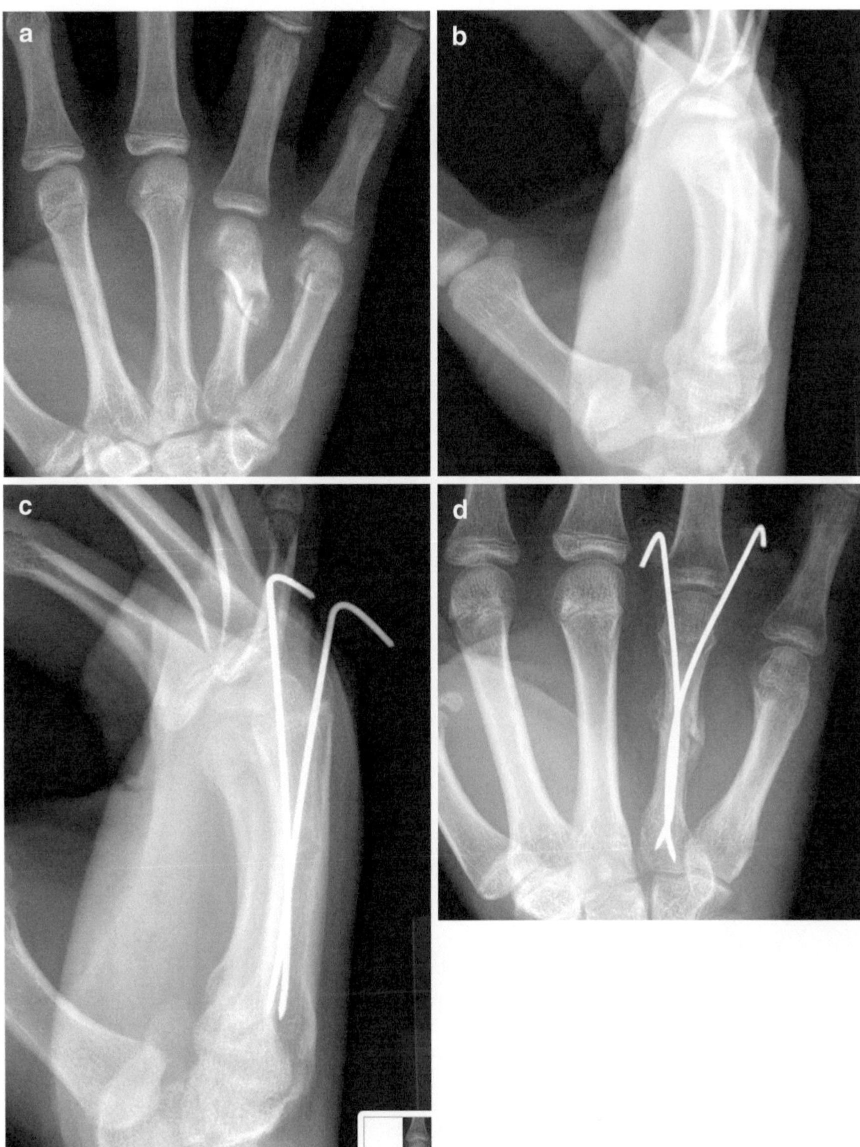

Fig. 3.3 A 16-year-old male presented to the orthopedic clinic 24 days following a hand injury. (**a**) AP and (**b**) lateral radiographs demonstrate a substantially displaced and angulated ring finger metacarpal shaft fracture with early fracture callus along with a healing small finger metacarpal neck fracture. (**c** and **d**) This injury was treated with percutaneous reduction and intramedullary pinning of the ring metacarpal fracture while the small metacarpal neck fracture was allowed to heal with acceptable alignment. (Images courtesy of Kevin J. Little, MD)

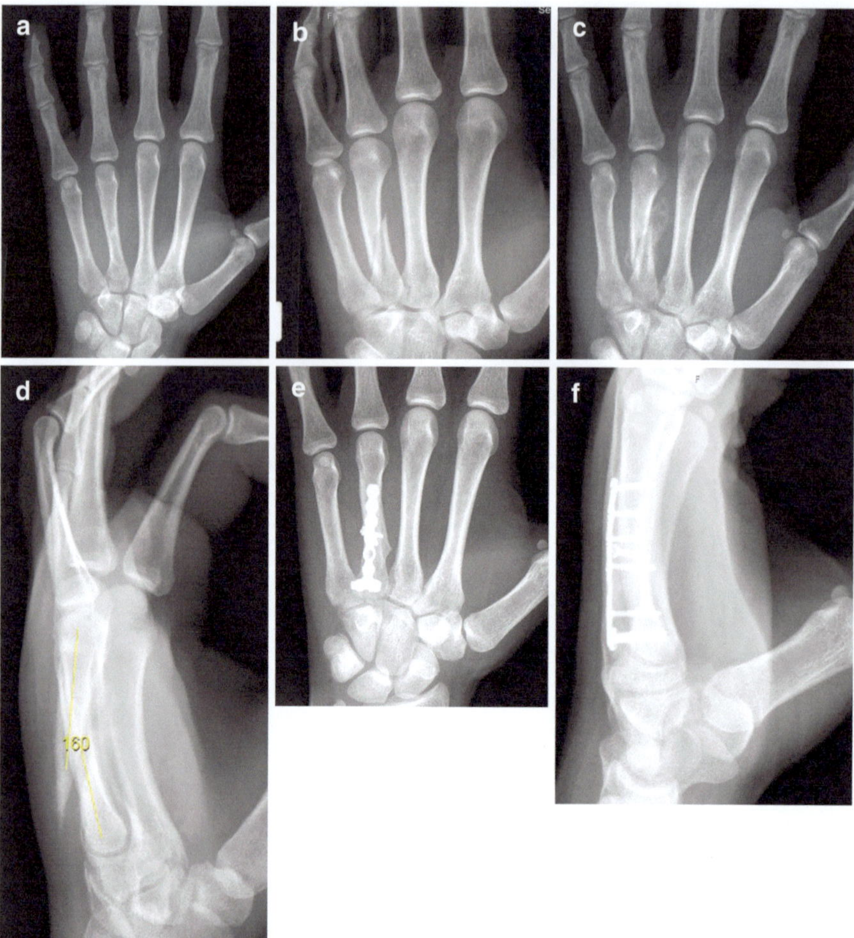

Fig. 3.4 A 14-year-old female presented with an acute ring finger injury sustained during a water polo match. (**a**) AP and (**b**) oblique radiographs show acceptable alignment; however (**c**) oblique and (**d**) lateral radiographs obtained following cast removal 4 weeks later showed a loss of alignment with shortening, flexion, and malrotation. The patient was taken to the operating room where ORIF was performed with full recovery of motion and (**e** and **f**) full radiographic healing at 1 year postoperatively. (Images courtesy of Kevin J. Little, MD)

x-ray, as well as in patients that are likely skeletally mature with an age of at least 17 years [16]. There is no consensus on what is acceptable angulation for these injuries. Some surgeons advocate for acceptance of increasing angulation as injuries occur in the more ulnar metacarpals. For example, one recommendation is to accept 10 degrees of angulation in the index finger, 20 degrees in the middle finger, 30 degrees in the ring finger, and 40 degrees in the small finger [14], while some advocate for acceptance of even greater angulation [17] and others advocate for less [18].

For fractures with acceptable angulation, immobilization for 3–4 weeks is all that is needed. There has been debate as to the best method of immobilization for nonoperative treatment. A recent randomized trial compared outcomes between a forearm-based and a hand-based ulnar gutter thermoplastic splint for fifth metacarpal neck fractures [19]. The authors found that the hand-based splint gave patients better early motion and grip strength, without differences in pain scores, functional outcomes, or union rates, even with lower treatment adherence rates. Among the group of metacarpal neck fractures that can be treated nonoperatively, there is uncertainty as to when a closed reduction should be pursued based on initial angulation. Lee et al. retrospectively reviewed their series of fifth metacarpal neck fractures and assessed the degree of angulation correction that was achieved and maintained at 35 days after reduction [20]. They determined that for fractures with 50 degrees or less of initial angulation, on average only a 4 degree improvement in angulation was maintained. For fractures with greater than 50 degrees of initial angulation, an average of 16 degrees of correction was maintained. This finding led them to conclude that closed reduction may not be indicated for fifth metacarpal neck fractures with less than 50 degrees of initial angulation, and that the fractures can be treated with immobilization in their initial position.

If the fracture is unstable or an acceptable reduction can be obtained or maintained, then surgical treatment can be considered. Depending on the patient's age and the status of the physis, percutaneous pinning with Kirschner wires can be considered versus intramedullary nail or screw fixation (Figure 3.5).

Physeal/Head

These are relatively rare injuries, and they may occur in the presence of a MCP dislocation [21]. One hypothesis for their relative rarity is that the collateral ligaments of the MCP joint act as a stabilizing force since they originate from the metacarpal metaphysis and epiphysis [22]. Findings on x-ray can be subtle, and correlation with the physical exam is crucial, especially in examining for an effusion. If clinical uncertainty remains, a CT scan can be considered (Fig. 3.6a–c). If a fracture is identified and it is truly nondisplaced, then nonoperative management can be pursued with casting for 3–4 weeks. If the fracture is displaced, then a reduction is required. When treating fractures through any physis, it is important to remember that multiple closed reduction attempts should be avoided in an attempt to limit damage to the growth plate and thereby trying to prevent causing premature physeal arrest. If an adequate closed reduction cannot be obtained, then open reduction should be performed, and some form of fixation either with Kirschner wires or screws should be considered (Fig. 3.6d, e). When open reduction is required, the possibility of a poor outcome is increased, with potential complications including stiffness, premature physeal closure and growth arrest, and even osteonecrosis [23–25].

Most patients with these injuries recover fully despite some persistent angulation. If appropriate treatment principles are followed, good outcomes can be

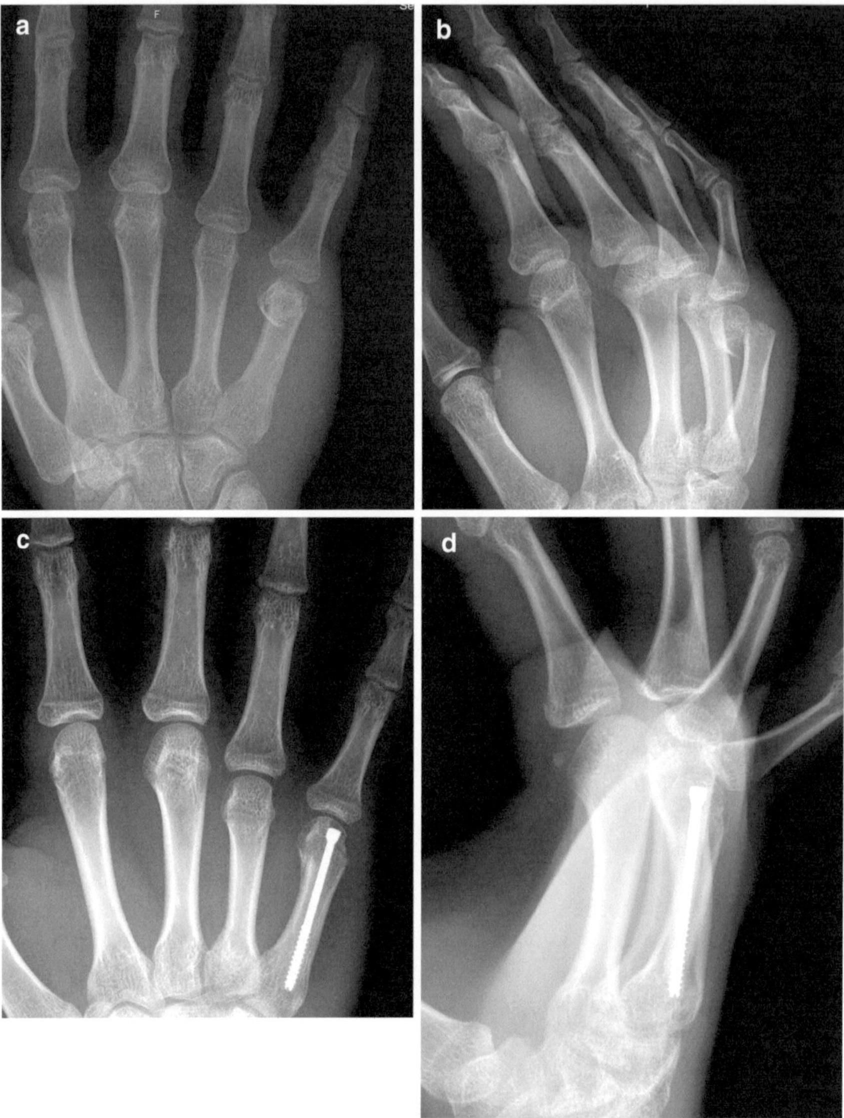

Fig. 3.5 A 15-year-old male sustained a substantial hand injury from an ATV accident. (**a**) AP and (**b**) oblique images demonstrate a completely displaced small finger metacarpal neck fracture and a displaced ring finger metacarpal base fracture. This was treated with closed reduction and intramedullary screw fixation, with full restoration of radiographic alignment noted 1 month postoperatively for both the ring and small finger fractures on (**c**) PA and (**d**) lateral radiographs. (Images courtesy of Kevin J. Little, MD)

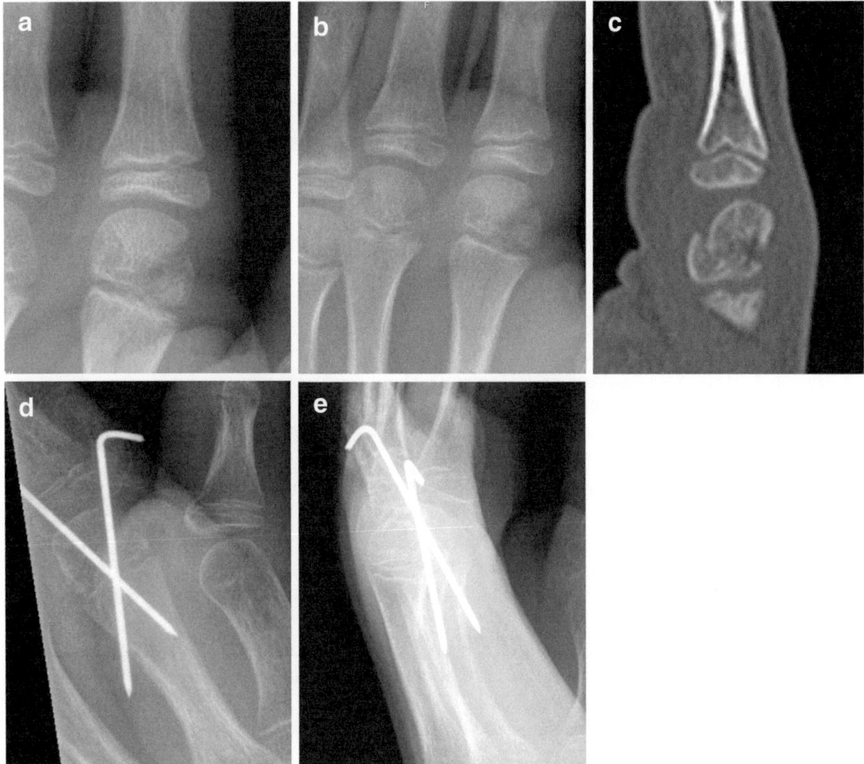

Fig. 3.6 A 10-year-old male sustained an index finger metacarpal neck fracture, which is subtly demonstrated on (**a**) AP and (**b**) oblique radiographs. (**c**) CT scan sagittal plane reformatted images show a substantial articular step off of the large osteochondral fragment without obvious physeal injury. (**d**) AP and (**e**) lateral radiographs demonstrate restored alignment 1 month following MCP joint capsulotomy and open reduction of the epiphyseal fragment. (Images courtesy of Kevin J. Little, MD)

expected and patients should return to full function and activities. The most common complication is refracture, not due to fracture treatment, but due to persistent activities that put the hand at risk of injury. Other complications include pseudo-clawing due to persistent flexion of the fracture [26], which leads to hyperextension contracture of the MCP joint and flexion contracture of the PIP joint. Other potential complications include malunion, nonunion, persistent malrotation, loss of joint motion, physeal arrest, and avascular necrosis.

Conclusion

While metacarpal fractures are relatively common injuries, it is important to remember that they most frequently occur in the neck region of the small finger and as a result rarely require surgical intervention. When the fractures occur in other metacarpals and in other locations within the bone it is important to consider the physical exam to determine if a reduction and/or surgical intervention is required. Fractures that result in severe shortening or finger overlap, as well as those involving the physis and metacarpal head are most concerning for sequelae if not adequately reduced and stabilized. Overall, though, most children with metacarpal fractures appear to do quite well with appropriate treatment.

References

1. Bhende MS, Dandrea LA, Davis HW. Hand injuries in children presenting to a pediatric emergency department. Ann Emerg Med. 1993;22(10):1519–23.
2. Rajesh A, Basu AK, Vaidhyanath R, Finlay D. Hand fractures: a study of their site and type in childhood. Clin Radiol. 2001;56(8):667–9.
3. Worlock PH, Stower MJ. The incidence and pattern of hand fractures in children. J Hand Surg Br. 1986;11(2):198–200.
4. Chung KC, Spilson SV. The frequency and epidemiology of hand and forearm fractures in the United States. J Hand Surg Am. 2001;26(5):908–15.
5. Rettig AC, Ryan R, Shelbourne KD, McCarroll JR, Johnson F Jr, Ahlfeld SK. Metacarpal fractures in the athlete. Am J Sports Med. 1989;17(4):567–72.
6. Vadivelu R, Dias JJ, Burke FD, Stanton J. Hand injuries in children: a prospective study. J Pediatr Orthop. 2006;26(1):29–35.
7. Landin LA. Epidemiology of children's fractures. J Pediatr Orthop B. 1997;6(2):79–83.
8. Chew EM, Chong AK. Hand fractures in children: epidemiology and misdiagnosis in a tertiary referral hospital. J Hand Surg Am. 2012;37(8):1684–8.
9. Gilsanz V, Ratib O. Hand bone age: a digital atlas of skeletal maturity. 1st ed. Berlin: Springer-Verlag; 2005. p. 98.
10. Limb D, Loughenbury PR. The prevalence of pseudoepiphyses in the metacarpals of the growing hand. J Hand Surg Eur Vol. 2012;37(7):678–81.
11. Lamraski G, Monsaert A, De Maeseneer M, Haentjens P. Reliability and validity of plain radiographs to assess angulation of small finger metacarpal neck fractures: human cadaveric study. J Orthop Res. 2006;24(1):37–45.
12. Strauch RJ, Rosenwasser MP, Lunt JG. Metacarpal shaft fractures: the effect of shortening on the extensor tendon mechanism. J Hand Surg Am. 1998;23(3):519–23.
13. Kiely AL, Griffin M, FHK J, Nolan GS, Butler PE. Phalangeal and metacarpal fractures in children: a 10-year comparison of factors affecting functional outcomes in 313 patients. J Hand Microsurg. 2021;15(2):124–32.
14. Cornwall R. Finger metacarpal fractures and dislocations in children. Hand Clin. 2006;22(1):1–10.
15. Tavassoli J, Ruland RT, Hogan CJ, Cannon DL. Three cast techniques for the treatment of extra-articular metacarpal fractures. Comparison of short-term outcomes and final fracture alignments. J Bone Joint Surg Am. 2005;87(10):2196–201.
16. Abzug JM, Chang T, Case AL, Dua K, Hara N. Variation amongst orthopedic surgeons when treating fifth metacarpal neck fractures in the pediatric population. Pediatrics. 2019;144(2 MeetingAbstract):800.
17. O'Brien E. Fractures of the hand and wrist region. In: Rockwood C, Wilkins K, King R, editors. Fractures in children. Philadelphia: JB Lippincott; 1984. p. 229–99.
18. Valencia J, Leyva F, Gomez-Bajo GJ. Pediatric hand trauma. Clin Orthop Relat Res. 2005;432:77–86.
19. Davison PG, Boudreau N, Burrows R, Wilson KL, Bezuhly M. Forearm-based ulnar gutter versus hand-based thermoplastic splint for pediatric metacarpal neck fractures: a blinded, randomized trial. Plast Reconstr Surg. 2016;137(3):908–16.

20. Lee SJ, Merrison H, Williams KA, Vuillermin CB, Bauer AS. Closed reduction and immobilization of pediatric fifth metacarpal neck fractures. Hand (N Y). 2022;17:416.
21. Light TR, Ogden JA. Complex dislocation of the index metacarpophalangeal joint in children. J Pediatr Orthop. 1988;8(3):300–5.
22. Bogumill GP. A morphologic study of the relationship of collateral ligaments to growth plates in the digits. J Hand Surg Am. 1983;8(1):74–9.
23. McElfresh EC, Dobyns JH. Intra-articular metacarpal head fractures. J Hand Surg Am. 1983;8(4):383–93.
24. Brown JE. Epiphyseal growth arrest in a fractured metacarpal. J Bone Joint Surg Am. 1959;41(3):494.
25. Prosser AJ, Irvine GB. Epiphyseal fracture of the metacarpal head. Injury. 1988;19(1):34–5.
26. Soldado F, Farr S. Chapter 10: finger metacarpal fractures. In: Cornwall R, Little KJ, editors. Pediatric hand trauma. Chicago, IL: American Society for Surgery of the Hand; 2020.

Pediatric Phalangeal Base and Shaft Fractures

4

Tristan B. Weir, Catherine C. May, and Joshua M. Abzug

Introduction

Pediatric hand fractures are very common, accounting for an estimated 1.5 million cases in United States emergency departments annually [1]. The clinical and radiographic evaluation of these injuries requires careful assessment to prevent long-term functional consequences. Understanding the differences between treating these injuries in pediatric and adult patients will enable the provider to achieve reliable clinical outcomes.

Phalangeal fractures are the most common hand injuries in children (excluding forearm injuries) accounting for 23% of cases, followed by metacarpal (18%) and carpal (14%) fractures. The fifth digit is the most commonly involved digit (53%), followed by the thumb (23%), ring (10%), index (8%), and middle finger (6%) [2]. Proximal phalanx fractures are the most common phalangeal fractures (63%, excluding the thumb), followed by the middle phalanx (19%) and distal phalanx (18%) [3].

The fracture location and mechanism of injury vary based on the patient's age. The incidence of hand fractures increases at the age of 11 years, with 14- and 15-year-olds being the peak age group. Distal phalanx and multiple hand fractures are more common in children under 9 years of age, while children over 12 years

Disclaimers: The views expressed in the submitted article are our own and not an official position of the institution.

T. B. Weir · C. C. May · J. M. Abzug (✉)
Department of Orthopedic Surgery, University of Maryland School of Medicine, Baltimore, MD, USA
e-mail: tweir@som.umaryland.edu; catherine.may@som.umaryland.edu; jabzug@som.umaryland.edu

J. M. Abzug et al. (eds.), *Pediatric and Adult Hand Fractures*,
https://doi.org/10.1007/978-3-031-32072-9_4

of age are more likely to sustain proximal phalanx fractures from sports-related activities [2]. A crush mechanism in smaller hands with digits in closer proximity may explain why multiple digits are more commonly involved in young children. The increased participation in contact sports for older children accounts for the higher incidence and mechanism of hand fractures in this age group [3, 4]. Also coinciding with greater participation in contact sports, males account for two-thirds of phalangeal fractures [3, 5]. Associated soft tissue injuries have been reported in 33% of patients, where 70–86% of toddlers and preschool children have such injuries, while only 22% of children over 10 years old have a soft tissue injury. This, again, can be explained by the crushing mechanism of injury in younger children.

This chapter focuses on the evaluation and treatment of pediatric phalangeal base and shaft fractures. Specifically focusing on the pathoanatomy, clinical and radiographic assessment, nonoperative and operative treatment, outcomes, and complications, this chapter aims to guide the medical provider caring for the hand to optimally manage these injuries.

Pathoanatomy

Understanding the unique anatomical differences in children is essential to the management of phalangeal base and shaft fractures. The phalangeal physis is located at the proximal end of the bone and is perpendicular to the longitudinal axis of the diaphysis. The physis is biomechanically weaker than the surrounding ligamentous structures and mineralized bone, making fractures through the physis more common than ligamentous injuries or diaphyseal fractures [6]. The ligamentous and tendinous insertions in relation to the physis can help explain the various fracture patterns and deforming forces.

Fractures of the base of the proximal phalanx are common in children. Al-Qattan et al. prospectively described the relative incidence and classification of these injuries in 100 consecutive patients [7]. They categorized fractures according to the Salter-Harris classification for physeal fractures and as juxta-epiphyseal or metaphyseal fractures for fractures not involving the physis. Juxta-epiphyseal fractures occur 1–2 mm distal to the physis and traverse the subchondral bone (type I juxta-epiphyseal fractures), but some may resemble the Thurstan-Holland fragment of Salter-Harris II fractures with a radial or ulnar corner metaphyseal fragment (Fig. 4.1). The authors reported that the juxta-epiphyseal type II fracture is the most common (53%), followed by Salter-Harris type II fractures (26%), and juxta-epiphyseal type I fractures (8%). All other Salter-Harris fractures occurred at a rate of 0–5%. The little finger was the most commonly injured digit (52%) and has been termed an "extra-octave" fracture due to the ulnar deviation assumed by the pull of the abductor digiti minimi and abduction force mechanism [8]. The term "extra-octave" was coined by Mercer Rang to describe the advantage a pianist would have to reach an "extra-octave" if the fracture was not reduced [9, 10]. Fractures of the

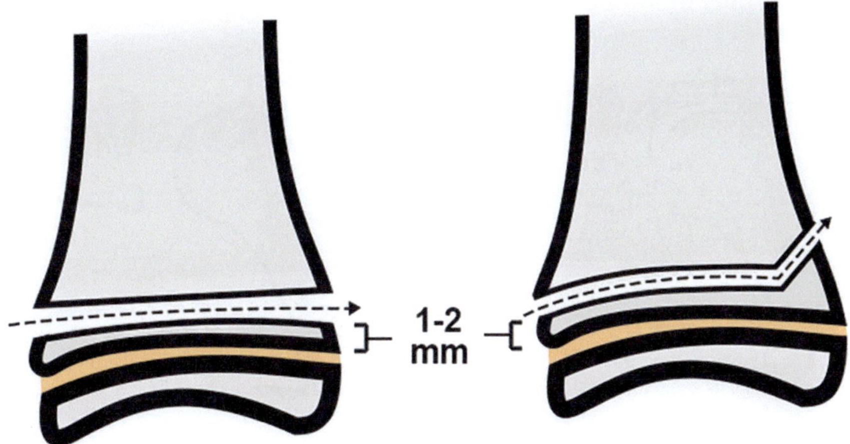

Fig. 4.1 The juxta-epiphyseal fracture classification. Type I juxta-epiphyseal fractures occur 1–2 mm distal to the physis and traverse the subchondral bone (left). Type II juxta-epiphyseal fractures are the same as type I, but have a Thurston-Holland fragment in the metaphysis at the radial or ulnar corner. (Courtesy of Tristan B. Weir, MD)

proximal phalanx usually have an apex volar deformity due to the dorsal pull of the distal fragment from the extensor mechanism and volar pull of the proximal fragment from the interossei attachments [11].

George Bogumill performed an anatomic study on fresh frozen amputated hands of a 10-year-old boy and a 13-year-old girl in 1983 to determine the relationship of the collateral ligaments of the digits to the physes [12]. At the metacarpophalangeal joint (MCPJ), the radial collateral ligament originates from the epiphysis, distal to the metacarpal physis (which is located at the distal metacarpal). Conversely, the ulnar collateral ligament of the MCPJ originates from the metacarpal epiphysis, but the accessory collateral portion extends proximally to the metacarpal shaft, thus inserting proximal to the level of the physis. The collateral ligaments of the MCPJ insert on the epiphysis of the proximal phalanx without distal extension to the metaphysis. At the proximal interphalangeal joint (PIPJ), the collateral ligaments extend from the proximal phalangeal neck to the epiphysis of the middle phalanx, extending beyond the growth plate to blend with the periosteum. Due to these anatomical considerations, Salter-Harris III fractures are more common at the MCPJ than the PIPJ given the stronger collateral ligaments can avulse the epiphysis from the weaker physis. At the PIPJ, the more distal insertion of the collateral ligaments makes Salter-Harris III fractures much less likely.

The fracture location in the middle phalanx determines the deforming forces that act on the fracture fragment. The flexor digitorum superficialis inserts on the volar shaft of the middle phalanx, while the central slip inserts on the dorsal epiphysis [6]. Fractures proximal to the flexor digitorum superficialis insertion will assume apex dorsal angulation, while those distal to the insertion have apex volar angulation. The

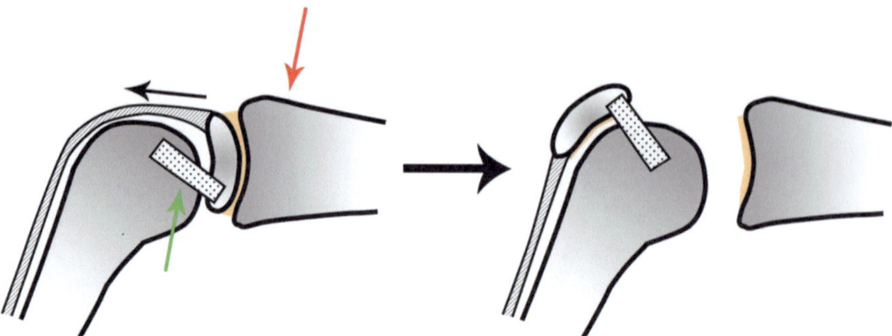

Fig. 4.2 The "jockeyed fracture" occurs when traction and shear forces result in the middle phalangeal epiphysis separating and being pulled proximally by the central slip. The left image shows the shear force from dorsal to palmar (red arrow), the traction force (black arrow), and the intact collateral ligament (green arrow). The image on the right shows the epiphysis of the middle phalanx has retracted, but the central slip and collateral ligaments are still intact. This resembles a jockey riding a horse, where the epiphysis is the jockey, the central slip is the reins, the collateral ligaments are stirrups, and the head of the proximal phalanx is the horse. (Courtesy of Tristan B. Weir, MD)

volar plate inserts on the epiphysis and metaphysis of the middle phalanx [13]. Hyperextension-type injuries to the proximal phalanx can lead to avulsion fractures of the middle phalanx epiphysis. It is important to distinguish these injuries from dorsal avulsions, which are due to the less common central slip avulsion. The central slip insertion on the dorsal aspect of the middle phalangeal epiphysis can act as a deforming force in Salter-Harris type I and III fractures of the middle phalanx. Keene et al. proposed a two-part mechanism for such injuries, involving both traction and shear forces on the epiphysis of the middle phalanx [13]. Hashizume and colleague termed such fractures "jockeyed" epiphyseal fractures because of the appearance of the retracted and rotated epiphysis attached to the central slip and intact collateral ligaments [14]. The epiphyseal fragment resembles a jockey (the epiphysis of the middle phalanx) on horseback (the proximal phalangeal condyle) holding reins (the central slip) with his legs in stirrups (the collateral ligaments) (Fig. 4.2). Finally, a less common mechanism of injury to the phalangeal epiphysis has been seen in adolescent rock climbers, resulting in a Salter-Harris III stress fracture [15, 16].

Clinical Evaluation

A careful history and clinical assessment of phalangeal base and shaft fractures is essential to determining the most appropriate treatment. As with any assessment, the history begins with the chief complaint, hand dominance, mechanism of injury,

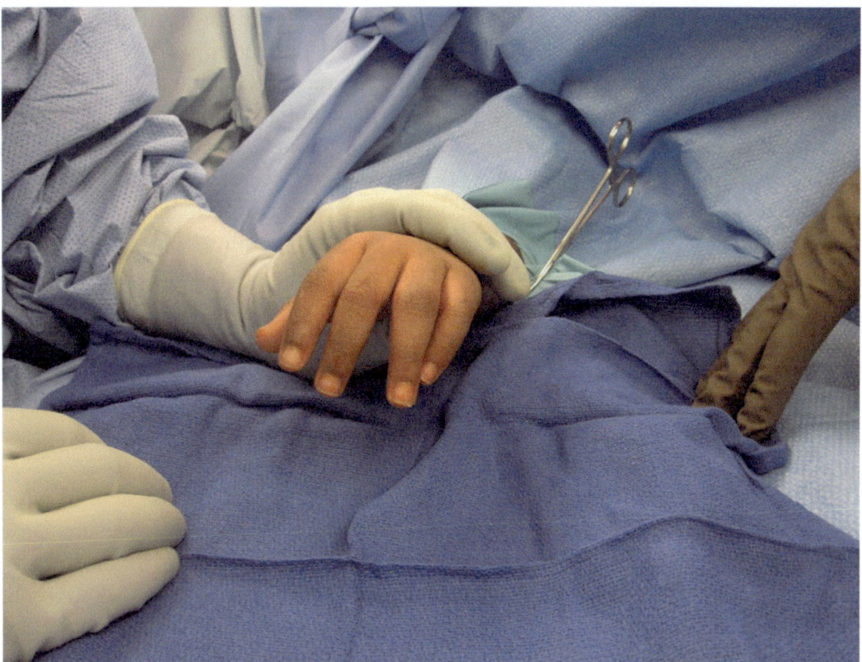

Fig. 4.3 Assessing for subtle or obvious rotational or angular deformities is essential to treating phalangeal base and shaft fractures. This patient has an obvious ring finger deformity with ulnar angulation, obvious scissoring, and malaligned nailbeds. (Image courtesy of Joshua M. Abzug, MD)

and timing of the injury. While hand fractures are rarely non-accidental, the provider should always consider this in at-risk patient populations and evaluate the patient holistically.

A careful physical examination is vital to establishing a proper diagnosis and treatment plan. Chew and Chong showed 16 of 204 (7.8%) hand fracture referrals to a tertiary hospital were misdiagnosed [3]. The physical examination contributed to the correct diagnosis in half of the misdiagnosed cases and 5 missed fractures were identified based on tenderness that correlated with radiographic findings. The hand care provider should first inspect the involved digit, assessing for swelling, obvious deformities, and skin abrasions or lacerations. Assessing the digital cascade and comparing it to the uninjured side can uncover subtle rotational or angular deformities that may alter the treatment plan [17] (Fig. 4.3). The nailbeds can also be used to assess rotation and should be in the same plane of rotation. The flexed index and middle fingers should point to the trapezium, while the flexed ring and small fingers should point to the scaphoid tubercle. The index finger is normally supinated slightly to help with pinch, which should be compared to the contralateral side. There is a normal slight overlap of the ring finger over the small finger, which can be compared to the uninjured side. Underlapping or overlapping of digits which is not symmetric to the uninjured side should be considered an angular deformity. Assessing active motion can be challenging depending on the patient age, pain level, and degree of swelling. Passive motion can be assessed with the tenodesis effect where the wrist is passively flexed and extended, causing the digits to extend and flex, respectively, if the tendons are intact. In young children, the volar forearm musculature can be compressed to flex the digits thus permitting an assessment of the digital cascade, assuming tendon integrity is present. Isolating the flexor digitorum superficialis and profundus tendon integrity may be challenging in the young patient, but should be attempted with active or passive motion. Especially when no or minor deformity is present, palpation of the digit will illicit pain in the fracture location. The surgeon should also palpate the entire extremity as well as the contralateral upper extremity to assess for concomitant injuries, starting at the shoulder and working distally to the digits.

The neurovascular examination is always important in the assessment of hand trauma. Capillary refill testing should be performed in all cases and should be repeated after any reduction or pinning procedure. Sensation testing can be especially difficult in young children and may require creative techniques. Comparing light touch in the median, radial, and ulnar nerve distributions of each hand and asking the child if they feel the same is the simplest way to assess sensation but may not be possible in young children [18, 19]. A recent study has shown that monofilament testing can be reliably performed in the majority of patients aged 4 years and above, while 2-point discrimination can be reliably performed in most children aged 6 years and older [20]. In younger patients, autonomic function can be tested with the *water basin* or *wrinkle test*, where the child's hand is submerged in warm water for 10 min [21]. A hand with normal sensation will produce wrinkled skin, while skin supplied by damaged peripheral nerves will remain smooth [22]. This test is not routinely performed as it requires a substantial amount of time and patient/parent cooperation. An alternative and faster option to assess autonomic function is the *sweat test* [23]. The examiner looks for the presence of sweating in a region supplied by a previously injured peripheral nerve. Sweating in that distribution indicates nerve regeneration, while dry skin indicates the peripheral nerve remains damaged.

Radiographic Evaluation

Radiographic evaluation with standard posteroanterior and lateral views of the hand is essential to establishing the correct diagnosis. Oblique view may be added to the series if an articular fracture is suspected [21]. Dedicated views of the injured digit are also helpful to improve visualization by reducing overlap with neighboring digits [24, 25]. Advanced imaging is typically not indicated in pediatric phalanx fractures [26].

While prior studies have assumed the phalangeal articular surface and physis in children are perpendicular to the diaphysis [27, 28], Krueger et al. showed this is not necessarily the case [29]. The authors assessed normal hand bone age radiographs to determine the normal articular and physeal angles to the diaphysis in the coronal plane. The articular and physeal angles differed from 90 degrees more than half the time and are never 90 degrees in the small finger PIPJ. There is a normal 6-degree radial tilt in the metaphysis of the small finger middle phalanx, accounting for the clinically normal slight overlap of the ring finger over the small finger. Additionally, the index and middle finger proximal phalangeal epiphyses are wedge-shaped, larger on the radial side, and become more symmetric as the child becomes older. This study highlights the importance of the clinical exam and comparison to the uninjured side, as radiographic findings are variable depending on the digit and patient age, and the physis and proximal articular surface are not always perpendicular to the diaphysis.

In fractures of the base of the proximal phalanx, "Campbell's line" can be used to assess the degree of displacement on initial evaluation, after reduction, and to assess remodeling during follow-up [8, 30]. A line is drawn from the center of the proximal phalangeal head, through the center of the proximal phalangeal metaphysis, and should intersect the center of the metacarpal head in a normal digit, regardless of digit flexion (Fig. 4.4) Displacement of proximal phalanx base fractures has been defined as "mild" if the line passes off-center of the metacarpal head, and "severe" if the line misses the metacarpal head altogether [8]. Al-Qattan et al. later defined the diaphyseal-head angle (DHA) as the angle formed between the proximal phalanx diaphysis and the center of the metacarpal head to better quantify displacement [31]. In normal digits, the DHA ranges from 177 to 180 degrees with moderate inter-observer reliability of 0.56 and good intra-observer reliability of 0.76. Therefore, the DHA is a reasonable alternative to the categorical method of quantifying fracture displacement in proximal phalanx base fractures (Fig. 4.4).

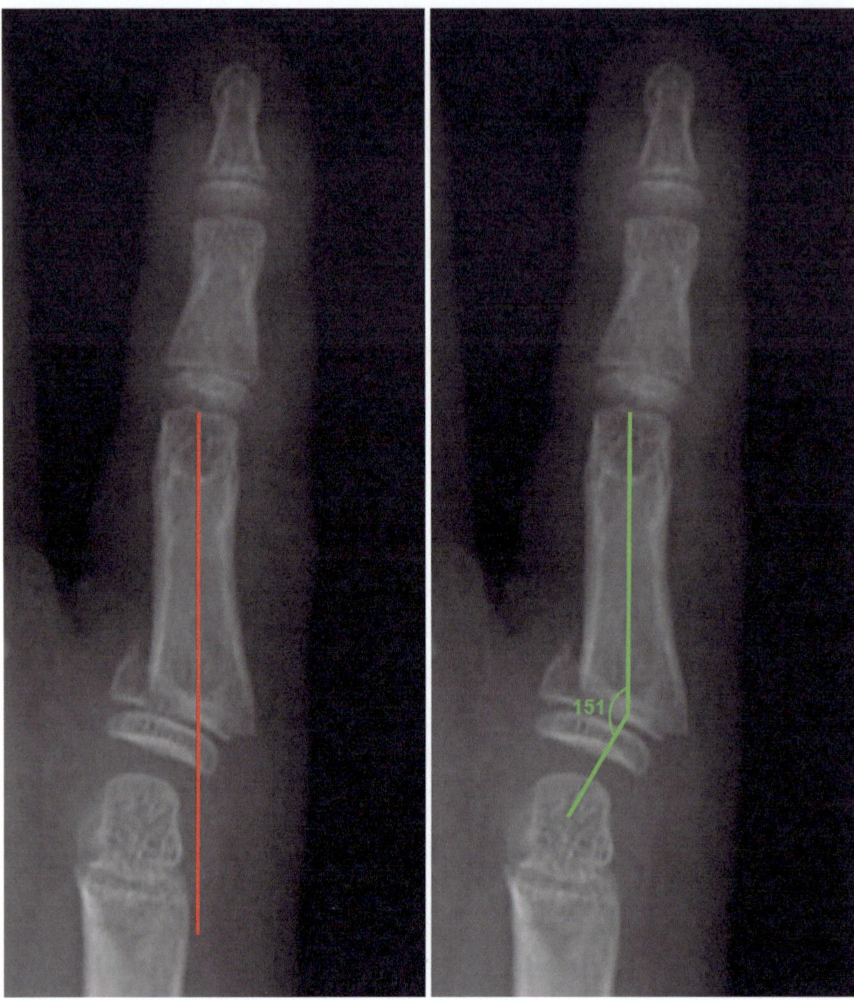

Fig. 4.4 Campbell's line (red line) is drawn from the center of the proximal phalangeal head through the center of the proximal phalangeal metaphysis. The line should intersect the center of the metacarpal metaphysis in the normal digit. Proximal phalangeal base fractures have "mild" displacement if the line intersects the metacarpal head off-center, whereas fracture with "severe" displacement will not intersect the metacarpal head at all (as in the radiograph shown). The diaphyseal-head angle (DHA) is shown by the green lines in the image on the right. The angle is formed between the proximal phalanx diaphysis and the center of the metacarpal head and normal values range between 177 and 180°. This patient's DHA of 151° requires a closed reduction. (Images courtesy of Joshua M. Abzug, MD)

Nonoperative Management

The decision to proceed with nonoperative management of pediatric phalangeal base and shaft fractures is based on clinical and radiographic findings. The most important radiographic factors that dictate management are the fracture location, orientation, and displacement [6]. Stable fracture patterns are generally transverse shaft fractures or metaphyseal extra-articular fractures, while oblique, spiral, or comminuted shaft fracture patterns are considered unstable [32]. Length stable fractures and those without articular involvement are generally amenable to a closed reduction and immobilization with buddy taping, casting, or splinting [33]. The success of nonoperative treatment based on fracture location was described by Hartley et al., where only 3.2% of fractures at the base of the phalanx required operative intervention and 20.7% of phalangeal shaft fractures required surgery [34]. This is due to the inherent stability of phalangeal base fractures compared with shaft fractures [35]. Importantly, fractures may appear radiographically innocuous, yet have substantial rotational deformity or deviation that would result in malunion and functional limitations if treated nonoperatively. This is because splints and casts can only control radial and ulnar deviation, flexion, and extension, but cannot control rotation or maintain length in a shortened fracture [33]. It is therefore vital to consider both the radiographic and clinical evaluation of the fracture to guide treatment.

Proximal Phalanx Fractures

Given the inherent stability and proximity to the physis for remodeling, extra-articular proximal phalangeal base fractures are typically treated with or without closed reduction and immobilization. Extra-octave fractures of the base of the small finger proximal phalanx are commonly reduced with the "pencil technique" described by Mercer Rang [9]. The pencil is placed in the fourth webspace to act as a fulcrum for the reduction and control the proximal fracture fragment, which enables the distal fragment to be radially deviated to reduce the fracture (Fig. 4.5a). While authors note that the pencil is exerting pressure at a point distal to the fracture, as the proximal phalanx extends more proximally than the web space would suggest, they have still found this to be an effective technique to obtain the reduction [31]. An alternative to this technique is the "90–90" method where the digit is flexed to 90° at the MCP and PIP joints, then radially deviating the small finger while applying a dorsal-to-palmar force on the metacarpal shaft and a palmar-to-dorsal force on the PIP joint [10] (Fig. 4.5b). One can attempt to stabilize the proximal fragment by holding it proximal to the fourth web space, but this is not typically necessary. Over-reduction of the digit can disrupt the robust periosteum that provides stability to these fractures [6]. Dorsally blocking the MCP joints helps correct the apex volar deformity, and rotation is assessed as described in the clinical evaluation section above.

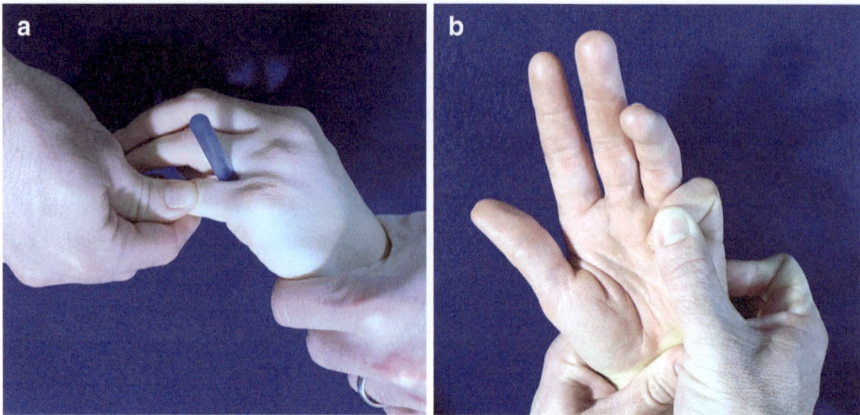

Fig. 4.5 (**a**) The "pencil" technique involves placing a pen or pencil in the webspace to act as a fulcrum for the reduction and control the proximal fracture fragment, which enables the distal fragment to be radially deviated to reduce the fracture. (**b**) The "90–90" technique is performed by flexing the digit to 90° at the MCP and PIP joints, then radially deviating the small finger while applying a dorsal-to-palmar force on the metacarpal shaft and a palmar-to-dorsal direction on the PIP joint. (Images courtesy of Tristan B. Weir, MD)

The radiographic parameters for obtaining an acceptable reduction depend on the fracture location and patient age. Extra-articular phalangeal base and shaft fractures with dorsal or palmar angulation of more than 25°, radial or ulnar deviation of more than 10°, or rotational deformities are considered unacceptable and warrant operative intervention after attempted reduction [36–38]. The amount of remodeling that occurs to correct residual deformity depends on the patient's age and proximity of the fracture to the physis [17, 39]. Extra-articular fractures near the physis have a greater ability to correct in the plane of motion of the adjacent joint. The MCP joint allows for flexion and extension, which makes remodeling in this plane possible if the patient has at least 2 years of remaining growth. Given the condyloid shape of the MCP joint, abduction/adduction is possible and allows for some remodeling in the coronal plane. There is more coronal plane motion in the more ulnar digits, making acceptable angulation in these digits more lenient than the radial digits.

Most evidence related to immobilization of phalangeal base and shaft fractures is limited to retrospective reports [8, 37, 40, 41]. Weber et al., however, performed a randomized controlled trial to assess the non-inferiority of buddy taping versus palmar splint immobilization for extra-articular phalangeal base and shaft fractures [38]. Patients were aged 4–16 years, and exclusion criteria included open fractures, multiple fractures on one hand, delayed presentation, and phalangeal neck fractures. Of the 99 patients (buddy taping, $n = 52$; splinting, $n = 47$) included in the study, secondary displacement occurred in 6.4% of the splinting patients and 1.9% of the buddy taping patients. The risk difference of 4.5% did not reach statistical significance, and the authors concluded that taping is not inferior to splinting. Of note, all secondary displacements occurred in fractures that required a reduction, and only one patient in the splint group required surgical intervention. While some authors note concerns with compliance of splinting and buddy taping [42], the authors of this study claim this was not an issue in their cohort.

Functional bracing of extra-articular proximal phalanx fractures aims to simultaneously promote bony healing while preserving motion [36]. Maintaining motion during healing is especially important in adults, but children tend to regain motion more readily. Nevertheless, multiple studies have sought to maintain motion during bony healing through more functional splinting methods to improve the child's ability to perform daily activities and writing in school. Regardless of the specific orthosis type, functional braces block MCP joint extension and allow PIP joint flexion [37]. This places tension on the extensor hood, advancing it over the proximal phalanx, and creates compression across the fracture with PIP joint flexion. The addition of buddy tape allows passive flexion of the injured digit by actively flexing an adjacent finger [43]. The indications for functional orthoses include intact soft tissues, an intact extensor hood, and a stable reduction without rotational or angular deformity. Franz et al. prospectively evaluated functional-conservative management of 75 extra-articular proximal phalanx fractures using a functional forearm orthosis or the Lucerne Cast (LuCa) [37]. The LuCa cast is a smaller hand-based cast/orthosis which allows for wrist and interphalangeal joint motion, dorsally blocking MCPJ motion to 70 to 90 degrees. The authors found the finger total arc of motion was no different at the time of orthosis removal, but the LuCa cast group had a better initial wrist arc of motion. There were no differences in motion at 3 months, and all fractures healed within 6 weeks without residual deformity. Overall, we believe the risk of secondary displacement outweighs the risk of stiffness in young patients and therefore cast immobilization for 3–4 weeks is preferred with weekly radiographic and clinical follow-up as necessary to assess for loss of reduction or malrotation [6, 44].

Middle Phalanx Fractures

Given the inherent instability of middle phalangeal fractures, more rigid immobilization is preferred to motion sparing options. All digits are included in the cast/orthosis, except for the thumb, with the MCP joints held in 70–90° of flexion and the PIP joints in 15–20° of flexion [17]. Acceptable radiographic criteria after closed reduction of middle phalanx fractures are comparable to proximal phalanx fractures in the sagittal plane, but coronal plane deformities are not tolerated well in the middle phalanx. Some have advocated nonoperative management for post-reduction dorsopalmar angulation of less than 30° in children under the age of 10 years, and less than 20° in children older than 10 years. Contrary to the MCP joint, however, the PIP joint is a true hinge joint and does not allow abduction or adduction, limiting the remodeling potential in the radial or ulnar plane for fractures of the middle phalanx. Like all phalangeal fractures, assessing rotational deformities and/or overlapping/underlapping of adjacent digits is essential as such deformities will not remodel adequately.

Other injuries may occur at the middle phalangeal epiphysis given the various soft tissue attachments. Hyperextension of the PIP joint can lead to avulsions of the volar plate from the palmar epiphysis. These injuries are treated with brief splinting of 1 week followed by early range of motion exercises to prevent stiffness [45]. Avulsions from the dorsal epiphysis have more variable injury patterns and treatment protocols. A fleck from the dorsal epiphysis with an intact Elson's test can be treated conservatively, while a central slip avulsion with palmar subluxation of the middle phalanx would necessitate operative intervention. Elson's test is performed by placing the patient's palm flat on the edge of a table or block, and flexing the PIP joint to 90° over the edge. The patient is asked to actively extend the PIP joint, and the examiner assesses the suppleness of the DIP joint. If the DIP joint remains supple, the central slip is intact. If the DIP joint is rigid, the central slip may be ruptured.

Radiographic Follow-Up

While close radiographic follow-up of many pediatric phalanx has been advocated by most authors, some have questioned their utility in some fractures. Vonlanthen et al. performed a retrospective review of extra-articular pediatric (<16 years old) phalangeal fractures to determine the subgroups that are stable and do not require follow-up radiographs [28]. Patients with index through small finger middle and proximal phalangeal base and shaft fractures were included. Of the 365 patients included in the study, 6.6% of the digits requiring a reduction had secondary displacement and no digits with minimal angulation (<10°) or displacement had secondary displacement. The authors concluded that follow-up radiographs were not indicated for fractures with minimally angulated or nondisplaced fractures, while those requiring a reduction are at greater risk of secondary displacement. In response to this study, Niddam et al. noted the broad inclusion criteria consisting of proximal and middle phalangeal base and shaft fractures, which have variable inherent stability [35]. The authors also pointed out that the study lacked statistical analysis to demonstrate the 10° cutoff, and the authors did not show which fracture types had secondary displacement. Our practice is to obtain weekly clinical and radiographic follow-up for 2 weeks for patients treated nonoperatively with a potentially unstable fracture or one that has undergone a reduction to assess for secondary displacement or angulation.

Operative Management

Proximal Phalanx Fractures

While most proximal phalangeal fractures are successfully managed nonoperatively, surgery is indicated for multiple reasons. Operative intervention should be considered for intra-articular fractures (i.e., Salter-Harris III and IV fractures or displaced epiphyseal Salter-Harris I fractures), length unstable fractures (spiral, oblique, or comminuted shaft fractures), fractures with rotational deformity, and fractures with greater than 25° of dorsal or palmar angulation or 10° of radial or ulnar angulation after attempted reduction. Additionally, patients may be indicated for surgery after attempted nonoperative management that demonstrates loss of reduction. In addition to the above operative criteria, proximal phalanx fractures may be irreducible by closed means for several reasons. Authors have reported multiple structures blocking a closed reduction, including flexor tendon entrapment at the fracture site, fibrous tissue interposition, extensor hood entrapment, collateral ligament disruption, and periosteum entrapment [6, 8, 45–49]. It is important to recognize that a fracture may not be reducible by closed means, and multiple attempts could damage the physis [33]. Despite these potential blocks to reduction, however, such reports are limited to case reports and small case series. Al-Qattan and colleagues showed blocks to closed reduction are rare, only reporting flexor tendon entrapment in 1 of 92 (1.1%) patients [31].

Middle Phalanx Fractures

Fractures of the middle and proximal phalanges have similar indications for operative intervention, but middle phalanx fractures have several unique considerations. Unlike the MCP joint, the PIP joint has minimal coronal plane motion. Therefore, any amount of radial or ulnar deviation is less likely to remodel to correct the deformity. Middle phalanx fractures are considered more unstable than proximal phalanx fractures and should be clinically and radiographically scrutinized [33, 35]. Additionally, the central slip insertion on the dorsal epiphysis of the middle phalanx can dorsally displace Salter-Harris I or III injuries, leading to PIP joint subluxation and requiring open reduction and internal fixation (ORIF) [13, 14, 45].

Surgical Technique

Most phalangeal base and shaft fractures requiring operative intervention can be treated with closed reduction and percutaneous pinning (CRPP), but occasionally an open reduction is required for irreducible or intra-articular fractures. Multiple methods of Kirschner wire (K-wire) fixation have been described and depend on the fracture configuration to maintain an adequate reduction.

Prior to the start of surgery, preoperative antibiotics may be given within an hour of the procedure, but this practice varies by surgeon and institution. Case et al. performed a survey study on the use of preoperative antibiotics among members of the Pediatric Orthopaedic Society of North America (POSNA) for upper extremity percutaneous procedures [50]. While 40% of providers did not feel preoperative antibiotics were needed for all percutaneous procedures, 80% of providers routinely order prophylactic antibiotics. The respondents felt the use of prophylactic antibiotics was less important the more distal the procedure is on the extremity. Despite this

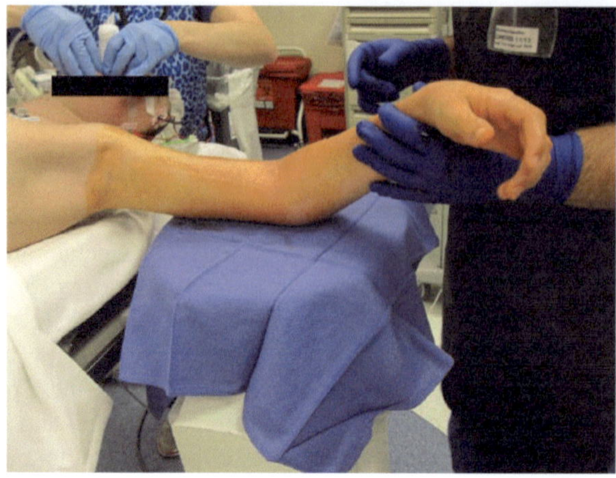

Fig. 4.6 This intraoperative example of the semisterile technique for upper extremity fractures uses the C-arm as an operative surface and only requires a sterile blue towel for draping. For phalangeal fractures, the mini C-arm is similarly used as the operating surface. (Image courtesy of Joshua M. Abzug, MD)

opinion, studies have shown that metacarpal and phalangeal fractures have higher pin site infection rates than distal radius fractures [51, 52]. Preoperative antibiotics have not been shown to affect infection rates in multiple soft tissue hand procedures, including carpal tunnel and trigger finger releases [53–55]. These studies were performed in adult patients, however, and no comparative studies have been performed in children undergoing percutaneous procedures to establish if prophylactic antibiotics are beneficial.

While a full preparation and draping is common practice, the "semisterile" technique has emerged as an option for percutaneous procedures of the upper extremity. The semisterile technique involves using a single chlorhexidine paint brush, or prepping agent of the surgeon's choice, to sterilize the operative site and a sterile towel is placed under the extremity. We prefer to perform the procedure using the mini C-arm as an operating surface. The surgeon and surgical technician wear sterile gloves, but do not wear sterile gowns (Fig. 4.6). Some surgeons do not wear surgical masks, which has not been shown to increase infection rates [56]. If an open reduction is necessary, the semisterile technique is aborted and a hand table with full sterile preparation and draping is used with administration of prophylactic antibiotics. Most studies evaluating the semisterile technique, however, are for supracondylar humerus fractures [56–58]. Abzug et al. evaluated the safety of percutaneous pinning procedures using the semisterile technique for pediatric upper extremity fractures, including 49 patients with phalangeal fractures (full preparation, $n = 21$; semisterile preparation, $n = 28$) [59]. Of the 219 patients included in the total cohort, only one infection occurred in the full preparation group. The authors concluded that the semisterile technique is safe and efficient and can potentially save hospital resources and reduce medical waste. Wilson et al. showed similar results in 1270 patients with supracondylar humerus fractures, where 0.34% of the patients in the full preparation group had a postoperative infection and no patients in the semisterile group had an infection [56]. With national adoption of the semisterile technique, the authors estimated an annual savings of $3.7 to $4.4 million of healthcare costs.

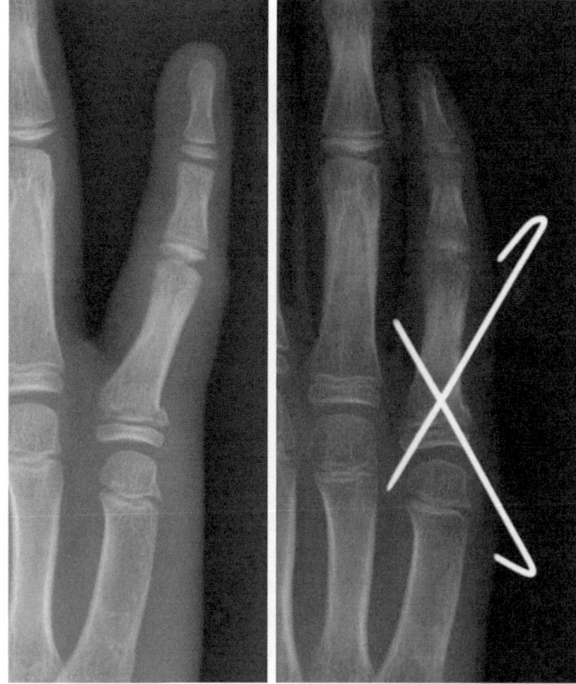

Fig. 4.7 Initial radiographs of an 11-year-old boy who sustained a juxta-epiphyseal type II fracture of the base of the small finger proximal phalanx with substantial angular deformity (left). Cross pinning restored the digital cascade and rotational deformity (right). Note that the pins do not cross at the fracture and have appropriate spread. (Images courtesy of Joshua M. Abzug, MD)

Multiple techniques have been described for percutaneous pinning of phalangeal base and shaft fractures. For base of the proximal phalanx fractures, Al-Qattan used a single retrograde K-wire passed from the proximal phalangeal head with the MCP and PIP joints held in 90° of flexion. The wire is driven through the base of the proximal phalanx, through the metacarpal head, and out the dorsal skin. The wire driver is switched to the proximal end of the wire to pull it out of the PIP joint [8]. Proponents of this technique note that it holds the MCP joint in flexion while allowing PIP joint motion. However, it should be noted that a single wire does not provide rotational stability. Alternatively, the wire can be passed antegrade through the metacarpal head and into the proximal phalanx [60]. Cross-pinning is another common technique for base of the proximal phalanx or transverse shaft fractures (Fig. 4.7). The wires can be passed antegrade or retrograde depending on the fracture location, starting the pin just lateral to the articular cartilage, and aiming so the pins have adequate spread to avoid intersection at the fracture site [44, 60]. Oblique and spiral fracture patterns are best pinned with at least two pins perpendicular to the fracture line to maintain length and rotational stability. Regardless of the technique utilized, care should be taken to avoid distraction at the fracture site while passing the K-wire [44]. A common mistake while passing K-wires is attempting to push the wire with force, which tends to displace the fracture. Drilling the K-wire at full speed without using force is the preferred technique in order to maintain the reduction. The pins are bent outside of the skin, cut with a wire cutter, a sterile dressing is applied, and all the digits are casted (excluding the thumb) in the intrinsic plus position.

If an open reduction is required, a volar, dorsal, or midlateral approach is appropriate depending on the location and morphology of the fracture. Indications for an open reduction include intra-articular fractures (Salter-Harris III or IV fractures) with joint incongruity, joint instability, or step-off of 1–2 mm, as well as blocks to a closed reduction, including entrapment of the flexor tendon, fibrous tissue, extensor hood, collateral ligaments, and/or periosteum [6, 8, 44–49]. A volar Brunner incision over the MCP or PIP joints is preferred to obtain a closed reduction for soft tissue interposition, while a dorsal curvilinear or volar approach can be used to obtain an anatomic reduction of the articular surface [44].

Outcomes

Malunion

Nascent malunions are not an uncommon presentation of pediatric phalangeal fractures. Given the robust periosteum in pediatric patients, a substantial amount of callus can form in 2–3 weeks and the patient may present without tenderness over the fracture site. Operative intervention is often required, and the surgeon should be prepared to percutaneously manipulate the fracture site under fluoroscopy with a K-wire to break up the callus (i.e., osteoclasis) [61]. This is typically accomplished from a dorsal-radial or dorsal-ulnar approach and a 0.9–1.6 mm K-wire (depending on the patient's age) is used with a sweeping motion from proximal-to-distal to mobilize the fracture. Pushing the K-wire by hand across the fracture can allow the palmar aspect of the proximal fragment to act as a fulcrum to lever the fragment to obtain a reduction [62].

Al-Qattan reported the degree of remodeling in eight patients who presented 4–6 weeks following the injury with malunion of the proximal phalanx base [63]. All patients had an inadequate post-reduction DHA ranging from 156° to 163° at the time of presentation and were offered operative intervention but refused surgery. The DHA remodeled to greater than 177° at 9–18 months following the injury in seven patients, while one patient had a DHA of 175° at 2 years. Al-Qattan and colleagues further showed that pediatric phalangeal base fractures can remodel about 10° of lateral deviation, but their later series illustrates that more remodeling is possible [31]. In patients who underwent percutaneous pinning for proximal phalangeal fractures, Boyer et al. reported no malunions in 105 patients, but 22.6% of patients had a coronal plane deviation of 5° (range, 3–13°) [64]. Coronal deviation, however, did not lead to worse outcomes. It should be noted that the authors included all proximal phalangeal fractures in this study, and coronal plane deviation was associated with subcondylar fractures. Despite the majority of these fractures involving the physis, physeal arrest is rare and is not thought to lead to progressive deformity [17, 45]. Such low rates of malunion should be considered in the context of the initial reduction, and close clinical and radiographic follow-up are needed to prevent missing rotational deformities that do not have the ability to remodel.

Al-Qattan reported the results of 34 juxta-epiphyseal fractures of the proximal phalanx in children [8]. Two patients had malunion in the flexion-extension plane that resulted in a "pseudoclaw" deformity characterized by MCP joint hyperextension and PIP joint flexion. The hyperextension at the MCP joint is attributed to the apex volar deformity at the base of the proximal phalanx. The PIP joint extensor lag is attributed to a relative bone-tendon discrepancy where shortening of the proximal phalanx from angular deformity leads to relative extensor tendon lengthening. In a cadaveric study, Vahey and colleagues showed apex volar angulations of 16°, 27°, and 46° led to PIP joint extension lags of 10°, 24°, and 66°, respectively. Given the proximity of these fractures to the physis and the deformity in the plane of motion, pseudoclaw deformity is a relatively rare sequalae from the base of the proximal phalanx fractures in children.

Stiffness

Stiffness is the most common complication following adult phalangeal fractures. Stiffness is not as problematic in children, but can still occur. Stickland et al. showed patients with extra-articular phalangeal fractures in the first two decades will regain 88% of their motion, while patients in the sixth and seventh decades only regain 60% of their motion [65]. Therefore, adult phalangeal fractures are typically immobilized for only 3 weeks to prevent stiffness and initiate early motion protocols [66]. Boyer and associates note that children are viewed differently from adults and the provider can immobilize phalangeal fractures for 4 weeks in a cast, as children are less likely to become stiff and are less compliant [64]. The authors showed stiffness still occurred in 53% of pediatric proximal phalanx pinning procedures, and 34% required formal therapy at a mean of 35 days postoperatively. Subcondylar fractures (33%) were significantly more likely to develop stiffness requiring therapy compared with phalangeal base fractures (6%), but there were no significant associations with the development of any amount of stiffness postoperatively. At final follow-up, all children had range of motion equal to the contralateral finger.

Pin Site Complications

Given the majority of pediatric phalangeal base and shaft fractures are treated non-operatively, there are few reports of complications related to percutaneous pinning. Boyer et al. reported 5 of 105 (4.8%) patients who underwent percutaneous pinning of proximal phalanx fractures had complications related to surgery [64]. Of these complications, all were observed in the base of the proximal phalanx fractures and no complications were seen in subcondylar fractures. Complications included pin migration (2 patients), pin site infection (1 patient), pin site infection and pin migration (1 patient), and pin migration with loss of reduction requiring revision surgery (1 patient). Of 34 juxta-epiphyseal fractures, Al-Qattan reported 6 patients required percutaneous pinning, none of which had pin-related complications [8]. There is a lack of evidence supporting various pin configurations for pediatric phalanx fractures.

Skin Complications

Few studies have assessed skin complications related to buddy taping in pediatric patients. Most studies related to skin complications from buddy taping and functional braces for hand fractures are in adults [67, 68]. In a survey study to surgeons treating adult patients with buddy taping of phalanx and toe injuries, 45% of respondents reported skin injuries related to the adhesive tape and 45% reported skin injuries between the injured and adjacent digit [42]. In pediatric patients randomized to buddy taping versus splint immobilization for extra-articular finger fractures, the authors reported no severe skin lesions that required further intervention or a change in the immobilization method [38].

Conclusion

Pediatric phalangeal base and shaft fractures of the proximal and middle phalanx are common injuries and can usually be treated with nonoperative management with or without a closed reduction and immobilization. The most important aspect in the management of these injuries is to recognize subtle rotational and/ or deviation deformities that will not correct with remodeling. Patients generally do well with nonoperative management, and stiffness is common but not permanent. Understanding the differences between pediatric and adult patients is important, as treatment strategies vary considerably, and children are not just small adults.

References

1. Chung KC, Spilson SV. The frequency and epidemiology of hand and forearm fractures in the United States. J Hand Surg Am. 2001;26(5):908–15. https://doi.org/10.1053/jhsu.2001.26322.
2. Vadivelu R, Dias JJ, Burke FD, Stanton J. Hand injuries in children: a prospective study. J Pediatr Orthop. 2006;26(1):29–35. https://doi.org/10.1097/01.bpo.0000189970.37037.59.
3. Chew EM, Chong AK. Hand fractures in children: epidemiology and misdiagnosis in a tertiary referral hospital. J Hand Surg Am. 2012;37(8):1684–8. https://doi.org/10.1016/j.jhsa.2012.05.010.
4. Landin LA. Fracture patterns in children. Analysis of 8,682 fractures with special reference to incidence, etiology and secular changes in a Swedish urban population 1950-1979. Acta Orthop Scand Suppl. 1983;202:1–109.
5. Worlock PH, Stower MJ. The incidence and pattern of hand fractures in children. J Hand Surg Br. 1986;11(2):198–200. https://doi.org/10.1016/0266-7681(86)90259-7.
6. Abzug JM, Dua K, Bauer AS, Cornwall R, Wyrick TO. Pediatric phalanx fractures. J Am Acad Orthop Surg. 2016;24(11):e174–e83. https://doi.org/10.5435/JAAOS-D-16-00199.

7. Al-Qattan MM, Al-Zahrani K, Al-Boukai AA. The relative incidence of fractures at the base of the proximal phalanx of the fingers in children. J Hand Surg Eur Vol. 2008;33(4):465–8. https://doi.org/10.1177/1753193408090146.

8. Al-Qattan MM. Juxta-epiphyseal fractures of the base of the proximal phalanx of the fingers in children and adolescents. J Hand Surg Br. 2002;27(1):24–30. https://doi.org/10.1054/jhsb.2001.0661.

9. Rang M. The extra-octave fracture of the little finger. Children's fractures. Philadelphia: Lippincott; 1983. p. 225–7.

10. Szymanski S, Zylstra M, Hull A. "One note higher": a unique pediatric hand fracture. Clin Pract Cases Emerg Med. 2021;5(2):270–2. https://doi.org/10.5811/cpcem.2021.3.51806.

11. Eladoumikdachi F, Valkov PL, Thomas J, Netscher DT. Anatomy of the intrinsic hand muscles revisited: part I. Interossei Plast Reconstr Surg. 2002;110(5):1211–24. https://doi.org/10.1097/01.PRS.0000024442.72140.56.

12. Bogumill GP. A morphologic study of the relationship of collateral ligaments to growth plates in the digits. J Hand Surg Am. 1983;8(1):74–9. https://doi.org/10.1016/s0363-5023(83)80059-8.

13. Keene JS, Engber WD, Stromberg WB Jr. An irreducible phalangeal epiphyseal fracture-dislocation. A case report. Clin Orthop Relat Res. 1984;186:212–5.

14. Hashizume H, Nishida K, Mizumoto D, Takagoshi H, Inoue H. Dorsally displaced epiphyseal fracture of the phalangeal base. J Hand Surg Br. 1996;21(1):136–8. https://doi.org/10.1016/s0266-7681(96)80030-1.

15. Chell J, Stevens K, Preston B, Davis TR. Bilateral fractures of the middle phalanx of the middle finger in an adolescent climber. Am J Sports Med. 1999;27(6):817–9. https://doi.org/10.1177/03635465990270062301.

16. Hochholzer T, Schoffl VR. Epiphyseal fractures of the finger middle joints in young sport climbers. Wilderness Environ Med. 2005;16(3):139–42. https://doi.org/10.1580/pr15-04.1.

17. Lindley SG, Rulewicz G. Hand fractures and dislocations in the developing skeleton. Hand Clin. 2006;22(3):253–68. https://doi.org/10.1016/j.hcl.2006.05.002.

18. Gellis M, Pool R. Two-point discrimination distances in the normal hand and forearm: application to various methods of fingertip reconstruction. Plast Reconstr Surg. 1977;59(1):57–63. https://doi.org/10.1097/00006534-197701000-00010.

19. Shiah YJ, Chang F, Tam WC. Recognition of tactile relief by children and adults. Percept Mot Skills. 2011;113(3):727–38. https://doi.org/10.2466/10.24.27.PMS.113.6.727-738.

20. Dua K, Lancaster TP, Abzug JM. Age-dependent reliability of Semmes-Weinstein and 2-point discrimination tests in children. J Pediatr Orthop. 2019;39(2):98–103. https://doi.org/10.1097/BPO.0000000000000892.

21. Abzug JM, Mehlman CT. The community orthopaedic surgeon taking trauma call: pediatric phalangeal fracture pearls and pitfalls. J Orthop Trauma. 2017;31(Suppl 6):S1–5. https://doi.org/10.1097/BOT.0000000000001013.

22. O'Riain S. New and simple test of nerve function in hand. Br Med J. 1973;3(5881):615–6. https://doi.org/10.1136/bmj.3.5881.615.

23. Wilgis EF. Techniques for diagnosis of peripheral nerve loss. Clin Orthop Relat Res. 1982;163:8–14.

24. Capo JT, Hastings H 2nd. Metacarpal and phalangeal fractures in athletes. Clin Sports Med. 1998;17(3):491–511. https://doi.org/10.1016/s0278-5919(05)70098-3.

25. Hastings H 2nd, Simmons BP. Hand fractures in children. A statistical analysis. Clin Orthop Relat Res. 1984;188:120–30.

26. Case AL, Hosseinzadeh P, Baldwin KD, Abzug JM. Hand fractures in children: when do I need to start thinking about surgery? Instr Course Lect. 2019;68:415–26.

27. Puckett BN, Gaston RG, Peljovich AE, Lourie GM, Floyd WE 3rd. Remodeling potential of phalangeal distal condylar malunions in children. J Hand Surg Am. 2012;37(1):34–41. https://doi.org/10.1016/j.jhsa.2011.09.017.

28. Vonlanthen J, Weber DM, Seiler M. Nonarticular base and shaft fractures of children's fingers: are follow-up X-rays needed? Retrospective study of conservatively treated proximal and

middle phalangeal fractures. J Pediatr Orthop. 2019;39(9):e657–e60. https://doi.org/10.1097/BPO.0000000000001335.

29. Krueger A, Qudsi R, Eckstein K, Cornwall R. Is a right angle the right angle? Normal coronal radiographic alignment in the pediatric finger phalanges. J Pediatr Orthop. 2021;41(8):e617–e23. https://doi.org/10.1097/BPO.0000000000001889.

30. Campbell RM Jr. Operative treatment of fractures and dislocations of the hand and wrist region in children. Orthop Clin North Am. 1990;21(2):217–43.

31. Al-Qattan MM, Al-Motairi MI, Al-Naeem HA. The diaphysial axis-metacarpal head angle in the management of fractures of the base of the proximal phalanx in children. J Hand Surg Eur Vol. 2013;38(9):984–90. https://doi.org/10.1177/1753193413480311.

32. Oetgen ME, Dodds SD. Non-operative treatment of common finger injuries. Curr Rev Musculoskelet Med. 2008;1(2):97–102. https://doi.org/10.1007/s12178-007-9014-z.

33. Nellans KW, Chung KC. Pediatric hand fractures. Hand Clin. 2013;29(4):569–78. https://doi.org/10.1016/j.hcl.2013.08.009.

34. Hartley RL, Lam J, Kinlin C, Hulin K, Temple-Oberle C, Harrop AR, et al. Surgical and nonsurgical pediatric hand fractures: a cohort study. Plast Reconstr Surg Glob Open. 2020;8(3):e2703. https://doi.org/10.1097/GOX.0000000000002703.

35. Niddam S, Bougie E, Mayoly A, Kachouh N, Witters M, Jaloux C. Nonarticular base and shaft fractures of children's fingers: are follow-up X-rays needed? Retrospective study of conservatively treated proximal and middle phalangeal fractures. J Pediatr Orthop. 2020;40(9):e898–e9. https://doi.org/10.1097/BPO.0000000000001589.

36. Franz T, Jandali AR, Jung FJ, Leclere FM, von Wartburg U, Hug U. Functional-conservative treatment of extra-articular physeal fractures of the proximal phalanges in children and adolescents. Eur J Pediatr Surg. 2013;23(4):317–21. https://doi.org/10.1055/s-0033-1333636.

37. Franz T, von Wartburg U, Schibli-Beer S, Jung FJ, Jandali AR, Calcagni M, et al. Extra-articular fractures of the proximal phalanges of the fingers: a comparison of 2 methods of functional, conservative treatment. J Hand Surg Am. 2012;37(5):889–98. https://doi.org/10.1016/j.jhsa.2012.02.017.

38. Weber DM, Seiler M, Subotic U, Kalisch M, Weil R. Buddy taping versus splint immobilization for paediatric finger fractures: a randomized controlled trial. J Hand Surg Eur Vol. 2019;44(6):640–7. https://doi.org/10.1177/1753193418822692.

39. Barton NJ. Fractures of the phalanges of the hand in children. Hand. 1979;11(2):134–43. https://doi.org/10.1016/s0072-968x(79)80025-x.

40. Ebinger T, Roesch M, Wachter N, Kinzl L, Mentzel M. Functional treatment of physeal and periphyseal injuries of the metacarpal and proximal phalangeal bones. J Pediatr Surg. 2001;36(4):611–5. https://doi.org/10.1053/jpsu.2001.22300.

41. Thomine JM, Gibon Y, Bendjeddou MS, Biga N. Functional brace in the treatment of diaphyseal fractures of the proximal phalanges of the last four fingers. Ann Chir Main. 1983;2(4):298–306. https://doi.org/10.1016/s0753-9053(83)80025-8.

42. Won SH, Lee S, Chung CY, Lee KM, Sung KH, Kim TG, et al. Buddy taping: is it a safe method for treatment of finger and toe injuries? Clin Orthop Surg. 2014;6(1):26–31. https://doi.org/10.4055/cios.2014.6.1.26.

43. Reyes FA, Latta LL. Conservative management of difficult phalangeal fractures. Clin Orthop Relat Res. 1987;214:23–30.

44. Wolfe SW, Pederson WC, Kozin SH, Cohen MS. Green's operative hand surgery. 8th ed. Philadelphia: Elsevier, Inc; 2021.

45. Cornwall R, Ricchetti ET. Pediatric phalanx fractures: unique challenges and pitfalls. Clin Orthop Relat Res. 2006;445:146–56. https://doi.org/10.1097/01.blo.0000205890.88952.97.

46. Harryman DT 2nd, Jordan TF 3rd. Physeal phalangeal fracture with flexor tendon entrapment. A case report and review of the literature. Clin Orthop Relat Res. 1990;(250):194–196.

47. Von R. Irreducible juxta-epiphysial fracture of a finger. J Bone Joint Surg Br. 1964;46:229.

48. Leonard MH, Dubravcik P. Management of fractured fingers in the child. Clin Orthop Relat Res. 1970;73:160–8.

49. Yamane T. Irreducible juxta-epiphyseal fracture due to entrapment of extensor hood: a case report. Hiroshima J Med Sci. 1999;48(3):99–100.
50. Case AL, Ty JM, Chu A, Ho CA, Bauer AS, Abzug JM. Variation among surgeons regarding the use of preoperative antibiotics in percutaneous pinning procedures of the upper extremity in the pediatric population. Hand (N Y). 2022;17(3):558–65. https://doi.org/10.1177/1558944720944259.
51. Hsu LP, Schwartz EG, Kalainov DM, Chen F, Makowiec RL. Complications of K-wire fixation in procedures involving the hand and wrist. J Hand Surg Am. 2011;36(4):610–6. https://doi.org/10.1016/j.jhsa.2011.01.023.
52. Ridley TJ, Freking W, Erickson LO, Ward CM. Incidence of treatment for infection of buried versus exposed Kirschner wires in phalangeal, metacarpal, and distal radial fractures. J Hand Surg Am. 2017;42(7):525–31. https://doi.org/10.1016/j.jhsa.2017.03.040.
53. Harness NG, Inacio MC, Pfeil FF, Paxton LW. Rate of infection after carpal tunnel release surgery and effect of antibiotic prophylaxis. J Hand Surg Am. 2010;35(2):189–96. https://doi.org/10.1016/j.jhsa.2009.11.012.
54. Johnson SP, Zhong L, Chung KC, Waljee JF. Perioperative antibiotics for clean hand surgery: a National Study. J Hand Surg Am. 2018;43(5):407–16 e1. https://doi.org/10.1016/j.jhsa.2017.11.018.
55. Tosti R, Fowler J, Dwyer J, Maltenfort M, Thoder JJ, Ilyas AM. Is antibiotic prophylaxis necessary in elective soft tissue hand surgery? Orthopedics. 2012;35(6):e829–33. https://doi.org/10.3928/01477447-20120525-20.
56. Wilson JM, Schwartz AM, Farley KX, Devito DP, Fletcher ND. Doing our part to conserve resources: determining whether all personal protective equipment is mandatory for closed reduction and percutaneous pinning of supracondylar humeral fractures. J Bone Joint Surg Am. 2020;102(13):e66. https://doi.org/10.2106/JBJS.20.00567.
57. Iobst CA, Spurdle C, King WF, Lopez M. Percutaneous pinning of pediatric supracondylar humerus fractures with the semisterile technique: the Miami experience. J Pediatr Orthop. 2007;27(1):17–22. https://doi.org/10.1097/bpo.0b013e31802b68dc.
58. Turgut A, Onvural B, Kazimoglu C, Bacaksiz T, Kalenderer O, Agus H. How safe is the semi-sterile technique in the percutaneous pinning of supracondylar humerus fractures? Ulus Travma Acil Cerrahi Derg. 2016;22(5):477–82. https://doi.org/10.5505/tjtes.2016.31614.
59. Dua K, Blevins CJ, O'Hara NN, Abzug JM. The safety and benefits of the semisterile technique for closed reduction and percutaneous pinning of pediatric upper extremity fractures. Hand (N Y). 2019;14(6):808–13. https://doi.org/10.1177/1558944718787310.
60. Henry MH. Fractures of the proximal phalanx and metacarpals in the hand: preferred methods of stabilization. J Am Acad Orthop Surg. 2008;16(10):586–95. https://doi.org/10.5435/00124635-200810000-00004.
61. Waters PM, Taylor BA, Kuo AY. Percutaneous reduction of incipient malunion of phalangeal neck fractures in children. J Hand Surg Am. 2004;29(4):707–11. https://doi.org/10.1016/j.jhsa.2004.03.007.
62. Matzon JL, Cornwall R. A stepwise algorithm for surgical treatment of type II displaced pediatric phalangeal neck fractures. J Hand Surg Am. 2014;39(3):467–73. https://doi.org/10.1016/j.jhsa.2013.12.014.
63. Al-Qattan MM. Fractures of the base of the proximal phalanx in children: remodeling of malunion in the radioulnar plane with a diaphyseal axis-metacarpal head angle of 156 degrees to 163 degrees. Ann Plast Surg. 2019;82(4):399–402. https://doi.org/10.1097/SAP.0000000000001816.
64. Boyer JS, London DA, Stepan JG, Goldfarb CA. Pediatric proximal phalanx fractures: outcomes and complications after the surgical treatment of displaced fractures. J Pediatr Orthop. 2015;35(3):219–23. https://doi.org/10.1097/BPO.0000000000000253.
65. Duncan RW, Freeland AE, Jabaley ME, Meydrech EF. Open hand fractures: an analysis of the recovery of active motion and of complications. J Hand Surg Am. 1993;18(3):387–94. https://doi.org/10.1016/0363-5023(93)90080-M.

66. Faruqui S, Stern PJ, Kiefhaber TR. Percutaneous pinning of fractures in the proximal third of the proximal phalanx: complications and outcomes. J Hand Surg Am. 2012;37(7):1342–8. https://doi.org/10.1016/j.jhsa.2012.04.019.
67. Geiger KR, Karpman RR. Necrosis of the skin over the metacarpal as a result of functional fracture-bracing. A report of three cases. J Bone Joint Surg Am. 1989;71(8):1199–202.
68. Nossaman BC, Rayan GM. Skin necrosis complicating functional bracing. Am J Orthop (Belle Mead NJ). 1998;27(5):371–2.

Pediatric Phalangeal Neck and Condylar Fractures

5

Logan Kolakowski, Catherine C. May, and Joshua M. Abzug

Phalangeal Neck Fractures

Thirteen percent of all pediatric fractures are fractures of the phalangeal neck [1]. A phalangeal neck fracture is a fracture that occurs distal to the collateral ligament recess of the proximal or middle phalanx [2]. This fracture has multiple pseudonyms including subcondylar, subcapital, cartilage cap, distal condylar, supracondylar, transcondylar, or bicondylar fracture [3]. Most phalangeal neck fractures will have apex volar angulation associated with sagittal and subcondylar malalignment [1, 4]. Phalangeal neck fractures have an elevated risk of malunion, proximal displacement, and decreased range of motion [4]. Therefore, they must be assessed shortly after the injury occurs in order to intervene prior to the rapid healing that occurs in pediatric patients [4]. Fractures treated beyond 1–2 weeks following the injury may require additional intervention in the form of osteoclasis and/or open reduction to restore acceptable alignment [4].

Clinical Presentation

Although phalangeal neck fractures are uncommon in the adult population, they are a relatively common injury in children ages 1–18 years [5]. Al Qattan identified a 1:10 ratio of adult to pediatric phalangeal neck fractures treated in a single hand

---

Disclaimer: The views expressed in the submitted article are our own and not an official position of the institution.

L. Kolakowski · C. C. May · J. M. Abzug (✉)
Department of Orthopedic Surgery, University of Maryland School of Medicine, Baltimore, MD, USA
e-mail: logan.kolakowski@som.umaryland.edu; catherine.may@som.umaryland.edu; jabzug@som.umaryland.edu

J. M. Abzug et al. (eds.), *Pediatric and Adult Hand Fractures*,
https://doi.org/10.1007/978-3-031-32072-9_5

center [5]. The mechanism of injury varies with age. Younger children often suffer crush injuries, such as a "door slam," in which the digit is trapped and subsequently withdrawn causing a separation of the diaphysis from the condyles of the phalanx [5]. Older children are more likely to injure their digit through sports, altercations, or falls from height [5].

The clinical presentation of a phalangeal neck fracture includes a swollen digit with tenderness at the fracture site [5]. The primary deformity is found in the sagittal plane (Fig. 5.1). However, it is important to note that radial or ulnar deviation may be present (Fig. 5.2) or the digit may be malrotated. Therefore, it is critical to assess for these. The use of the tenodesis effect is helpful when assessing the digital cascade, especially in young children who may not cooperate with performing active motion. Depending on the mechanism of injury, there may be concomitant skin lacerations present [5]. Evaluation of the digit must also include an assessment for damage to the tendons and neurovascular structures [5].

During the injury, the adjacent interphalangeal joint hyperextends which causes the volar cortex to fail in tension leading to apex volar angulation of the fracture. The resulting volar spike (distal extent of the proximal fragment) can impede flexion [2]. The distal fragment displaces dorsally, making the subcondylar fossa nonexistent (Fig. 5.1) [6]. With increasing displacement, the phalangeal head loses

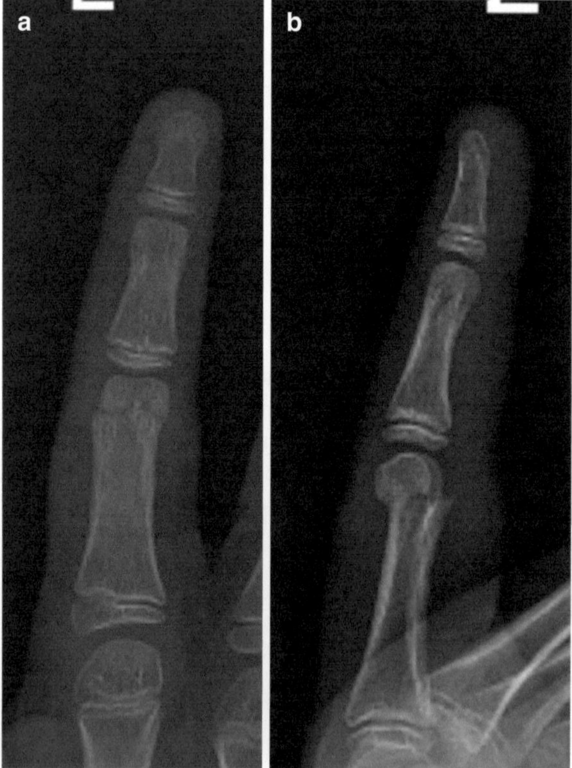

Fig. 5.1 Radiographs of a displaced P1 phalangeal neck fracture in an 11-year-old male who injured his index finger when he fell from a dirt bike. Note the mild angulation in the coronal plane but the substantial displacement in the sagittal plane. (**a**) PA and (**b**) lateral views. (Courtesy of Joshua M. Abzug, MD)

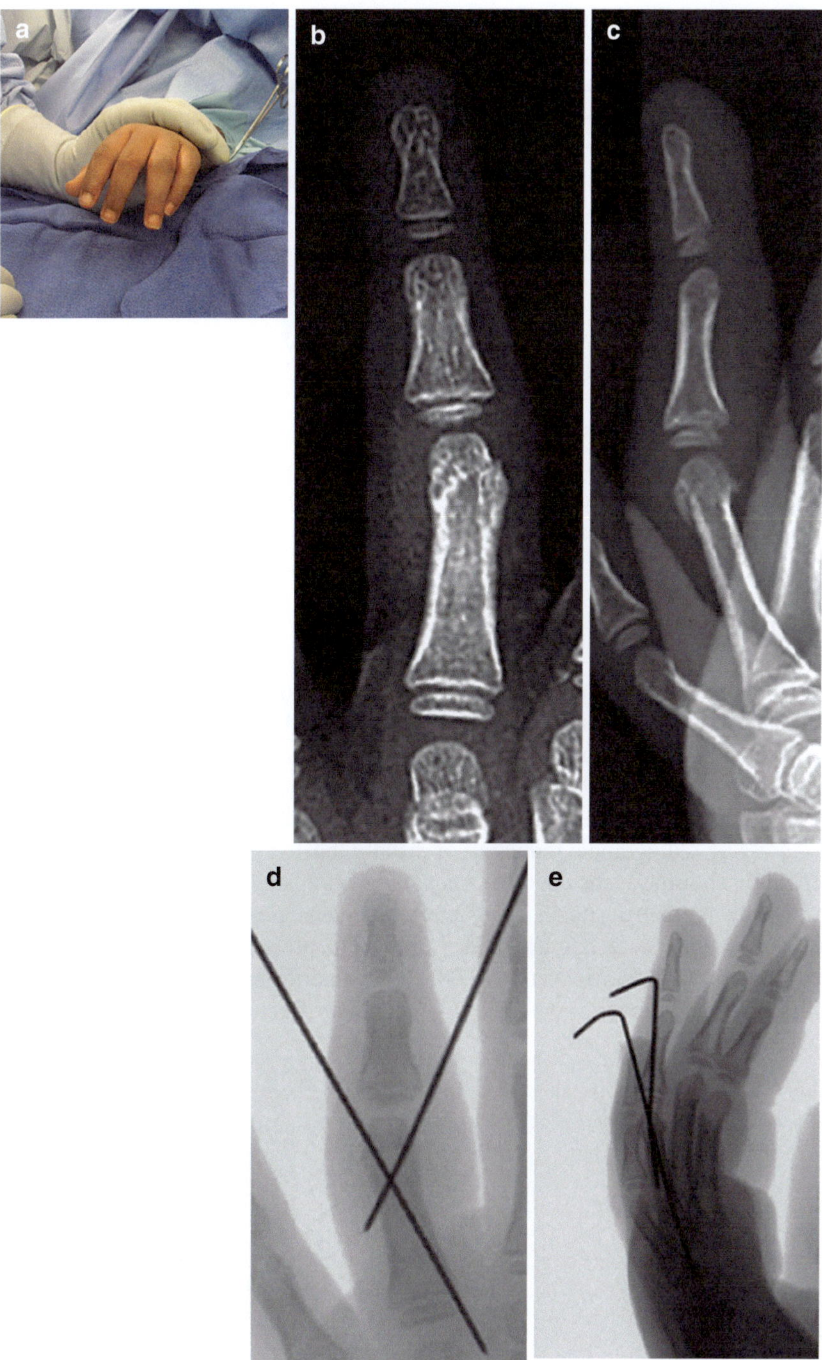

Fig. 5.2 (**a**) Clinical photograph of a phalangeal neck fracture with substantial ulnar deviation in a 5-year-old male who caught his left ring finger in a door. Preoperative (**b**) PA and (**c**) lateral views. Intraoperative (**d**) PA and (**e**) lateral views demonstrating correction and stabilization of the fracture utilizing a closed reduction and percutaneous pinning of the fracture. (Courtesy of Joshua M. Abzug, MD)

more periosteal connections. However, the phalangeal head is primarily cartilaginous without tendinous attachments, and the periosteum is the main blood supply. Therefore, there is an increased risk of avascular necrosis with phalangeal neck fractures, especially ones that are substantially displaced [7]. It is important to document concurrent injuries to the neurovascular bundles, which may be determined through observation of capillary refill and pulse oximetry [5].

Classification

Phalangeal neck fractures are described using the Al Qattan classification system which is somewhat analogous to the modified Gartland classification system for supracondylar humerus fractures (Table 5.1). A type I fracture is nondisplaced and considered to be "stable" [3, 5]. A type II fracture is displaced with some cortical contact maintained [3, 5]. Type III fractures are displaced with a rotational deformity, implying no intact cortex [8]. According to Al Qattan, the relative incidence of type I, II, and III fractures is 19%, 71%, and 10% respectively [5].

Imaging

Plain radiographs are used to confirm the diagnosis of a phalangeal neck fracture. The hand should be positioned to allow isolation of the affected digit for increased visualization of the fracture site [3]. Proper diagnosis should be made with posterior-anterior (PA) and lateral radiographs of the involved digit (Fig. 5.1). The lateral view will be used to determine the degree of dorsal displacement [3].

Assessing radiographic reduction of distally located phalangeal fractures can be difficult in children as the condyles may not be completely ossified [9]. Abzug et al. proposed a predictive model using the volar phalangeal line (VPL) as a tool to assess phalangeal neck fracture reduction [9]. The process is analogous to the technique described by Herman et al. in which the anterior humeral line (AHL) is used to assess the alignment of pediatric supracondylar fractures [9, 10]. On the lateral

Table 5.1 Al Qattan classification system of phalangeal neck fractures

Classification		Description
Type I		Stable, nondisplaced
Type II	II_a	Displaced with transverse fracture lines
	II_b	Displaced with oblique fracture lines
	II_c	Displaced with dorsal or dorso-lateral bony flanges present, which aid in maintaining the stability of the displaced fracture
	II_d	Displaced with small distal fragments, which increase difficulty of achieving a closed reduction
Type III	III_a	Displaced with phalangeal head rotation of 90°
	III_b	Displaced with phalangeal head rotation of 180°
	III_c	Open injury with partial amputation of the digit in the dorsal direction
	III_d	Open injury with partial amputation of the digit in the volar direction

Fig. 5.3 Radiographs demonstrating volar phalangeal line (VPL) measurements. (**a**) Patient under 8 years of age showing the VPL intersect the volar third of the condyles. (**b**) Patient over 8 years of age showing the VPL intersect the middle third of the condyles. (Courtesy of Joshua M. Abzug, MD)

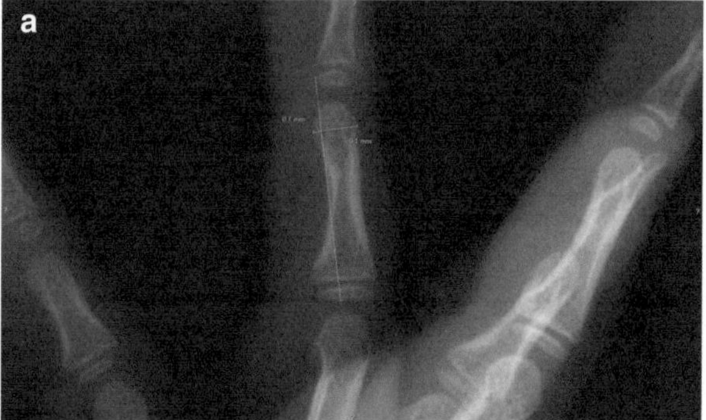

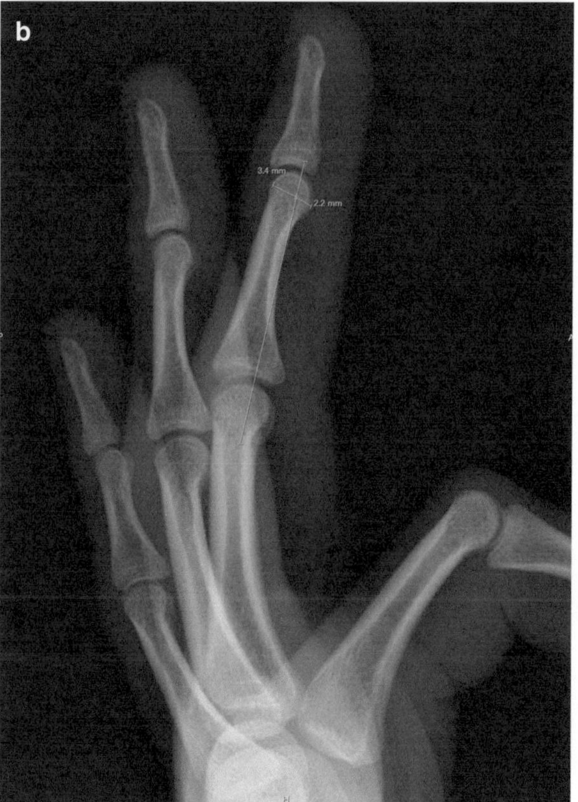

radiograph, the VPL is drawn along the volar aspect of the phalangeal shaft [9]. This line along the volar cortex of the phalanx predictably intersects the phalangeal condyles based on age and thereby reflects anatomic alignment (Fig. 5.3) [9]. Below the age of 8, the VPL typically intersects the anterior third of the phalangeal condyles [9]. Children will experience a rapid growth period between ages 8 and 9 after which the VPL will intersect the middle third of the phalangeal condyles [9]. This predictive model may be used as both a preoperative and intraoperative radiographic tool for clinicians to use in addition to their physical examinations.

Treatment

Management of pediatric phalangeal neck fractures is dependent on the amount of fracture displacement [3]. Type I, nondisplaced fractures are treated nonoperatively with 3–4 weeks of immobilization [3, 11, 12]. Often, this includes short arm mitten cast placement but can also be accomplished with buddy taping and placement in a splint to immobilize the affected digit [13]. Fracture alignment should be monitored weekly for at least 2 weeks with a repeat clinical evaluation and repeat radiographs to ensure there is no loss of alignment [13].

Displaced phalangeal neck fractures are unstable in nature and typically present with dorsal displacement of the distal fragment due to the tendinous attachments [3, 4]. This dorsal displacement can result in the subcondylar fossa becoming nonexistent, thus leading to a mechanical block in finger flexion [3, 4]. Therefore, displaced and angulated phalangeal neck fractures warrant operative intervention [3]. Additional indications for surgical intervention include joint incongruency, coronal angulation, and/or complete lack of cortical contact [1].

The preferred operative intervention is a closed reduction and percutaneous pinning (CRPP) (Fig. 5.4) [3]. Reduction may be aided by hyperflexion of the adjacent interphalangeal joint. Multiple Kirschner wire (K-wire) configurations can be used for satisfactory fracture stabilization. Our preferred technique is to follow the technique proposed by Strauch et al. which permits K-wire placement while flexing the adjacent joint (Fig. 5.5) [14]. After flexion of the adjacent joint, a K-wire is placed retrograde through the head of the fractured phalanx, exiting the skin dorsally, to hold provisional reduction [15]. The K-wire is advanced retrograde until the distal tip of it is in the affected phalangeal condylar region. During this process, the K-wire exits the skin of the dorsal hand. Subsequently, the adjacent interphalangeal joint is extended and the K-wire can be advanced antegrade, exiting out the fingertip [15]. Ultimately, the wire should be lying within the affected phalanx and exiting out the fingertip. To achieve increased stability, an additional K-wire may be used [15].

Matzon and Cornwall outlined a stepwise algorithm for the surgical management of Type II phalangeal neck fractures in pediatric patients [13]. The recommended starting point is a CRPP [3]. If the CRPP is unsuccessful, a percutaneous reduction and pinning, with or without an osteoclasis, may be performed with the help of an intrafocal K-wire, which is used as a lever to push the fracture into place (Fig. 5.6) [3, 4]. If this also fails, the age and nature of the fracture is assessed to determine the following course of treatment [4]. Although the potential for remodeling decreases as the fracture is further from the physis, several studies report the correction of phalangeal neck fracture deformities in the sagittal plane [6, 16]. Cornwall and Waters outlined criteria for remodeling which includes no rotational or coronal malalignment, congruency of the adjacent interphalangeal joint, bony union of the fracture site, and substantial growth potential [6]. If the criteria are met, the fracture may be left to remodel and will continue to be evaluated periodically [4, 6]. It is important for the patient and family to understand that the remodeling process can take 2 years or even longer [9].

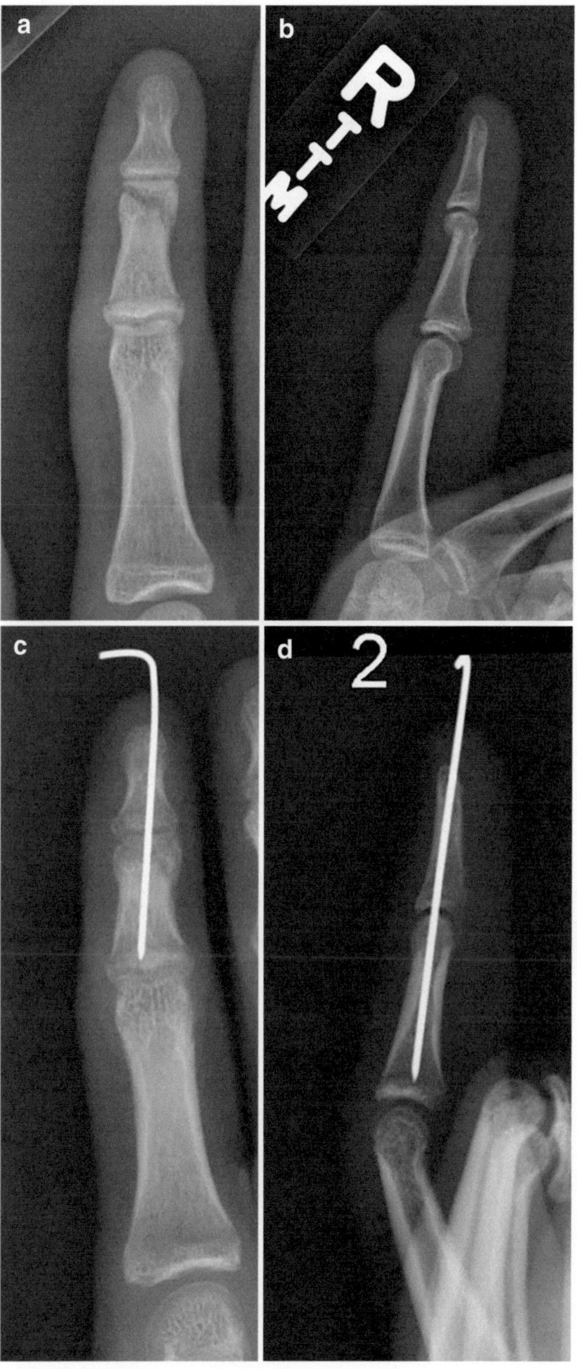

Fig. 5.4 Radiographs of a P2 phalangeal neck fracture in a 13-year-old male who injured his index finger while playing football. Preoperative (**a**) PA and (**b**) lateral views. Postoperative (**c**) PA and (**d**) lateral views following a closed reduction and percutaneous pinning. (Courtesy of Joshua M. Abzug, MD)

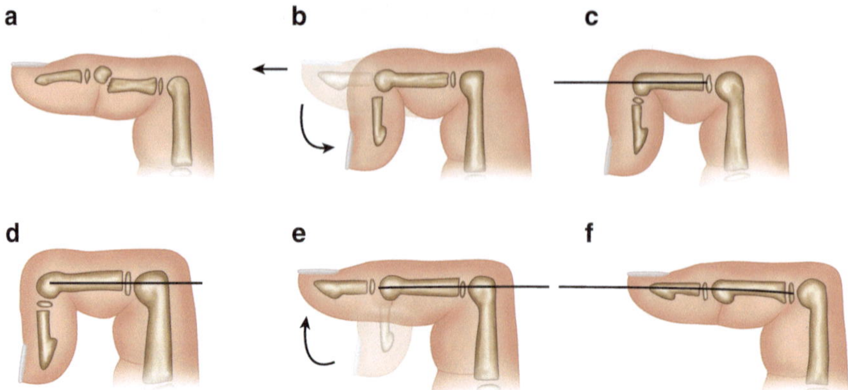

Fig. 5.5 Illustration of the CRPP technique that permits hyperflexion of the adjacent interphalangeal joint to aid in reduction. A displaced phalangeal neck fracture is present (Panel A). Once the adjacent joint is hyperflexed, the fracture reduces as shown in panel B. The K-wire can then be driven retrograde to stabilize the fracture (Panel C). The K-wire is advanced further to exit the dorsal aspect of the digit while maintaining fixation across he fracture site just deep to the phalangeal head (Panel D). The adjacent interphalangeal joint can now be extended and the K-wire can be advanced antegrade to exit the tip of the digit (Panel E). The K-wire is then brought out the tip of the digit further to allow the most proximal extent of the wire to lie in the base of the fractured phalanx (Panel F). (Courtesy of Catherine C. May, BS)

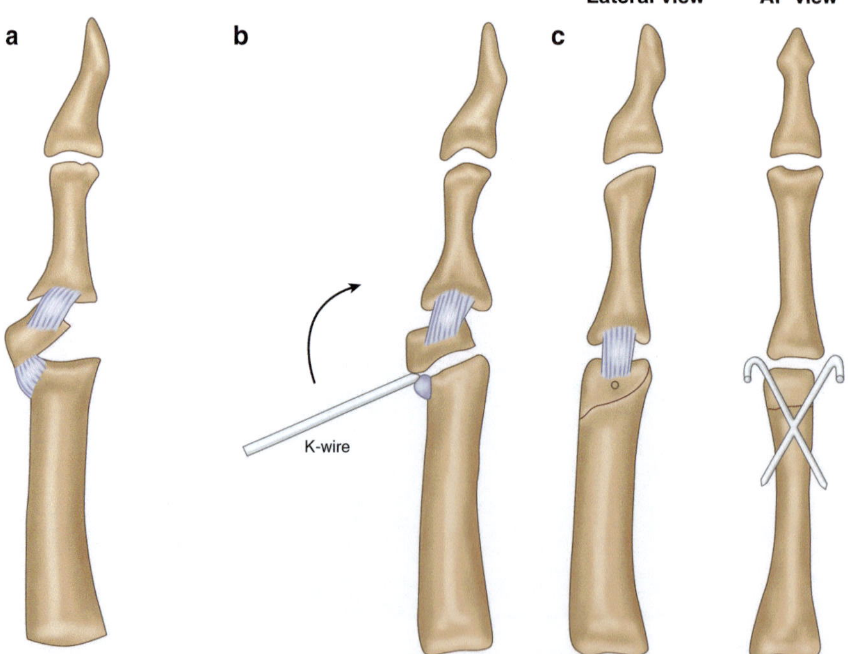

Fig. 5.6 Illustration of the use of an intrafocal K-wire to achieve percutaneous reduction after osteoclasis. (**a**) Bony callus is present at the fracture site. (**b**) An intrafocal K-wire is used to break up the aging fracture and as a lever arm to obtain anatomical alignment. (**c**) Reduction is achieved and pins are placed across the fracture site to provide stabilization. (Courtesy of Catherine C. May, BS)

Fractures which do not meet the aforementioned criteria and/or are greater than 2 weeks old require additional intervention through an osteoclasis and/or open reduction (Fig. 5.7) [4]. The intrafocal K-wire used during the initial CRPP attempt may be used to break up the aging fracture, thus performing an osteoclasis (Fig. 5.6) [4, 6]. If the osteoclasis is unsuccessful, an open reduction/osteotomy and percutaneous pinning is performed [4].

Outcomes

Liao et al. compared clinical and radiographic outcomes of pediatric phalangeal neck fractures treated with cast immobilization and removable orthoses [17]. In this study, 47 patients were managed nonoperatively [17]. Nine of the fractures were classified as Type I fractures and the other 38 were classified as Type II fractures [17]. Of these fractures, 40% were placed in a short arm cast and 60% were placed in a removable splint [17]. No differences in clinical or radiographic outcomes between the two treatment groups were observed [17]. While there are known benefits to splinting, including comfort, convenience, and improved hygiene, it is often

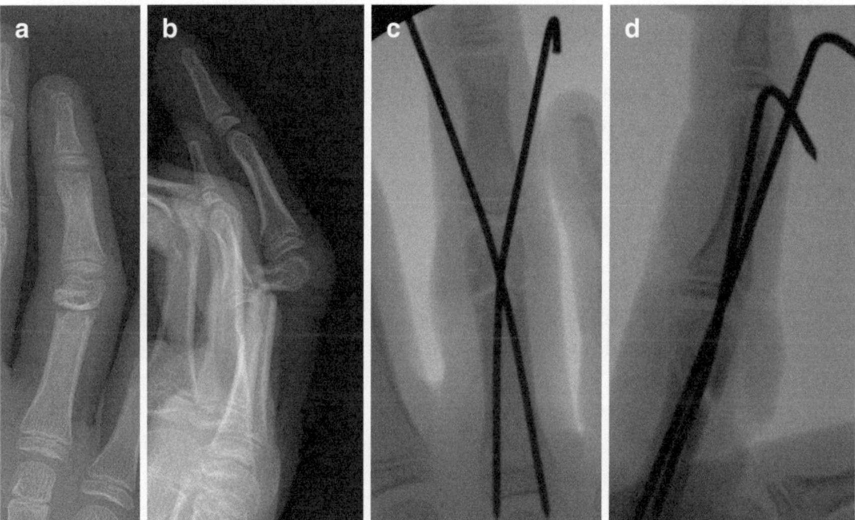

Fig. 5.7 Radiographs of an 8-year-old female who underwent an open reduction and internal fixation of a right ring finger P1 phalangeal neck fracture that was unable to be reduced into acceptable alignment following attempts at closed reduction. Preoperative (**a**) PA and (**b**) lateral views. Intraoperative (**c**) PA and (**d**) lateral views. (Courtesy of Joshua M. Abzug, MD)

difficult to ensure patient compliance with splinting guidelines, especially in young children. However, the authors did not find a high rate of noncompliance with splinting [17]. Therefore, both splinting and casting may be considered when determining the best course of treatment for nondisplaced or minimally displaced fractures. It is imperative that the treatment is individualized to the patient to account for patient and parent preferences [17].

Park et al. compared outcomes of phalangeal neck fractures treated nonoperatively with reduction, buddy taping, and a short arm splint to fractures treated operatively with CRPP [12]. Overall, outcomes were similar between both treatment groups, suggesting the possibility of treating certain type II fractures nonoperatively and allowing for bony remodeling [3, 12]. This is founded in evidence that type II fractures can remodel to some extent in the sagittal plane allowing patients to obtain full range of motion [16]. Successful remodeling is more likely to occur in dorsally displaced fractures (sagittal plane deformities) as compared to those with coronal malalignment [9]. Malrotation will not remodel. According to Liao et al., good candidates for nonoperative treatment are patients with fractures that have "minimal coronal plane finger deformity and no scissoring" [17]. Sagittal plane deformities have more remodeling potential; therefore, coronal malalignment is thought to be better suited for reduction and fixation.

In the study conducted by Matzon and Cornwall, 61 patients with phalangeal neck fractures were treated using the algorithm described previously [13]. Initial CRPP was successful in 80% of patients, while the other 20% required an additional percutaneous reduction and pinning [13]. Patients treated with percutaneous reduction and pinning received treatment over 2 weeks after the initial injury [13]. Outcomes were considered to be good to excellent in 92% of patients [13]. This included successful fracture union, range of motion greater than 50 degrees at the DIP joint and greater than 90 degrees at the PIP joint, no residual deformity, and normal digital function [13].

Wallace et al. performed a retrospective review to determine the factors which impact management and outcomes of pediatric phalangeal neck fractures [18]. Fifteen patients, with an average age of 6 years, were reviewed. The small finger was the most commonly injured digit. The fractures were classified as type I (27%), type IIa (33%), type IIb (33%), and type IIc (7%) fractures [18]. Patients were treated with a cast ($N = 1$), a closed reduction ($N = 9$), a closed reduction and percutaneous pinning ($N = 2$), and an open reduction and internal fixation ($N = 3$) [18]. Clinical outcomes were considered to be good to excellent in 12 patients, while the remaining three patients experienced fair outcomes [18]. Those with fair outcomes had a delay in treatment with an average of 14 days following the initial injury [18]. The best predictors of post reduction stability were fracture geometry and the amount of initial displacement [18]. Early intervention should be performed in order to obtain stability of the fracture [18].

A notable risk factor associated with worse outcomes is vascular injury [19]. In a study by Al Qattan et al., outcomes of 13 phalangeal neck fractures presenting with concomitant vascular injury were reviewed [19]. All 13 cases failed to achieve an "excellent" outcome [19]. Compared to a phalangeal neck fracture without vascular injury where excellent outcomes occurred in 75% of cases, this outcome is very poor [19].

Boyer et al. compared outcomes following surgical management of displaced phalangeal neck fractures to other types of phalangeal fractures [20]. Phalangeal neck fractures were more likely to develop stiffness that required therapy and have a persistent deformity after surgery [20]. While there was a difference in scores for digit appearance and stiffness, phalangeal neck fractures did not differ significantly in pain, strength, or final range of motion [20].

Complications

Common complications associated with phalangeal neck fractures include joint stiffness, malunion, deformity, and avascular necrosis/osteonecrosis [21, 22]. Compared to patients with nondisplaced proximal phalangeal neck fractures, patients with displaced and/or nonreduced proximal phalanx phalangeal neck fractures are more likely to experience joint stiffness, coronal plane deviation, and poor aesthetics [3, 21]. Joint stiffness is a result of decreased flexion of the adjacent interphalangeal joint [21]. Anatomic reduction, early mobilization, and therapy may be used to minimize the onset of joint stiffness [20].

Patients who experience malunion or nonunion of their affected digit may be treated by allowing for bone remodeling, although the potential for remodeling decreases as the distance from the fracture site to the physis increases [3]. If remodeling is unlikely to correct the deformity, an osteotomy (uniplanar or biplanar) may be performed (Fig. 5.8). However, corrective osteotomy procedures increase the risk for osteonecrosis development due to the limited collateral blood supply [3]. It is imperative that the collateral ligaments remain intact during this procedure [3].

An additional technique used to correct a malunion is a subcondylar fossa reconstruction. The goal of the reconstruction is to recreate the volar concavity of the subcondylar recess through a palmar approach. This procedure is uncommon but has been reported to increase flexion by an average of 41.7 degrees [23].

Risk of avascular necrosis remains high with both treatment options following a malunion, as the blood supply to a mature phalangeal head is through the collateral ligaments [24]. Radiographically, sclerosis can be seen in the phalangeal head, while clinically, the interphalangeal joint becomes stiff. Avascular necrosis can be managed conservatively if the joint is in a functional position [5].

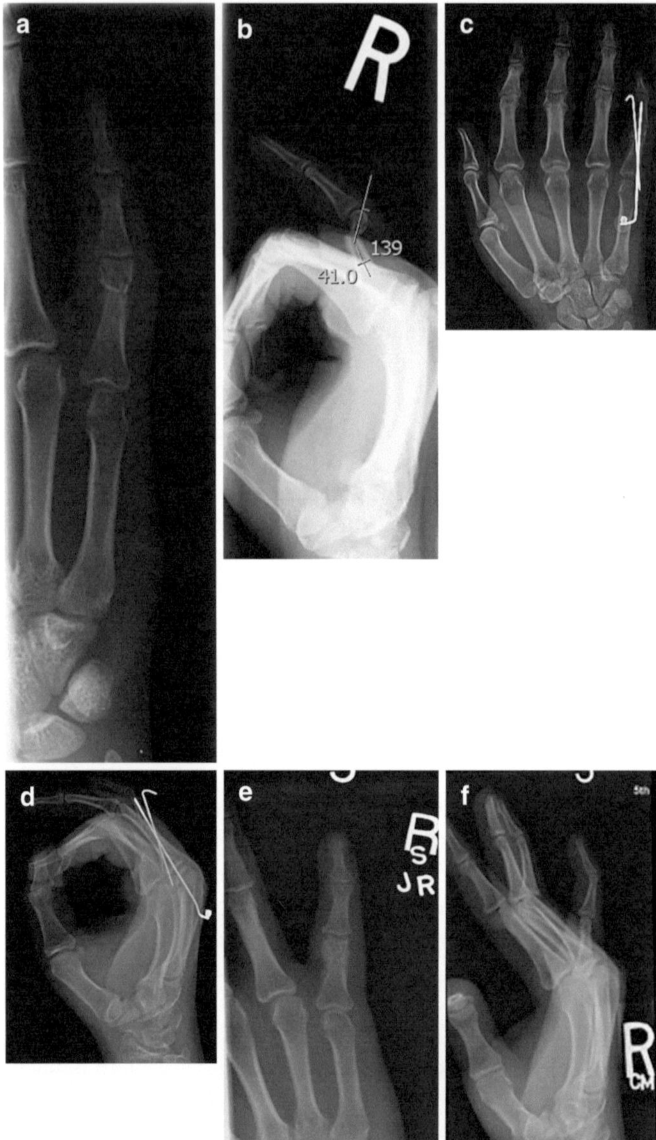

Fig. 5.8 Radiographs of a 15-year-old male who underwent correction of a right small finger P1 nascent malunion. Preoperative (**a**) PA and (**b**) lateral views. Postoperative (**c**) PA and (**d**) lateral views. Final follow-up (**e**) PA and (**f**) lateral views. (Courtesy of Joshua M. Abzug, MD)

Phalangeal Condylar Fractures

Introduction

Fractures of the phalangeal condyles are relatively uncommon in children. Phalangeal condyle fractures encompass a wide variety of fracture morphologies including unicondylar, bicondylar, lateral avulsion, and subcondylar shearing patterns with or without associated joint subluxation or dislocation [3]. Often, phalangeal condylar fractures are difficult to manage due to their frequent late presentation [2, 3]. Repairing of the small articular fragments becomes more technically challenging as time progresses [3]. In pediatric patients, this is increasingly difficult as the bony fragments are much smaller than in adults and can be primarily composed of articular cartilage (Fig. 5.9) [2, 3].

Clinical Presentation

While specific mechanisms of injury are not well established, phalangeal condyle fractures occur during direct axial compression, avulsion forces, or subchondral shearing from the underlying phalangeal shaft [2, 3, 25]. If the axial load is high energy and centralized to the bone, the fracture may present as bicondylar with buckling of the articular surface (Fig. 5.10) [25]. Due to the common oblique fracture pattern, phalangeal bicondylar fractures are unstable and require stabilization for their treatment [25]. Often, comminution of the fracture is present making it more difficult to manage [3].

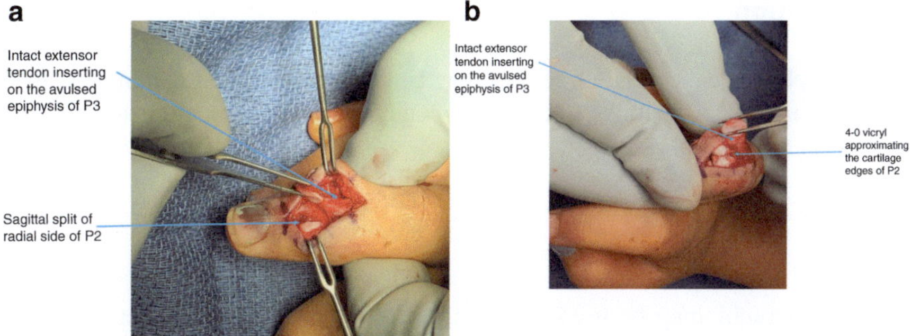

Fig. 5.9 Intraoperative photographs of a right intra-articular P2 condylar fracture with a concomitant avulsion fracture of the P3 epiphysis in a 10-year-old female who injured her middle finger when she fell from a horse. (**a**) Note the P2 condylar fracture fragment is almost entirely cartilaginous in nature. (**b**) Note the suture utilized to stabilize the cartilaginous condylar fracture of P2. (Courtesy of Joshua M. Abzug, MD)

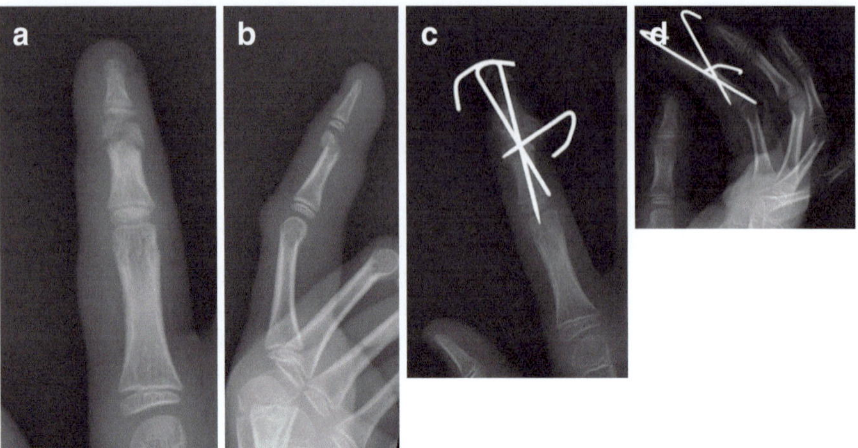

Fig. 5.10 Radiographs of a P2 bicondylar phalanx fracture in a 7-year-old female who injured her index finger when she tripped and fell. Preoperative (**a**) PA and (**b**) lateral views. Postoperative (**c**) PA and (**d**) lateral views. Note the K-wire stabilizing the radial and ulnar condyles together to then permit the articular surface (both condyles) to be stabilized to the remainder of the phalanx. (Courtesy of Joshua M. Abzug, MD)

Table 5.2 London classification system of phalangeal condyle fractures

Classification	Description
Type 1	Unicondylar; nondisplaced
Type II	Unicondylar; displaced
Type III	Bicondylar; fragmented

Classification

Pediatric phalangeal condyle fractures may be described by the London classification system, which separates fractures by condyle involvement and degree of displacement (Table 5.2) [26].

Imaging

Plain radiographs may be used to identify a phalangeal condyle fracture. These fractures may appear normal on PA radiographs; therefore lateral and oblique images are necessary to obtain an accurate diagnosis. A double density sign may be seen on a true lateral image which represents displaced offset of the condyles relative to each other (Fig. 5.11) [2, 27]. This indicates a condylar fracture that is both displaced and malrotated [15]. Misdiagnosis of this injury commonly leads to a delay in receiving appropriate treatment.

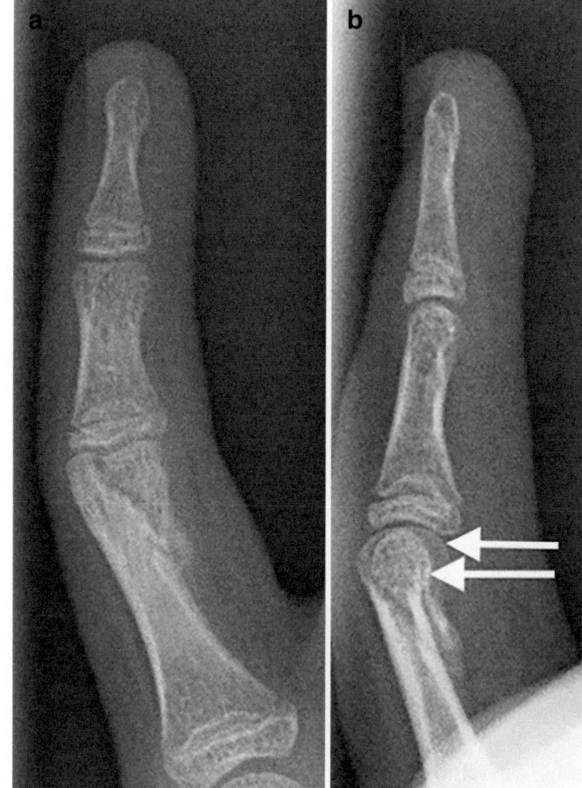

Fig. 5.11 Radiographs of a phalangeal condyle fracture in an 11-year-old female. (**a**) PA and (**b**) lateral views. Note the proximal displacement of the fracture fragment causing a step-off at the articular surface on the PA view and the double density sign present on the lateral view indicating the presence of displacement and malrotation. (Courtesy of Joshua M. Abzug, MD)

Treatment

The course of treatment is determined by the degree of fracture displacement and the ability to perform a closed reduction. Delays greater than 1 week following the injury may substantially impede the ability to obtain a closed reduction [4]. Nondisplaced fractures may be treated nonoperatively through 4 weeks of immobilization of the affected digit. Phalangeal condyle fractures with displacement greater than 1.5–2 mm and angulation greater than 5 degrees warrant operative intervention [28]. Due to the involvement of the articular surface, management of the fracture displacement is crucial to avoid increased risk of accelerated development of osteoarthritis.

Closed reduction and percutaneous pinning is the preferred operative intervention to preserve the blood supply to the fracture fragment(s) [3]. A towel clip or Kirschner wire joystick may be used to achieve anatomical reduction of the fracture [2, 3, 15]. One or two 0.035–0.045 mm Kirschner wires can then be placed percutaneously for fixation of the fracture fragment(s) [3]. The hand is immobilized for

4 weeks, after which the K-wires are removed [3]. Following the immobilization period, the patient may begin early active range of motion exercises to prevent joint stiffness [3].

Internal fixation may also be achieved using a single lag screw via a lateral approach [25]. In this technique, an incision is made in the vertical retinacular fibers to visualize the collateral ligament [25]. Proximal to the condyle, the periosteum is incised and elevated [25]. The condyle is then exposed, and the reduction is performed to obtain anatomical alignment of the fracture. A single 1.2 or 1.4 mm self-tapping lag screw is placed into the condyle [25]. Using a 5-0 absorbable suture, both the periosteum and the vertical retinacular fibers are repaired [25]. The incision is closed, and the digit is placed in sterile dressings [25]. A bicondylar fracture may be treated in a similar method using a bilateral approach in which the longer fragment is fixed to the diaphysis first, and the shorter fragment is subsequently attached to the fixed longer fragment [25].

In a study conducted by Sirota et al., outcomes of 13 phalangeal intra-articular unicondylar fractures in cadaver models treated with either one 1.5 mm headless compression screw, one 1.5 mm lag screw, two 1.1 mm smooth K-wires, or one 1.1 mm K-wire were compared [29]. No significant differences were found between the displacement of the fractures treated with the various methods described previously. This suggests that the techniques are biomechanically equivalent allowing surgeons to choose the implant that best fits each fracture [29].

Open reduction should only be used if absolutely necessary. Since the blood supply of the condyles enters through the collateral ligament, there is a high risk for osteonecrosis [3]. To protect the soft tissue envelope and prevent periosteal stripping, a careful dissection should be performed [3]. The subcondylar fossa is debrided to remove mechanical blocks to flexion [3]. After reduction and fixation are achieved, condylar fractures should be immobilized for 4 weeks (Fig. 5.12).

Outcomes

Shewring et al. examined the outcomes of 74 patients with condylar fractures of the proximal and middle phalanges [25]. The average age of the patient was 27 years (range: 11–56 years), with 13 patients under the age of 16 [25]. Seven patients were treated nonoperatively through immobilization of the affected digit in a thermoplastic splint with adhesion to the neighboring digit [25]. All seven patients experienced no complications and regained a full range of motion by 12 weeks following the injury [25]. Sixty-seven patients were treated surgically using a mid-lateral approach [25]. Twenty-seven of these patients regained full range of motion when treated within 2 weeks of the injury [25]. The most common surgical complications were fixed flexion at the PIP joints and extensor lag in the DIP joints [25]. Fifty-seven percent of patients treated operatively experienced a loss of extension of an average of 10 degrees [25].

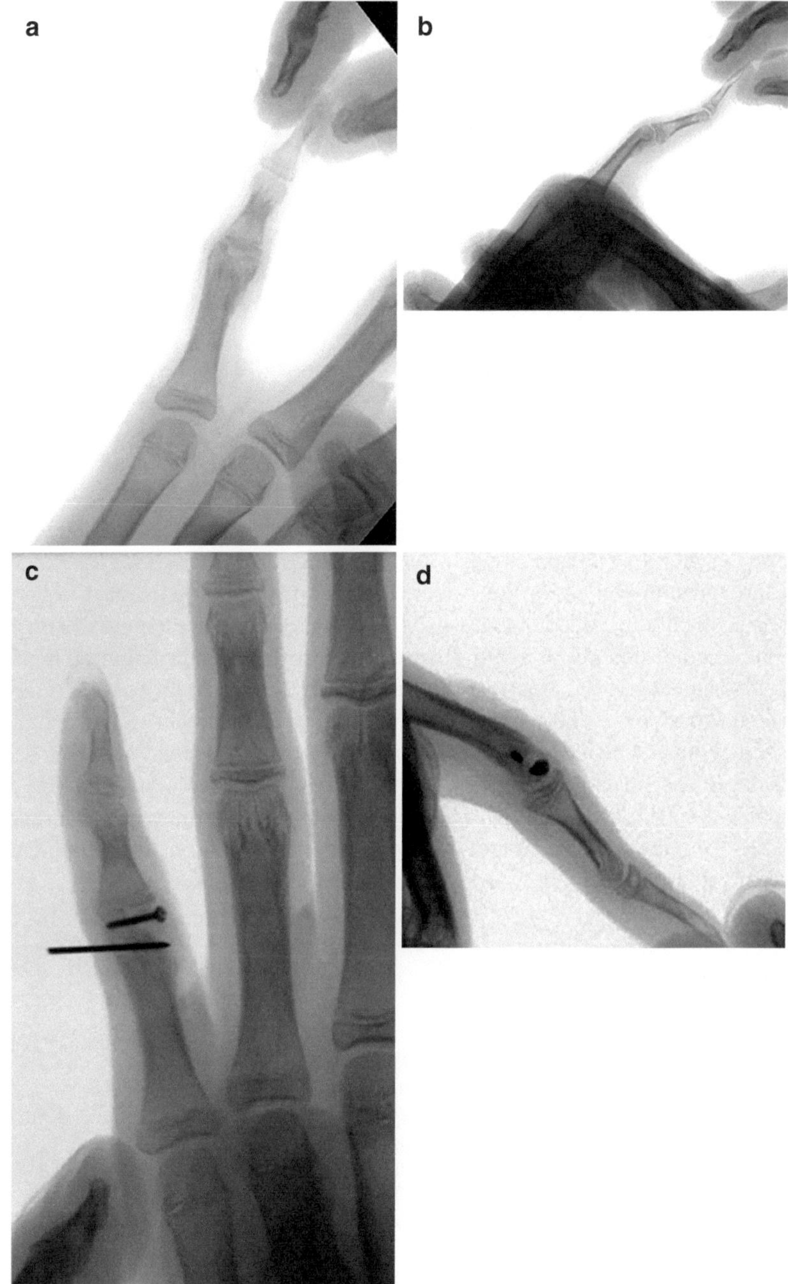

Fig. 5.12 Intraoperative fluoroscopic images of a phalangeal condyle fracture in a 13-year-old female who injured her small finger while playing soccer. The fracture was treated with an open reduction and internal fixation while preserving the vascular supply to the condyles. Preoperative (**a**) PA and (**b**) lateral views. Postoperative (**c**) PA and (**d**) lateral views. (Courtesy of Joshua M. Abzug, MD)

Complications

Pediatric phalangeal condyle fractures are at risk for developing long-term complications including joint stiffness, pain, instability, degenerative arthritis, and avascular necrosis. These risks are elevated when there is a comminuted intra-articular fracture or a concomitant fracture dislocation is present. Following a phalangeal condyle fracture, the potential for bone remodeling is low; therefore, there is high risk for malunion if the fracture is not treated early and appropriately. A corrective osteotomy to restore articular congruity may be considered for patients with a substantial malunion [27]. Patients treated with a corrective osteotomy experience a greater risk of avascular necrosis because there is limited blood supply to the phalangeal condyles [3].

Conclusion

Phalangeal neck fractures are fractures distal to the collateral ligament recess of the proximal or middle phalanx. Nondisplaced phalangeal neck fractures may be managed through immobilization for 4 weeks, while displaced phalangeal neck fractures are typically managed operatively with a CRPP. It is important to identify and treat the fracture quickly to avoid displacement, stiffness, and malunion development. Phalangeal condyle fractures are fractures involving the articular surface and may be unicondylar, bicondylar, lateral avulsion, or subcondylar shearing patterns with or without associated joint subluxation or dislocation. Depending on the degree of displacement, phalangeal condyle fractures may be treated nonoperatively with immobilization or operatively with a CRPP. Open reduction may be necessary but increases the risk of complications. Complications include joint stiffness, instability, accelerated development of osteoarthritis, and avascular necrosis.

References

1. Kang HJ, Sung SY, Ha JW, Yoon HK, Hahn SB. Operative treatment for proximal phalangeal neck fractures of the finger in children. Yonsei Med J. 2005;46(6):491–5.
2. Nellans KW, Chung KC. Pediatric hand fractures. Hand Clin. 2013;29(4):569–78.
3. Abzug JM, Dua K, Bauer AS, Cornwall R, Wyrick TO. Pediatric phalanx fractures. J Am Acad Orthop Surg. 2016;24(11):e174–83. https://doi.org/10.5435/JAAOS-D-16-00199.
4. Case AL, Hosseinzadeh P, Baldwin KD, Abzug JM. Hand fractures in children: when do I need to start thinking about surgery? Instr Course Lect. 2019;68:415–26.
5. Al-Qattan MM, Al-Qattan AM. A review of phalangeal neck fractures in children. Injury. 2015;46(6):935–44.
6. Cornwall R, Waters PM. Remodeling of phalangeal neck fracture malunions in children: Case report. J Hand Surg Am. 2004;29(3):458–61.
7. Graham TJ, Waters PM. Fractures and dislocations of the hand and carpus in children. In: Beaty JH, Kasser JR, editors. Rockwood and Wilkins' fractures in children, ed 5. Philadelphia, PA: Lippincott, Williams & Wilkins; 2001. p. 269–379.
8. Al-Qattan MM. Phalangeal neck fractures in children: classification and outcome in 66 cases. J Hand Surg Br. 2001;26(2):112–21.

 9. Dua K, O'Hara NN, Shusterman I, Abzug JM. Ossification of the proximal and middle phalangeal condyles: radiographic aid in phalangeal neck fracture reduction. J Pediatr Orthop. 2019;39(3):e222–6. https://doi.org/10.1097/BPO.0000000000001255.
10. Herman MJ, Boardman MJ, Hoover JR, et al. Relationship of the anterior humeral line to the capitellar ossific nucleus: variability with age. J Bone Joint Surg Am. 2009;91:2188–93.
11. Campbell RM Jr. Operative treatment of fractures and dislocations of the hand and wrist region in children. Orthop Clin North Am. 1990;21(2):217–43.
12. Park KB, Lee KJ, Kwak YH. Comparison between buddy taping with a short-arm splint and operative treatment for phalangeal neck fractures in children. J Pediatr Orthop. 2016;36(7):736–42.
13. Matzon JL, Cornwall R. A stepwise algorithm for surgical treatment of type II displaced pediatric phalangeal neck fractures. J Hand Surg Am. 2014;39(3):467–73.
14. Karl JW, White NJ, Strauch RJ. Percutaneous reduction and fixation of displaced phalangeal neck fractures in children. J Pediatr Orthop. 2012;32(2):156–61. https://doi.org/10.1097/BPO.0b013e3182423124.
15. Abzug JM, Mehlman CT. The community orthopaedic surgeon taking trauma call: pediatric phalangeal fracture pearls and pitfalls. J Orthop Trauma. 2017;31(Suppl 6):S1–5. https://doi.org/10.1097/BOT.0000buddy000000001013.
16. Puckett BN, Gaston RG, Peljovich AE, Lourie GM, Floyd WE 3rd. Remodeling potential of phalangeal distal condylar malunions in children. J Hand Surg Am. 2012 Jan;37(1):34–41. https://doi.org/10.1016/j.jhsa.2011.09.017.
17. Liao JCY, Huan SKW, Tan RES, Lim JX, Chong AKS, Das DS. A comparison of casting versus splinting for nonoperative treatment of pediatric phalangeal neck fractures. J Pediatr Orthop. 2021 Jan;41(1):e30–5. https://doi.org/10.1097/BPO.0000000000001687.
18. Wallace R, Topper SM, Eilert RE. Management of phalangeal neck fractures in children. Mil Med. 2006;171(2):139–41.
19. Al-Qattan MM. Phalangeal neck fractures with concurrent vascular injury. J Hand Surg Eur Vol. 2009;34(1):104–9.
20. Boyer JS, London DA, Stepan JG, Goldfarb CA. Pediatric proximal phalanx fractures: outcomes and complications after the surgical treatment of displaced fractures. J Pediatr Orthop. 2015;35(3):219–23.
21. Leonard MH, Dubravcik P. Management of fractured fingers in the child. Clin Orthop Relat Res. 1970;73:160–8.
22. Al-Qattan MM. Nonunion and avascular necrosis following phalangeal neck fractures in children. J Hand Surg Am. 2010 Aug;35(8):1269–74. https://doi.org/10.1016/j.jhsa.2010.03.038; Epub 2010 June 17.
23. Simmons BP, Peters TT. Subcondylar fossa reconstruction for malunion of fractures of the proximal phalanx in children. J Hand Surg Am. 1987;12(6):1079–82.
24. Yousif NJ, Cunningham MW, Sanger JR, Gingrass RP, Matloub HS. The vascular supply to the proximal interphalangeal joint. J Hand Surg Am. 1985;10(6 pt 1):852–61.
25. Shewring DJ, Miller AC, Ghandour A. Condylar fractures of the proximal and middle phalanges. J Hand Surg Eur Vol. 2015;40(1):51–8. https://doi.org/10.1177/1753193413508514.
26. Kiral A, Erken HY, Akmaz I, et al. Pins and rubber band traction for treatment of comminuted intra-articular fractures in the hand. J Hand Surg Am. 2014;39(4):696–705.
27. Cornwall R, Ricchetti ET. Pediatric phalanx fractures: unique challenges and pitfalls. Clin Orthop Relat Res. 2006;445:146–56.
28. Williams AA, Lochner HV. Pediatric hand and wrist injuries. Curr Rev Musculoskelet Med. 2013;6(1):18–25.
29. Sirota MA, Parks BG, Higgins JP, Means KR Jr. Stability of fixation of proximal phalanx unicondylar fractures of the hand: a biomechanical cadaver study. J Hand Surg Am. 2013;38(1):77–81. https://doi.org/10.1016/j.jhsa.2012.09.026.

Seymour Fractures and Bony Mallet Fractures in the Pediatric Population

Catherine C. May and Joshua M. Abzug

Introduction

Pediatric hand fractures are responsible for 2.3% of all visits to the emergency room and 20% of all pediatric fractures [1, 2]. Most pediatric hand fractures occur in the phalanges and commonly present in children ages 9–12 with males more commonly affected [1, 2]. These injuries often occur due to a crushing mechanism and/or during sports-related activities. Fractures of the distal phalanx may be classified as mallet finger injuries when there is a fracture that is near the extensor tendon insertion adjacent to the distal interphalangeal (DIP) joint [3, 4].

Seymour Fractures

Twenty to thirty percent of all pediatric fractures involve the physeal region [5]. A Seymour fracture is a juxta-epiphyseal fracture of the distal phalanx with a concomitant nail bed laceration [6]. Due to the nail bed laceration, these injuries are considered open fractures and as such, must be treated accordingly in order to mitigate soft tissue infection and/or osteomyelitis [6]. An imbalance between the extensor tendon—which inserts on the epiphysis—and the flexor digitorum profundus tendon—which inserts into the metaphysis—creates a flexed posture of the injured digit (Fig. 6.1) [5]. The appearance of the finger may cause the fracture to be

---

Disclaimer: The views expressed in the submitted article are our own and not an official position of the institution.

C. C. May · J. M. Abzug (✉)
Department of Orthopedic Surgery, University of Maryland School of Medicine, Baltimore, MD, USA
e-mail: catherine.may@som.umaryland.edu; jabzug@som.umaryland.edu

J. M. Abzug et al. (eds.), *Pediatric and Adult Hand Fractures*,
https://doi.org/10.1007/978-3-031-32072-9_6

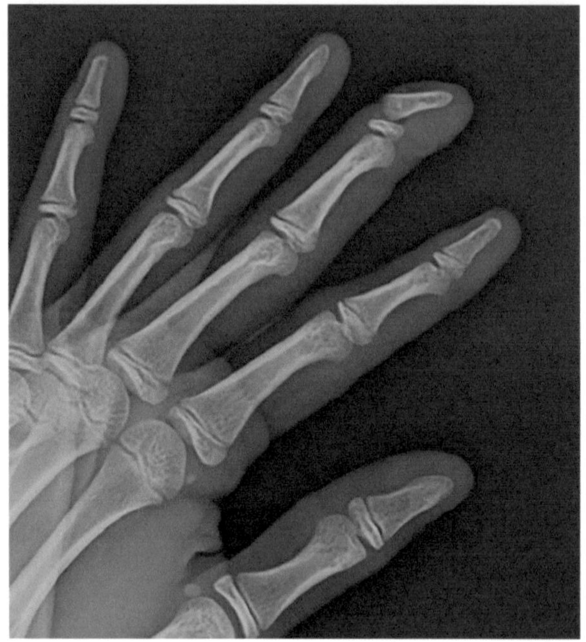

Fig. 6.1 Oblique radiograph of a Seymour fracture demonstrating a flexed posture of the digit following displacement through the physis of the long finger distal phalanx. (Courtesy of Joshua M. Abzug, MD)

misidentified as a bony mallet fracture [5, 6]. However, unlike bony mallet fractures, there is no disruption of the extensor mechanism in a Seymour fracture [5]. Instead, the disruption will occur at the site of the fracture near the physis due to the biomechanically weak nature of the physeal region [5]. The exact location of the fracture is determined by the biomechanical weakness of the physis, the difference in angulation between the epiphysis and diaphysis of the distal phalanx, and the direction and magnitude of force during the time of injury [5].

Clinical Presentation

Seymour fractures commonly occur through crushing mechanisms such as entrapment in doors, falls from a height, or compression by heavy objects [7]. Al-Qattan reported on the presentation and treatment of 25 Seymour fractures in children and adolescents [8]. Of these fractures, the most common mechanisms of injury were entrapment of the digit in a door or swing (52%), falls from height (12%), and collision with a heavy object (36%) [8]. Most of these cases occurred in the middle finger (48%) and the thumb (24%) and in children under the age of 12 (60%) [8].

The clinical presentation of a Seymour fracture includes a flexed posture of the distal phalanx and an associated nail bed injury [5, 8]. Typically, the nail plate rests superficial to the eponychial fold following dorsal displacement [5, 7]. However, some patients experience torn nail beds and breaks in the cuticle seal resulting in an open fracture [6]. Patients may have eschar about the proximal extent of the nail

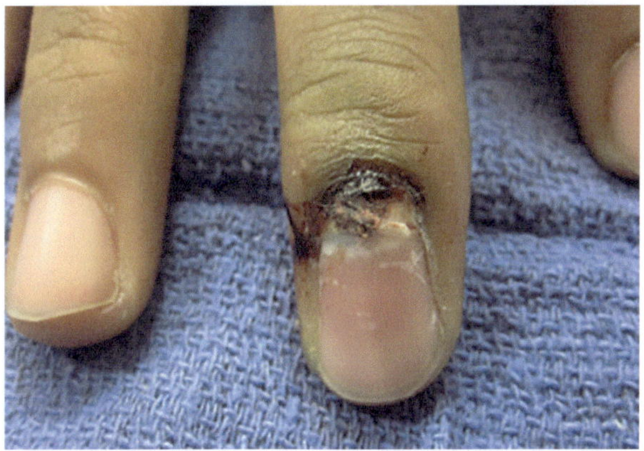

Fig. 6.2 Clinical photograph of a Seymour fracture in a 12-year-old male who crushed his finger in a car door. Note that the proximal nail plate is superficial to the eponychial fold and eschar is present. (Courtesy of Joshua M. Abzug, MD)

complex making the assessment difficult; however suspicion should be high for a nail complex injury when such eschar is present (Fig. 6.2). Concomitant injuries, other than nail bed lacerations, are somewhat rare because the surrounding areas are biomechanically stronger than the physis [6].

Classification

Seymour originally included Salter Harris type I or type II fractures, and/or metaphyseal fractures 1–2 mm distal to the epiphyseal plate in the description of a Seymour fracture [2, 5]. A Salter Harris type I fracture passes through the growth plate separating the epiphysis from the metaphysis, while a Salter Harris type II fracture extends through the physis into the metaphysis [2, 6]. Confirmation of the diagnosis is obtained through radiographic imaging [2].

Imaging

Plain radiographs can confirm the suspected diagnosis of a Seymour fracture. It is important to note that radiographs of the injured digit in the posteroanterior (PA) plane may appear normal. A true lateral view is essential to assess for physeal widening and/or displacement of the epiphysis, characteristic of a Seymour fracture (Fig. 6.3) [5, 6].

Treatment

Displaced distal phalangeal physeal fractures that do not have an associated nail bed laceration are managed nonoperatively via a closed reduction and subsequent placement of a splint [6]. Patients are monitored with weekly radiographs to assess the fracture alignment and for potential loss of reduction [6]. Patient compliance is

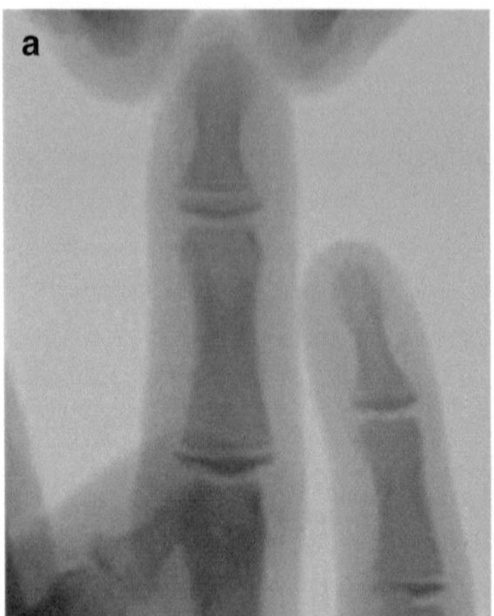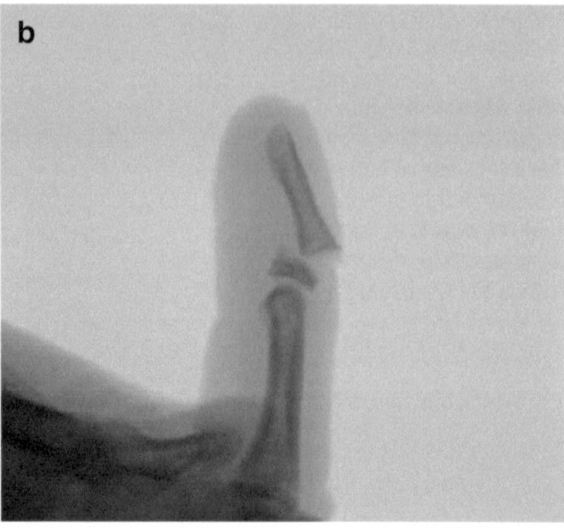

Fig. 6.3 a. Posteroanterior fluoroscopic image which appears normal. **b**. Lateral fluoroscopic image demonstrating physeal widening and displacement of the epiphysis characteristic of a Seymour fracture. (Courtesy of Joshua M. Abzug, MD)

necessary for optimal healing. Therefore, it is necessary to be cognizant that in pediatric patients, it is more difficult to ensure splint instructions are being followed. One option to overcome this concern is to place a cast over the splint and adjacent uninjured digits; however, it is then difficult to obtain radiographs free of obstruction by the other digits to assess alignment [6]. Therefore, if this treatment is undertaken, one can remove the cast weekly to obtain the radiographs and then reapply the cast.

Seymour fractures, which are an open fracture by definition, are treated operatively to manage the laceration and displacement of the fracture [5]. The procedure can be performed in the emergency department if feasible or in the operating room. Regardless of location, the digit should be prepped through typical sterile protocols including cleansing and draping of the digit [5]. Surgeons may choose to use either a digital tourniquet or a pneumatic forearm/arm tourniquet to restrict blood flow during the procedure [5]. A digital block, regional anesthetic and/or general anesthetic can be utilized to provide the necessary anesthesia.

At the start of the procedure, the nail plate is removed atraumatically by a blunt instrument such as a Freer elevator and a hemostat [5, 6]. During this process it is imperative that the attachments of the paronychial folds to the nail plate are gently elevated off, as a lack of care will lead to tearing of the paronychia. Once the nail plate is removed, the fracture site can often be accessed through a transverse laceration in the germinal matrix of the nail bed [5, 6]. Further visualization may be obtained by creating one- to two-centimeter oblique incisions directed proximally towards the DIP joint at the junction of the eponychial and paronychial folds and then reflecting the eponychial fold proximally (Fig. 6.4) [5, 6]. Hyperflexion of the distal phalanx can also aid in exposing the fracture site (Fig. 6.5). Any interposed soft tissue within the fracture site should be identified and extracted to prevent difficulty during the reduction and future physeal arrest [5, 6]. While doing so, one must be careful not to damage the terminal extensor tendon attachment on the

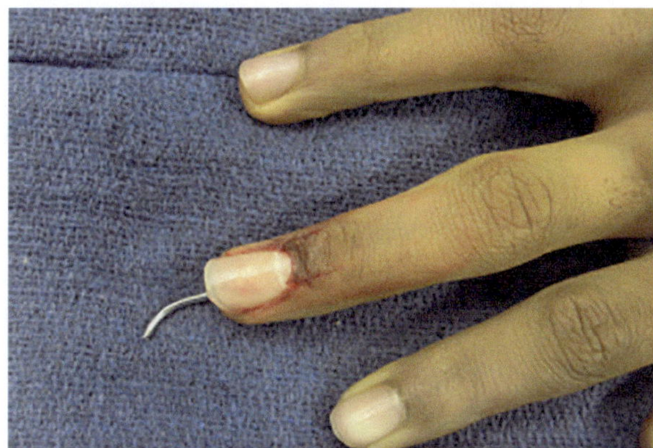

Fig. 6.4 Clinical photograph of the patient from Fig. 6.2 following I&D of the fracture site, nail bed repair, reduction of the fracture, and replacement of the nail plate. Note the two proximal incisions used to aid in visualization of the fracture site. (Courtesy of Joshua M. Abzug, MD)

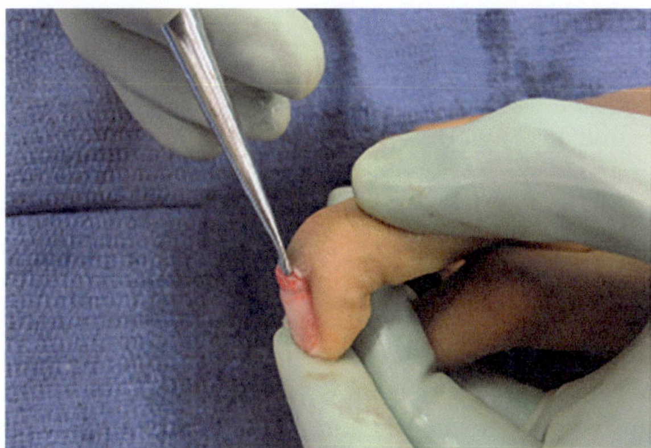

Fig. 6.5 Clinical photograph of the patient from Fig. 6.2 demonstrating hyperflexion to aid in visualization during irrigation and debridement of the fracture site. (Courtesy of Joshua M. Abzug, MD)

epiphysis of the distal phalanx [5]. A gentle irrigation and debridement of the fracture site should be performed. Subsequently, the distal phalanx is extended to reduce the fracture and align the physis [5, 6]. Fluoroscopy is used throughout the procedure to ensure proper anatomical alignment [5]. After appropriate alignment is achieved, a 0.035 in. or 0.045 in. Kirschner wire is driven in a retrograde fashion into the fingertip across the fracture site and DIP joint [5, 6]. Alternatively, one can simply splint the digit in full extension. The nail bed laceration is then repaired using a 6-0 or 7-0 absorbable suture [5–7]. Any additional incisions made during the procedure are repaired using simple interrupted absorbable sutures [5]. The digit is then dressed with sterile nonadhesive dressings and placed in a short-arm mitten cast to protect the surgical site [5, 6]. Patients are given IV antibiotics prior to the start of the procedure and continued on oral antibiotics for 5–7 days subsequently [6].

Outcomes

A study by Ganayem and Edelson examined outcomes following the treatment of seven pediatric patients with Seymour fractures [9]. All seven patients were injured through crush injuries or digital entrapment and four of the cases involved the middle finger [9]. Six of the seven patients had open fractures with concomitant lacerations to the nail matrix [9]. Therefore, these six patients were treated operatively akin to the surgical procedure described above [9]. The remaining patient had a closed injury which was treated nonoperatively [9]. At 18 months of follow-up, all patients experienced fracture healing and no complications were reported [9].

Reyes and Ho (2017) identified a greater risk of infection when treatment of Seymour fractures was either delayed or incomplete [10]. Patients who received proper irrigation and debridement (I&D), fracture reduction, and antibiotic administration within 24 h of the injury experienced no complications [10]. The group who received treatment within 24 h of the injury but lacked either I&D, fracture reduction, or antibiotic administration experienced an infection rate of 15% [10]. Those who received treatment after 24 h from the injury had the poorest outcomes with an infection rate of 45% [10].

Complications

Failure to recognize and treat a Seymour fracture can increase the chance of suboptimal outcomes. It is important to administer antibiotics appropriately as they may serve as a protective factor against lack of fracture healing [11]. Osteomyelitis has been shown to occur in approximately 50% of patients who had a delay in treatment [10]. Additional complications can occur including physeal arrest and nail growth abnormalities. To minimize the chances of a physeal arrest, it is imperative to perform any debridement in a very gentle manner and ensure that no interposing tissue remains when the fracture is reduced. Nail growth abnormalities are minimized by reducing the fracture in a near-anatomic manner and by performing a meticulous near-anatomic repair of the nail bed laceration.

Bony Mallet Fractures

A bony mallet fracture is a fracture with an associated disruption of the extensor mechanism about the DIP joint due to an avulsed intra-articular fracture at the attachment site of the extensor tendon on the epiphysis (Fig. 6.6) [2, 6]. If there is further extension of the fracture to or through the metaphysis of the distal phalanx, the fracture may be classified as a Salter-Harris type IV fracture [6]. Disruption of the extensor mechanism causes an imbalance between the proximal interphalangeal (PIP) joint and the DIP joint, which must be treated shortly after the injury to avoid future deformity [12].

Clinical Presentation

Bony mallet fractures are caused by forced flexion of the DIP joint of an extended finger [2, 6, 12]. Typically, this fracture is a result of an axially directed load on the

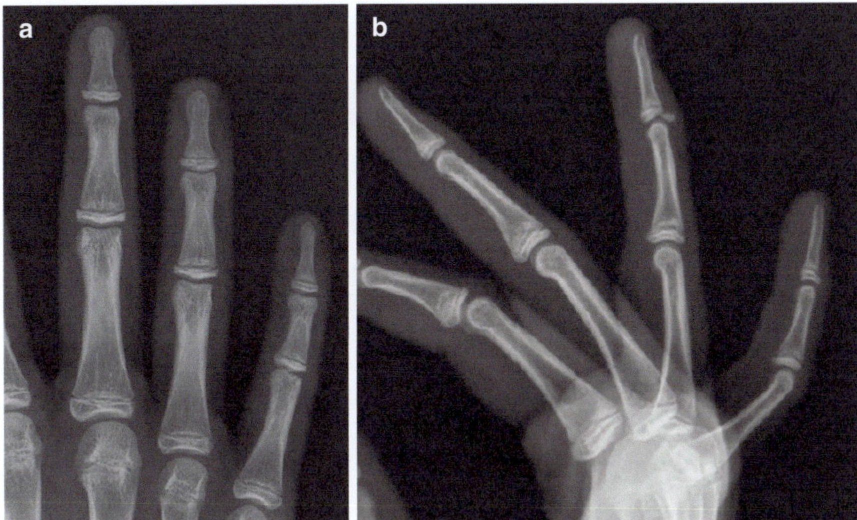

Fig. 6.6 Radiographs of a 14-year-old male who jammed his finger while playing basketball and sustained a bony mallet fracture. (**a**) PA and (**b**) lateral view. (Courtesy of Joshua M. Abzug, MD)

Table 6.1 Wehbe and Schneider classification system

Classification	Description
Type	
Type I	No subluxation of the DIP joint
Type II	Subluxation of the DIP joint
Type III	Injury to the epiphysis and physis
Subtype	
Type A	< 1/3 articular surface involvement
Type B	1/3 to 2/3 articular surface involvement
Type C	> 2/3 articular surface involvement

extended finger [6]. These fractures are most commonly seen in male patients and athletes [12]. Often, the fracture is present in the dominant hand (74%) and in one of the three ulnar digits (90%) [12]. Athletes who experience forceful contact to the fingertips may describe their injury as a "jammed finger" [12]. Ultimately, the resultant clinical deformity is flexion of the DIP joint with or without substantial swelling of the distal extent of the digit.

Classification

There are several ways to classify bony mallet fractures, the most common of which is the Wehbe and Schneider classification system [6, 12]. In this system, bony mallet fractures are divided into three main types of injury, then further divided into three subtypes based on the extent of articular involvement (Table 6.1) [6, 12]. The different types of fractures warrant their own treatment protocols, as those with a greater

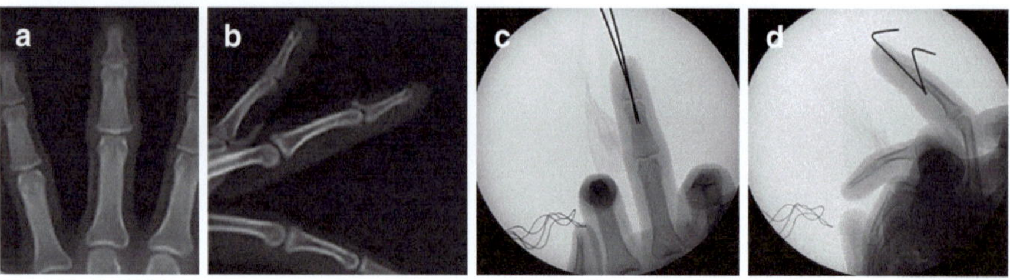

Fig. 6.7 A 15-year-old male with a bony mallet fracture after jamming his long finger while playing basketball. Preoperative (**a**) PA and (**b**) lateral views. Postoperative (**c**) PA and (**d**) lateral fluoroscopic views following extension block pinning. (Courtesy of Joshua M. Abzug, MD)

Table 6.2 Doyle classification system

Classification		Description
Type I		Closed injury, may or may not have avulsion fracture
Type II		Open injury (superficial) with tendon discontinuity
Type III		Open injury (deep) reaching the tendon
Type IV	IV_A	Transepiphyseal fracture
	IV_B	Hyperflexion with 20–50% articular involvement
	IV_C	Hyperextension with >50% articular involvement

degree of articular involvement are more likely to be treated operatively (Fig. 6.7) [12].

Patel and Gerberman divided bony mallet fractures into two separate groups: acute and chronic injuries [6, 12, 13]. Acute injuries present within 4 weeks of the injury, while chronic injuries present after 4 weeks from the time of injury [6, 12, 13]. Doyle developed another classification system based on the mechanism of injury and soft tissue damage (Table 6.2) [14].

Imaging

Plain radiographs are used to confirm the diagnosis of a bony mallet fracture. The PA view may appear normal and therefore it is mandatory to obtain a true lateral view of the digit to assess for the injury. An oblique view may be obtained to provide additional information regarding the fracture fragment; however the lateral radiograph will optimally depict the avulsion of the distal phalanx epiphysis characteristic of this fracture (Fig. 6.8).

Treatment

Many methods to treat bony mallet fractures have been described ranging from splinting to various surgical techniques. However, currently there is persisting

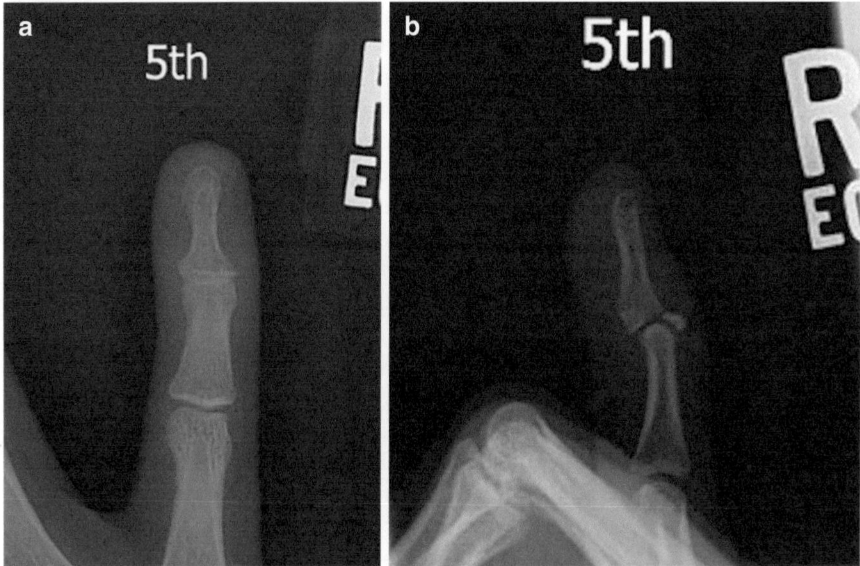

Fig. 6.8 Radiograph of a bony mallet fracture in a 17-year-old male who injured his finger during an altercation. (**a**) PA and (**b**) lateral views. (Courtesy of Joshua M. Abzug, MD)

controversy surrounding the preferred treatment type for each bony mallet fracture variation [6, 12]. Literature guiding the treatment of pediatric patients is further limited [6]. Each method of treatment shares a common goal of maintaining joint stability and avoiding extensor lag and swan neck deformities [6].

Noninvasive methods may be used to treat patients with bony mallet fractures affecting less than one third of the articular surface [6]. A splint or cast is used to immobilize the DIP joint in full extension [6, 12]. Patients should maintain the full extension immobilization for 4–6 weeks, after which they may utilize the splint only at nights for 2–4 weeks [6]. Physicians should inform patients of proper hygiene and care of the splint to prevent skin breakdown, ischemia, and/or joint dysfunction [6, 12]. Complications may arise if the patient fails to comply with the splinting protocol.

Operative interventions are performed on patients with injuries affecting greater than one third of the articular surface, those not experiencing cortical bone contact after reduction, and those patients that have repeated volar subluxation [6, 12]. In addition, surgery may be recommended for patients who are unable to maintain splinting and/or do not identify improvements following a period of splinting [6, 12].

Bony mallet fractures are commonly reduced through the percutaneous extension-block pinning technique first described by Ishiguro [15]. In this procedure, patients are given either digital or metacarpal block anesthesia and/or general anesthesia [16]. The PIP and DIP joints are held in maximum flexion while fluoroscopic imaging is used to visualize the fracture site [16]. Two Kirshner wires (K-wire) are percutaneously inserted to reduce and stabilize the fracture and DIP joint [16]. The first

K-wire is placed through the extensor tendon 1–2 mm dorsal and proximal to the fracture fragment into the middle phalanx [16]. To reduce the fracture, the distal phalanx is then extended and adjusted distally [16]. An additional K-wire is placed through the DIP joint obliquely and palmar to the fracture site or directly retrograde from the tip of the finger [16]. The digit is cleaned and placed into a splint with the DIP joint held in full-time extension for 4–8 weeks followed by 2–4 weeks of splinting at night [6, 16]. Radiographs obtained after 4–6 weeks will be assessed for proper healing to determine whether or not the wires are ready to be removed [16].

Additional techniques include K-wire fixation, hook plating, tension band wiring, pin fixation, internal suturing, bone anchoring, and umbrella handle k-wire fixation [6, 12, 14]. The hook plating technique is selected for patients who are unable to tolerate exposed pins and/or patients who have avulsion fractures involving more than 30% of the joint surface [17]. In this operation, a 0.5 cm Lazy-Y incision is made proximal to the DIP crease [18]. To prevent extension lag of the DIP joint and damage to the germinal matrix, the skin is carefully dissected from the extensor tendon [18]. Subsequently, the region is prepared for implant placement by elevating the germinal matrix approximately 3 to 4 mm [18]. The 1.7 mm hook plate is placed proximal to the terminal extensor tendon and distally beneath the elevated germinal matrix [18]. While maintaining contact between the hook plate and the distal phalanx with a Kelly clamp, the avulsion fracture may be reduced [18]. The plate should not interfere with the DIP joint and should maintain a fracture gap less than 1 mm [18]. A 1.0 mm K-wire is placed through the DIP joint to temporarily maintain full joint extension [18]. An additional K-wire, called the pilot wire, is placed into the screw hole to establish appropriate screw access [18]. To increase bony purchase length, the screw axis is arranged obliquely towards the fingertip [18]. Throughout the procedure, fluoroscopy is used to visualize the position of the hook plate, the reduction of the avulsion fracture, and the alignment of the pilot K-wire. If acceptable alignment is achieved, the K-wire is removed and replaced by a 1.7 mm screw driven into the distal phalanx [18]. The wound is then irrigated and closed using 5-0 absorbable sutures. The digit is splinted for at least 2 weeks following the procedure [18]. At the 2-week postoperative period, the patient begins rehabilitation which includes active and passive motion of the DIP joint. Follow-up continues monthly until the bone is fully healed [18].

Outcomes

Clinical outcomes and treatment may be assessed through the Crawford evaluation criteria, which identifies flexion-extension movement, DIP joint mobility, and indications of pain [14]. According to this criteria, a "perfect" score would include patients with normal flexion and extension of the DIP joint and no pain [14]. Patients who lose zero to ten degrees of extension, have normal flexion, and no pain are considered "good" [14]. Those with ten to twenty-five degrees of extension loss, any flexion loss, and no pain are classified as "moderate" while those with greater than 25 degrees of extension loss and any reported pain are considered "bad" [14].

The outcomes are often determined by the extent of terminal extensor tendon shortening or lengthening, as each millimeter of extensor tendon lengthening leads to twenty-five degrees of extensor lag, and each millimeter of extensor tendon shortening leads to limited joint flexion [6]. Through surgical treatment, patients often experience five to ten degrees of extensor lag and mild loss of range of motion, although they report no change in patient satisfaction [6, 12].

Pegoli et al. conducted a retrospective review of 65 patients with bony mallet fractures treated through the Ishiguro extension block pinning technique [16]. Based on the Webhe and Schneider classification system, the fractures consisted of 27 type IB, 19 type IIB, 17 type IA, and 2 type IIA fractures [16]. The K-wires were removed on average of 36 days following the procedure [16]. One patient developed an infection, resulting in an earlier removal of the K-wires [16]. The outcomes were evaluated based on the Crawford evaluation criteria. Results identified 30 "perfect," 21 "good," 13 "moderate," and 1 "bad" outcomes [16]. "Moderate" outcomes were due to poor fracture reduction leading to decreased range of motion [16]. The "bad" outcome was a result of a nail bed deformity and angular deformity [16]. The overall complication rate was 5%, which is considered acceptable given the number of "perfect" and "good" outcomes [16].

Orhun et al. monitored outcomes of 34 patients with bony mallet fractures which were unable to undergo successful closed reduction [14]. Each patient was subsequently treated through an open reduction and K-wire fixation an average of 1.3 days following the injury [14]. Thirty-one patients achieved successful anatomic reductions [14]. Three patients experienced a malunion, three patients had loss of 10 degrees of flexion, and four patients had a loss of 5 degrees of extension [14]. According to the Crawford evaluation criteria, results were "perfect" in 27 patients, "good" in 4 patients, and "moderate" in 3 patients [14].

Wang et al. observed the outcomes of 16 bony mallet fractures treated through the hook plating technique [18]. Although the patients were ages 18–51 years, the mechanisms and classification of injuries were similar to those found in children. There were 9 fractures classified as type IB fractures, 2 type IC fractures, and 5 types IIB and IIC fractures [18]. The mean DIP extension lag and flexion in patients following treatment was 0 degrees (range: 0–30 degrees) and 60 degrees (range: 40–90 degrees), respectively [18]. The treatment outcomes were evaluated according to the Crawford criteria. Outcomes were considered to be "perfect" in 9 patients, "good" in 5 patients, "moderate" in 1 patient, and "bad" in 1 patient [18]. Within this group, 88% of patients were satisfied with their treatments [18]. Overall, the hook plating procedure had a complication rate of 18% [18]. There were three total complications in three unique patients including 2 nail deformities and 1 implant that loosened [18].

Complications

While the extension block pinning technique is commonly used to treat bony mallet fractures which include more than one third of the articular surface, the ideal treatment method remains disputed [14]. This technique is quicker and less invasive than other procedures and the use of fluoroscopic imaging helps to achieve proper reduction and fixation [14]. However, the potential shortcomings of this technique include damage to the articular cartilage, delayed bone union, pin tract infection, and nail deformity [14].

In the study conducted by Wang et al., there were four identified "pitfalls" of the hook plating technique [18]. The first complication was operative wound skin necrosis [18]. Using incisions other than the Lazy-Y resulted in a limited surgical field and the development of transient skin flap ischemia [18]. Therefore, the authors chose to incorporate the Lazy-Y incision into the surgical procedure to improve the surgical field and increase blood supply to the skin flap [18]. As a result, there were no cases of necrosis in the sixteen patients included in the study [18]. The second complication was a nail deformity due to iatrogenic germinal matrix injury during soft tissue exposure [18]. By elevating the germinal matrix by approximately 3–4 mm, the surgeons could place the hook plate underneath it [18]. Ultimately, this eliminated nail deformities after the procedure was corrected by the researchers [18]. The third complication was terminal tendon laxity with postoperative extension lag [18]. This is often due to screw loosening, loss of reduction, and/or over-dissection of the terminal tendon-to-bone structure [18]. Consequently, it is imperative to carefully perform the dissection and monitor the digit using fluoroscopy imaging [18]. The fourth complication was a loss of reduction [18]. In the study, one patient experienced a loss of reduction due to screw loosening [18]. This may be avoided through adjustments in the surgical technique when the fracture involves more than 40% of the articular surface [18]. Adjustments include the addition of an extra pin, drilling of another K-wire into the screw hole to ensure proper screw axis, and modifying the strength and/or length of the screw [18].

Regardless of the treatment approach, it is important to quickly identify and treat bony mallet fractures. A study performed by Kootstra et al. examined outcomes following delayed treatment of bony mallet fractures over 21 days from the initial injury [17]. Outcomes in 27 patients with an average time to surgical intervention of 35 days were reviewed [17]. Following treatment, 67% of patients experienced limited range of motion, and 33% of patients had persisting stiffness [17]. Eleven percent of patients developed infections which required antibiotic treatment [17]. However, there was a relatively low complication rate of 15% [17]. Literature surrounding surgical interventions of pediatric bony mallet fractures is limited and requires further study. However, it is important to treat the fracture optimally to avoid loss of motion and the development of a swan neck deformity.

Conclusion

Seymour fractures are juxta-epiphyseal fractures of the distal phalanx with an associated nail bed laceration. Operative intervention is necessary to extract any interposed soft tissue and reduce the fracture site. It is important to treat these fractures quickly and appropriately to prevent infection, physeal arrest, and nail bed deformity. Bony mallet fractures are intra-articular avulsion fractures at the site of attachment of the extensor tendon on the epiphysis. Depending on the degree of articular involvement, bony mallet fractures may be treated nonoperatively through splinting or operatively through techniques such as extension block pinning or hook plating. Management of bony mallet fractures should aim to prevent loss of reduction, extensor lag, and development of bony deformities.

References

1. Nellans KW, Chung KC. Pediatric hand fractures. Hand Clin. 2013;29(4):569–78. https://doi. org/10.1016/j.hcl.2013.08.009.
2. Case AL, Hosseinzadeh P, Baldwin KD, Abzug JM. Hand fractures in children: when do I need to start thinking about surgery? Instr Course Lect. 2019;68:415–26.
3. Bendre AA, Hartigan BJ, Kalainov DM. Mallet finger. J Am Acad Orthop Surg. 2005;13(5):336–44.
4. Bandi S, Drone E, Vera A, Ganti L. Seymour fracture in a pediatric patient: a case report. Cureus. 2020;12(9):e10687. https://doi.org/10.7759/cureus.10687.
5. Abzug JM, Kozin SH. Seymour Fractures. J Hand Surg Am. 2013;38(11):2267–70. https://doi. org/10.1016/j.jhsa.2013.08.104.
6. Abzug JM, Dua K, Bauer AS, Cornwall R, Wyrick TO. Pediatric phalanx fractures. J Am Acad Orthop Surg. 2016;24(11):e174–83. https://doi.org/10.5435/JAAOS-D-16-00199.
7. Goodell PB, Bauer A. Problematic pediatric hand and wrist fractures. JBJS Rev. 2016;4(5):e1. https://doi.org/10.2106/JBJS.RVW.O.00028.
8. Al-Qattan MM. Extra-articular transverse fractures of the base of the distal phalanx (Seymour's fracture) in children and adults. J Hand Surg. 2001;26(3):201–6. https://doi.org/10.1054/jhsb.2000.0549.
9. Ganayem M, Edelson G. Base of distal phalanx fracture in children: a mallet finger mimic. J Pediatr Orthop. 2005;25(4):487–9. https://doi.org/10.1097/01.bpo.0000158813.37225.fa.
10. Reyes BA, Ho CA. The high risk of infection with delayed treatment of open Seymour fractures: salter-Harris I/II or juxta-epiphyseal fractures of the distal phalanx with associated nailbed laceration. J Pediatr Orthop. 2017;37(4):247–53. https://doi.org/10.1097/BPO.0000000000000638.
11. Samade R, Lin JS, Popp JE, Samora JB. Delayed presentation of Seymour fractures: a single institution experience and management recommendations. Hand (N Y). 2021;16(5):686–93. https://doi.org/10.1177/1558944719878846.
12. Alla SR, Deal ND, Dempsey IJ. Current concepts: mallet finger. Hand (N Y). 2014;9(2):138–44. https://doi.org/10.1007/s11552-014-9609-y.
13. Patel MR, Desai SS, Bassini-Lipson L. Conservative management of chronic mallet finger. J Hand Surg Am. 1986;11(4):570–3. https://doi.org/10.1016/s0363-5023(86)80202-7.
14. Orhon H. Open reduction and K-wire fixation of mallet finger injuries: mid-term results. Acta Orthop Traumatol Turc. 2009;43(5):395–9. https://doi.org/10.3944/AOTT.2009.395.
15. Ishiguro T. A new method of closed reduction for mallet fracture using extension-block Kirschner wire. Cent Jpn J Orthop Trauma Surg. 1988;6:413–5.
16. Pegoli L, Toh S, Arai K, Fukuda A, Nishikawa S, Vallego I. The Ishiguro extension block technique for the treatment of mallet finger fracture: indications and clinical results. J Hand Surg. 2003;28(1):15–7. https://doi.org/10.1054/jhsb.2001.0733.
17. Kootstra TJM, Keizer J, van Heijl M, Ferree S, Houwert M, van der Velde D. Delayed extension block pinning in 27 patients with mallet fracture. Hand (N Y). 2021;16(1):61–6. https://doi.org/10.1177/1558944719840749.
18. Wang W-C. Functional outcomes and complications of hook plate for bony mallet finger: a retrospective case series study. BMC Musculoskelet Disord. 2021;22:281.

Fingertip Injuries and Tuft Fractures in the Pediatric Population

7

Hilton P. Gottschalk and Grant McHorse

Introduction

Hand injuries are the most common injuries in the pediatric population, and the phalanges are the most commonly injured bones in the hand [1]. Younger children use their hands to explore the environment, which when combined with poorly developed motor skills and absence of fear predisposes to fingertip injuries [2]. Older adolescents may also sustain fingertip injuries during athletic participation or manual labor [2]. The fingertip has been defined as the portion of the finger distal to the insertion of the extensor mechanism and flexor digitorum profundus (FDP) tendons [3]. Fingertip injuries can take the form of nail bed injuries, distal phalanx fractures, amputations, or partial amputations, as well as flexor digitorum profundus avulsions.

Though most fingertip injuries in the pediatric population are associated with excellent outcomes, poor outcomes are possible and more likely when the severity of the initial injury is underestimated [2]. The importance of early diagnosis and proper management makes it critical that frontline providers are comfortable evaluating and treating fingertip injuries. Treatment should prioritize restoring function, eliminating and preventing pain, and preserving protective sensation in the digit [4].

The unique anatomy of the fingertip, including the paucity of soft tissue and the presence of the nail plate, as well as the presence of physes in pediatric patients, further complicates fingertip injury diagnosis and management.

H. P. Gottschalk (✉)
Department of Surgery and Perioperative Care, Dell Medical School, The University of Texas at Austin, Austin, TX, USA

Central Texas Pediatric Orthopedics, Austin, TX, USA

G. McHorse
Central Texas Pediatric Orthopedics, Austin, TX, USA

J. M. Abzug et al. (eds.), *Pediatric and Adult Hand Fractures*,
https://doi.org/10.1007/978-3-031-32072-9_7

109

Evaluation

The initial evaluation of fingertip injuries must be thorough, as the risk of poor outcomes increases when the severity of the initial injury is underestimated [1, 2]. It is important for non-hand surgeon providers to be comfortable evaluating fingertip injuries, as children may present to urgent care facilities or adult emergency rooms, especially when the fingertip injury is severe such as an amputation or open fracture.

Patient history should include the mechanism of injury, hand dominance if it has developed, and time since injury, as those repaired within 24 h have lower chance of infection. As with clinical evaluation of most musculoskeletal injuries, the evaluation should begin with careful observation of the skin, nail bed complex, and finger movement. Evaluation of the skin should include an examination for any abrasions, ecchymosis, and/or swelling, as well as turgor and dryness. If lacerations are present, care should be taken to ensure no foreign bodies are present in the wound before treatment, as they may not appear on plain radiographs. The nail plate should be assessed for subungual hematoma (Fig. 7.1), as well as eschar at the base of the nail, subluxation of the proximal nail plate, and/or other nail plate damage which may signify an underlying nail bed laceration [1, 4, 5]. The nail may appear longer than neighboring or contralateral nails if it has subluxated from beneath the eponychial fold [6]. If nail bed damage is clearly present in a pediatric patient, it is important to rule out an underlying physeal fracture which would signify a Seymour fracture (Fig. 7.2) that requires antibiotics and specific management. A digital nerve block or conscious sedation may be necessary to obtain an adequate evaluation in younger children, though such intervention may limit assessment of neurologic structures and tendon integrity. Midazolam or intranasal fentanyl may also be used to help calm children in order to conduct a thorough exam [5].

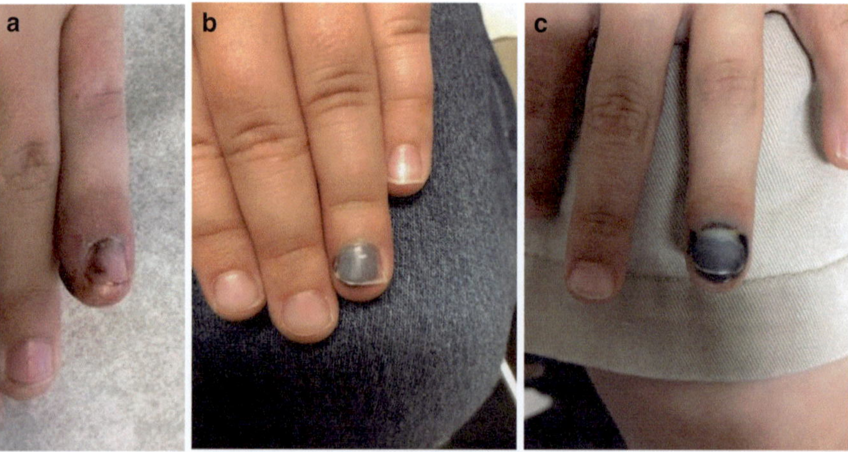

Fig. 7.1 Variations on subungual hematoma. (**a**) Clinical photograph of a subungual hematoma encompassing one third of the radial subungual area of small finger. (**b**) Clinical photograph of a subungual hematoma involving nearly the entire subungual area. (**c**) Clinical photograph of a subungual hematoma extending beyond the subungual margins

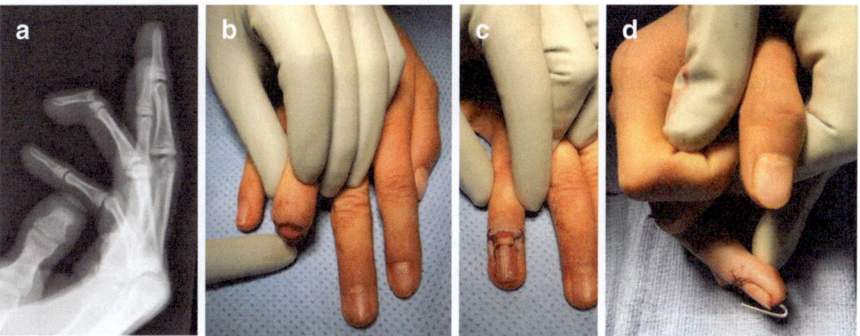

Fig. 7.2 Seymour fracture—physeal fracture of the distal phalanx. (**a**) Lateral radiograph of the right ring finger showing open displaced distal phalanx physeal fracture. (**b**) Exposed bone of the distal phalanx. (**c**) Open wound evident and skin marked for corner incisions to aid in the reduction of the fracture and freeing the germinal matrix. (**d**) Post-reduction and pinning

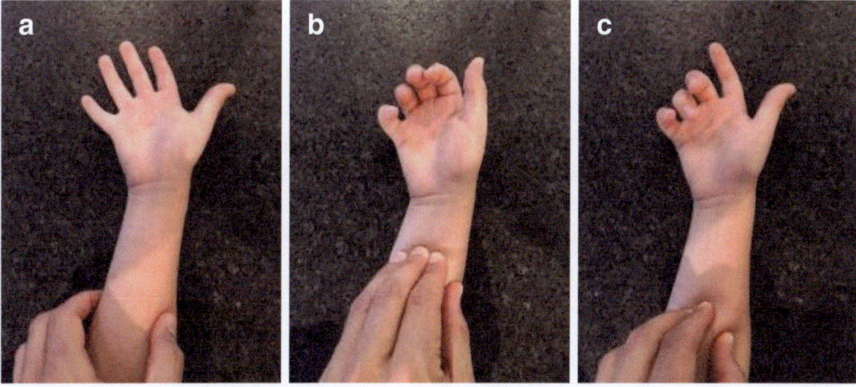

Fig. 7.3 Forearm compression test. (**a**) Fingers are extended. (**b**) Compression is placed over the flexor tendons in the forearm and the fingers flex appropriately. (**c**) Notice the index finger does not flex despite compression, suggesting a possible tendon injury

Vascular status may be grossly assessed with capillary refill testing. Nerve injury may be assessed by observing for dry, cracking skin on one side of the digit ("the sweat test"), which is indicative of nerve injury, or with two-point discrimination in older children, generally starting at age six [1]. Nerve injuries may also be investigated via the "wrinkle test" by soaking the injured fingertip in water for 10–20 min and observing for the development of wrinkles, which will only be present if the nerve is intact. The alignment of the phalanges should also be observed to evaluate for any underlying displaced fractures.

Observation of finger movement, or the digital cascade, can provide information regarding the continuity of tendons and malrotation or angulation of the phalanges, and may be more easily observed than formal range of motion testing in younger children [1]. Comparison to the contralateral side is often useful. Tendon function (Fig. 7.3) may also be investigated by assessing the tenodesis effect of the fingers with wrist extension and flexion, or forearm compression [5, 7].

Further evaluation should include palpation starting from the shoulder and moving distally to assess for other points of tenderness. Isolating the distal interphalangeal (DIP) joint by grasping the joint on the radial and ulnar sides and asking the patient to flex and extend their fingertip should also be attempted to determine the integrity of the flexor digitorum profundus tendon insertion.

Evaluation of fingertip injuries often necessitates the use of plain radiographs to diagnose phalangeal fractures, as up to half of fingertip injuries have associated or underlying fractures [8]. We recommend 3 views of the affected area: posteroanterior, oblique, and lateral views. The oblique views are helpful in discerning articular involvement. Radiographs of the entire hand are useful when multiple digits are injured [1].

Specific Injuries: Nail Bed Injuries

Epidemiology

Nail bed injuries are the second most common form of fingertip injuries and have been reported in up to 24% of fingertip injuries [9, 10]. Up to 50% of nail bed injuries may be associated with fractures of the distal phalanx (Fig. 7.4), with the most common being tuft fractures [4, 11]. Fingertip injuries most frequently occur on the third digit after the finger is crushed, commonly by a door in younger patients or after a laceration, machine injury, or sports participation in older patients [9].

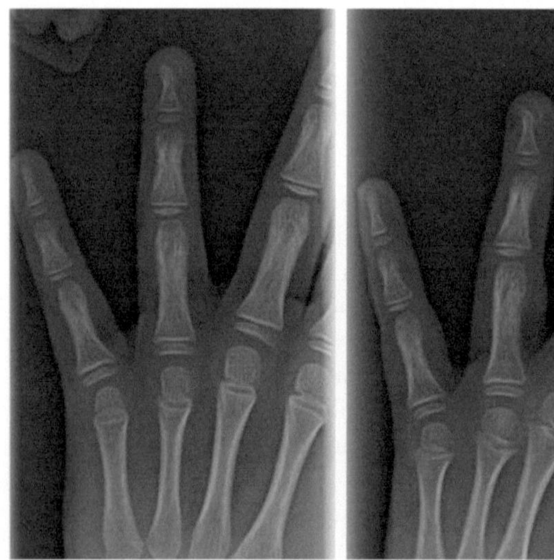
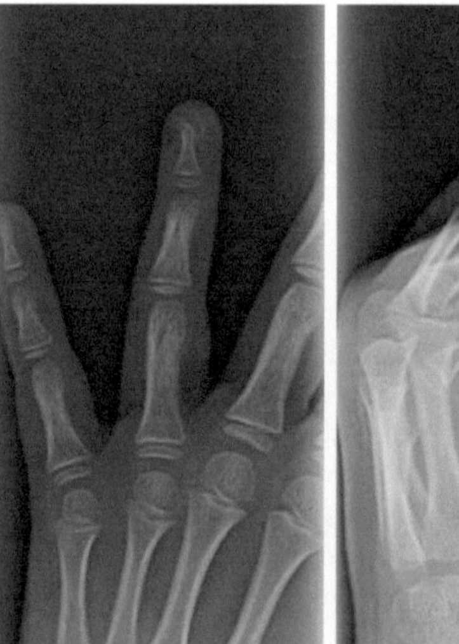
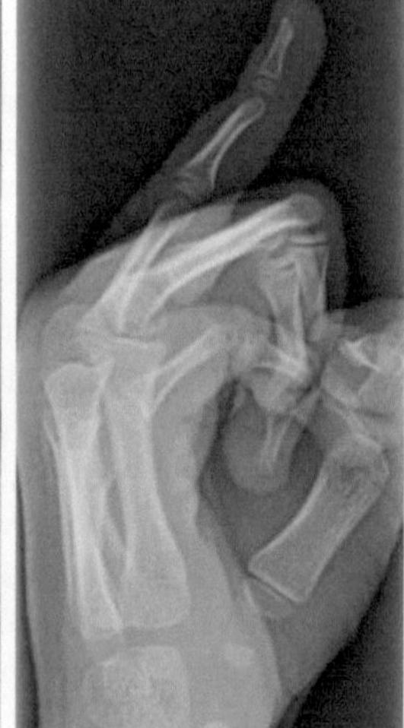

Fig. 7.4 Posteroanterior, oblique, and lateral views of a left hand showing a distal phalanx tuft fracture

The fingernail provides both protection and support to the fingertip, plays a role in tactile sensation, and also provides a counterforce when grasping small objects [4, 11]. In addition to functional consequences, a nail bed injury may have long-term cosmetic consequences [11].

Nail bed injuries can be classified into subungual hematomas, simple or stellate lacerations, crush injuries, or avulsions [12]. Subungual hematomas result from bleeding beneath the nail plate, while nail bed lacerations are the result of compression of the germinal or sterile matrix between the overlying nail plate and underlying distal phalanx [10]. The Van Beek classification of nail bed injuries differentiates between sterile and germinal matrix injuries, as well as based on the presence and size of a subungual hematoma, an underlying distal phalanx fracture, and/or a nail matrix avulsion [13].

Clinical Evaluation

Accurate diagnosis of nail bed injuries at the initial presentation is important, as delayed interventions, or secondary interventions after the initial treatment, often result in unsatisfactory outcomes. When taking the patient's history, understanding the mechanism of injury may inform the need for debridement and/or antibiotics. It is also important to clarify if the nail plate subluxated from the eponychial fold. Upon examination, signs of a nail bed injury may range from nail plate splitting to obvious nail bed laceration and/or nail plate subluxation. Evaluation should also include ruling out any underlying fractures and an evaluation of tendon and neuro-vascular integrity. The use of a digital block may be needed to allow for a thorough examination of the injured nail bed.

Previous studies have demonstrated that subungual hematoma size may be predictive of nail bed injuries. Sixty percent of patients with hematoma covering at least 50% of the nail plate have nail bed lacerations greater than 3 millimeters requiring repair. If an underlying fracture is present, the prevalence of a substantial nail bed laceration rose to 95% [14]. However, if the eponychial fold is intact, removal of the nail plate may not be necessary to definitely delineate the presence of a nail bed laceration [11]. The current practice at our institution is to leave the nail plate in place if there is no obvious skin laceration or break in the nail folds. However, experience has demonstrated that large subungual hematomas (Fig. 7.5) tend to be quite painful for these patients, and trephination of the nail plate in the appropriate setting or removal of the nail plate completely may be needed for pain relief. Ideally, this should be done within 24 h of the injury, as it becomes harder to release the hematoma after this time.

Plain radiographs are needed to evaluate for underlying fractures which should alert the examiner to the likely presence of a nail bed laceration and can result in differing management plans. Seymour fractures are important to rule out because of their unique management, including difficulty of reduction, and unique complications including physeal arrest, infection, and nonunion (see Chap. XX).

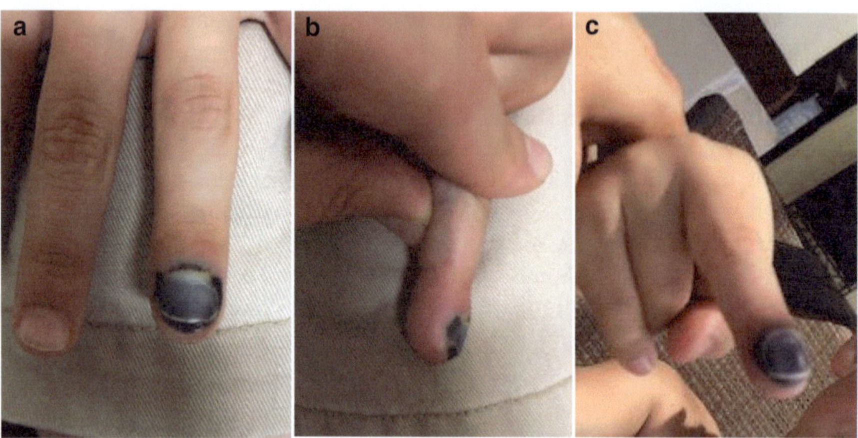

Fig. 7.5 Expansile hematoma: (**a**) and (**b**) 2 days after getting the finger caught in a door. (**c**) 7 days after the injury, note the increased size of the hematoma

Antibiotics

Prophylactic antibiotics, although traditionally indicated for larger wounds and open fractures of long bones, may not be needed following nail bed injuries or open fractures of the distal phalanx. Both a randomized controlled trial consisting of pediatric and adolescent patients and a meta-analysis of four larger trials found no difference in infection rates following open fractures of the distal phalanx with or without the use of prophylactic antibiotics [15, 16]. The initial focus should instead be towards prompt irrigation and debridement of the injury, which can often be done using a digital block in the emergency room setting [16]. Important exceptions include bite injuries, grossly contaminated wounds, and delayed presentation, all of which were excluded from the aforementioned studies and may still require prophylactic antibiotics. Tetanus prophylaxis should be administered if indicated following determination of vaccination status.

Repair (Emergency Department Vs. Operating Room)

Isolated nail bed injuries, or those associated with underlying tuft fractures, are often amenable to repair in the emergency room setting following a digital block [16]. Conscious sedation may also be used for young children unable to tolerate repair even with a digital block. Repair in the emergency room with local anesthesia allows for timeliness of the repair and avoids delays associated with operating room availability as well as the need for general anesthesia. If the presence of an underlying fracture is unclear, or if reduction and fixation of an underlying fracture is required, debridement in the operating room may be required.

Technique

Nail bed repair technique should be guided by the extent of the injury. If the nail plate and bed remain intact, the matter of nail removal and nail bed repair remains a matter of debate, though recent research suggests isolated trephination to relieve pressure from the subungual hematoma may be adequate [11, 17]. Trephination, with a needle or microcautery device, may reduce pain from the hematoma by relieving pressure, and allows the underlying nail bed to heal without further disruption. Trephination has been shown to produce similar results to nail removal and nail bed repair at lower cost, even in the presence of a nondisplaced tuft fractures [11, 17].

If the nail bed is disrupted or the nail plate is subluxated, the nail plate should be removed, and the nail bed laceration should be repaired. A small finger tourniquet may be used to reduce bleeding but should not be applied for more than 2 h, and the duration of tourniquet application should be minimized [18]. The nail plate can be removed from the underlying bed with a freer elevator, scissors, mosquito hemostat, and/or other small instrument, generally starting from the free edge/hyponychia region, and should be retained for replacement following nail bed repair (Fig. 7.6). The injury should be irrigated with sterile saline before the edges of the underlying laceration are reapproximated and repaired using 6-0 chromic suture [4, 19]. *Nonabsorbable sutures should be avoided! Again, nonabsorbable sutures should be avoided* (Fig. 7.7). The removed nail

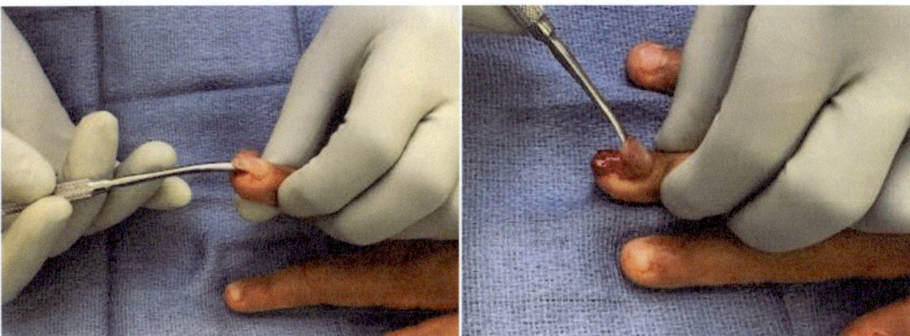

Fig. 7.6 Use of a freer elevator to lift the nail plate. Gradual pressure and side to side motion will allow for less traumatic nail plate removal

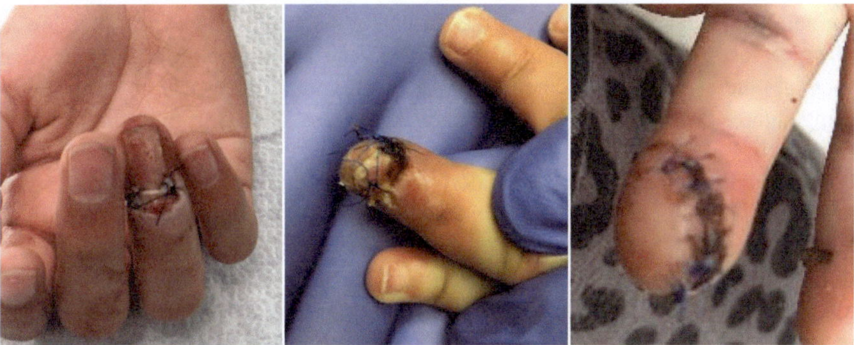

Fig. 7.7 Examples of nonabsorbable sutures in the fingertips. These cause pain and increase trauma to the patient on removal and should be avoided

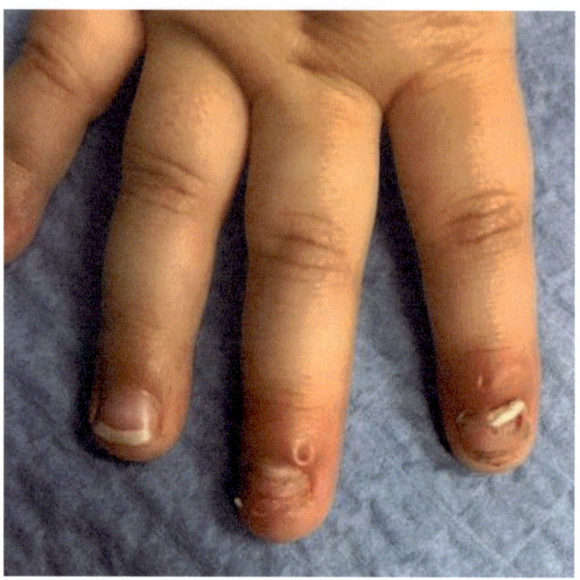

Fig. 7.8 Inflamed tissue from retained suture in the eponychium of the middle and index fingers

plate can then be replaced over the repaired nail bed and inserted below the nail folds to serve as a native dressing. Some providers may opt to create holes in the nail plate to allow drainage or fix the nail plate in place using small sutures in a U or X configuration. We prefer not to suture the nail plate in place as we have seen more problems with the new nail growing under the old nail and infection from retained sutures in the eponychium [19] (Fig. 7.8). Though most providers choose to replace the nail plate to decrease postoperative pain and prevent adhesion between the eponychial fold and nail bed, studies have found no difference in outcomes whether the nail plate is replaced or not following nail bed repair [19, 20]. Other wounds on the fingertip should be closed with 4-0 or 5-0 absorbable suture.

Recent randomized controlled trials, including one in the pediatric population, have demonstrated that 2-octylcyanoacrylate (OCA) produces safe results with good cosmetic and functional outcomes, and may be faster than sutures for nail bed repair [21, 22]. However, care must still be taken to ensure meticulous alignment of the nail bed prior to application of the surgical glue, and the glue must be allowed to dry before replacing the nail plate [4, 21]. The authors caution providers that surgical glue is not a replacement for good, meticulous repair of a fingertip injury using sutures. Some wounds are not amenable to this as seen in this case example (Fig. 7.9).

If the nail plate is avulsed with underlying nail bed attached, small deficits can be repaired with suture and nail plate replacement while larger defects may require nail bed grafting [19]. Small deficits in the nail bed may be able to heal with replacement of the nail plate, which provides support for nail bed healing via secondary intention, whereas larger deficits, such as those greater than 3 by 3 millimeters, may require nail bed grafts [12, 23]. Split thickness nail bed grafts in pediatric patients are often obtained from the injured digit or from the great toe [19]. The graft can be

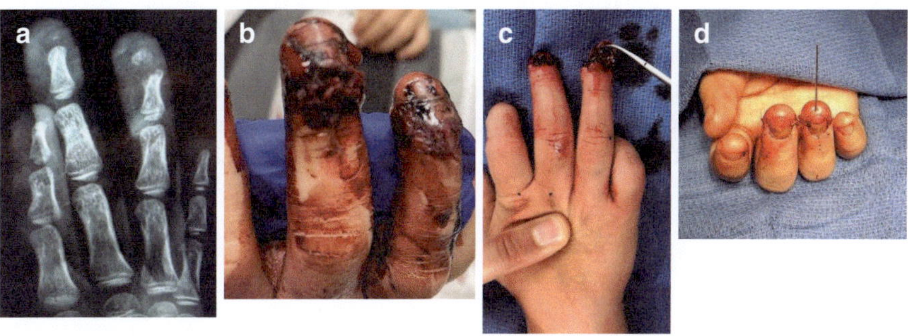

Fig. 7.9 Case example of an 8-year-old male who had their hand crushed by a rock. (**a**) Oblique radiograph of the hand showing distal phalanx fractures of the middle and ring fingers. (**b**) Clinical photograph of the hand after the outside facility and provider attempted to "glue" the wounds closed. (**c**) Clinical photograph obtained in the operating room demonstrating that these were clearly open displaced fractures requiring surgery. (**d**) Clinical photograph in the operating room post-reduction and nail bed repair with 6-0 chromic suture

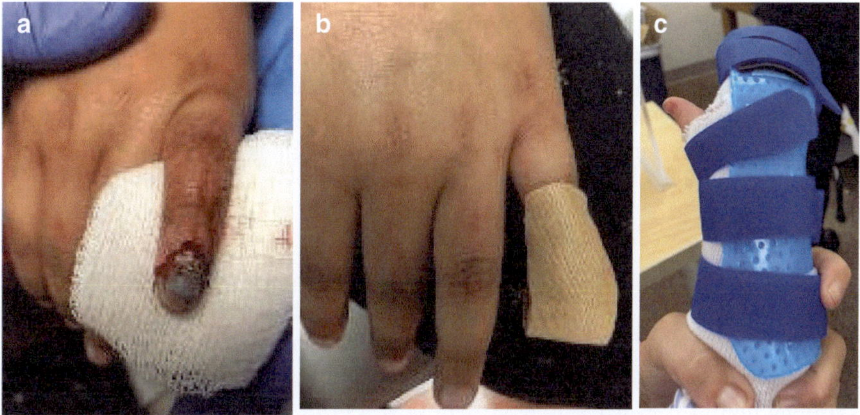

Fig. 7.10 (**a**) Fingertip injury of the small finger with an associated subungual hematoma (**b**) The area was cleaned and repaired in the ED with 6-0 chromic sutures and then a band-aid applied. (**c**) In the office an ulnar gutter orthosis was fabricated to protect the area for 2 weeks. The family can change the band-aid every other day for the first week

sutured into place, and the nail plate replaced for protection and comfort. Full-thickness grafts are avoided due to the potential donor site morbidity, but may be needed for large germinal matrix defects [19].

Post-op Care

After the repair of nail bed injuries, steri-strips may be applied to help hold the nail plate in place. Although it has been described to place sterile gauze, with or without antibiotic ointment, over the repair, the authors have found that this usually causes more pain at the time of removal. Therefore, our recommendations and current practice include the following: placement of a band-aid over the repaired nail complex injury (Fig. 7.10) before then wrapping a sterile gauze over the digit.

This prevents the gauze and xeroform from pulling at the sutures as well as sticking to the injured digit and pulling off any eschar that has formed. We recommend urgent care/emergency care providers place a splint over the area and then follow up with our team within a week, where an orthosis can be fabricated for the child. Another very acceptable approach is to place the young child into a cast for 2 weeks.

Outcomes

Nail bed injuries, when properly managed, can result in excellent outcomes, though patients and families should be counseled regarding potential cosmetic and functional complications, including disrupted or abnormal nail growth and scarring, especially during the 12 months immediately following the injury [11]. The risk of cosmetic or functional problems increases with severity of the injury: simple nail bed lacerations can be expected to heal without substantial sequelae, whereas nail bed injuries with associated open fractures or amputations are more likely to lead to latent nail or fingertip deformities. One study comparing nail bed trephination to surgical repair following nail bed injury in 52 children reported no functional or cosmetic complications in either group [24], while another reported "good to excellent" outcomes in 90% of nail bed injuries [25], suggesting that while the majority of simple nail bed injuries will recover well, complications may still occur in more substantial injuries.

Complications

Nail plate deformity and nail growth issues are common complications following a nail bed injury [4]. Nail ridges, caused by uneven repair of the nail bed, is the most common deformity, and can be treated with removal of nail and excision of the matrix and nail ridge [4]. Split nails may form following disruption of the germinal matrix if scar tissue is present or if a bridging scar between the dorsal nail fold and germinal matrix is present. Excision of the scar with repair of the germinal matrix may alleviate the deformity. Hook nails may form if there is loss of volar support for the nail plate, leading to volar curving of the nail plate (Fig. 7.11). Hook nails are not only cosmetically distressing but may also be a source of pain.

It is also important to counsel patients and their families that nail growth may be stunted or paused for up to 3 weeks after the injury, before accelerating for a period. This disruption in nail plate growth may lead to temporary nail deformities that resolve over time [11]. If the nail plate is replaced following the nail bed repair, patients should be counseled that it will be displaced by the growing nail over the following 1–3 months.

Adequate debridement is important to prevent infection, though patients should be counseled to return to clinic if they experience increasing pain and/or continued drainage from the wound.

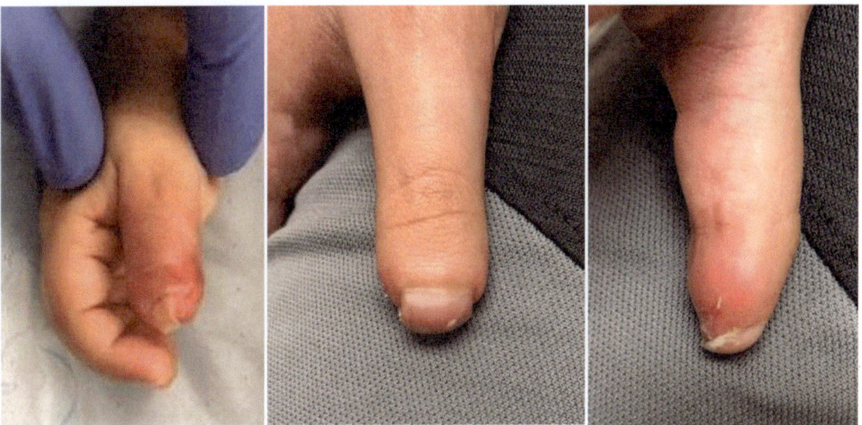

Fig. 7.11 Examples of hook nail deformities

Tuft Fracture (Distal Phalanx)

Epidemiology

Fractures of the nonarticular and nonphyseal portion of the distal phalanx, also known as tuft fractures, are common hand injuries in children as they explore [1]. Distal phalanx fractures have been reported to account for up to half of all hand fractures, and up to 80% of hand fractures in toddlers and preschool aged children [6, 26]. The most commonly involved finger is the long finger, given its distal position and the nature of crush injuries [26]. Tuft fractures can be seen in the setting of nail bed injuries and may be open or closed fractures. It is not uncommon for a child to sustain an accompanying laceration to the pulp or nail bed.

Tuft fractures are often comminuted, but diaphyseal fractures of the distal phalanx may also be oblique or transverse following crush injuries or axial forces [26]. Though tuft fractures may appear benign at presentation, distal phalanx fractures require early diagnosis and intervention to reduce morbidity and complications [6].

Clinical Evaluation

Evaluation of the hand following fingertip injuries should include careful inspection for swelling and ecchymosis which may signify underlying osseous injury. The digit should also be inspected for abrasions or lacerations, the presence of foreign bodies, and associated injuries to the pulp or nail bed. If a laceration is present, the depth of the laceration should be explored, often with the aid of a digital block and/ or conscious sedation (Fig. 7.12). Tuft fractures are commonly associated with nail

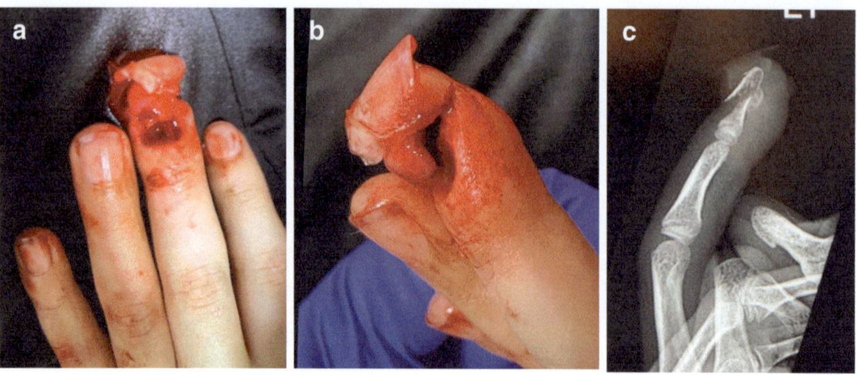

Fig. 7.12 (**a**) and (**b**) Left middle finger crush injury with obvious open wound and deformity. (**c**) Lateral radiograph showing the extent of the bony injury. This was treated with surgical fixation/pinning of the distal phalanx and closure of the soft tissues

bed injuries, and care should be taken to evaluate for an underlying fracture, if a nail bed injury is present [4]. Palpation of the digits may identify point tenderness, and capillary refill can provide information regarding the vascular status of the digit distal to the zone of injury.

Observation of the digital cascade as the patient makes a fist can reliably demonstrate malalignment of the digits, as the tips of the index through small finger should point towards the scaphoid tubercle [26]. Malalignment or divergence of the fingertips may signify an underlying fracture. The integrity of the FDP tendon and extensor mechanism insertions onto the distal phalanx may also be assessed during movement, and the DIP joint may be isolated to further investigate these structures.

PA and lateral views of plain radiographs should be obtained following a fingertip injury to identify any underlying tuft fractures, as well as to rule out fractures involving the physis or articular surface. Oblique views can be helpful to identify minimally displaced fractures or further delineate any joint involvement.

Antibiotics

As with nail bed injuries, recent randomized trials and a meta-analysis have suggested that antibiotics may not be necessary for open fractures of the distal phalanx, though certain exceptions are important to note [15, 16]. The studies do suggest that prompt irrigation and debridement of the open wound is more important for preventing infections. Digital blocks allow for expeditious irrigation and debridement in the emergency room setting. It is thought that antibiotics are not needed for open hand fractures, as compared to open long bone fractures, because of the hand's rich vascular supply, lack of periosteal stripping in most fractures, and ability to promptly debride injuries with digital blocks [16].

Patients may require prophylactic antibiotics if the open fracture is secondary to an animal bite, the wound is grossly contaminated, and/or if the patient presents in a delayed manner (>24 h after injury) [15, 16]. Regardless of antibiotic administration, patients should receive tetanus prophylaxis when indicated following ascertainment of the patient's vaccination status.

Repair (Reduction)

Technique

The management of tuft fractures rarely requires operative treatment as even comminuted fractures are stabilized by the fibrous septae in the distal fingertip [4]. If the fracture is displaced, often in the form of transverse or oblique fractures, closed reduction can often be accomplished. Closed fractures rarely require significant reduction or internal fixation because of the associated soft tissue support and the considerable remodeling potential in children [6]. Young children may require a mitten case, while adolescents can be immobilized in a clamshell or cap splint for several weeks [1]. Though immobilization is only needed for a period of weeks, it is important to recognize that plain radiographs may demonstrate an unchanged appearance for a substantially longer period of time as fibrous union is achieved prior to osseous union, requiring patience from the provider and patient [6, 27]. The combination of young age and relatively short period of immobilization render formal hand therapy an infrequently required intervention after the splint is discontinued [6].

Although closed injuries rarely require surgical intervention, open fractures require irrigation and debridement. The fracture can then be stabilized via suturing of the disrupted skin, and internal fixation is infrequently required [1]. Wound repair, and thus fracture stabilization, is often possible in the emergency department using a digital block, and conscious sedation when necessary, rather than requiring a trip to the operating room [1, 16]. Sutures placed in the hand should be absorbable, such as 5-0 or 6-0 chromic, to avoid the need for subsequent suture removal. The injured digit can then be dressed with nonadherent dressings and immobilized in a splint or cast, much like closed injuries.

In the rare instance when internal fixation of the fracture is required (Fig. 7.13), open versus closed reduction with percutaneous pinning through the distal fingertip using longitudinal k-wires can be employed [27].

Post-op Care

Outcomes

It is important to counsel patients that although immobilization is generally discontinued after 3–4 weeks, full recovery may take months and radiographic findings may lag behind functional outcomes [4, 6, 28].

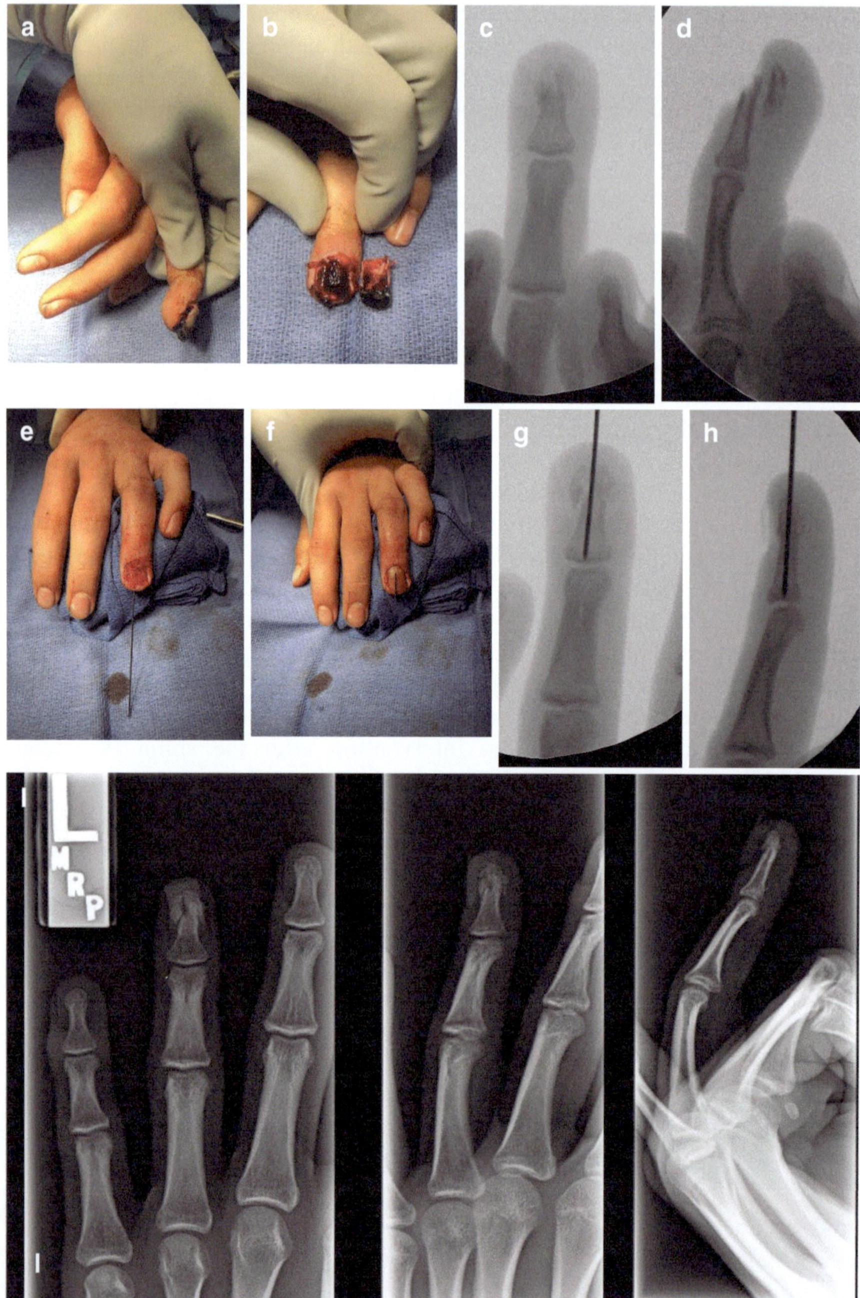

Fig. 7.13 (**a**) and (**b**) A 16-year-old with left ring finger crush injury and displaced distal phalanx fracture. (**c**) and (**d**) Posteroanterior and lateral fluoroscopic images showing translated and displaced distal phalanx fracture of the left ring finger. (**e**) The nail plate was removed, and the fracture reduced by open means and then pinned. (**f**) Nail plate was replaced without sewing it in. (**g**) and (**h**) Posteroanterior and lateral fluoroscopic images showing the fracture reduced and stabilized with a pin. (**i**) Posteroanterior, oblique and lateral radiographs at 2 months post fixation

Complications

Despite their benign appearance, tuft fractures are associated with morbidities and complications that patients should be counseled on. Malunion or nonunion can lead to pain and limited range of motion of the digit, and fractures disrupting the physis can lead to growth arrest in the digit [2, 29]. In the setting of a nonunion, cortical miniscrews or headless screws have been described as hardware options that can be utilized to address the nonunion [27]. Other common complications following tuft fractures include disruption of sensation in the form of numbness or temperature sensitivity [4]. Fine motor movement may also be disrupted. Following open fractures or surgical intervention, infection is a possible sequelae though prophylactic antibiotics are usually not indicated [16].

Amputations

Epidemiology

Although amputations or partial amputations of the fingertip remain relatively rare events overall, males under the age of five have the highest rate of fingertip amputations in the United States, which has been cited at a rate of 18.8/100,000 [12]. Amputations most commonly occur following entrapment or crush injuries in door frames, though other common mechanisms include cutting or piercing injuries and injuries secondary to machinery including lawn mowers, home exercise equipment, and bike chains [30]. It is important for providers to recognize differences in the principles of amputation management between adults and pediatric patients, including the use of composite grafts [30].

Clinical Evaluation

After advanced cardiovascular life support (ACLS) protocols have been followed, evaluation of pediatric patients following amputation injuries involves examination of both the detached fingertip as well as the remainder of the involved digit. It is important to gather a history which includes the mechanism of injury, which may inform contamination concerns, and time since the injury, which informs both treatment and prognosis. If the amputated portion is present, it should be wrapped in gauze dampened with saline, placed into a bag, and placed on ice (Fig. 7.14).

Size, location, and direction of the injury should be noted as these factors may determine treatment modality. Osseous involvement is common, and finger or hand radiographs should be performed. However, it is important to note that ossification of the distal phalanx may not be complete in very young children and careful inspection of the wound and amputated portion should be undertaken to further evaluate for any skeletal involvement [31]. Physicians should also evaluate for gross contamination of the wound but must be careful to avoid further damage which may

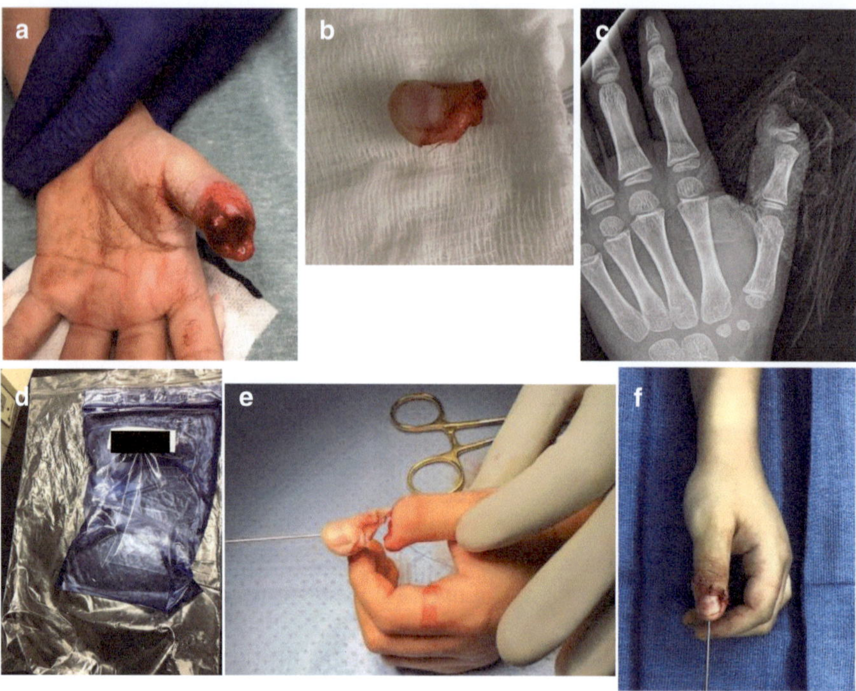

Fig. 7.14 (**a**) A 6-year-old with a thumb amputation after getting it caught on a cord from a blind. (**b**) Clinical photograph of the thumb tip that was brought to the hospital. (**c**) Posteroanterior radiograph showing the thumb injury near the level of the growth plate of the distal phalanx. (**d**) Thumb tip placed into bag and then placed on ice. (**e**) Intraoperative fixation with pin. (**f**) Clinical photograph following repair of the amputated thumb soft tissues, including the tendons

have deleterious effects on replantation efforts. Both gross and two-point sensation and vascular supply of the distal phalanx should be assessed if a partial amputation is present.

The amputation may be described by several classification systems. The Allen classification, first described in 1980, describes the injury using the level of amputation, with those in the first group being considered the most distal without distal phalanx involvement, and those falling into the fourth group involving almost the entire distal phalanx [32]. Though some authors consider the Allen classification the most useful for treatment decisions, others cite the Tamai classification system as more informative because of its basis on the blood supply [4, 33]. Under the Tamai classification, zones I and II involve the fingertip, with zone I being the area distal to the lunula and zone II including the area from the DIP to the nail matrix [33]. Other classifications include the pulp, nail, and bone (PNB) classification, which assigns scores to the involvement of the respective components to generate a three digit score [34], and the Ishikawa classification, which describes only the distal phalanx and is based on the fingernail [12, 35].

Classification system	Classes
Allen	Type I—fingertip pulp only
	Type II—fingertip pulp and nail bed
	Type III—partial loss of distal phalanx
	Type IV—injury proximal to lunula
Tamai	Zone I—distal to lunula
	Zone II—area from DIP to nail matrix
Pulp, nail, and bone	Pulp score:
	0 No injury
	1 Laceration
	2 Crush
	3 Loss—distal transverse
	4 Loss—palmar oblique partial
	5 Loss—dorsal oblique
	6 Loss—lateral
	7 Loss—complete
	Nail score:
	0 No injury
	1 Sterile matrix laceration
	2 Germinal and sterile matrix laceration
	3 Crush
	4 Proximal nail bed dislocation
	5 Loss—distal one third
	6 Loss—distal two thirds
	7 Loss—lateral
	8 Loss—complete
	Bone score:
	0 No injury
	1 Tuft fracture
	2 Comminuted nonarticular fracture
	3 Articular fracture
	4 Displaced basal fracture
	5 Tip exposure
	6 Loss—distal half
	7 Loss—tendon insertions preserved/subtotal
	8 Loss—complete
Ishikawa	Type Ia—beyond distal edge of nail
	Type Ib—between midnail and distal edge of nail
	Type II—between midnail and eponychium
	Type III—midway between eponychium and DIP joint
	Type IV—between type II and DIP joint

Antibiotics

The need for prophylactic antibiotics following fingertip amputations in pediatric patients remains unclear. Rubin et al.'s small randomized controlled trial in adults found no difference in infection rates following fingertip amputation in adult patients; however all patients underwent treatment in the operating room [36]. Altergott found no difference in superficial infection rates following distal fingertip injuries in the setting of adequate wound care, though the small number of amputations and partial amputations included in the study made it difficult to draw conclusions for these specific injuries [15]. Based on these findings, it may be reasonable to hypothesize that prophylactic antibiotics may not be needed for amputations which are not grossly contaminated, the result of animal bites, and present within the first 24 h; however many providers may still provide a short course of prophylactic antibiotics.

Repair (Emergency Department Vs. Operating Room)

Treatment of distal fingertip amputations in pediatric patients depends on a variety of factors ranging from injury severity and location to patient age, and can vary from local wound care to microvascular repair and replantation [11].

Partial amputations consisting of only soft tissue loss without bone exposure can be treated with local wound management in the form of primary closure, healing via secondary intention, or completion of amputation for some partial amputations. Primary closure is preferable in most cases as distal injuries allowed to heal by secondary intention may have associated nail deformities secondary to loss of volar support in up to 25% of cases [4, 32]. Primary closure is generally achieved using 5-0 or 6-0 absorbable sutures to avoid possible traumatic suture removal in young children.

When primary closure is not possible, conservative treatment with healing by secondary intention can reliably be achieved within a few weeks. Studies have also demonstrated acceptable aesthetic and functional results, as well as improved sensation following healing via secondary intention compared to other surgical treatments, though studies have focused on adults [5, 37]. Some authors propose that secondary intention should be reserved for Ishikawa Type I and II amputations without bone or tendon exposure, both of which can inhibit healing via secondary intention [5, 38]. Exposed bone requires tissue coverage to prevent osteomyelitis.

Though less commonly utilized in the pediatric population, skin grafting has been employed to treat partial amputations in the adult population. Well-vascularized wounds are required to achieve successful graft, and the dorsal surface of the finger is generally more amenable to grafting because of its thinness [4]. Grafting, however, fails to provide substantial subcutaneous padding, and cannot be placed directly onto bone or tendon, further limiting its applicability for distal fingertip injuries [4]. Full thickness skin grafts may better prevent wound contracture but require the donor site to be closed primarily. Split thickness grafts can heal by secondary intention and require less preparation of the recipient site but are more prone to contracture.

Flap reconstruction of the fingertip may be required when there is a need for soft tissue coverage and exposed bone is present. Both local and distal flaps are options, and flap selection depends on the digit injured and characteristic of the soft tissue loss (transverse, volar oblique, dorsal oblique).

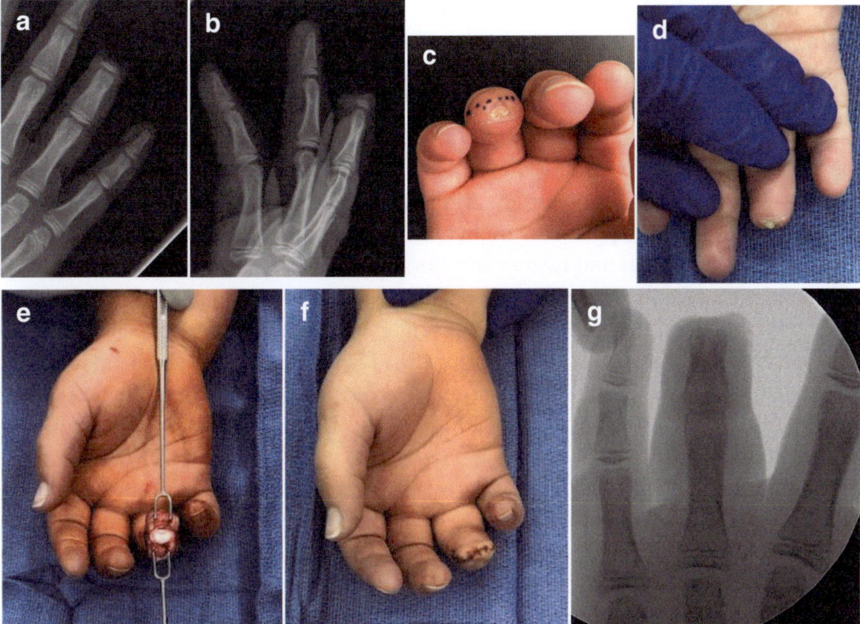

Fig. 7.15 An 8-year-old female with a right ring finger amputation at the distal phalanx growth plate level. (**a**) and (**b**) Posteroanterior and lateral radiographs of the digit. (**c**) and (**d**) The area was allowed to granulate and heal with secondary intention, but nail deformity and pain developed. (**e**) and (**f**) A "fish mouth" approach was used to address the complications, and the remaining distal phalanx was removed. The flexor and extensor tendons were released and not sutured to avoid a quadriga phenomenon. (**g**) Posteroanterior fluoroscopic image showing the distal phalanx has been resected

Lastly, some partial amputations may require completion of the amputation, as replantation distal to the DIP joint is technically difficult due to the small caliber of the vessels. In some cases, completion of amputation may require debridement of the injury to allow for primary closure, including partial removal of distal phalanx to allow for soft tissue coverage (Fig. 7.15). If completion of the amputation is needed, the physician should ensure the nail bed is ablated, hemostasis is achieved, and digital nerves are transected proximally to limit the chance of symptomatic neuroma formation [4].

Partial Amputations

When primary closure is not achievable and allowing the wound to heal via secondary intention is unfeasible, the use of flaps may allow for closure of the wound. Flap options include local flaps, when tissue from the same finger is advanced distally, regional flaps, when tissue from other fingers or the hand is used to temporarily cover the wound, and distant or island flaps, which involve the use of tissue from the groin, contralateral arm, or abdomen [4]. Flap choice is generally dictated by wound size and location, though patient preference and surgeon experience also factor into the decision.

Local flaps, or V-Y flaps, are commonly used to treat distal fingertip amputations that are unable to be primarily closed [17]. Local flap options include the Atasoy flap, the Kutler-Lateral flap, and the Moberg flap. The Atasoy flap has been shown to reliably produce adequate closure in children without dehiscence or infection, be employed on all digits, and restore sensation in up to 67% of patients, though it is commonly associated with hook nail deformities and lower pulp sensitivity [5, 38]. Care must be taken not to detach the vascular supply during flap elevation, which can increase the risk of complications [5]. The Kutler flap, which is typically employed for injuries with volar tissue loss, has a limited distance which it can advance due to the desire to avoid crossing the DIP joint proximally, while the Moberg flap is used for the thumb [4, 33].

Regional flaps, which involve utilizing tissue from the adjacent finger, may be used to cover larger defects but require prolonged immobilization of the finger as well as a second operation to release the flap. The cross finger flap may be used to cover volar tissue loss on any digit, but it is important to consider that skeletally immature children may experience growth restriction from scarring following flap creation [5]. The most common complication following cross finger flaps is dorsal hyperpigmentation, and children have been shown to have little to no postoperative stiffness or numbness following the procedure [5]. Thenar and hypothenar flaps are another option for the treatment of relatively larger pulp defects following amputation injuries. Studies have demonstrated that pediatric thenar flaps, which are generally used for the radial two digits, produce near full range of motion and two-point discrimination of 7 mm [5, 39]. Thenar flaps are generally divided and finalized after 2 weeks, and children rarely experience postoperative stiffness [39]. Island flaps, or sensory flaps, may be used for the thumb and index finger when concern for restoring sensation is heightened; however most children's developing nervous systems render sensory flaps unnecessary as most flaps develop at least protective sensation [5].

Complete Amputations

Treatment considerations for complete amputations should begin immediately, though initial attention should be directed towards patient stability before considering replantation. Once the patient is stabilized and ACLS protocols have been followed, attention can be turned towards management of the injured digit.

Care for both the amputated segment and wound bed is important to consider from the time of injury in order to preserve the chance for replantation. During the initial management of the wound, emergency personnel should avoid applying a clamp directly on an exposed vessel, as the force of the clamp may damage the vessel and make future anastomosis more difficult [30]. Rather, a tourniquet should be applied proximal to the site of injury if bleeding does not resolve with direct pressure. The amputated part should be wrapped in saline moistened gauze and placed into a bag, which can then be placed into a container with ice or an ice-water slush. The amputated portion should not be placed directly on ice, nor on dry ice, both of which can induce frostbite injuries and limit replantation success [30]. Emergency room personnel should avoid exposing both the amputated portion and the injury site, as repeated inspections may lead to further damage. Emergency department management should instead focus on resuscitation of the patient and timely administration of antibiotics (first generation cephalosporin, with the addition of penicillin for contaminated injuries) [30].

If the amputated portion of the finger is available and clean, reconstruction may be attempted either via replantation or composite grafting. Although replantation distal to the DIP joint is technically challenging due to the small size of vessels which must be repaired, complete amputation of the fingertip is one of the best indications for replantation [4]. Replantation should involve the anastomosis of at least one artery, and attempts should be made to reconnect at least one vein [33]. Systematic reviews have demonstrated an 86% success rate with increased odds when at least one vein is repaired [40]. If vessels are unable to be repaired, interventions to prevent venous congestion, such as heparin-soaked gauze and prophylactic periungual incisions, may be used to facilitate venous drainage and improve replantation outcomes [4]. Though earlier replantation is preferred, case reports have demonstrated successful replantation following greater than 24 hours of cold ischemia [41]. Crush injuries have been shown to decrease the chance of a successful replantation [42]. The replanted digit may require a substantial immobilization period following surgery when compared to other treatment options, which should be considered in older adolescents.

Composite Grafting

An alternative to replantation in the pediatric population is composite grafting, or the non-microsurgical reattachment of the amputated soft tissue [43, 44] (Fig. 7.16). Composite grafting is a reliable alternative to replantation, especially in children under the age of 3 years old and when the amputation is distal to the DIP joint [30]. Even if the composite graft is ultimately nonviable, the graft works as a biologic dressing which may help prevent painful dressing changes in small children and can reduce donor site morbidity. Therefore, amputated fingertips may be placed, with appropriate patient counseling, as composite grafts even if there is a high chance of failure [43]. Composite grafting also preserves the ability to undertake other reconstructive options at a later date, regardless of the degree of success of the graft [43]. While performing a composite graft, which is often achieved with small caliber absorbable sutures, it is important to repair the nail bed before replacing the nail plate, which will reduce complications related to nail

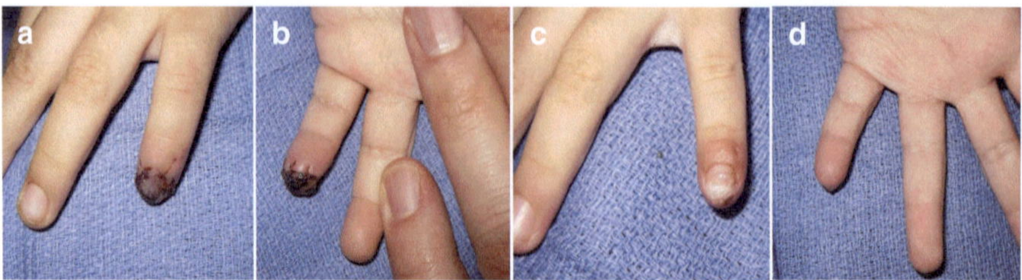

Fig. 7.16 Composite grafting with secondary healing in a 6-year-old patient. (**a**) and (**b**) 1 week out from composite graft sutured on with 6-0 chromic suture to the small finger. (**c**) and (**d**) Clinical photographs 6 weeks later of the same finger

bed injuries such as nail plate deformities [4]. Despite the lack of microvascular repair, composite grafts should still be completed in a timely manner, as previous studies have found increased success rates when composite grafts were placed within 5 h and no survival after 24 h [35, 45]. Other studies also indicate that patients under the age of four have a greater chance of successful composite graft take [45].

When discussing composite grafts with patients and families, it is important to counsel the family that partial necrosis of the graft is common. This necrosis should not be debrided, but rather can continue to serve as a biological dressing under which healing via secondary intention will occur.

Regardless of whether replantation or composite grafting is being attempted, any fracture of the distal tuft should be addressed at the time of treatment. Oftentimes, sutures alone, placed during replantation or composite grafting, provide adequate reduction. If additional fixation is required, K-wires or 18 gauge needles placed through the fingertip may provide internal fixation and can be removed at a later date [4].

Post-op Care

Following surgical treatment of amputation, many physicians have recommended a dressing which includes antibiotic ointment, bismuth-petroleum gauze (xeroform), sterile gauze, and an overlying gauze wrap which should extend to the hand and wrist [5]. However, the authors have stopped this practice in the ED, as experience has taught us that this just leads to more pain when the dressing is removed (Fig. 7.17). Instead, our current practice is to apply a very small amount of antibiotic ointment and then apply a band-aid. This prevents the gauze from sticking to the sutures and being pulled off as an eschar. Following this, gauze may then be placed, and the entire digit and hand splinted or casted as needed. Larger wraps may provide extra padding, while also preventing young children from placing their injured hand in their mouth, which may contaminate the wound [5].

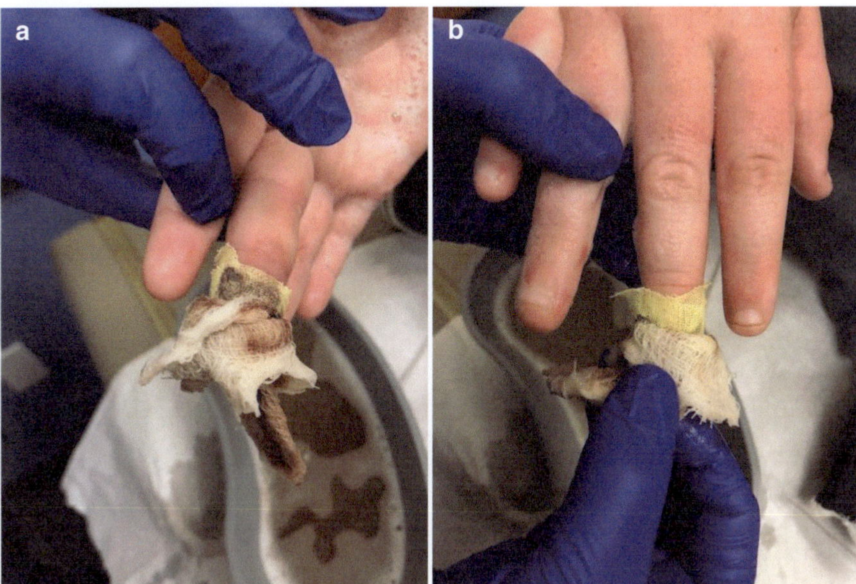

Fig. 7.17 (**a**) and (**b**) A middle finger injury with xeroform and gauze. The combination of blood and sutures creates a "conglomerated mess" that requires extensive time and patience to remove in clinic, while the patient is in tears and pain

Outcomes

Replantation of the distal fingertip has been shown to be successful, with systematic reviews demonstrating success rates in 80–90% of patients [40, 46]. Success rate increased when venous repair was accomplished, as well as in injuries that were cutting in nature [40]. Previous studies have also demonstrated 100% patient and parent satisfaction following replantation [47].

Composite graft outcomes are often divided into three outcomes—no graft take, partial take, and complete take. Recent reviews demonstrate that 50–60% of patients have partial graft take following composite grafting, while 20–30% have no take and 7–16% demonstrated complete take [43–45]. Up to 10% of children may require revision procedures [43, 44]. Long-term functional outcomes are good despite the relatively low rate of complete graft success.

Common complications following treatment of partial and complete amputations include cold intolerance, neuroma formation, nail bed deformity (i.e., hook nail), and fat atrophy [4, 45]. Cold intolerance is typically the result of a radial digital nerve injury and may occur regardless of management technique [4, 45]. Neuromas may form if the digital nerve is not transected, especially in completion of partial amputations, and the nerve is continually exposed to distal fingertip forces [4]. Nail bed deformities are the result of loss of volar support, and can occur following completion of amputation and replantation or composite grafting if the nail bed is not properly repaired [4, 45]. Healing by secondary intention may increase the risk of nail plate deformity in up to 25% of cases [4]. Lastly, the fingertip may also experience fat atrophy following the loss of vascular support, which can lead to cosmetic concerns and occasionally functional problems [4]. Other complications common to lacerations, including infection, may also occur following amputation injuries of the distal fingertip.

FDP Avulsion

Epidemiology

Flexor digitorum profundus (FDP) avulsion fractures, also known as "jersey fingers" are generally the result of forced extension of the digit when the finger is in a flexed position [48]. The resulting force leads to an avulsion of the volar base of the distal phalanx [49]. Flexor tendon injuries are rare injuries in the pediatric population, occurring at a rate of 0.036 per 1000 children with a peak age of 3 years; however most flexor tendon injuries are tendon injuries rather than avulsion fractures [50]. Further, studies have reported avulsion fractures represent only 8% of flexor tendon injuries, while zone II injuries account for over 50% of flexor tendon injuries [51]. The treatment of FDP avulsion fractures in children pose a difficult challenge due to the smaller anatomy and inconsistent postoperative rehabilitation.

Clinical Evaluation

FDP avulsion fractures often present following forced extension of the digit, and patient histories may include injury during a sporting event. The motor exam is critical to the evaluation of potential jersey finger injuries. It may be easy to miss FDP avulsions if careful attention is not paid to distal fingertip movement while asking the patient to make a fist, or if the provider incorrectly assumes lack of motion is secondary to pain or swelling. If flexion at the DIP joint is unclear, the examiner may isolate the DIP joint by stabilizing the PIP joint and instructing the patient to flex their finger. Lack of motion signifies likely FDP tendon disruption or FDP avulsion. If there is concern for flexor tendon injury, plain radiographs of the finger or hand should be used to evaluate for bone fragments avulsed from the distal phalanx.

FDP avulsion fractures are further described by the Packer and Leddy Classification which informs treatment decisions [52]. Type I Packer and Leddy FDP avulsions occur when the avulsed FDP tendon retracts to the palm after the vinculum ruptures. Early repair, within 7 days, is required for type I injuries due to the disruption of vascular supply to the tendon. Type II injuries occur when the FDP tendon retracts to the PIP joint, whereas type III injuries signify the retraction of the FDP tendon to the DIP joint, where the bony fragment is caught in the distal sheath. Type IV injuries are those in which the tendon also separates from the bony fragment displaced from the volar distal phalanx. Antibiotics should be given based on the presence of open fractures as described above.

Repair

Technique

Treatment of FDP avulsion fractures depends on displacement of the tendon and bone fragment. Conservative, nonoperative management may be pursued in minimally displaced avulsion fractures that remain in acceptable alignment, while displaced fractures require surgical fixation.

FDP Avulsions

FDP avulsion fractures requiring surgical management may be repaired with a variety of options including screws, plates, anchor suture, and pullout button sutures [53]. Though a recent cadaveric study found corkscrew anchors had a higher load to failure level than suture anchor and suture buttons for FDP avulsions [54], studies investigating outcomes following zone I and II flexor tendon injuries suggest suture technique is not as important in children as in adults when outcomes are dependent on number of sutures passing the disruption [50, 55]. The authors' preferred technique is to do a suture anchor into the metaphyseal midline of the distal phalanx and use a suture button (Fig. 7.18). We follow a standard protocol for return of motion setup by the Brigham and Women's Hospital [56, 57].

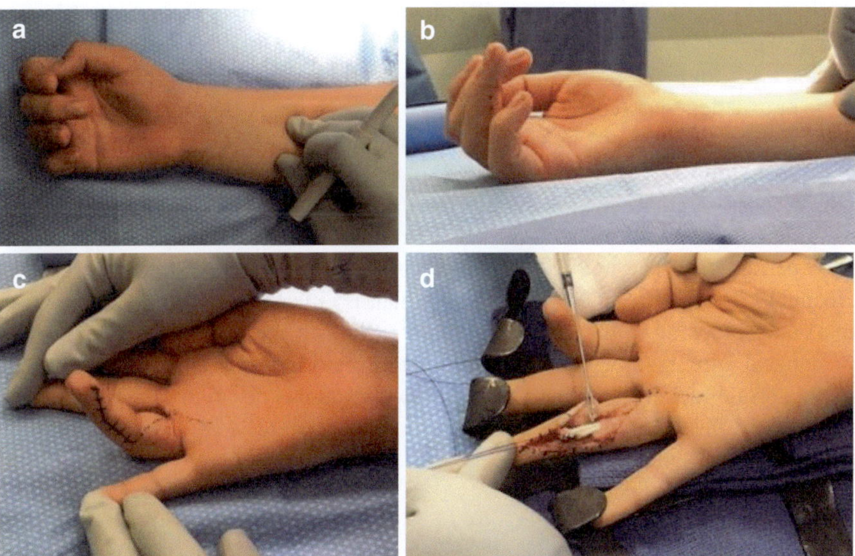

Fig. 7.18 A 15-year-old male with a flexor digitorum profundus (FDP) avulsion after getting the finger caught in another player's jersey. (**a**) and (**b**) Compression forearm test demonstrates FDP rupture as the distal interphalangeal joint does not flex. (**c**) Incision for repair. (**d**) Exposed FDP tendon. (**e**) Fluoroscan image showing placement of the suture anchor in the distal phalanx. (**f**) Position of the digit following repair of the FDP tendon with suture button in place. The button stays in place for 6 weeks

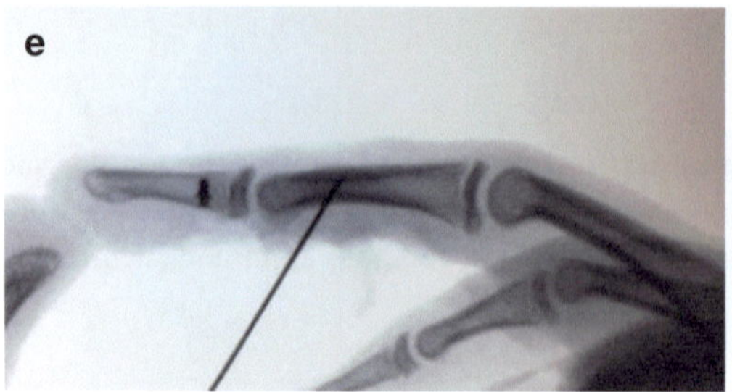
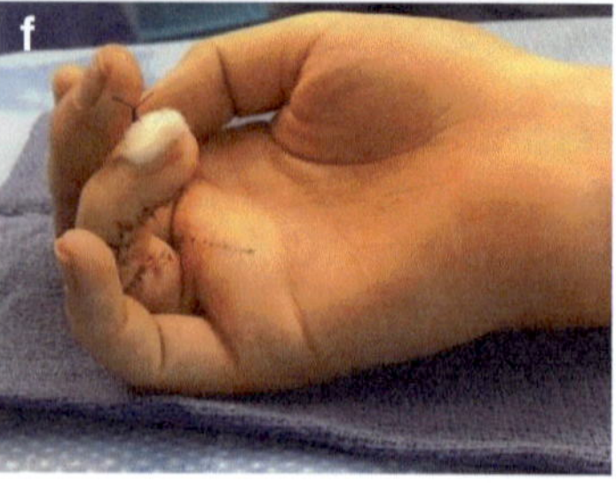

Fig. 7.18 (continued)

Local Vs General Anesthesia

Though the use of wide-awake local anesthesia no tourniquet (WALANT) surgery is increasing and is prevalent in the adult population, its use remains somewhat limited in pediatric patients. Generally, patients under the age of eight receive general anesthesia to avoid patient movement during surgery, whereas patients older than eight commonly receive a combination of local and general anesthetic [51].

Post-op Care

Following surgical fixation of FDP avulsion fractures or repair of flexor tendon injuries, children may either proceed with popular early motion protocols, such as the Kleinert protocol, or be immobilized with a cast or splint. Though the Kleinert protocol has been a popular choice in some studies evaluating the outcome of flexor tendon repair in pediatric patients, splint or cast immobilization has also resulted in good or excellent outcomes [51]. In contrast to adults, early postoperative mobilization may be unnecessary in young children, and may even expose the repair to excessive strain in patients unlikely to adhere to a structured therapy plan [55]. However, any immobilization should not extend beyond 4 weeks, as past studies have demonstrated detrimental effects if immobilization is continued beyond this time period [58]. The authors follow the protocol set by Brigham and Women's Hospital [56, 57]. The first 3 weeks the patient is either in a cast (based on age) or in a dorsal blocking splint. A separate finger splint is placed holding the distal interphalangeal joint in 45 degrees of flexion. At 3 weeks the wrist is brought to neutral in the dorsal blocking splint and the DIP flexion splint is discontinued. By 5 weeks, the splint is discontinued, and therapy is continued weekly. By 8 weeks, resistive exercises are progressed.

Outcomes/Complications

The literature is varied on results of zone I flexor injuries. Published reports demonstrate good outcomes as low as 53% [59], but other studies demonstrate good or excellent results in 80–94% of cases [55, 60]. Fortunately, children tend to fare better than adults, secondary to increased healing ability likely from better blood supply and remodeling of scars and adhesions [55]. In addition, zone I flexor tendon injuries have better total active motion results compared to zone

II injuries. Isolated zone I results were excellent in 87% percent of cases following early ROM and 91% following immobilization [55]. Timely surgical intervention increases the likelihood of a better outcome. We recommend an outer limit for primary fixation of a flexor digitorum profundus rupture of 6 weeks. Even at this period, the surgery is more complicated and takes longer, and we have found that the rehabilitation takes longer and results in some residual flexion contracture. There is no consensus about repair technique [50], but our preference is to try for 2-stranded braided or monofilament core sutures and a suture anchor. Per Elhassan, suture technique is not as important in children as it is in adults [54].

Conclusion

Fingertip injuries, ranging from nail bed lacerations to amputations, are common injuries in the pediatric and adolescent population. Early diagnosis and proper management of these injuries reduces complications and contributes to improved outcomes and quicker recovery. Frontline providers should be comfortable diagnosing and managing fingertip injuries, though some injuries may require referral to a hand surgeon. Many injuries may be treated in the emergency department; however those with greater tissue damage may require operative management. Treatment should focus on restoring function of the fingertip and addressing cosmetic concerns while working to prevent the development of known complications.

References

1. Abzug JM, Mehlman CT. The community orthopaedic surgeon taking trauma call: pediatric phalangeal fracture pearls and pitfalls. J Orthop Trauma. 2017;31(Suppl 6):S1–5.
2. Huelsemann W, Singer G, Mann M, Winkler FJ, Habenicht R. Analysis of sequelae after pediatric phalangeal fractures. Eur J Pediatr Surg. 2016;26(2):164–71.
3. Fassler PR. Fingertip injuries: evaluation and treatment. J Am Acad Orthop Surg. 1996;4(1):84–92.
4. Lee DH, Mignemi ME, Crosby SN. Fingertip injuries: an update on management. J Am Acad Orthop Surg. 2013;21(12):756–66.
5. Loewenstein SN, Adkinson JM. Pediatric fingertip injuries. Hand Clin. 2021;37(1):107–16.
6. Nellans KW, Chung KC. Pediatric hand fractures. Hand Clin. 2013;29(4):569–78.
7. Havenhill TG, Birnie R. Pediatric flexor tendon injuries. Hand Clin. 2005;21(2):253–6.
8. Satku M, Puhaindran ME, Chong AKS. Characteristics of fingertip injuries in children in Singapore. Hand Surg. 2015;20(3):410–4.
9. Yorlets RR, Busa K, Eberlin KR, Raisolsadat MA, Bae DS, Waters PM, et al. Fingertip injuries in children: epidemiology, financial burden, and implications for prevention. Hand (N Y). 2017;12(4):342–7.
10. Patel L. Management of simple nail bed lacerations and subungual hematomas in the emergency department. Pediatr Emerg Care. 2014;30(10):742–5.
11. Gellman H. Fingertip-nail bed injuries in children: current concepts and controversies of treatment. J Craniofac Surg. 2009;20(4):1033–5.
12. Venkatesh A, Khajuria A, Greig A. Management of pediatric distal fingertip injuries: a systematic literature review. Plast Reconstr Surg Glob Open. 2020;8(1):e2595.

13. Van Beek AL, Kassan MA, Adson MH, Dale V. Management of acute fingernail injuries. Hand Clin. 1990;6(1):23–35; discussion 37–38.
14. Simon RR, Wolgin M. Subungual hematoma: association with occult laceration requiring repair. Am J Emerg Med. 1987;5(4):302–4.
15. Altergott C, Garcia FJ, Nager AL. Pediatric fingertip injuries: do prophylactic antibiotics alter infection rates? Pediatr Emerg Care. 2008;24(3):148–52.
16. Metcalfe D, Aquilina AL, Hedley HM. Prophylactic antibiotics in open distal phalanx fractures: systematic review and meta-analysis. J Hand Surg Eur Vol. 2016;41(4):423–30.
17. Martin-Playa P, Foo A. Approach to fingertip injuries. Clin Plast Surg. 2019;46(3):275–83.
18. Cox C, Yao J. Tourniquet usage in upper extremity surgery. J Hand Surg. 2010;35(8):1360–1.
19. Tos P, Titolo P, Chirila NL, Catalano F, Artiaco S. Surgical treatment of acute fingernail injuries. J Orthop Traumatol. 2012;13(2):57–62.
20. O'Shaughnessy M, McCann J, O'Connor TP, Condon KC. Nail re-growth in fingertip injuries. Ir Med J. 1990;83(4):136–7.
21. Langlois J, Thevenin-Lemoine C, Rogier A, Elkaim M, Abelin-Genevois K, Vialle R. The use of 2-octylcyanoacrylate (Dermabond(®)) for the treatment of nail bed injuries in children: results of a prospective series of 30 patients. J Child Orthop. 2010;4(1):61–5.
22. Strauss EJ, Weil WM, Jordan C, Paksima N. A prospective, randomized, controlled trial of 2-octylcyanoacrylate versus suture repair for nail bed injuries. J Hand Surg. 2008;33(2):250–3.
23. Rohard I, Subotic U, Weber DM. Primary reconstruction of fingernail injuries in children with split-thickness nail bed grafts. Eur J Pediatr Surg. 2012;22(4):283–8.
24. Brown RE. Acute nail bed injuries. Hand Clin. 2002;18(4):561–75.
25. Zook EG, Guy RJ, Russell RC. A study of nail bed injuries: causes, treatment, and prognosis. J Hand Surg. 1984;9(2):247–52.
26. Gaston RG, Chadderdon C. Phalangeal fractures: displaced/nondisplaced. Hand Clin. 2012;28(3):395–401, x.
27. Meals C, Meals R. Hand fractures: a review of current treatment strategies. J Hand Surg. 2013;38(5):1021–31; quiz 1031.
28. DaCruz DJ, Slade RJ, Malone W. Fractures of the distal phalanges. J Hand Surg Edinb Scotl. 1988;13(3):350–2.
29. Leclercq C, Korn W. Articular fractures of the fingers in children. Hand Clin. 2000;16(4):523–34, vii.
30. Abzug JM, Kozin SH. Pediatric replantation. J Hand Surg. 2014;39(1):143–5.
31. Stuart HC, Pyle SI, Cornoni J, Reed RB. Onsets, completions and spans of ossification in the 29 bone-growth centers of the hand and wrist. Pediatrics. 1962;29:237–49.
32. Allen MJ. Conservative management of finger tip injuries in adults. Hand. 1980;12(3):257–65.
33. Peterson SL, Peterson EL, Wheatley MJ. Management of fingertip amputations. J Hand Surg. 2014;39(10):2093–101.
34. Evans DM, Bernardis C, Bernadis C. A new classification for fingertip injuries. J Hand Surg Edinb Scotl. 2000;25(1):58–60.
35. Borrelli MR, Dupré S, Mediratta S, Bisquera A, Greig A. Composite grafts for pediatric fingertip amputations: a retrospective case series of 100 patients. Plast Reconstr Surg Glob Open. 2018;6(6):e1843.
36. Rubin G, Orbach H, Rinott M, Wolovelsky A, Rozen N. The use of prophylactic antibiotics in treatment of fingertip amputation: a randomized prospective trial. Am J Emerg Med. 2015 May;33(5):645–7.
37. Lee LP, Lau PY, Chan CW. A simple and efficient treatment for fingertip injuries. J Hand Surg Edinb Scotl. 1995;20(1):63–71.
38. Haehnel O, Plancq M-C, Deroussen F, Salon A, Gouron R, Klein C. Long-term outcomes of Atasoy flap in children with distal finger trauma. J Hand Surg. 2019;44(12):1097.e1–6.
39. Barr JS, Chu MW, Thanik V, Sharma S. Pediatric thenar flaps: a modified design, case series and review of the literature. J Pediatr Surg. 2014;49(9):1433–8.
40. Sebastin SJ, Chung KC. A systematic review of the outcomes of replantation of distal digital amputation. Plast Reconstr Surg. 2011;128(3):723–37.

41. Lin C-H, Aydyn N, Lin Y-T, Hsu C-T, Lin C-H, Yeh J-T. Hand and finger replantation after protracted ischemia (more than 24 hours). Ann Plast Surg. 2010;64(3):286–90.
42. Li J, Guo Z, Zhu Q, Lei W, Han Y, Li M, et al. Fingertip replantation: determinants of survival. Plast Reconstr Surg. 2008;122(3):833–9.
43. Eberlin KR, Busa K, Bae DS, Waters PM, Labow BI, Taghinia AH. Composite grafting for pediatric fingertip injuries. Hand (N Y). 2015;10(1):28–33.
44. Murphy AD, Keating CP, Penington A, McCombe D, Coombs CJ. Paediatric fingertip composite grafts: do they all go black? J Plast Reconstr Aesthet Surg. 2017;70(2):173–7.
45. Butler DP, Murugesan L, Ruston J, Woollard AC, Jemec B. The outcomes of digital tip amputation replacement as a composite graft in a paediatric population. J Hand Surg Eur Vol. 2016;41(2):164–70.
46. Berlin NL, Tuggle CT, Thomson JG, Au A. Digit replantation in children: a nationwide analysis of outcomes and trends of 455 pediatric patients. Hand (N Y). 2014;9(2):244–52.
47. Cheng GL, Pan DD, Zhang NP, Fang GR. Digital replantation in children: a long-term follow-up study. J Hand Surg. 1998;23(4):635–46.
48. Halát G, Negrin L, Erhart J, Ristl R, Hajdu S, Platzer P. Treatment options and outcome after bony avulsion of the flexor digitorum profundus tendon: a review of 29 cases. Arch Orthop Trauma Surg. 2017;137(2):285–92.
49. Henry SL, Katz MA, Green DP. Type IV FDP avulsion: lessons learned clinically and through review of the literature. Hand (N Y). 2009 Dec;4(4):357–61.
50. Nietosvaara Y, Lindfors NC, Palmu S, Rautakorpi S, Ristaniemi N. Flexor tendon injuries in pediatric patients. J Hand Surg. 2007;32(10):1549–57.
51. Huynh MNQ, Ghumman A, Agarwal A, Malic C. Outcomes after flexor tendon injuries in the pediatric population: a 10-year retrospective review. Hand (N Y). 2022;17:278.
52. Leddy JP, Packer JW. Avulsion of the profundus tendon insertion in athletes. J Hand Surg. 1977;2(1):66–9.
53. Fa-Binefa M, Pérez-López G, Almenara M, Lamas C. Hook plate as a treatment for flexor Digitorum Profundus avulsion types II and III. Hand (N Y). 2021;16(4):551–6.
54. Putnam JG, Adamany D. Biomechanical comparison of flexor Digitorum Profundus avulsion repair. J Wrist Surg. 2019;8(4):312–6.
55. Elhassan B, Moran SL, Bravo C, Amadio P. Factors that influence the outcome of zone I and zone II flexor tendon repairs in children. J Hand Surg. 2006;31(10):1661–6.
56. Brigham and Women's Hospital. Flexor tendon repair protocol zone 1 [internet]. Brigham and Women's Hospital, Department of Rehabilitation Services; 2007. https://www.brighamandwomens.org/assets/BWH/patients-and-families/rehabilitation-services/pdfs/hand-flexor-tendon-repair-pt-protocol-zone-1-bwh.pdf
57. Brigham and Women's Hospital. Flexor tendon repair protocol zone 2–5 [internet]. Brigham and Women's Hospital, Department of Rehabilitation Services; 2007. https://www.brighamandwomens.org/assets/BWH/patients-and-families/rehabilitation-services/pdfs/hand-flexor-tendon-repair-pt-protocol-zone-2-5-bwh.pdf
58. O'Connell SJ, Moore MM, Strickland JW, Frazier GT, Dell PC. Results of zone I and zone II flexor tendon repairs in children. J Hand Surg. 1994;19(1):48–52.
59. Sikora S, Lai M, Arneja JS. Pediatric flexor tendon injuries: a 10-year outcome analysis. Can J Plast Surg. 2013;21(3):181–5.
60. Grobbelaar AO, Hudson DA. Flexor tendon injuries in children. J Hand Surg Edinb Scotl. 1994;19(6):696–8.

Pediatric Thumb Fractures

Theresa O. Wyrick and Sean Morell

Background

Ossification

The thumb is different from the other digits in several ways including ossification timing and pattern, osseous anatomy, and soft tissue anatomy. In the metacarpals of the digits, there are secondary ossification centers located at the distal ends of the index, long, ring, and small fingers but the secondary ossification center for the thumb metacarpal is located proximally. Secondary ossification of the epiphyses within the hand occurs in a predetermined order. The majority of proximal phalangeal epiphyses are apparent on plain radiographs between 10 and 24 months. The process occurs in an anterograde fashion with more proximal structures ossifying prior to distal structures. The secondary ossification centers in the phalanges appear in girls around 10–15 months of age and in boys around 15–24 months of age. The closure of these secondary ossification centers occurs in girls around 14 years of age and 16 years of age in boys. The secondary ossification centers in the metacarpals of the fingers are seen first around 12–17 months of age in girls and 18–27 months in boys. Uniquely, the proximal thumb metacarpal secondary ossification center appears 6–12 months after the secondary ossification centers in the fingers. The closure of the secondary ossification centers in the metacarpals occurs between 14 and 16 years of age in girls and boys [1, 2]. The epiphysis of the thumb distal phalanx first appears in boys at 1.51 years of age and in girls at 0.99 years of age. The proximally located thumb metacarpal epiphysis first appears in boys at 2.59 years of age and in girls at 1.5 years of age. Lastly, the thumb proximal phalanx epiphysis first appears in boys at 3 years of age and in girls at 1.71 years of age [1, 2]. The

T. O. Wyrick (✉) · S. Morell
Orthopaedic Surgery, University of Arkansas for Medical Sciences, Arkansas Children's Hospital, Little Rock, AR, USA
e-mail: towyrick@uams.edu; smorell@uams.edu

J. M. Abzug et al. (eds.), *Pediatric and Adult Hand Fractures*,
https://doi.org/10.1007/978-3-031-32072-9_8

thumb is unique in that the metacarpal epiphysis does not ossify until approximately 2 years of age when all other fingers show signs of ossification up to 1 year earlier. The thumb metacarpal is unique in that pseudoepiphyses are common radiographic findings in young children. These "false physes" are located at the metacarpal head and neck and can be mistaken for fractures. The pseudoepiphysis does not provide any appreciable longitudinal growth within the thumb metacarpal [3]. A working knowledge of all of these ossification patterns is imperative when assessing skeletally immature patients for thumb and digital fractures [1–3].

Anatomy

The soft tissue anatomy of the pediatric thumb is not different from that seen in adults. An intimate knowledge of anatomy within the skeletally immature hand is imperative to appropriate diagnosis along with treatment of the complex fractures. One must understand both the ligamentous and tendinous insertions in relation to the physes to fully treat these fractures. Tendon insertions vary between flexor tendons and extensor tendons. The flexor pollicis longus inserts along the metaphysis of the distal phalanx while the extensor pollicis longus inserts on the dorsal epiphysis. The extensor pollicis brevis inserts along the dorsal epiphysis of the proximal phalanx. The abductor pollicis longus has a broad insertion that spans the proximal portion of the metacarpal. The adductor has a broad insertion along the proximal and ulnar portion of the proximal phalanx. The collateral ligaments located on the radial and ulnar aspects of the metacarpophalangeal joint originate from the metacarpal head and insert on the epiphysis of the proximal phalanx. The epiphyseal insertion site can lead to either Salter-Harris 3 type injuries of the proximal phalanx with an associated collateral ligament injury or less commonly a purely ligamentous injury [4, 5].

Due to laxity in the pediatric volar plate at the thumb metacarpophalangeal joint seen in young children, this joint can dislocate dorsally with trauma and is the most common metacarpophalangeal joint dislocation seen in children [6]. In skeletally immature patients with a significant traumatic radial or ulnar force across the collateral ligaments at the metacarpophalangeal joint, an epiphyseal fracture can be seen. The physis at the thumb proximal phalanx generally closes centrally first leaving adolescents particularly vulnerable to sustaining this type of "bony skier's thumb" which is typically a Salter-Harris III fracture pattern [4, 5].

Incidence

Chew et al. found that in hand fractures, the thumb proximal phalanx is the most commonly fractured bone in the thumb representing 16% of all hand fractures. Fractures of the thumb distal phalanx and metacarpal are seen much less frequently representing 3% and 2% respectively [7]. The most common mechanisms of injury resulting in pediatric thumb fractures are similar to the causes of other pediatric hand trauma including crushing door-related injuries at home, sports-related injuries, lawnmower injuries, All-Terrain Vehicles, and, rarely, nonaccidental trauma. Fireworks injuries are particularly damaging to the thumb and first webspace as the adolescent patient is injured typically while holding the firework in their hand while it is ignited and discharged. This creates a blast injury to the thumb and first webspace which is seen in 84% of the fireworks injuries affecting the hand with soft tissue damage, fractures, and joint dislocations commonly seen [8].

Specific Injury Patterns

Carpometacarpal Fracture Dislocations

Pediatric thumb carpometacarpal fractures and dislocations are uncommon injuries. These injuries are usually associated with higher energy mechanisms in adolescents who are skeletally mature. These can be correlated with other basilar thumb fractures (Bennett, Rolando, etc.). The ligamentous insertion at the base of the thumb is mostly epiphyseal which can lead to a Salter-Harris III pattern at the volar ulnar corner consistent with a Bennett type fracture. The goal of treatment in these injuries is re-establishing the position of the thumb metacarpal on the trapezium with reduction to facilitate healing. This is usually done under closed means and carpometacarpal pinning. Pins are kept in place for four to six weeks while the fracture and surrounding ligamentous restraints heal. There have been reports of successful nonoperative treatment for these injuries if a stable reduction can be achieved and maintained in a cast with close weekly follow-up to monitor for loss of alignment and operative intervention if needed [9, 10].

Thumb Metacarpal Base Fractures

Metacarpal base fractures are very common and usually associated with higher energy mechanisms seen in adolescents but can also be seen in younger children. Most of these fractures involve the physis with one study showing a 72% incidence of SH-2 fracture at the base of the thumb [11].

The general consensus is that metacarpal angulation <30 degrees is necessary for successful closed treatment of thumb metacarpal base fractures. Pediatric patients have the benefit of tremendous remodeling potential and usually have no significant long-term problems with closed treatment of these injuries. The large amount of mobility within the thumb ray and the carpometacarpal joint along with the remodeling potential allow for very successful closed treatment. Patients less than ten years of age have a greater remodeling potential and can remodel even severe angulation with minimal long-term deficits. Physeal arrest secondary to trauma is very rare due to the resilience of metacarpal and phalangeal physes.

If surgery is indicated, closed reduction and percutaneous pinning is usually successful. In most cases, two retrograde Kirschner wires are placed through the metacarpal and across the carpometacarpal joint to prevent displacement of the fracture and subluxation of the joint [12].

Thumb Metacarpal Shaft and Neck Fractures

Thumb metacarpal shaft fractures and neck fractures do not have the same remodeling potential as base fractures. One concern with metacarpal shaft fractures is the rotational deformity that can occur with the injury pattern and lead to long-term functional issues. Assessment of rotation and overall clinical alignment is a key component in treating these fractures. It is helpful to inspect the contralateral side. Metacarpal neck fractures should be treated in instances of significant angular deformity due to the inability of that area to remodel. It is also important to keep in mind the existence of the metacarpal pseudoepiphysis which can lead to misdiagnosis as a fracture.

It is the author's preference to treat the majority of these minimally displaced metacarpal shaft fractures with thumb spica casting for four weeks. If surgery is required, successful closed reduction and percutaneous pinning is the preferred method. If open reduction is required, internal fixation with a small 1.5 mm or 2.0 mm plate and screws can be used. Postoperative joint stiffness is rarely encountered in the pediatric patient and therefore early mobilization is not a priority in most cases.

In the case of metacarpal neck fractures, there is minimal tolerance for angulation due to the lack of a physis in the area. This area has minimal remodeling potential and angular deformity is common and should be addressed. Closed reduction and percutaneous pinning is usually adequate in treating these patterns with minimal concern for postoperative stiffness [13].

Proximal Phalanx Fractures

Proximal phalanx fractures are treated very differently based on the location of the fracture within the phalanx. The pediatric equivalent of a "skier's thumb" or "game keeper's thumb" is usually associated with an avulsion fracture from the insertion on the ulnar epiphysis of the proximal phalanx. Salter-Harris II fracture patterns in the thumb proximal phalanx are quite common and often angulated. Fractures of the diaphysis are uncommon but should be treated in the same fashion as the fingers. Fractures of the phalangeal neck have the same risk of angular deformity, tendon dysfunction, and avascular necrosis seen in similar fractures seen in the fingers.

Truly ligamentous disruptions at the metacarpophalangeal joint are rare in skeletally immature patients. In younger pediatric patients, a Salter-Harris I or II fracture of the proximal phalanx is often seen in this setting. In preadolescents and adolescents, ulnar collateral ligament injuries most commonly result in a Salter-Harris III fracture at the base of the proximal phalanx. The central portion of the proximal phalanx physis closes first leaving the peripheral portion of the physis still prone to fracture creating this injury pattern. These injuries should be treated with a high amount of suspicion for the need for surgical intervention. Minimally displaced fractures can be treated in a closed fashion with immobilization in a thumb spica cast for 4 weeks with good results. Displacement >1–2 mm or fractures that involve a large portion of the joint surface should be treated with open reduction if needed and fixation to ensure congruent joint surface alignment and restore integrity of the ulnar collateral ligament [4].

In some cases, these can be adequately reduced by closed means and fixed using two percutaneously placed small k wires in a divergent fashion. In the case of a displaced fracture, the author's preferred treatment is a small curvilinear incision along the dorsal ulnar portion of the metacarpophalangeal joint. Careful dissection should be conducted down to the extensor hood to avoid damage to the superficial radial sensory nerve branches which can be seen immediately subcutaneous to the incision. Following this, the extensor hood/aponeurosis should be incised dorsally at the ulnar border of the EPL tendon. The hood can then be reflected to identify the joint capsule and fracture. Care should be taken to maintain healthy soft tissue layers for future repair. As with the adult UCL avulsion, the fragment can be found superficially with the adductor aponeurosis interposed. Fixation varies on the skeletal maturity of the child and the size of the bony fragment. Usually, two small Kirschner wires are utilized to hold the fracture in place. An additional pin across the metacarpophalangeal joint for rigid stability in the cast may be used. Soft tissue layers are then closed using absorbable suture and pins are removed at four weeks.

The Salter-Harris II fracture of the thumb proximal phalanx is a commonly seen injury pattern in children. Often these fractures are angulated and require a closed reduction under digital block or other method of anesthesia. The majority of these fractures are stable in a cast after closed reduction and do not require pin fixation. However, as with other displaced phalangeal fractures, close follow-up with repeat radiographs one week after the reduction is recommended to evaluate for redisplacement. Due to the physeal location of these fractures, there is significant potential for remodeling of deformity in skeletally immature patients with years of growth remaining.

Diaphyseal phalangeal fractures of the thumb should be treated in the same fashion as in the other digits. Malrotation and significant shortening and angulation should be addressed to prevent dysfunction. Closed reduction and percutaneous fixation is the author's preferred method of treatment with subsequent pin removal after four weeks.

Phalangeal neck fractures should be treated with diligence. Significant angulation can lead to joint stiffness and deformity. These should be promptly treated to prevent malunion as there is less remodeling potential in this area of the phalanx. The author's preferred treatment is closed reduction and percutaneous pinning. A variety of pin configurations can work in this setting including placing a pin through the distal phalanx and across the thumb interphalangeal joint when needed for very distal fragments. Pins are left outside of the skin and the patient is immobilized for four weeks with pins removed in clinic at that time. Open reduction of these fractures is rarely necessary and if undertaken, dissection around the origin of the collateral ligaments proximally is not recommended so as to avoid the complication of avascular necrosis of the phalangeal head as can be seen in digital phalanx fractures [14, 15].

Distal Phalanx Fractures

Distal phalanx fracture mechanism of injury, fracture patterns, and treatment are very similar to those seen in the fingers. This injury is often seen in younger patients and is the result of a crush injury from doors and drawers. There is often an associated nail bed injury or laceration of the nail fold or pulp of the finger. Physeal fractures can be seen with associated nail bed injury and interposed nail matrix consistent with a Seymour lesion and must be addressed in the same way as in the fingers with extraction of the interposed nail matrix, fracture reduction, and nail bed repair +/− pinning of the distal phalanx fracture depending on stability of the reduction [16].

Conclusion

An understanding of the ossification patterns and timing in the thumb, soft tissue anatomy, and injury patterns is critical in evaluating traumatic injuries of the thumb. There are some similarities in evaluating and treating thumb fractures to those seen in the other digits. There are unique injury patterns in the thumb that require special attention including the Salter-Harris III fracture of the thumb proximal phalanx with associated incompetence of the ulnar collateral ligament. Most pediatric thumb fractures can be successfully treated either by cast immobilization alone, closed reduction and casting or closed reduction with percutaneous stabilization using temporary Kirschner wires, and good outcomes are achieved with few long-term complications seen.

References

1. Stuart HC, Pyle SI, Cornoni J, et al. Onsets, completions, and spans of ossification in the 29 bone-growth centers of the hand and wrist. Pediatrics. 1962;29:237–49.
2. Garn SM, Rohmann CG, Silverman FM. Radiographic standards for postnatal ossification and tooth calcification. Med Radiogr Photogr. 1967;43:41–66.
3. Limb D, Loughenbury PR. The prevalence of pseudoepiphyses in the metacarpals of the growing hand. J Hand Surg Eur Vol. 2012;37(7):678–81.
4. Kozin SH. Fractures and dislocations along the pediatric thumb ray. Hand Clin. 2006;22(1):19–29.
5. White GM. Ligamentous avulsion of the ulnar collateral ligament of the thumb of a child. J Hand Surg Am. 1986;11(5):669–72.
6. Kozin SH, Waters PM. Fractures and dislocations of the hand and carpus in children. In: Beaty JH, Kasser JR, editors. Rockwood and Wilkins' fractures in children. 6th ed. Philadelphia: Lippincott Williams & Wilkins; 2006. p. 257–336.
7. Chew EM, Chong AK. Hand fractures in children: epidemiology and misdiagnosis in a tertiary referral hospital. J Hand Surg Am. 2012;37(8):1684–8.
8. Sandvall BK, Keys KA, Friedrich JB. Severe hand injuries from fireworks: injury patterns, outcomes, and fireworks types. J Hand Surg Am. 2017;42(5):385.e1–8.
9. Nusem I, Lklec F, Wientroub S, Ezra E. Isolated dislocation of the thumb carpometacarpal joint in a child. J Pediatr Orthop B. 2001;10(2):158–60.

10. Soldado F, Mascarenhas V, Rr J. Paediatric trapeziometacarpal dislocation: a case report. J Hand Surg Eur Vol. 2016;41(9):999–1000.
11. Jehanno P, Iselin F, Frajman J, Pennecot G, Glicenstein J. Fractures of the base of the first metacarpal in children: role of k-wire stabilization. Ann Chir Main. 1999;18(3):184–90.
12. Lindley SG, Rulewicz G. Hand fractures and dislocations in the developing skeleton. Hand Clin. 2006;22(3):253–68.
13. Wood V. Fractures of the hand in children. Orthop Clin North Am. 1976;7(3):527–42.
14. Karl JW, White NJ, Strauch RJ. Percutaneous reduction and fixation of displaced phalangeal neck fractures in children. J Pediatr Orthop. 2012;32(2):156–61.
15. Waters PM, Taylor BA, Kuo AY. Percutaneous reduction of incipient malunion of phalangeal neck fractures in children. J Hand Surg Am. 2004;29(4):707–11.
16. Lankachandra M, Wells CR, Cheng CJ, Hutchison RL. Complications of distal phalanx fractures in children. J Hand Surg Am. 2017;42(7):574.e1–6.

Pediatric Hand Fractures: Rehabilitation and Orthoses

9

Ritu Goel, Catherine C. May, and Joshua M. Abzug

Introduction

The hand is the most common place of injury in the pediatric and adolescent population [1–3]. It is used for exploration in younger children and for sports activities as children grow into adolescence, making the hand and fingers more susceptible to injury [2].

Pediatric patients are typically casted following an injury and/or surgery to the hand due to poor compliance and decreased likelihood of developing postoperative stiffness and adhesions [2, 3]. However, understanding the risks and benefits of cast versus orthosis use is to the treating physician and therapists' advantage. A variability in compliance exists that may not correspond with the child's age; therefore an individualized treatment plan should be considered with this population when determining the most appropriate modality for treating the injury and the child [4].

While casting, the typical preference for fracture stabilization, ensures compliance and immobilization, potential complications may include odor, skin maceration, and/or skin irritation [5]. Thermoplastic orthoses, however, provide improved comfort, satisfaction, and permit removal for hygiene, yet they are also associated with potential for skin breakdown, pressure sores, and improper fit [5]. Consideration of the child's age, activity level, and reason for use when ordering and fabricating orthoses is beneficial for healing and compliance. This chapter aims to outline and discuss the orthoses and therapy associated with various common pediatric hand fractures.

Disclaimer: The views expressed in the submitted article are our own and not an official position of the institution.

R. Goel · C. C. May · J. M. Abzug (✉)
Department of Orthopedic Surgery, University of Maryland School of Medicine, Baltimore, MD, USA
e-mail: ritu.goel@som.umaryland.edu; catherine.may@som.umaryland.edu; jabzug@som.umaryland.edu

Therapy Considerations

Formal therapy is typically not indicated for pediatric patients following a hand fracture, as the patients typically regain their motion with activity, such as play and sports, following cast removal. When a child has a finger injury, therapists will often use play activities to engage the patient. Treatment through play activity will encourage digit use without the child's focus on the injury, but rather on the activity. Oftentimes, pediatric and adult patients will avoid use of their injured digit and perform fine motor tasks with other fingers. In therapy, treatment will encourage injured digit use rather than avoidance. Activities incorporated in treatment of a finger or hand injury include fine motor coordination tasks, such as writing and coloring, as well as picking up small objects, such as pegs and marbles. These activities may be graded by incorporating various sized tweezers to pick up objects, placing small objects in mouthed containers, or cutting paper with scissors if age appropriate. It is beneficial to incorporate activities that can easily be replicated in the home environment for the patient to continue progressing with their family's assistance when not in therapy. Additionally, video games and computer use are useful modalities to encourage active hand use for sustaining holding and pushing buttons.

Pediatric hand injuries occasionally cause decreased sensation and/or hypersensitivity to touch following cast removal, which may necessitate desensitization and/or sensory re-education to the involved area. Desensitization involves tactile stimulation with various objects from smooth and soft to textured and rough. Children with hypersensitivity are often hesitant to do any type of tactile stimulation to the affected area. Allowing the child to perform their own desensitization with sensory sticks (Fig. 9.1) may increase their comfort. Furthermore, desensitization and sensory re-education may be done as an activity with sensory bins filled with rice, corn, Waterbeads™, or sand (Fig. 9.2), where the child may not be aware of the tactile stimulation when engaged in an activity. The patient may either simply play in the sensory bins with the involved hand or objects may be hidden in the filling for the patient to find and remove. Waterbeads™ are colorful, light, water-based beads that make a fun sensory modality most children are comfortable attempting to play with. Pegs, large marbles, and plastic coins can all be placed in the sensory bin with Waterbeads™ for the patient to find, encouraging both active hand use and desensitization. Kinetics Sand™ and Play-Doh™ are desensitization modalities children enjoy playing with at the table to create different shapes with their affected hand or using molds. Sand has a rougher texture than water; therefore Waterbeads™ should be used prior to Kinetics Sand™ when developing a sensory re-education program.

Decreased functional use can lead to atrophy and a decrease in strength of the affected extremity. Limitations in grip and pinch strength often result following a hand injury; however in the pediatric population, children often regain their strength without focused hand strengthening. When developing a strengthening program, the child's age, baseline strength and activity level, and functional limitations should be considered. At a young toddler age, strengthening is not required as the child will initiate weight bearing for balance and stability independently, using pain as their

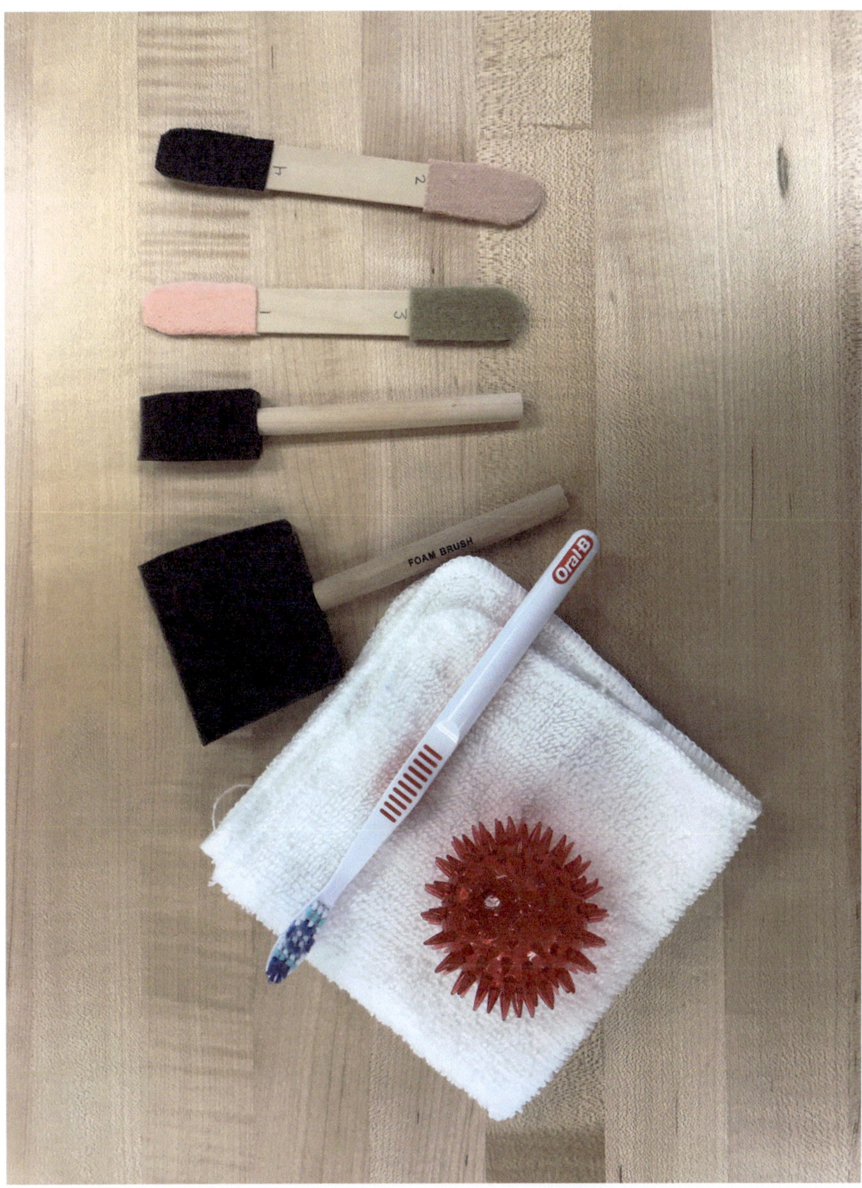

Fig. 9.1 Desensitization tools, sensory sticks (Courtesy of Ritu Goel, MS, OTR/L)

guide. Young children may regain strength and endurance of their dominant hand through writing, coloring, and other play activities. Adolescent patients returning to a competitive sport may require formal therapy to regain their strength, endurance, and/or coordination skills to prevent a reinjury upon return. In these situations, therapy will focus on fine motor coordination skills as well as regaining grip and pinch

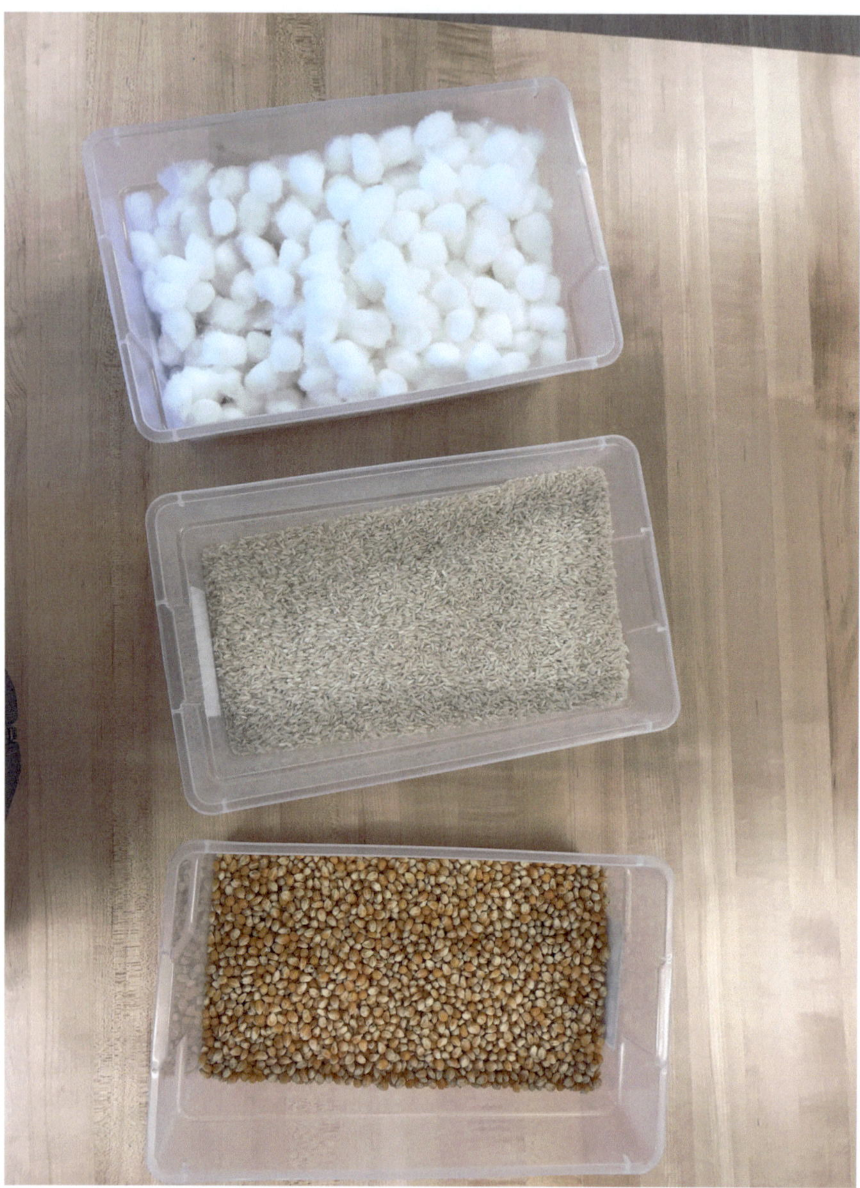

Fig. 9.2 Sensory bins (Courtesy of Ritu Goel, MS, OTR/L)

strength, weight bearing, and wrist strengthening in all planes. For example, a patient returning to tennis will require grip strengthening to sustain holding of the racket and to absorb impact of the ball upon contact. Grip and pinch strengthening may consist of theraputty, various hand grippers, and resistive clothespins. Ball toss with weighted balls and upper extremity strengthening with theraband and weighted cable units may be used to prepare the patient for return to the sport as well as assist with sustaining grip with push and pull motions. The patient may also be asked to bring their racket to therapy for practice in bouncing a tennis ball for endurance and coordination skills. As the patient is returning to sport activity, the preference is to play without adaptive equipment or durable medical equipment use; however, if taping, buddy loops, or bracing is needed, it would be assessed and discussed with the referring physician during this phase of treatment.

Specific Fractures

Metacarpal Fractures

Metacarpal fractures are more prevalent in the adolescent age group and typically present more in boys than girls [6]. Eighty percent of metacarpal fractures involve the fifth metacarpal neck [4], occurring from an axial load and rotation at a flexed metacarpophalangeal (MCP) joint, as in a punch or fall [6]. Initial treatment typically involves closed reduction with a mitten cast for 3 weeks, positioning the MCP joint in full extension [7]. In a study by Lee et al. (2020), fifth metacarpal neck fractures with less than 50 degrees of angulation were treated with closed treatment without fracture reduction, resulting in adequate results [6]. Benefits of treatment without closed reduction in the pediatric population include decreased analgesia and less radiographs, thus decreasing exposure to radiation and cost [6].

Davidson et al. (2016) found comparable results between a forearm-based plaster splint compared to a hand-based thermoplast orthosis (Fig. 9.3) for nonoperative treatment of pediatric (<16 years of age) fifth MCP fractures in a group of 36 patients [8]. Results showed comparable results at 12-week follow-up in both groups, specifically regarding range of motion (ROM), fracture union, grip strength, pain, and functional outcome scores [8]. The benefits of hand-based orthosis use included decreased stiffness as well as equivalent grip strength between both hands at three- and six-week follow-up [8]. Patients demonstrated increased compliance with plaster splint wear as compared to the removable thermoplast orthosis; however easy removal allows for improved patient comfort and hygiene [8].

Case Example
A 19-year-old left-hand-dominant male sustained a right little finger comminuted metacarpal shaft fracture secondary to a gunshot wound. The patient underwent surgical repair of the little finger metacarpal shaft with open reduction and internal fixation (ORIF) and distal radius autogenous bone graft. The patient was immobilized in a postoperative ulnar gutter splint in which the MCP joints were kept free. At 9 days post-surgery, the patient was transitioned to a short arm cast. At three and a half weeks post-surgery, the short arm cast was removed and the patient was referred to occupational therapy (OT) for transition to a thermoplast ulnar gutter orthosis in neutral pronation/supination with the MCP joints free. OT was initiated for ROM at the time of orthosis fabrication. The patient presented with limited ring and small finger MCP joint ROM as well as limited small finger extension.

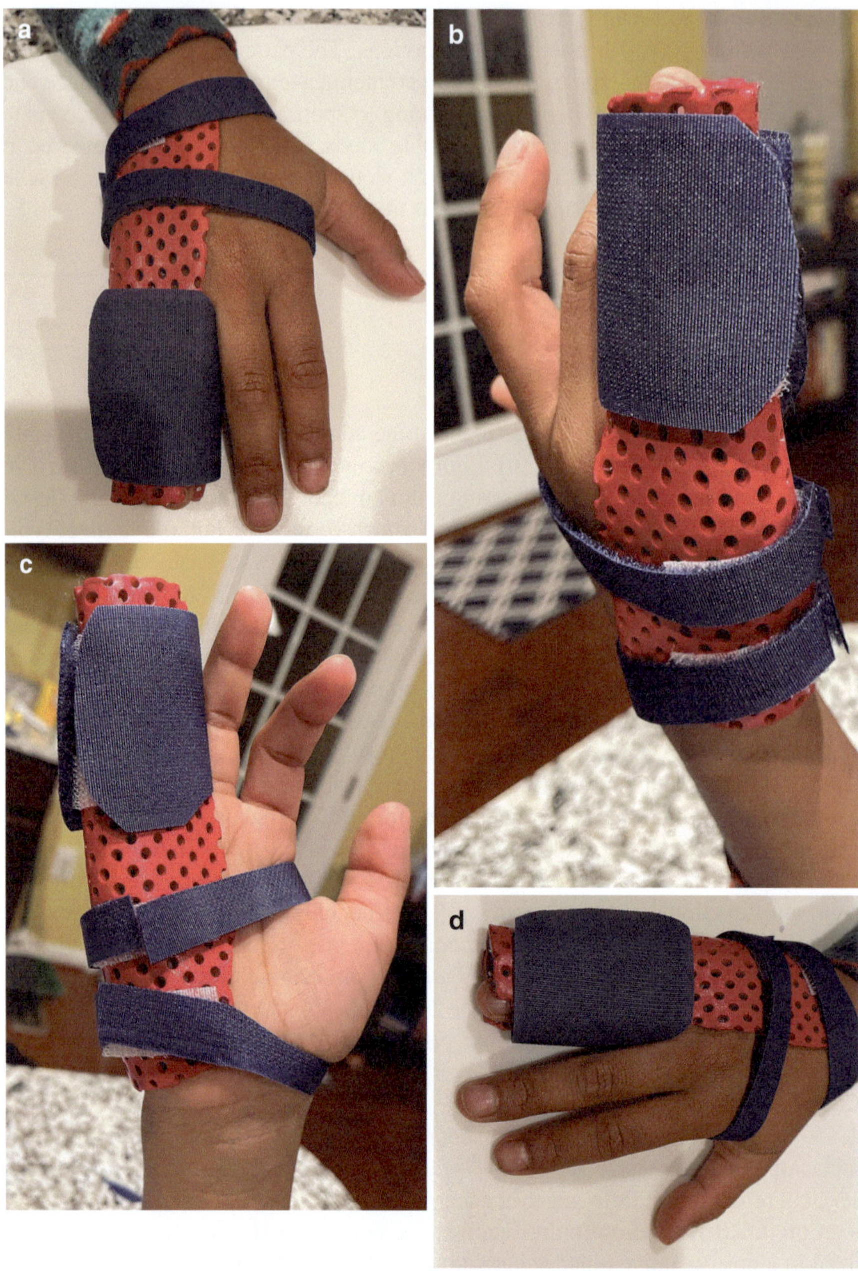

Fig. 9.3 Hand-based ulnar gutter orthosis (**a**) dorsal view (**b**) dorsal ulnar view (**c**) volar view and (**d**) dorsal radial view. (Courtesy of Ritu Goel, MS, OTR/L)

Table 9.1 Range of motion before and after treatment of a 19-year-old male patient with a right small finger metacarpal neck fracture secondary to a gunshot wound

Visit	Ring finger	Small finger
Initial evaluation	MP[a] -20-60 PIP[b] 0–95 DIP[c] 0–50	MP[a] -25-30 PIP[b] -55-90 DIP[c] -25-60
Re-evaluation *10 visits*	MP[a] 0–80 PIP[b] 0–90 DIP[c] 0–50	MP[a] 0–80 PIP[b] 0–90 DIP[c] 0–50

[a]Metacarpophalangeal joint
[b]Proximal phalangeal joint
[c]Distal phalangeal joint

Table 9.2 Baseline strength of patient from Table 9.1

Baseline strength (pounds)	Left hand	Right hand (affected)
Jamar grip: II	95	50
Pinch: lateral	20	14
Pinch: 2 point	9	7
Pinch: 3 point	15	11

Treatment focused on right hand tendon gliding, scar management, as well as place and hold exercises to regain composite motion. The patient was issued buddy loops at his fourth visit to assist with regaining composite motion. Within 10 visits, full active ROM of the right hand digits, in both flexion and extension planes, was achieved (Table 9.1). Upon follow-up with the referring physician, the ulnar gutter orthosis was discontinued and the patient was cleared to initiate strengthening. A strengthening program was initiated in therapy and the patient was issued a home exercise program for forearm to hand strengthening with free weights and red theraputty (Table 9.2).

The patient attended a total of 11 visits with substantial improvement in right hand ROM and improving strength. Unfortunately, the patient was lost to follow-up and discharge measurements were not obtainable.

Phalanx Fractures

Phalanx fractures account for the majority of hand fractures in children, typically of the distal phalanx in toddlers and younger children, compared to the middle and proximal phalanges in older children and adolescents [1–3]. The most common mechanisms of injury for proximal and middle phalanx fractures include sports and falls, whereas distal phalanx fractures are typically the result of crush injuries, such as a finger caught in a doorway [3, 4].

The degree of displacement and fracture orientation often dictate the treatment [1]. Minimally or nondisplaced fractures of the phalanges are typically treated with cast immobilization with or without a closed reduction or buddy taping with placement of an orthosis, followed by active ROM exercises [1–3, 9]. Closed reduction and percutaneous pinning (CRPP) or open reduction and internal fixation (ORIF) is

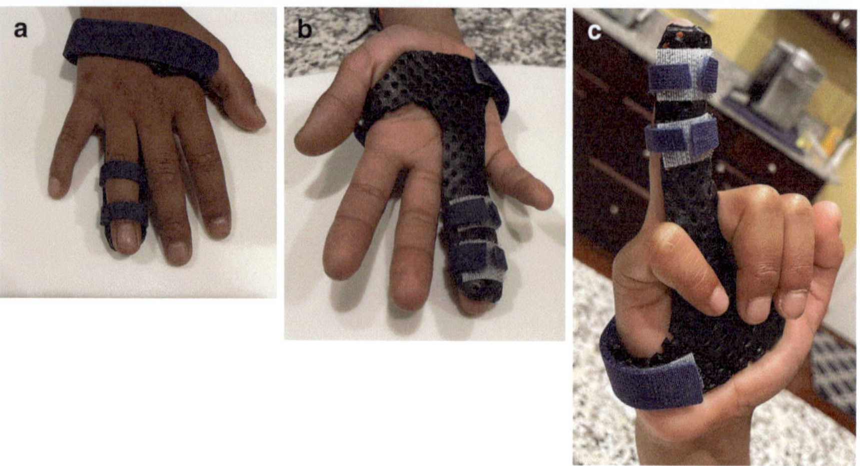

Fig. 9.4 Hand-based RF digit extension orthosis (**a**) dorsal view (**b**) volar view and (**c**) volar radial view. (Courtesy of Ritu Goel, MS, OTR/L)

reserved for displaced fractures [1, 3, 9]. It is important to note that the assessment of proximal phalanx fractures should be performed with the digits in mid-flexion to identify malrotation or scissoring, which may be missed when assessing the digit resting in extension [4].

Immobilization for nonoperative and postoperative cases is often accomplished with a short arm mitten cast. The immobilization period often varies by the degree of fracture displacement and the treating provider's protocol. In a retrospective study by Boyer et al. (2015), 105 patients with a mean age of 11 years presented with a proximal phalanx fracture treated with CRPP and cast immobilization for 4 weeks [3]. Following cast removal, 53% of patients regained full motion and 34% required formal therapy due to residual stiffness [3].

The majority of patients achieve full, pain-free functional use and aesthetics following operative treatment of a proximal phalanx fracture [3]. However, postoperative complications do occur and may include pin site infection, malunion, and/or residual stiffness [4]. To address residual stiffness, patients presenting with a proximal interphalangeal (PIP) joint extension lag may benefit from a nighttime, hand-based digit extension orthosis (Fig. 9.4) to assist in regaining motion, as well as to provide additional protection during play activity as needed.

Case Example

A 10-year-old right hand dominant male child sustained a right ring finger P1 fracture secondary to a fall off a swing. After failing to initially seek medical attention, the patient developed a malunion, which was surgically treated with an osteotomy and fixation with postoperative cast immobilization for 4 weeks. Upon cast removal, the child was transitioned to a hand-based ulnar gutter orthosis (Fig. 9.3), which was fabricated in the intrinsic plus position. The patient initiated OT, with substantial limitations of the ring and small finger interphalangeal (IP) joints, specifically no

Table 9.3 Range of motion before and after treatment of a 10-year-old male with right ring finger P1 fracture sustained during a fall from a swing

Visit	Ring finger		Small finger	
	Before treatment	After treatment	Before treatment	After treatment
Initial evaluation	MP[a] 0–80 PIP[b] -35-35 DIP[c] 0–0	MP[a] 0–80 PIP[b] -25-55 DIP[c] 0–20	MP[a] 0–80 PIP[b] 0–40 DIP[c] 0–0	MP[a] 0–75 PIP[b] 0–85 DIP[c] 0–45
Re-evaluation *12 visits* *4 weeks*	MP[a] +20–80 PIP[b] -20-60 DIP[c] 0–30	MP[a] +20–80 PIP[b] –20-70 DIP[c] 0–45	MP[a] +20–80 PIP[b] 0–80 DIP[c] 0–60	NT
Discharge *18 visits* *8 weeks*	MP[a] +20–85 PIP[b] -15–80 DIP[c] 0–75	MP[a] 0–80 PIP[b] -15-90 DIP[c] 0–70	WNL	NT

[a]Metacarpophalangeal joint
[b]Proximal phalangeal joint
[c]Distal phalangeal joint

motion at the ring finger PIP or DIP joints, as well as small finger limitation at the PIP joint and no motion at the DIP joint.

Therapy focused on ROM (active, active-assisted, passive) for tendon gliding, blocked IP exercises, and differential gliding. Buddy loops were issued to assist with regaining composite motion, and a compression sleeve was issued for swelling management. Modalities utilized included moist heat packs prior to treatment as well as kinetic sand and theraputty for regaining composite motion and grip strength. At discharge, full composite flexion with a slight ring finger PIP extension lag was achieved (Table 9.3).

The ulnar gutter orthosis was used for approximately two weeks, at which point the orthosis was self-discharged by the patient and family. Unfortunately, the patient experienced a slight setback due to a re-injury of the operative digit when he was sledding without his orthosis in place 2 weeks after initiating therapy. The patient was subsequently diagnosed with a contusion and was cleared to initiate passive motion with continued orthosis wear for an additional 2 weeks. Upon the ulnar gutter orthosis discharge, the patient was issued a hand-based ring finger PIP extension orthosis (Fig. 9.4) for nighttime wear, which was periodically re-molded for increased PIP joint extension.

Phalangeal Neck Fractures

Phalangeal neck fractures are rather unique to the pediatric population [4, 10, 11]. The typical mechanism of injury in younger children is a finger caught in a closed door, whereas in older children it is often related to sports or falls [10, 11]. Phalangeal neck fractures occur at the distal end of the proximal or middle phalanges, and can be identified on radiographs as a bony spike or apex volar angulation with dorsal displacement of the phalangeal head, where the volar spike is found to impede flexion [1, 4, 9, 12].

This fracture type is typically classified as problematic and unstable with poor remodeling potential due to the increased distance of the phalangeal neck from the physis [2, 4, 10, 11, 13]. Al-Qattan (2001) published a classification system for pediatric phalangeal neck fractures based on the "degree and type of displacement of the distal fragment" (p. 112) [14]. According to this classification system, type I fractures are nondisplaced, type II fractures are displaced with some bone-to-bone contact between the distal and proximal fragments, and type III fractures are displaced with no bone-to-bone contact between the distal and proximal fragments and rotational deformity [14].

Type I, nondisplaced, phalangeal neck fractures are treated with cast or orthosis immobilization for 3–6 weeks, followed by active ROM exercises [1, 11]. In the younger child a forearm-based orthosis should be considered due to their impeccable ability to independently remove orthoses; however older children may be treated with a digit- or hand-based orthosis. Most phalangeal neck fractures, however, commonly present as a displaced type II or type III fracture, which often requires pin fixation for stabilization via CRPP with or without percutaneous osteoclasis, followed by cast application for 3–4 weeks [11, 12].

Although surgical fixation has traditionally been the recommended treatment for displaced fractures, recent studies demonstrate successful fracture healing with adequate alignment nonoperatively [5, 11, 13]. Park et al. (2016) studied type II and type III phalangeal neck fracture treatment options, comparing buddy taping with an orthosis versus surgical fixation [13]. The results showed that buddy taping with a short arm orthosis ($n = 19$) yielded full ROM, and similarly the surgical group ($n = 18$) also regained full ROM and function except for two patients experiencing a limitation in flexion and/or extension. Tan et al. (2020) investigated the outcomes of nonsurgical management of type II displaced phalangeal neck fractures in 35 patients with a mean age of 12 years [11]. The authors concluded that type II phalangeal neck fractures may successfully be treated nonoperatively without significant further displacement during healing with an overall angulation and translation improvement [11]. Liao and colleagues (2021) studied outcomes of nonoperative management of type I and type II phalangeal neck fractures in 47 children (mean age 10 years) [5]. Patients were provided with either a forearm-based intrinsic plus cast or a custom-fabricated finger- or hand-based orthosis (Figs. 9.5 and 9.6) for an immobilization period of 3–4 weeks [5]. Results showed that all patients regained full, pain-free ROM and returned to all activity without a significant difference in outcomes between groups [5]. The authors concluded that when treating displaced phalangeal neck fractures, cast or orthosis immobilization may be a "safe" option; however "treatment should be individualized," considering the type of fracture, the patient's age, and healing potential [5].

Although full ROM and functional use for return to sport and activity have been established following phalangeal neck fracture treatment, complications can occur impeding function and causing pain. Factors that may impact successful outcomes include avascular necrosis, substantial stiffness, and/or residual deformity that impedes function [14].

Fig. 9.5 Finger-based interphalangeal joint extension orthosis (Courtesy of Ritu Goel, MS, OTR/L)

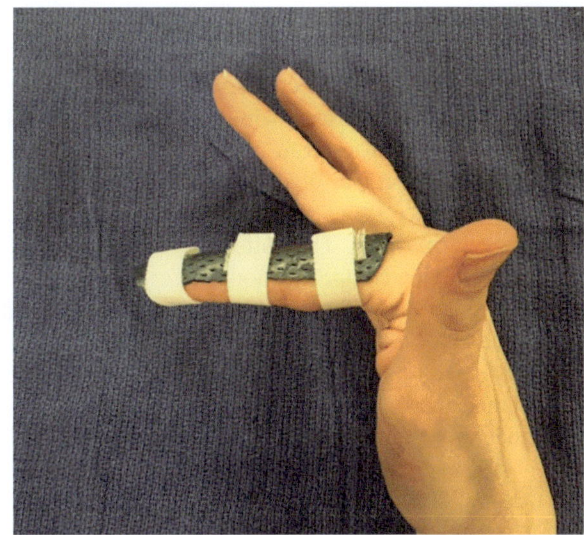

Fig. 9.6 Hand-based ulnar gutter intrinsic plus, IP included (Courtesy of Ritu Goel, MS, OTR/L)

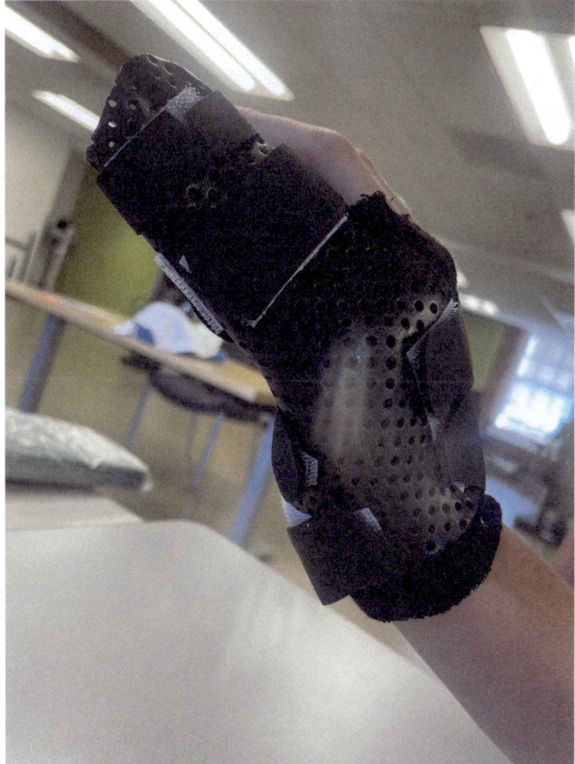

Case Example

An eight-year-old right hand dominant male child sustained a right index finger P1 phalangeal neck fracture secondary to a jammed finger when playing football. The patient was initially treated with an aluma foam splint issued in the emergency department, which was worn for 2 months. Upon consulting with the orthopedic surgeon, the patient was diagnosed with a healed right index finger P1 phalangeal neck fracture. The splint was discontinued and the patient was noted to have mild stiffness with no pain. The patient was referred to occupational therapy (OT) to assist in regaining composite motion.

The therapy focused on ROM (active, active-assisted, passive) including tendon gliding and blocked interphalangeal (IP) exercises (Table 9.4). Pegboards (grooved pegboard, small pegs, and resistive easy grip pegs) were used to regain two-point (2 pt) pinch and encourage right index finger use for fine motor skills, such as writing. Additionally, theraputty and kinetic sand were used to regain composite motion and grip strength. Pinch strength was achieved with resistive clothespin use and digiflex implementation.

Bony Mallet Fracture

A mallet finger is the result of an excessive flexion force through the distal phalanx causing damage to the extensor mechanism at the DIP joint [15]. In contrast, a bony mallet fracture occurs when there is damage to the extensor mechanism at the DIP joint due to an avulsion fracture at the extensor tendon attachment site on the epiphysis [1]. Bony mallet fractures result from an axial load on an extended digit [1, 2]. Treatment of bony mallet fractures in the pediatric population often follows the same principles used to treat adults, which aim to prevent extensor lag or swan neck deformity [1].

Table 9.4 Range of motion before and after treatment of an 8-year-old male patient with a right index finger P1 phalangeal neck fracture who jammed his finger while playing football

Visit	Index finger	
	Before treatment	After treatment
Initial evaluation	MP[a] 0–90	MP[a] 0–90
	PIP[b] -10-70	PIP[b] -5-75
	DIP[c] 0–60	DIP[c] 0–60
1 week	MP[a] 0–90	MP[a] 0–90
	PIP[b] -5-80	PIP[b] 0–85
	DIP[c] 0–75	DIP[c] 0–75
3 weeks	MP[a] 0–90	MP[a] 0–80
	PIP[b] -5-80	PIP[b] 0–90
	DIP[c] 0–75	DIP[c] 0–70
6 weeks	MP[a] 0–85	MP[a] 0–90
	PIP[b] 0–80	PIP[b] 0–90
	DIP[c] 0–75	DIP[c] 0–85

[a]Metacarpophalangeal joint
[b]Proximal phalangeal joint
[c]Distal phalangeal joint

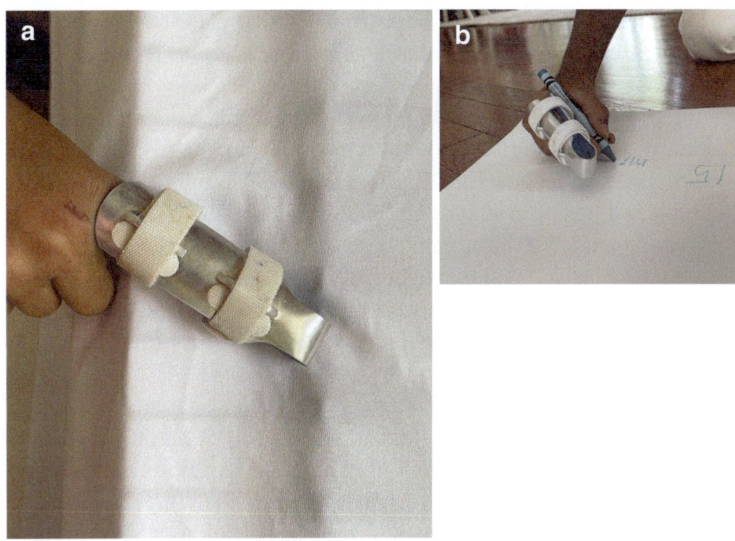

Fig. 9.7 Aluma foam splint (**a**) dorsal view and (**b**) dorsal radial view. (Courtesy of Ritu Goel, MS, OTR/L)

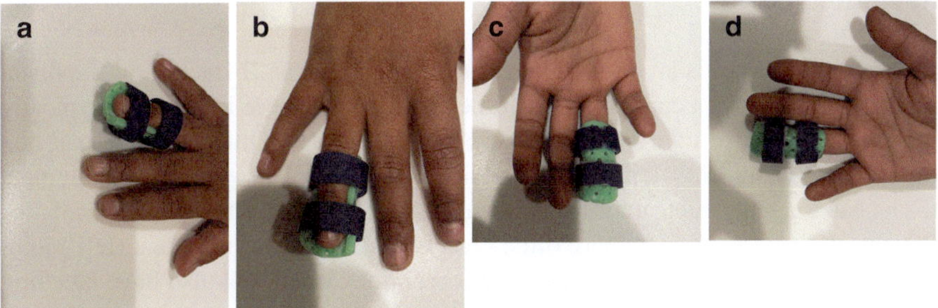

Fig. 9.8 DIP extension orthosis (**a**) dorsal radial view (**b**) dorsal view (**c**) volar view and (**d**) volar ulnar view. (Courtesy of Ritu Goel, MS, OTR/L)

Nonsurgical treatment involves immobilization with a DIP extension orthosis such as a Stack™ splint, an aluma foam splint (Fig. 9.7), or a custom thermoplast orthosis (Fig. 9.8), all of which have been found to result in similar outcomes [15]. A full-time immobilization period of 6–8 weeks plus an additional nighttime wear schedule for 2–4 weeks is recommended for bony mallet fractures [1]. Lin and Samora (2018) examined nonsurgical treatment of pediatric mallet fingers with splint immobilization in 99 mallet fingers, 79 of which presented with bony mallet injuries [15]. The results showed a residual extension lag in 11% of patients and minimal complications such as skin issues (20%), prominence over the DIPJ (18%), and deformity (13%) [15]. It should be noted that 93% of patients were compliant with immobilization in this study and the mean age of included patients was 13.7 years [15]. Therefore, it should be recognized that these conclusions are appropriate for older children and adolescents as opposed to younger aged patients.

Cast application or surgical intervention may be considered, specifically in children with potentially poor compliance with orthosis wear [2, 15]. In younger patients where compliance is a concern, DIP extension orthosis application covered with a long arm club cast has been suggested; however due to the potential for skin breakdown, it is recommended to have patients return for weekly cast changes and skin checks [16]. Factors for surgical management include joint incongruence, persistent distal phalanx volar subluxation, a fracture fragment comprising greater than one-third of the articular surface, irreducible injuries, and/or poor orthosis compliance [1, 2, 4].

Aside from orthosis fabrication and educating patients and parents, no formal therapy is typically indicated for bony mallet fractures in the pediatric population. If the patient presents with residual stiffness following cast or orthosis removal that is not resolved with return to activity prior to next physician follow-up, they may be referred to therapy to assist with regaining ROM, desensitization, and/or strength as needed.

Seymour Fracture

A Seymour fracture is an open Salter-Harris type I or type II fracture of the distal phalanx physis with a concomitant nail bed laceration. These injuries are typically the result of a crush injury at the distal phalanx level [1]. Oftentimes the nail bed injury is not visible due to proximal avulsion of the nail plate, causing the nail plate to appear longer, which may result in nail plate deformity if left untreated [4]. Patients with a Seymour fracture often present in distal interphalangeal (DIP) joint flexion, similar to a mallet deformity; however, they often will also have bleeding around the nail bed due to a laceration [2].

Treatment of Seymour fractures requires nail plate removal, irrigation and debridement (I&D), nail bed repair, fracture reduction, and nail plate replacement to ensure fracture stability [2, 4]. The injured digit is often stabilized with an orthosis for 4 weeks; however if compliance and fracture stability are of concern, surgical K-wire fixation through the DIP joint with cast application is recommended for 4 weeks [2, 4, 9].

Early intervention and diagnosis are imperative with Seymour fractures to reduce the risk of infection, osteomyelitis, growth arrest, and/or nail plate deformity [1, 12, 16]. Due to the infection risk associated with this injury, in addition to an I&D, patients are prescribed a course of antibiotics in an effort to prevent a soft tissue infection and/or osteomyelitis [2]. Growth arrest is a complication that may be difficult to correct, resulting in potentially altered finger length and/or aesthetic deformity [12]. Patients typically have a good outcome following appropriate treatment of a Seymour fracture; however it should be noted that closed treatment has a higher incidence of complications as compared to operative management [16].

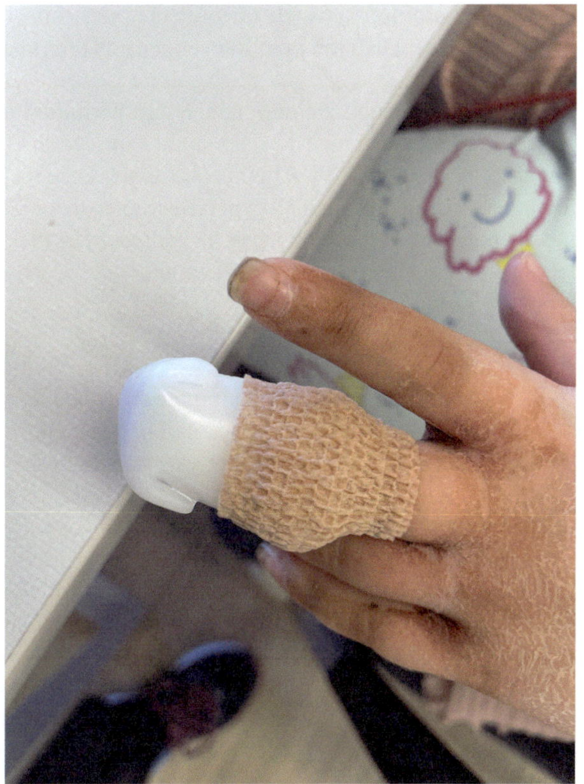

Fig. 9.9 Clamshell tip protector orthosis (Courtesy of Ritu Goel, MS, OTR/L)

Following cast or postoperative splint removal, patients may be referred to therapy for a custom cap or tip protector orthosis (Fig. 9.9) to provide additional protection as the patient returns to activity. Other treatment needs may include sensory re-education due to hypersensitivity or decreased sensation. Patients may also present with stiffness or fear of moving the digit following the injury, which may be resolved with play activity focusing on fine motor coordination skills. Oftentimes, however, educating the patient and family on techniques that may be incorporated in the home environment may be sufficient to regain functional deficits.

Tuft Fracture

Tuft fractures are common to the pediatric population at the toddler and preschool age, typically resulting from a crush injury of the fingertip, such as a finger caught in a doorway or stepped on [4, 9]. This injury may present with a nailbed laceration and/or soft tissue injury alongside the distal phalanx tuft fracture [1]. Open injuries are often addressed with an I&D and laceration closure followed by antibiotic administration [1]. Closed injuries, however, are often treated nonoperatively with immobilization for 2–3 weeks [1, 9]. Digits are immobilized with either a mitten cast or low-profile clamshell tip protector orthosis (Fig. 9.9) that restricts distal interphalangeal (DIP) joint motion yet permits proximal interphalangeal (PIP) joint motion [1, 9].

Following immobilization, patients are permitted to initiate active motion and are referred to a therapist for cap splint fabrication (Fig. 9.9) to protect sensitive fingertips as needed [1, 9]. Patients may experience residual sensory limitations following a tuft fracture such as hypersensitivity to cold, hyperesthesia, and/or numbness [1]. Sensory limitations may be addressed in therapy with desensitization and sensory re-education activities. Limitations in sensation often resolve within 6 months of the injury [1].

Case Example

A 14-year-old right hand dominant male sustained a right index finger P3 open tuft fracture with an associated complex nail bed laceration secondary to the digit being slammed in a doorway. The patient was treated in the emergency department with nail plate removal, an I&D, repair of the nailbed laceration, and replacement of the nail plate, followed by cast application for 4 weeks. Upon cast removal, the patient was referred to therapy for a cap or tip protector orthosis, which was recommended to be removed for AROM and hygiene. Upon follow-up with the referring physician, the patient was informed to wean from the orthosis and a referral to therapy for ROM and desensitization was made.

The patient was seen for only the initial evaluation. The treatment focused on active ROM including tendon gliding (full fist and hook fist) and blocked IP exercises (Table 9.5). The patient was educated on a home program for hand hygiene, ROM exercises, orthosis discontinuation, and desensitization exercises at the distal tip due to compromised sensation. Desensitization tools included the use of a washcloth, a toothbrush, and foam brushes. Although the patient was recommended to continue a course of therapy, he only attended the evaluation. However, during the initial visit, substantial ROM gains were achieved.

Table 9.5 Range of motion before and after treatment of a 14-year-old male patient with a right index finger P3 open tuft fracture with associated nailbed laceration after slamming the digit in a doorway

	Index finger	
Visit	Before treatment	After treatment
Initial evaluation	MP[a] 0–70	MP[a] 0–70
	PIP[b] -10-65	PIP[b] -8-90
	DIP[c] 0–30	DIP[c] 0–40

[a]Metacarpophalangeal joint
[b]Proximal phalangeal joint
[c]Distal phalangeal joint

Conclusion

When treating children and adolescent hand injuries, an understanding of the injury, bony development, and treatment protocol is beneficial. Therapy offers various age-appropriate modalities to assist with regaining motion and sensation. Orthoses immobilize the injury site, forearm-based for younger children and possibly hand- or finger-based for older children. Although pediatric hand therapy is available, this population's impeccable healing ability may prevent them from needing therapy following cast or orthosis removal. However, patient and parent education are often beneficial to provide a safe and timely re-integration into sports and daily life activities.

References

1. Abzug JM, Dua K, Bauer AS, Cornwall R, Wyrick TO. Pediatric phalanx fractures. J Am Acad Orthop Surg. 2016;24:e174–83. https://doi.org/10.5435/jaaos-d-16-00199.
2. Cornwall R, Ricchetti ET. Pediatric phalanx fractures: unique challenges and pitfalls. Clin Orthop Relat Res. 2006;445:146–56. https://doi.org/10.1097/01.blo.0000205890.88952.97.
3. Boyer JS, London DA, Stepan JG, Goldfarb CA. Pediatric proximal phalanx fractures: outcomes and complications after the surgical treatment of displaced fractures. J Pediatr Orthop. 2015;35(3):219–23. https://doi.org/10.1097/BPO.0000000000000253.
4. Liao JCY, Chong AKS. Pediatric hand and wrist fractures. Clin Plastic Surg. 2019;46:425–36. https://doi.org/10.1016/j.cps.2019.02.012.
5. Liao JCY, Huan SKW, Tan RES, Lim JX, Chong AKS, De SD. A comparison of casting versus splinting for nonoperative treatment of pediatric phalangeal neck fractures. J PediatrOrthop. 2021;41(1):e30–5. https://doi.org/10.1177/1558944720942890.
6. Lee SJ, Merrison H, Williams KA, Vuillermin CB, Bauer AS. Closed reduction and immobilization of pediatric fifth metacarpal neck fractures. Hand (N Y). 2020;17:416. https://doi.org/10.1177/1558944720942890.
7. Kocher MS, Waters PM, Micheli LJ. Upper extremity injuries in the paediatric athlete. Sports Med. 2000;30(2):117–35. https://doi.org/10.2165/00007256-200030020-00005.
8. Davidson PG, Bondreau N, Burrows R, Wilson KL, Buzuhly M. Forearm-based ulnar gutter versus hand-based thermoplastic splint for pediatric metacarpal neck fractures: a blinded, randomized trial. Plast Reconstr Surg. 2016;137(3):908–16. https://doi.org/10.1097/01.prs.0000479974.45051.78.
9. Nellans KW, Chung KC. Pediatric hand fractures. Hand Clin. 2013;29(4):569–78. https://doi.org/10.1016/j.hcl.2013.08.009.
10. Al-Qattan MM, Al-Qattan AM. A review of phalangeal neck fractures in children. Injury. 2015;46:935–44. https://doi.org/10.1016/j.injury.2015.02.018.
11. Tan RES, Lim JXL, Chong AKS. Outcomes of phalangeal neck fractures in a pediatric population. J Hand Surg Am. 2020;45(9):880.e1–6. https://doi.org/10.1016/j.jhsa.2020.02.019.
12. Cornwall R. Pediatric finger fractures: which ones turn ugly? J Pediatr Orthop. 2012;32(1):S25–31. https://doi.org/10.1097/bpo.0b013e31824b2582.
13. Park KB, Lee KJ, Kwak YH. Comparison between buddy taping with a short-arm splint and operative treatment for phalangeal neck fractures in children. J Pediatr Orthop. 2016;36(7):736–42. https://doi.org/10.1097/bpo.0000000000000521.

14. Al-Qattan MM. Phalangeal neck fractures in children: classification and outcome in 66 cases. J Hand Surg Br. 2001;26B(2):112–21. https://doi.org/10.1054/jhsb.2000.0506.
15. Lin JS, Samora JB. Outcomes of splinting in pediatric mallet finger. J Hand Surg Am. 2018;43(11):1041.e1–9. https://doi.org/10.1016/j.jhsa.2018.03.037.
16. Goodell PB, Bauer A. Problematic pediatric hand and wrist fractures. J Bone Joint Surg. 2016;4(5):e1–9. https://doi.org/10.2106/jbjs.rvw.o.00028.

Nicholas D. D'Antonio and Praveen G. Murthy

Physical Examination of the Adult Hand

As with any body system, physical examination of the hand proceeds in systematic fashion. The examination typically includes the following elements: inspection, palpation, range of motion, stability, tendon/muscle function, and neurovascular examination.

Examination begins by observing the appearance of the hand. The presence of swelling and ecchymosis can immediately provide clues to the location of injury. The examiner should make note of any wounds, which may or may not indicate the presence of an open fracture and/or other associated soft tissue injury. Finally, evaluation of deformity is critical in determining treatment for hand fractures. In particular, the fingers should be scrutinized for any evidence of angulation or malrotation.

Angular deviation of the finger resulting from a phalangeal fracture is relatively clear by observation alone. Angulation in the metacarpals can be harder to assess by observation alone. The examiner may note diminished dorsal prominence of the metacarpophalangeal joint, or loss of the knuckle. Malrotation is suspected when the orientation of the nail is asymmetric to the adjacent nails (Fig. 10.1) and becomes more clear as the fingers are brought down into a composite fist (Fig. 10.1).

Tenderness to palpation is critical in the examination of an injured hand. When radiographic findings are not obvious, or if chronicity of an injury is

N. D. D'Antonio
Sidney Kimmel Medical College, Thomas Jefferson University Hospital, Philadelphia, PA, USA

P. G. Murthy (✉)
Philadelphia Hand to Shoulder Center, Thomas Jefferson University Hospital, Philadelphia, PA, USA
e-mail: pgmurthy@handcenters.com

© The Author(s), under exclusive license to Springer Nature Switzerland AG 2023
J. M. Abzug et al. (eds.), *Pediatric and Adult Hand Fractures*,
https://doi.org/10.1007/978-3-031-32072-9_10

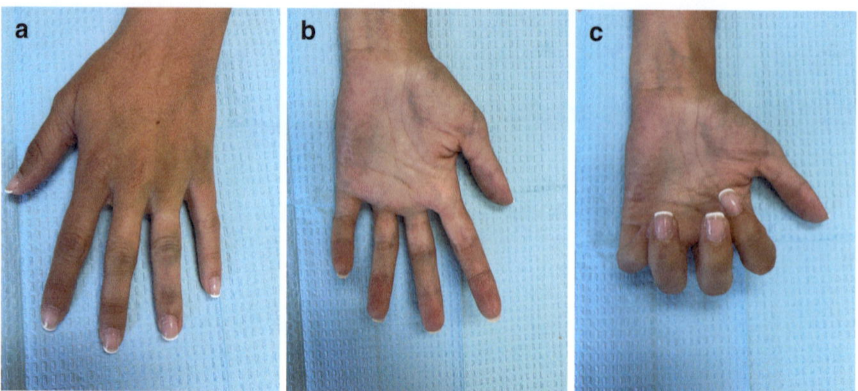

Fig. 10.1 Malrotation. In extension, the direction of the ring fingernail (**a**) and finger pulp (**b**) is asymmetric to the adjacent nails. In flexion, the ring finger is no longer pointing to the scaphoid tubercle, and there is crossover of the ring finger with respect to the small finger (**c**)

unclear, tenderness provides an excellent guide to determine the location and acuity of a fracture. Tenderness can also raise suspicion for additional unrecognized injuries. The examination should proceed in a systematic manner, beginning away from the suspected zone of injury, and examining the fractured finger last.

Range of motion is examined next. Motion is often limited in the setting of a fractured hand; however, even a limited motion exam can provide critical information to guide treatment of a metacarpal or phalangeal fracture. First, the patient is instructed to attempt making a composite fist, and the fingers are scrutinized for evidence of malrotation. In a normal hand, all fingers should point toward the scaphoid tubercle as they come down into the palm. Abnormal digital cascade and crossover of the fingers indicates malrotation through the fracture and is typically an indication for surgical repair (Fig. 10.1).

Next, the patient is instructed to fully extend the fingers. Here, the examiner scrutinizes the injured finger for any evidence of extensor lag or pseudoclawing. Extensor lag, or lack of full extension with respect to the adjacent uninjured fingers, typically results from shortening of the metacarpal. Pseudoclawing results from metacarpal or phalangeal base fractures with significant volar angulation, typically greater than 30°. Imbalance in the extensor mechanism leads to hyperextension at the metacarpophalangeal (MCP) joint and flexion at the proximal interphalangeal (PIP) joint.

Specific fracture patterns should then be examined for certain hallmark features that help to guide treatment. Metacarpal fractures often present with loss of the knuckle and volar prominence of the metacarpal head, owing to volar angulation at the fracture site. In addition, volar angulation may lead to extensor lag and pseudoclawing as described above. The degree of extensor lag should be assessed carefully to determine whether surgical repair is indicated. Finally, malrotation must be evaluated in the setting of metacarpal fractures, as any malrotation is typically an indication for surgical repair.

Phalangeal fractures should be similarly evaluated for angulation and malrotation. Extensor lag should also be noted, as volar angulation and shortening in the phalanges can often produce more dramatic extensor lag than in the metacarpals. Extra-articular phalangeal base fractures should be scrutinized for MCP hyperextension and pseudoclawing.

Ligamentous avulsion fractures in the MCP and PIP joints should be examined for stability. The MCP joints of the fingers are typically tested by applying varus and valgus stress with the joint positioned in 90° of flexion, while the thumb MCP joint is tested in 0° and 30° of flexion. The PIP joint is tested in full extension. Avulsion fractures with associated joint instability may necessitate surgical intervention.

Tendon dysfunction should also be recognized in the setting of tendon avulsion injuries. At the PIP joint, the central slip should be examined using the Elson test. The PIP joint is flexed to 90° and the patient is instructed to extend the middle phalanx against resistance. In a central slip avulsion injury, there will be weak PIP extension and the DIP joint will be rigid, as the entire force of the extensor mechanism is now applied to the DIP joint alone.

At the distal interphalangeal (DIP) joint, terminal extensor tendon avulsion injuries (mallet finger) should be examined for extensor lag. Isolated active DIP joint flexion should be tested if there is any concern for flexor digitorum profundus tendon avulsion (Jersey finger). Finally, patients with distal phalangeal tuft fractures should be examined for any evidence of subungual hematoma and/or nail plate avulsion. This helps to determine the extent of the underlying nail bed injury and the need for surgical repair.

Finally, neurovascular examination is routinely performed. This is of particular importance in the setting of open injuries with involvement of multiple tissue layers. Sensation is examined at the fingertip to ensure that both radial and ulnar digital nerves are intact. If there is any abnormality in sensation, two-point discrimination can be utilized to quantify the deficit. Fingertip perfusion is assessed by appearance and capillary refill. Poorly perfused fingers demonstrate discoloration, loss of skin turgor, and delayed capillary refill. Pulse oximetry can be utilized to clarify the degree of vascular compromise.

Radiographic Examination of the Adult Hand

Standard radiographic examination of the hand includes posteroanterior (PA), lateral, and oblique projections (Fig. 10.2). Additional special views can be utilized depending on the pathology suspected on physical examination. Regardless of pathology, radiographic evaluation must always be performed in systematic fashion. We prefer to begin proximally at the carpometacarpal joints and progress distally along each ray toward the phalanges.

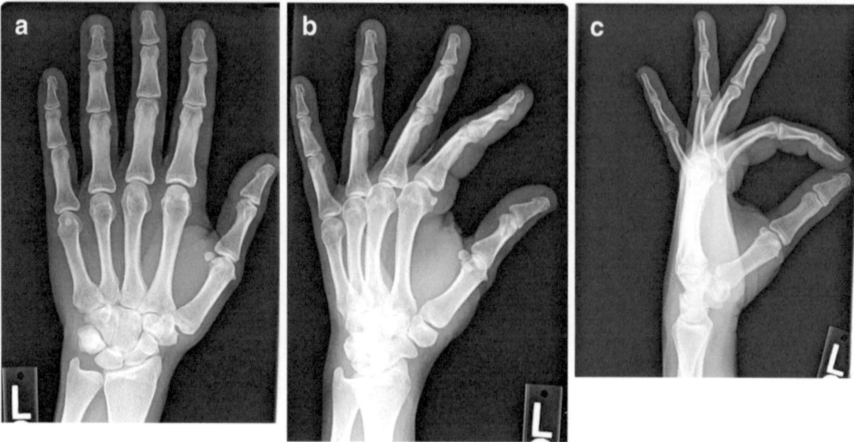

Fig. 10.2 Standard radiographic series of the hand, consisting of (**a**) posteroanterior or PA, (**b**) oblique, and (**c**) lateral projections

Fig. 10.3 The carpometacarpal (CMC) articulations of the second through fifth CMC joints create parallel M-shaped lines. Disruption in these lines suggests an abnormality involving the CMC joint

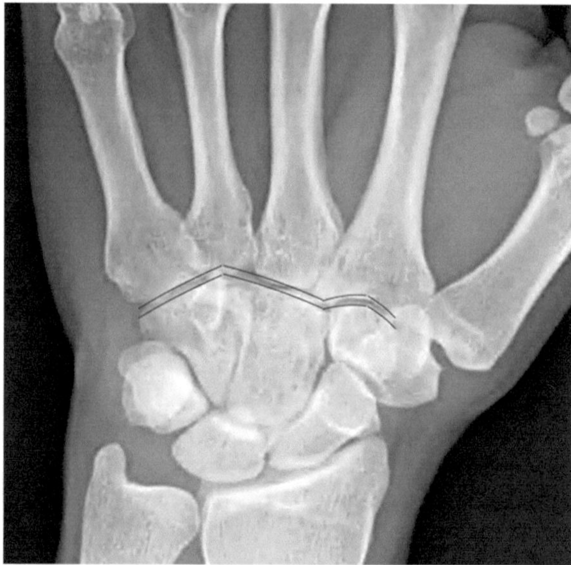

Carpometacarpal Joints

When viewed on the PA radiograph, the carpometacarpal (CMC) articulations of the second through fifth joints normally create parallel M-shaped lines (Fig. 10.3). The proximal line follows the distal articular surfaces of the trapezoid, capitate, and hamate. The distal line follows the parallel proximal articular surfaces of the second through fifth metacarpals. The width of the CMC joints normally measures 1–2 mm. Any loss of parallelism or joint space congruity suggests an abnormality in that joint.

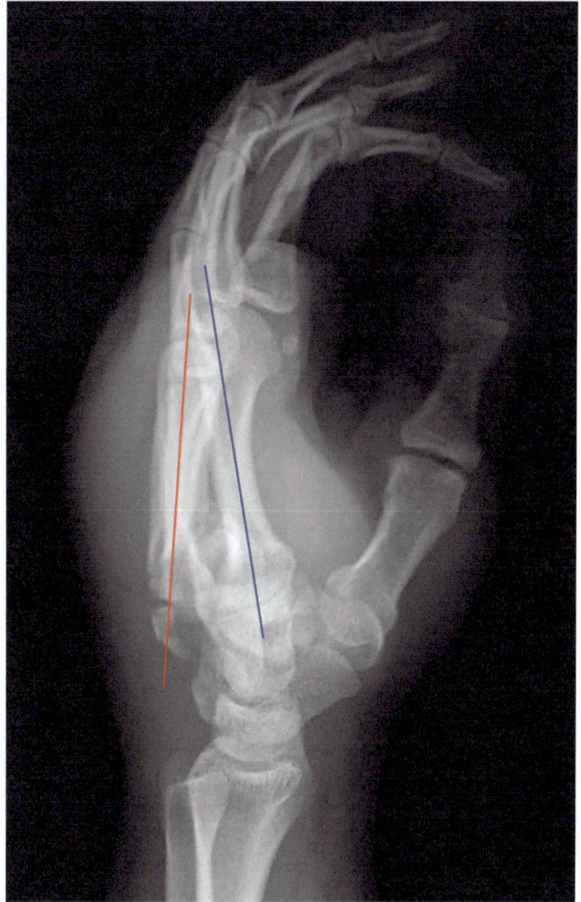

Fig. 10.4 On the lateral projection of a carpometacarpal fracture dislocation, the longitudinal axis of the affected metacarpal(s) (red line) will no longer be parallel to that of the unaffected metacarpal(s) (blue line)

On the lateral radiograph, the second through fifth metacarpals should be parallel. In a dislocation or fracture dislocation at the carpometacarpal joint, the longitudinal axis of the affected metacarpal(s) no longer parallels that of the unaffected metacarpals (Fig. 10.4). Supinated and pronated oblique radiographs should be utilized to obtain better visualization of the radial and ulnar carpometacarpal joints, respectively. When supinated or pronated from the neutral position, these oblique views allow for better evaluation of sagittal plane abnormalities without overlap of the adjacent metacarpals.

The CMC articulation between the trapezium and the thumb metacarpal base (trapezio metacarpal joint) is a saddle joint supported by 16 ligaments. The volar oblique ligament and the dorsal ligament complex are essential for resisting dorsoradial displacement of the metacarpal base. Thumb metacarpal base fractures that involve the CMC articulation (Bennett and Rolando fractures) can result in dorsoradial subluxation of thumb base, varus malalignment, and narrowing of the first web space. These are evaluated using PA, lateral, and oblique radiographs. A true

Fig. 10.5 Roberts view of the thumb CMC joint, which is acquired by hyper-pronating the wrist and resting the dorsum of the thumb on the X-ray plate

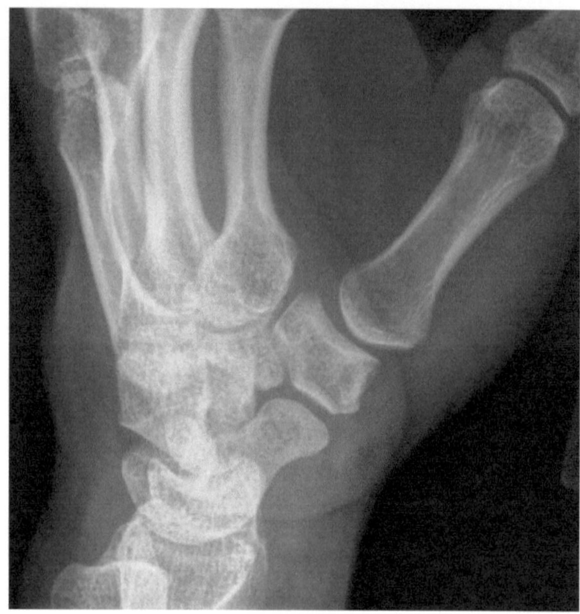

anteroposterior (AP) radiograph, or a Robert's view, is also helpful to evaluate fractures at the thumb base. The Roberts view is acquired by hyper-pronating the wrist and resting the dorsum of the thumb on the X-ray plate (Fig. 10.5) [1].

Metacarpals

The metacarpal bones form the palm of the hand. The base of each metacarpal articulates with the carpus, forming the CMC joints, while the head of each metacarpal articulates with the proximal phalanges, forming the metacarpophalangeal (MCP) joints. The first metacarpal, which is shorter and thicker than the second through fifth metacarpals, forms a saddle-like articulation with the trapezium. The shaft for the first metacarpal is set at a right angle relative to the plane of the second through fourth metacarpals such that the axis of thumb flexion and extension is perpendicular to the flexion and extension axes of the phalanges. The second and third metacarpals are fixed relative to the carpus, while the fourth and fifth metacarpals have a flexion-extension arc of motion of 15–25° at the carpometacarpal joint [2]. The metacarpal heads are cam-shaped and form condyloid joints with the proximal phalanges. The second and third metacarpal heads are typically similar in height, while the fourth and fifth metacarpals are each successively shorter, such that a tangential line drawn from the third to fifth MCP joints should also pass through the fourth MCP joint. This provides a reference point to determine the degree of shortening in the context of metacarpal fractures.

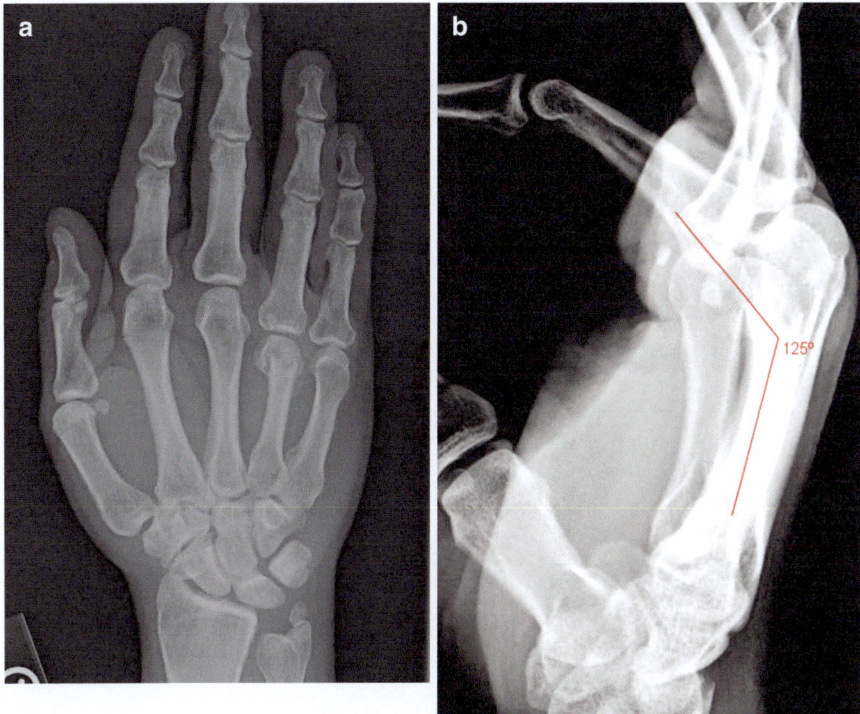

Fig. 10.6 Metacarpal neck fracture of the ring finger (**a**), with volar angulation measured at 55° on the lateral radiograph (**b**)

Metacarpal fractures are the most common fracture of the hand and typically result from direct trauma, axial loading, or rotational injury [3, 4]. Three standard radiographic views—PA, lateral, and oblique of the hand—are utilized for the diagnosis of metacarpal fractures. Fracture lines may be transverse, oblique, spiral, or comminuted. Shortening, which may be apparent on physical examination, is best quantified radiographically and is more common in second or fifth metacarpal fractures due to lack of intermetacarpal ligament support. Angulation is also best evaluated radiographically. Most commonly, metacarpal fractures are found to have volar angulation due to the pull of the interosseous muscles. Volar angulation is quantified on the lateral view and helps to guide treatment (Fig. 10.6) [5].

If standard radiographs fail to detect fracture of the metacarpal neck or head but clinical suspicion remains high, a Brewerton view can be obtained. The Brewerton view is useful to detect occult fractures and is obtained by placing the phalanges flat on the X-ray plate, flexing the MCP joints to 65° from the surface of the plate, and then angling the beam at 15° to the ulnar side of the hand [6].

Fractures of the first metacarpal base are classified and diagnosed separately from fractures of the second through fifth metacarpals. The standard radiographic

Fig. 10.7 Bett's view

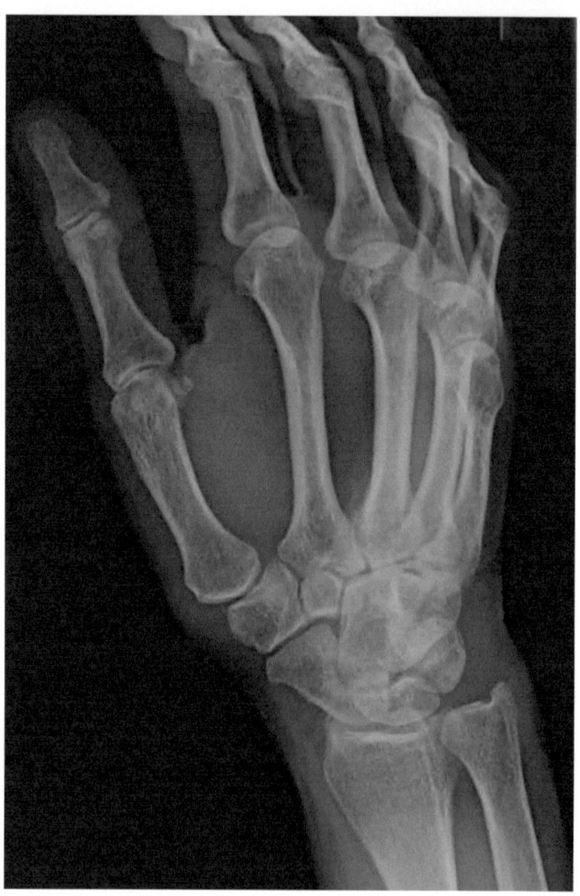

series can be supplemented with a true AP radiograph or Robert's view, as well as a true lateral radiograph known as Gedda or Bett's view. This is obtained by placing the palm in 15–30° of pronation and angling the X-ray beam obliquely in a distal to proximal direction (Fig. 10.7) [1].

Metacarpophalangeal Joints

The metacarpophalangeal (MCP) joints are condyloid joints formed by the articulations between the asymmetric, cam-shaped metacarpal heads and the shallow, concave surface of the proximal phalanges. The capsule of the MCP joint extends from the metacarpal neck to the base of the proximal phalanx and is supported by multiple ligaments. The proper collateral ligaments, which originate from the dorsal metacarpal head and insert on the volar proximal phalangeal base, are the primary stabilizers of the MCP joint.

MCP joint dislocations occur as a result of joint hyperextension or hyperflexion. The first and second MCP joints are most commonly affected, and dorsal dislocations are more common than volar dislocations due to the weak ligamentous support of the dorsal aspect of the MCP joint [7]. These injuries are classified as simple or complex. Complex dislocations are defined by avulsion and interposition of the volar plate into the MCP joint space. A standard series including AP, lateral, and oblique radiographs is obtained for the diagnosis of all MCP joint dislocations. Dorsal or volar displacement of the proximal phalanx is best appreciated on the lateral radiograph. Radiographic widening of the joint space should raise suspicion for volar plate interposition within the joint. If present, radiographic evidence of a sesamoid bone within a widened joint space of the second through fifth digit MCP joints is diagnostic of a complex dislocation as the sesamoids are normally embedded within the volar plate. Similarly, in the thumb, the sesamoid of the conjoint tendon can become entrapped in the MCP joint [8].

Phalanges

The index through small fingers each contain a proximal, middle, and a distal phalanx, while the thumb is comprised of only a proximal and distal phalanx. A 2:1 ratio of length between the proximal and middle phalanges of the index through small fingers is typically observed on radiographs. The proximal and middle phalanges are anatomically divided from proximal to distal into a base, shaft, neck, and head. The distal phalanx is anatomically divided into a base, shaft, and tuft [9]. The tuft of the distal phalanx is a crescent-shaped ridge of bone that provides support to the nail complex.

The concave base of the proximal phalanx articulates with the head of the metacarpal bone to form the MCP joint. The base of the middle phalanx articulates with the head of the proximal phalanx to form the proximal interphalangeal (PIP) joint, while the base of the distal phalanx articulates with the head of the middle phalanx to form the distal interphalangeal (DIP) joints. The heads of the proximal and middle phalanges are defined by radial and ulnar condyles that serve to stabilize the PIP and DIP joints, both through their bony architecture and by serving as attachment points for the collateral ligaments.

Phalangeal fractures are the second most common fracture of the hand. A standard series of three radiographic views—PA, lateral, and oblique of the affected finger—is typically obtained for the evaluation of phalangeal fractures (Fig. 10.8). In general, bending forces typically result in transverse fractures of the phalanx shaft, while rotational and angular forces result in spiral and oblique fractures. Comminuted fractures are typically seen after crush injuries. Axial loading forces are responsible for most articular fractures and dislocations, though rotational forces can also cause small avulsion fractures involving the interphalangeal joints. Radiographs should be scrutinized for the fracture pattern, angulation, intra-articular involvement, and joint congruity.

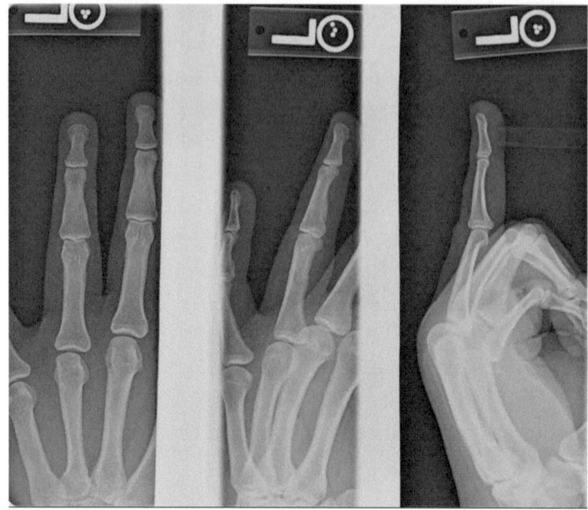

Fig. 10.8 Standard radiographic series of the finger, consisting of (from left to right) posteroanterior or PA, oblique, and lateral projections

Fractures of the proximal phalanx shaft are generally found to have apex volar angulation, as the interosseous muscles pull the proximal segment into flexion and extensor mechanism pulls the distal segment into extension [10]. The lateral view is best to appreciate the degree of angulation, which is important to consider in management of the injury. Fractures of the middle phalanx are generally found to have apex dorsal angulation if they occur proximal to the flexor digitorum superficialis (FDS) insertion, as the central slip pulls the proximal segment into extension and FDS tendon pulls the distal segment into flexion. Conversely, fractures distal to the FDS insertion typically present with apex volar angulation. Radiographs should also be scrutinized for intra-articular involvement and incongruity of the PIP joint.

Fractures of the distal phalanx are classified as fractures of the base, shaft, or tuft [11]. Fractures of the base and shaft may be found to have volar or dorsal angulation depending on their relation to the flexor digitorum profundus (FDP) tendon insertion. Angulation is again best discerned on the lateral radiograph. Tuft fractures are commonly seen after a crush injury and typically demonstrate a comminuted pattern at the tip of the distal phalanx. Tuft fractures visualized on radiographs should raise suspicion for associated nail bed injury.

Interphalangeal Joints

The PIP and DIP joints are both hinge joints and permit flexion and extension in the sagittal plane [12]. The PIP and DIP joint capsules are both stabilized by proper and accessory collateral ligaments, which provide resistance against radial and ulnar deviation at these joints. The proper collateral ligaments of the PIP and DIP joints originate from the condyles of the proximal and middle phalangeal heads and insert on the volar aspect of the middle and distal phalangeal bases, respectively. The accessory collateral ligaments of the PIP and DIP joints insert into the volar plate of each respective joint. The fibrocartilaginous volar plates of the PIP and DIP joint capsules stabilize the palmar aspect of the joints and prevent joint hyperextension. The PIP joint is further stabilized by the central slip dorsally and the FDS tendon volarly, and the DIP joint is further stabilized by the terminal extensor tendon dorsally and FDP tendon volarly [13].

Interphalangeal joint injuries are evaluated using a standard series of three radiographic views—PA, lateral, and oblique projections of the affected finger. A perfect lateral radiograph must be obtained and scrutinized for congruity of the interphalangeal joints. In cases where static radiographs are inadequate to determine the congruity and stability of the joint, examination of the affected digit under fluoroscopy is highly useful to obtain a complete characterization of the injury.

The lateral radiograph is critical in the diagnosis of PIP joint dislocations and fracture-dislocations. The lateral view can be evaluated to determine the direction of the dislocation, the degree of subluxation or dislocation, and the presence and extent of an associated fracture. With even subtle dorsal subluxation, the contour of the dorsal aspect PIP joint may appear as a "V" shape on the lateral radiograph, indicating incongruity of the joint and need for intervention (Fig. 10.9). Dorsal

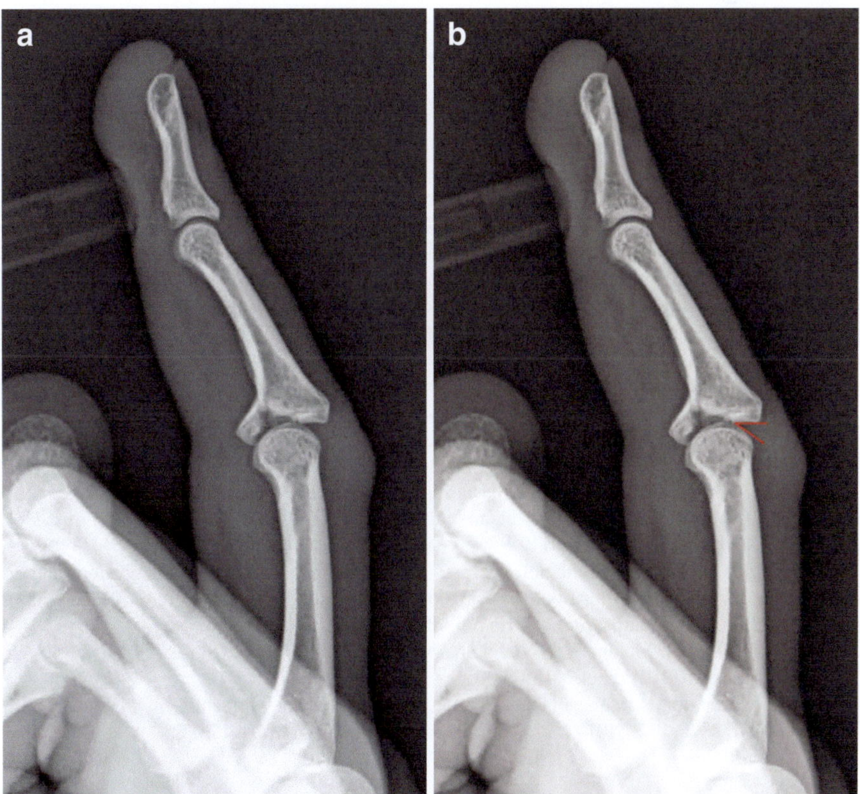

Fig. 10.9 Proximal interphalangeal (PIP) joint fracture dislocation (**a**), with dorsal "V" sign demonstrated on the lateral view (**b**)

dislocations can be associated with small volar plate avulsion fractures (as a result of hypertension injury), or with larger fractures of the volar base of the middle phalanx (as a result of axial loading injury). Volar dislocations, while less common than dorsal dislocations, are caused by PIP joint hyperflexion and subsequent rupture of the central slip of the extensor mechanism [12]. Volar dislocations can be associated with central slip avulsion fractures of varying size. Lateral dislocations are best visualized on the PA radiograph, which may also reveal associated small avulsion fractures.

DIP joint injuries should be scrutinized for two hallmark fractures on the lateral radiograph. Mallet injuries may be associated with terminal extensor tendon avulsion fracture from the dorsal lip of the distal phalanx base. Jersey finger injuries may be associated with FDP avulsion fracture from the volar lip of the distal phalanx base.

Radiographs of the finger should also be scrutinized for small avulsion fractures of the PIP and DIP joints. These subtle fractures can provide clues to the presence of a ligamentous injury and possibly instability of the joint. If the stability of the joint is in question, varus and valgus stress views may be obtained to confirm the diagnosis. In addition, live fluoroscopy can be invaluable in confirming joint congruity through a full range of motion.

References

1. Brown MT, Rust PA. Fractures of the thumb metacarpal base. Injury. 2020;51(11):2421–8. https://doi.org/10.1016/j.injury.2020.07.053.
2. Chin SH, Vedder NB. MOC-PS(SM) CME article: metacarpal fractures. Plast Reconstr Surg. 2008;121(1S):1–13. https://doi.org/10.1097/01.prs.0000294704.48126.8c.
3. Kollitz KM, Hammert WC, Vedder NB, Huang JI. Metacarpal fractures: treatment and complications. Hand. 2014;9(1):16–23. https://doi.org/10.1007/s11552-013-9562-1.
4. Gould JS, Nicholson BG. Capsulectomy of the metacarpophalangeal and proximal interphalangeal joints. J Hand Surg. 1979;4(5):482–6. https://doi.org/10.1016/s0363-5023(79)80048-9.
5. Hussain MH, Ghaffar A, Choudry Q, et al. Management of fifth metacarpal neck fracture (boxer's fracture): a literature review. Cureus. 2020;12(7):e9442. https://doi.org/10.7759/cureus.9442.
6. Lane CS. Detecting occult fractures of the metacarpal head: the Brewerton view. J Hand Surg. 1977;2(2):131–3. https://doi.org/10.1016/s0363-5023(77)80098-1.
7. Minami A, An K-N, Cooney WP, Linscheid RL, Chao EYS. Ligament stability of the metacarpophalangeal joint: a biomechanical study. J Hand Surg. 1985;10(2):255–60. https://doi.org/10.1016/s0363-5023(85)80117-9.
8. Patel MR, Bassini L. Irreducible palmar metacarpophalangeal joint dislocation due to junctura tendinum interposition: a case report and review of the literature. J Hand Surg. 2000;25(1):166–72. https://doi.org/10.1053/jhsu.2000.jhsu025a0166.
9. Panchal-Kildare S, Malone K. Skeletal anatomy of the hand. Hand Clin. 2013;29(4):459–71. https://doi.org/10.1016/j.hcl.2013.08.001.
10. Wahl EP, Richard MJ. Management of metacarpal and phalangeal fractures in the athlete. Clin Sport Med. 2020;39(2):401–22. https://doi.org/10.1016/j.csm.2019.12.002.

11. Gaston RG, Chadderdon C. Phalangeal fractures displaced/nondisplaced. Hand Clin. 2012;28(3):395–401. https://doi.org/10.1016/j.hcl.2012.05.032.
12. Elfar J, Mann T. Fracture-dislocations of the proximal interphalangeal joint. J Am Acad Orthop Surg. 2013;21(2):88–98. https://doi.org/10.5435/jaaos-21-02-88.
13. Rozmaryn LM. The collateral ligament of the digits of the hand: anatomy, physiology, biomechanics, injury, and treatment. J Hand Surg. 2017;42(11):904–15. https://doi.org/10.1016/j.jhsa.2017.08.024.

Adult Metacarpal Base and CMC Dislocations Fractures

11

Anthony L. Logli and Sanjeev Kakar

Background

Metacarpal base and carpometacarpal (CMC) fracture-dislocations are relatively uncommon injuries in hand trauma [1]. While seeming to occur infrequently, they may also be underreported or underdiagnosed given subtle radiographic findings or the presence of other, more obvious concomitant injuries. Unfortunately, failure to accurately recognize and properly treat these injuries may lead to considerable long-term morbidity with deleterious effects on grip strength, motion, and dexterity [2–5]. Adverse sequelae of posttraumatic osteoarthritis, tendon rupture, instability, and/or poor cosmesis are also associated with missed injuries [2–5]. Due to the rarity of metacarpal base and CMC fracture-dislocations, no clear consensus on management exists [1, 6]. However, several guiding principles, gleaned from retrospective series and collective surgeon experience, can be followed in order to increase the likelihood of a successful outcome. As always, in order to develop a sound understanding of the guiding principles for metacarpal base and CMC fracture-dislocation management, one must first have a detailed understanding of the relevant anatomy.

Anatomy

There is generally robust, inherent stability to the second through fifth CMC joints due to the surrounding soft tissue anatomy. The dorsal and palmar CMC ligaments, interosseous ligaments, and capsule serve as static restraints to joint motion, while the tendinous insertions of the ECRL, ECRB, and ECU on the second, third, and

A. L. Logli (✉) · S. Kakar
Department of Orthopedic Surgery, Mayo Clinic, Rochester, MN, USA
e-mail: logli.anthony@mayo.edu; kakar.sanjeev@mayo.edu

fifth metacarpal bases, respectively, afford an element of dynamic stability during wrist extension, deviation, or gripping maneuvers [1, 7]. The hypothenar musculature is thought to confer an additional element of stability to the fifth CMC joint it traverses [7].

Dorsal CMC ligaments are stronger than palmar ligaments [8]. There are two dorsal ligaments for every CMC joint with the exception of the third, which has three dorsal ligamentous strips. There is also one palmar CMC ligament for every joint with the exception of the third, which has four ligamentous strips [9]. A discrete intra-articular ligament located between the third and fourth metacarpal and another between the capitate and hamate has also been identified. These ligaments seem to impart robust CMC joint stability even in the absence of functionally competent palmar and dorsal ligaments [9].

Inspection of the articulation of the second and third metacarpal bases demonstrates greater joint surface area and concavity with the trapezoid and capitate, respectively. This bony relationship inherently confers more joint constraint and stability compared to the fourth and fifth CMC joints that have less congruent geometry [8]. This may explain why the ulnar CMC joints require lower mechanisms of injury to incur dislocation [8] (Fig. 11.1). The ulnar fourth and fifth CMC joints also have a lower threshold to injury because the strength of the static CMC restraints incrementally decreases from radial to ulnar and allows more inherent mobility in the fourth and fifth CMC joints [10].

While dynamic CMC joint stabilizers typically resist motion across the CMC joint, they also may generate a forceful pull and impart a displacing force. An avulsion fracture injury, occurring when the muscular pull at its tendinous insertion overcomes the strength of the dorsal metaphyseal bone of the proximal metacarpal, is an excellent example of this paradox. One of the most commonly observed metacarpal base fractures is an intra-articular fracture of the fifth metacarpal. A strong pull from the ECU tendon can cause an avulsion fracture that mirrors a Bennett fracture of the thumb and is thus sometimes referred to as a "reverse Bennett fracture" or "baby Bennett fracture" [11]. In this type of metacarpal base fracture, the fifth metacarpal shaft migrates proximally and ulnarly with the pull of the ECU and hypothenar muscle, respectively, while the radial condyle remains attached to the fourth metacarpal through the strong intermetacarpal ligament and flexor carpi ulnaris (FCU) attachments volarly [12, 13].

While a reverse Bennett injury is one of the most common examples of a metacarpal base fracture, other more unusual case reports have been published. Avulsed fracture fragments of the second metacarpal due to the pull of the ECRL on the radial condyle have been found in the carpal tunnel region [14], in the forearm [4], impinging under the extensor pollicis longus (EPL) tendon in the anatomic snuffbox [5], and having sharply transected the EPL tendon [2]. Conversely, the radial condyle of the index metacarpal may remain in place, stabilized by the ECRL and intermetacarpal ligament to the thumb metacarpal, and the ulnar condyle or entire second metacarpal can dislocate [15, 16]. Avulsion fractures of the ECRB are even more rare and may occur with the bony fragment attached [3, 17, 18] or with the

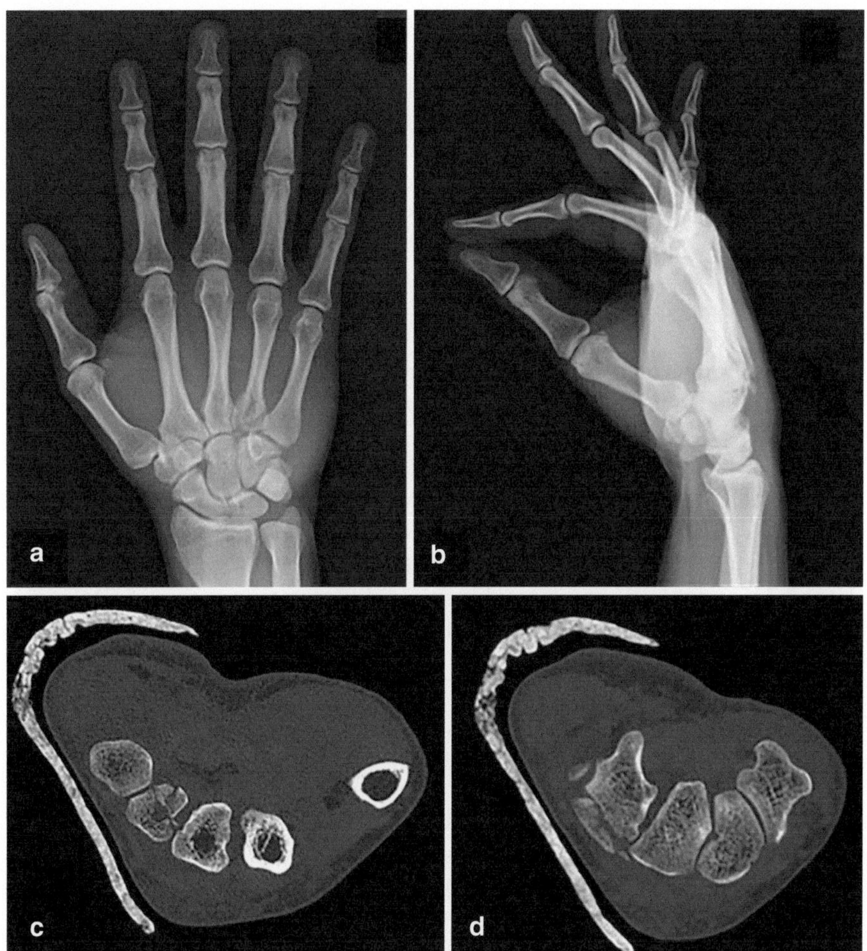

Fig. 11.1 A 36-year-old right hand dominant male struck a wall with a closed fist. He sustained a fourth and fifth CMC fracture-dislocation injury. AP radiograph of the right wrist shows a comminuted, intra-articular fracture of the fourth metacarpal base and a frank dislocation of the fifth metacarpal with superimposition of the metacarpal base over the hamate (**a**). Lateral radiograph shows a cortical irregularity dorsal to the hamate suggestive of fracture (**b**). The patient was reduced and splinted in the emergency department. Post-reduction CT demonstrates interval reduction of the fifth CMC joint and the fourth metacarpal base fracture in better detail (**c**), as well as confirmation of a dorsal hamate fracture (**d**)

bony fragment completely free [19]. In a 2008 review article on metacarpal base fractures, the authors identified only seven total cases of ECRB avulsion fractures in the literature [1].

Normal motion at the second and third CMC joints is more limited in flexion-extension (11°, 7°), radial-ulnar deviation (2°, 4°), and pronation-supination (5°, 5°) when comparted to the fourth and fifth CMC joints (20°, 27°; 7°, 13°; 27°,

22°, respectively) [10]. While less constrained, the fourth and fifth metacarpals resist an abduction moment due to their tether to the relatively immobile third metacarpal via the transverse intermetacarpal ligament [10]. The axis of rotation for digital flexion-extension lies within the metacarpal base of all respective CMC joints. Conversely, radial-ulnar and pronation-supination axes of rotation lie within the associated distal carpal bone; the third CMC joint is an exception with the center axis of rotation instead lying within the metacarpal base [10]. The fourth CMC joint includes articulations with the hamate and capitate 86% of the time. There are also four different reported morphologies of the fourth metacarpal base with various facet configurations [9, 20]. A fourth CMC fracture-dislocation in isolation occurs very uncommonly; bony articulations with adjacent third and fifth CMC joints, strong supporting ligaments, and absence of a muscular insertion to impose a deforming force at time of injury are thought to account for this finding [21].

The foundation for the fourth and fifth CMC joints is the hamate. The hamate represents a saddle surface with reasonably deep concavity for the fifth metacarpal while a flatter radial facet for the fourth metacarpal [7]. Motion of the fifth CMC joint is dependent on and contributed by the freedom of motion of the fourth CMC joint [10]. In a three-dimensional kinematic analysis of CMC joint motion, El-shennawy et al. found total flexion-extension motion to be reduced by 40% when the fourth CMC joint was immobilized experimentally by pin fixation [10].

When thinking about CMC injuries, we find it useful to consider the uncommonly discussed anatomic parallel found in the midfoot. The tarsometatarsal (TMT) joint, or Lisfranc joint, bears striking similarities and is also much more commonly injured and studied in the foot and ankle literature. For example, the native surrounding bony and ligamentous anatomy of the second and third TMT joints make for a more constrained articulation allowing little to any motion, while the fourth and fifth TMT joints have up to 10° of motion in the frontal and sagittal planes [22]. These differences in joint mobility have implications on treatment and the incidence of downstream sequelae as they do in the CMC joints of the hand. Discussion and treatment of TMT joint fracture-dislocations are often guided by a three column paradigm consisting of the medial column (navicular, medial cuneiform, and first metatarsal), the middle column (second and third metatarsals and intermediate and lateral cuneiforms), and the lateral column (fourth and fifth metatarsals and cuboid). Thinking of fractures surrounding the CMC joints in a similar fashion may present a useful construct by which to work with, study, and discuss these injuries. Therefore, the construct we propose is as such: radial column (thumb metacarpal, trapezium, and scaphoid), central column (second and third metacarpal, trapezoid, and capitate), and the ulnar column (fourth and fifth metacarpal and hamate) (Fig. 11.2).

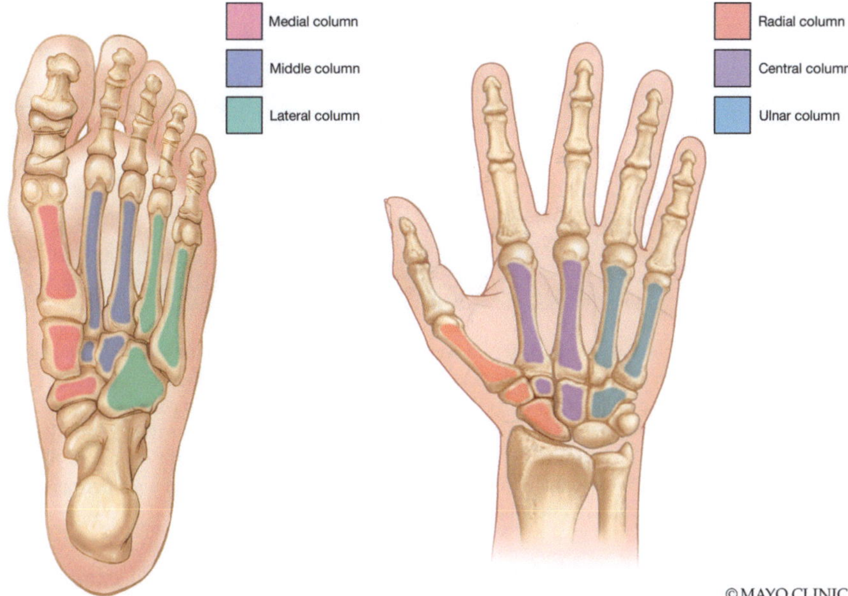

Fig. 11.2 Illustration depicting similarities between the tarsometatarsal or Lisfranc articulation in the foot to the carpometacarpal joints of the hand. The former is typically discussed in terms of three columns: medial, middle, and lateral. We propose a similar construct composed of a radial, central, and ulnar columns be considered for the hand. (Used with permission of Mayo Foundation for Medical Education and Research. All rights reserved)

Diagnosis and Imaging

History and Mechanism of Injury

As is the case with the majority of hand trauma, there is a higher incidence in the young and active population. Injuries tend to occur when fingers are in a position of flexion and a violent load is transmitted down the longitudinal axis of the metacarpal in a distal to proximal direction. A clenched fist striking an unyielding object such as with a punch is a common example of this [7, 23] (Fig. 11.1). Other proposed mechanisms of injury include a downward-directed force onto the dorsum of the hand during wrist flexion, enough to force dorsal dislocation or distraction of the metacarpal bases; or, a direct blow or vigorous force targeted at the palm of the hand, resulting in dorsal translation of the metacarpal bases [24]. Motorcycle or automobile collisions, a fall from height, or striking an object with a clenched fist are other mechanisms of injury [24]. The relatively greater inherent mobility of the ulnar column makes injury to this region more likely to occur by lower energy mechanisms [25]. Due to the difficultly in detecting an injury on radiographs, metacarpal base and CMC fracture-dislocation injuries can easily be overlooked at initial presentation causing a delay in diagnosis, an increase in complications, and poorer

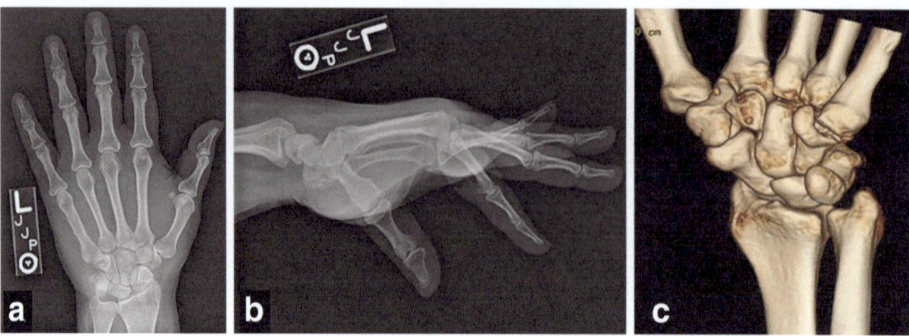

Fig. 11.3 A 58-year-old right hand dominant patient slipped and fell onto her outstretched left hand while at work. In the emergency department, AP (**a**) and lateral (**b**) X-rays of left wrist were initially read as negative. Patient presents for repeat evaluation 6 months later with continued pain and a CT was obtained. A three-dimensional rendering from this study demonstrated chronic volar dislocation of the fifth CMC joint with impaction into the hamate (**c**). Careful review of her presenting radiographs demonstrates the volar fifth CMC dislocation. ((**c**): Used with permission of Mayo Foundation for Medical Education and Research. All rights reserved)

long-term outcomes [24, 25] (Fig. 11.3). A comprehensive physical examination and careful assessment of appropriate imaging is therefore critical.

Physical Examination

Length, alignment, and rotation of the columns of the hand should be critically assessed as they are key to detecting a CMC dislocation or fracture-dislocation. Localized swelling, bruising, point tenderness in the CMC area, and/or a dorsal prominence are helpful signs of injury. In some instances, shortening or malrotation of the metacarpals is observed. Metacarpal shortening causes increased laxity to the extrinsic tendons that traverse the joint and may manifest as an extensor lag or difficulty with finger flexion [8]. The close anatomic proximity of the distal motor and sensory branches of ulnar nerve in the hand to the ulnar column can lead to acute numbness or weakness after a fracture-dislocation injury that should not be missed on physical examination prior to and after any attempted reduction maneuver [25]. Due to the higher energy mechanisms commonly seen in these injuries, patients should also be closely monitored for acute carpal tunnel syndrome that may develop at the time of presentation or even a few days after the inciting injury [24]. Finally, while less helpful in the acute setting, wrist motion and grip and pinch strength may be affected when patients are seen back after a missed injury.

Imaging

A standard radiographic series consisting of a PA, lateral, and two oblique views of the hand is routinely ordered when evaluating a traumatic hand injury. Abnormal overlapping of the CMC articular surfaces, a disruption in the distal Gilula's line

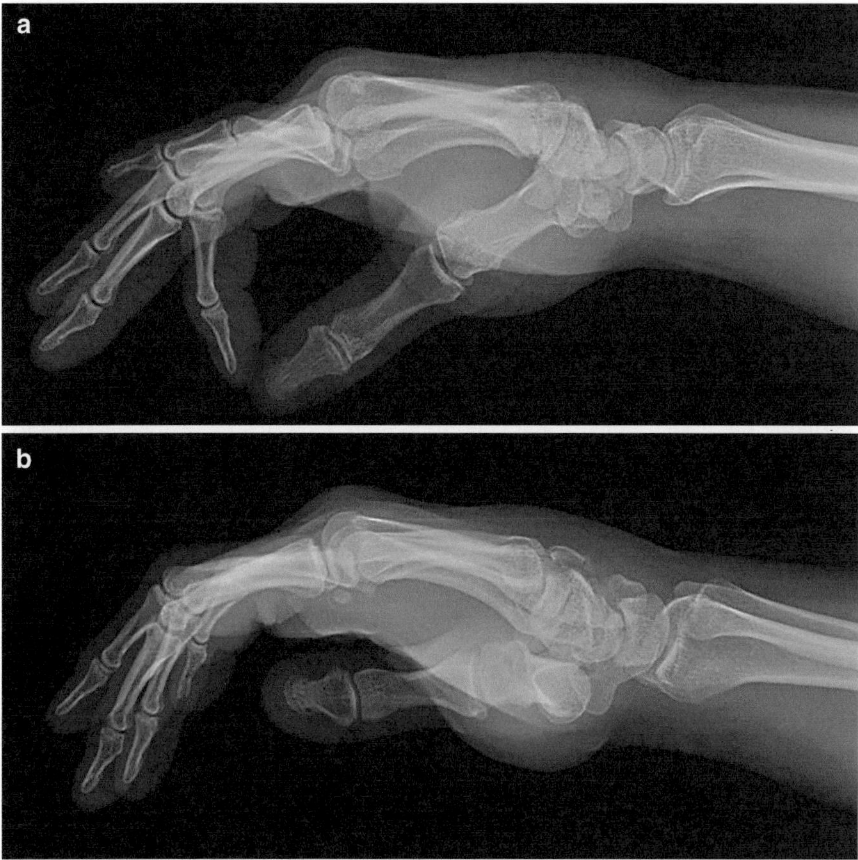

Fig. 11.4 Right wrist radiographs of a 35-year-old patient who punched an object. Due to bony overlap, it is difficult to discern a fracture on the true lateral view of the wrist (**a**). A 45° pronated oblique view of the same wrist portrays an acute comminuted fracture of the dorsal hamate (**b**)

[26], or shortening of the capitate may be gleaned from this standard series and be indicative of an injury in the CMC region. Unfortunately, on these routine views, the CMC joints are often obscured by bony overlap and subtle fracture or dislocation injuries may be missed [7]. Therefore, should history or physical examination be suggestive of CMC involvement, supplemental views may be helpful. A 30–45° pronated oblique view of the hand, for example, is useful in detecting and assessing the degree of displacement or dislocation of an intra-articular fracture of the fourth and/or fifth CMC joint [7, 27] (Fig. 11.4). McDonald et al. proposed the "intermeta-carpal angle screening test" for the diagnosis of fourth and fifth CMC joint fracture-dislocations [28]. The screening test is performed by measuring the angle between the index or middle finger's metacarpal shaft and that of the small finger. When an angle greater than 10° is obtained, these authors found reliable correlation to the presence of a CMC joint injury [28].

While substantial information may be gleaned from reviewing plain films, computed tomography (CT) is extremely valuable in understanding fracture characteristics, assessing articular congruency, and for treatment planning. Particularly if multiple joints are involved or significant fracture comminution is present, a post-reduction CT is helpful [29].

Classification Systems

In order to be useful, classification systems should be logical and comprehensive, have high inter- and intra-observer reliability, and guide clinical treatment. Due to the rarity of metacarpal base and CMC fracture-dislocation injuries, we are not aware of a classification system that has been described to characterize injuries involving the CMC joints of the central column. Conversely, many classification systems have been described for CMC fracture-dislocations of the ulnar column. Cain et al. described four patterns of injury characterized predominantly by the fracture of the hamate (Table 11.1).

Using CT scans, Kim and Shin as well as Lee et al. independently proposed classification systems with the intention of providing better guidance for surgeon decision making [29, 30]. These classification systems are more inclusive in that they

Table 11.1 Classification of hamatometacarpal fracture-dislocation injuries

Cain et al.		Possible treatment
Type I	Fifth MC base subluxation/dislocation and concomitant fourth metacarpal base fracture	Closed reduction and cast vs. CRPP[a]
A	Dorsal CMC ligament disruption	Closed reduction and cast vs. CRPP[a]
B	Dorsal hamate rim avulsion fracture	ORIF[b]
Type II	Type 1 + dorsal hamate comminution	ORIF
Type III	Type 1 + coronal split of hamate	ORIF
Lee et al.[c]		**Possible treatment**
Type I	<1/3 intra-articular hamate fracture	CRPP
Type II	>1/3 intra-articular hamate fracture	ORIF
Type III	Coronal split of the hamate	ORIF
A	No MC base fracture	
B	Fourth MC base fracture	
C	Fifth MC base fracture	
D	Fourth and fifth MC base fractures	

CMC carpometacarpal, *MC* metacarpal
[a] These injuries were closed reduced and tested for stability. If stable, casting alone was used. Unstable lesions underwent CRPP
[b] Occasionally, the fracture fragment was large enough to permit closed reduction and percutaneous pinning
[c] Each injury is assigned a type and letter

remove the need for a metacarpal fracture (i.e. hamate fracture with pure dislocation of fourth and/or fifth metacarpals) while also providing the possibility of a hamato-metacarpal fracture-dislocation injury that does not involve a fracture of the fourth metacarpal base [29, 30] (Table 11.1).

Dislocated, intra-articular base of the fifth metacarpal fractures, aka reverse Bennett fractures, has been classified into four unique fracture patterns [31–33]. First described by Niechajev et al., these are as follows: type I—oblique radial fracture; type II—Y- or T-shaped fracture similar to the Rolando fracture of the thumb metacarpal; type III—comminuted fracture with separate intermediary intra-articular fragment; type IV—avulsion fracture with small fragment attached to the intermetacarpal ligament [33].

Treatment

Due to the infrequency with which metacarpal base and CMC fracture-dislocation injuries occur, no consensus exists regarding their optimal treatment. However, regardless of the treatment strategy, what has certainly been demonstrated is that the time to definitive intervention is of utmost importance for a successful outcome [7, 34].

Nonoperative

Nonoperative treatment consisting of a closed reduction and splint or cast application is reserved for CMC fracture-dislocations and metacarpal base fractures with minimal or no displacement. If the injury meets these criteria and is a stable fracture injury with low risk of secondary displacement, then nonoperative treatment may be considered. Some authors advocate for closed reduction and intraoperative assessment of stability as a first attempt for these injuries [35]. Plans for open intervention with internal fixation are then dictated by a failed attempt at closed reduction under general anesthesia [35]. Residual joint displacement, joint subluxation, or an incongruent reduction warrants an open reduction to reduce the risk of ongoing pain, posttraumatic CMC arthritis, stiffness, and weakness of grip strength.

If nonoperative treatment is elected, the applied splint starts distal to the elbow and may be volarly, dorsally, or volarly and dorsally based. The wrist is immobilized in approximately 30° of extension, and the MCP joints are left unimpeded until the fracture heals [12]. The semi-extended wrist position is thought to minimize the deforming pull of the extensor tendons on the proximal aspect of the metacarpal. A nonoperative treatment pathway may also be considered for those patients who are extremely low demand or medically ill. It is critical that these patients are followed closely with accurate radiographic imaging to ensure the CMC joints remain anatomically aligned.

Crinchlow and Hoskinson as well as Jessa and Hodge each separately described nonoperative treatment for ECRL avulsion fractures [36, 37]. Two of the three patients treated with plaster immobilization in the Crinchlow and Hoskinson series had a "satisfactory" result with full recovery of wrist motion and strength, while one patient developed a symptomatic dorsal CMC boss that underwent surgical removal [36]. These authors suggest that the inherent lack of motion in the second CMC joint makes restoration of the articular surface less critical and ECRL retraction is unlikely to occur as long as the intermetacarpal ligaments and ligamentous slips to the thumb and third metacarpal all remain intact. Jessa and Hodge discuss nonoperative treatment of two patients but do not report any outcome results [37]. Treble and Arif [5] agree that joint surface restoration is less important in second CMC fracture-dislocations but still advocate for an open reduction to avoid retraction of the avulsed bony fragment and such sequelae as loss of grip strength, wrist extension strength, and motion [4], or less likely, an EPL tendon rupture [2].

Petrie and colleagues reported on the outcome of 23 cases of reverse Bennett fractures treated with early active mobilization and found minimal deficits in grip strength, an average of 3 weeks missed work, and only one patient with residual pain [13]. These authors acknowledge the inability to comment on the risk of subsequent osteoarthritis. In a retrospective study of 37 largely military personnel, Lundeen and Shin treated patients with an initial reduction consisting of 5 kg of longitudinal traction and finger traps on the ring and small fingers followed by digital pressure dorsally over the metacarpal base as well as extension of the metacarpal shaft [32]. Patients were then immobilized in a short arm cast with aluminum outriggers maintaining the ring and small finger MCP joints at 70° of flexion. Twenty of the 22 patients treated in this manner returned for follow-up at a mean 43-months and had excellent or good results, 98% grip strength compared to the contralateral side, and return to full duty by a mean of 6 weeks. While the long-term development of osteoarthritis was again not captured by this study, 13 had none, and 9 had mild arthrosis at final follow-up [32].

Despite reports of success with closed reduction and immobilization for reverse Bennett fractures, others have found decreased grip strength, progressive displacement, non-anatomic alignment, ongoing pain, and risk of delayed osteoarthritis with nonoperative treatment [7, 31, 38]. Therefore, some authors advocate for CRPP for these injuries [33, 38].

Operative

The mainstay of second to fifth CMC fracture-dislocations is anatomic reduction with percutaneous or internal fixation of the metacarpal base and/or carpal component. This can be done under fluoroscopic control with care taken to ensure an anatomic reduction. If any doubt exists as to the quality of the reduction, an open reduction should be performed. Once the skin is incised, care must be taken to identify and protect cutaneous nerve branches. The extensor tendons are then retracted to the either side of the joint and the cortical bone is approached through the elevation of full-thickness subperiosteal flaps. Fracture hematoma is debrided until all fracture edges can be easily visualized. Various methods of operative fixation have been described. Kirschner wires (K-wires) or Steinmann pins may be placed across the CMC joint or traversing multiple metacarpals. Plate and screw fixation including spanning plates have also been used [34]. When implanted, percutaneous K-wires are typically left in place for 4–6 weeks, while buried K-wires may remain until the soft tissues and fractures are completely healed. Plate and screw fixation constructs are left indefinitely (except for spanning plates which are removed after fracture union) unless they became symptomatic or strong patient desire for implant removal.

As noted above, closed reduction and percutaneous K-wires can be used to treat single or multiple CMC fracture-dislocations providing an anatomic reduction is obtained. In passing the K-wires, care must be paid to the close anatomic proximity of the flexor and extensor tendons, Guyon's canal, and the deep motor and sensory branches of the ulnar nerve to avoid iatrogenic injury. This is of utmost importance when performing pin fixation of the ulnar column. Some authors have attempted to describe guiding principles to ensure safe pin fixation into the hamate [39, 40]. Saing et al. reported three cases of deep motor branch of the ulnar nerve injury after using the "traditional trajectory of pin placement toward the base of the hook of the hamate" during closed reduction and percutaneous pinning of a fourth and fifth CMC joint [40]. Based on their experience, these authors suggest a more midaxial K-wire starting point on the proximal metacarpal and aiming instead at the center of the hamate body to decrease the likelihood of penetrating the volar cortex of the hamate and causing an iatrogenic nerve injury [40]. To provide more specific recommendations for safe placement of a retrograde K-wire across the fifth CMC joint, Mozaffarian et al. performed a cadaveric study assessing possible damage to the ulnar neurovascular bundle, flexor, and extensor tendons [39]. These authors found a safe corridor to most reliably be achieved when the K-wire starts 2 cm distal to the metacarpal base in the midaxial part of the fifth metacarpal with a 20–30° trajectory in the coronal plane and in the range of 10° volar to dorsal to 20° dorsal to volar in the sagittal plane [39].

Internal fixation is another option to consider especially with the advent of contemporary low profile, fragment-specific, and anatomically designed plate and screw options. Tay et al. described their experience using a low profile, 1.5 mm dorsal buttress plate to span the fourth and/or fifth CMC joints. This procedure relies on monocortical locking screw fixation in the hamate and none distally, thereby allowing the CMC joint continued mobility postoperatively [21]. This technique was originally described by Tan et al. [41]. In their cohort of 11 patients, mean time to union was 48 days, grip strength was 79% of the contralateral side, and all fingers achieved full range of motion without scissoring at median of 34 weeks follow-up. Five of 11 patients had removal of implants due to plate breakage, pain, or cold intolerance. These authors suggest that for fractures where there is clearly a proximally and dorsally directed deforming force, such as the fourth and/or fifth CMC joints, buttress plate fixation is a viable option allowing early motion postoperatively. Iwata et al. employed a similar technique in a case report of fracture-dislocation of the fifth CMC joint with avulsion fracture of the hamate [42]. These authors used a 2.3 mm locking T-plate spanning the capitohamate articulation with monocortical screw fixation in the capitate alone as an adjunct to percutaneous K-wire pinning of the fourth and fifth CMC joints fractures. In patients with comminuted fracture-dislocations that are not amenable to K-wire stabilization or plate fixation, we may consider a temporary spanning plate locked proximally and distally to stabilize the injury.

While there has been some success with nonoperative treatment of second and third CMC fracture-dislocation injuries, these injuries on the whole seem to be do better with surgical treatment. Their inherent relative rigidity compared to the ulnar column may be more forgiving to minor articular malreductions, but restoration of the insertion and function of the avulsed ECRL and ECRB tendons and their contribution to wrist motion and strength seems to be a major advantage of open reduction and internal fixation for these injuries [1]. In their 2008 review of literature, Bushnell et al. captured 17 total cases of surgically treated metacarpal base fractures due to ECRL ($n = 10$) and ECRB avulsions ($n = 7$) of the second and third metacarpals, respectively [1]. With the exception of only one case of an ECRL avulsion fracture in which the insertion was incompletely restored and led to deficits in strength and motion [4], all patients with second metacarpal base fractures were described as returning to normal function after open reduction and K-wire fixation [1]. Similarly, in the seven cases of ECRB avulsion fractures treated with surgery, all had good outcomes with the exception of one patient with some residual loss of grip strength at 7 months postoperatively [19] and another that required hardware removal for symptomatic implants [43]. A number of alternative surgical techniques have been employed for third metacarpal base fractures including tension band wire constructs [3, 17, 43], sutures through bone tunnels [17], lag screws [18, 19, 44, 45], and suture anchors [18, 19, 44, 45].

Some authors advocate for surgical intervention for reverse Bennett fractures [33, 38]. More specifically, they recommend CRPP for simple base of the fifth metacarpal fractures and ORIF for those that are comminuted with the goal of restoring articular congruity. In the series by Niechajev, 23 patients treated in this manner, 21 of 23 patients were available at a mean of 18 months postoperatively, and all of them had returned to work by 2–3 months after surgery. Further, 62% of patients were asymptomatic, while the remaining patients had local tenderness, occasional rest pain, slight weakness in grip, and residual swelling at the fracture site recorded at final follow-up [33].

To avoid sequelae of internal fixation—symptomatic hardware, adhesions and stiffness—while also benefiting from the advantages of K-wire fixation—less invasive, transient hardware—Miyamoto et al. reported on a technique that involves locked fixation of percutaneously placed K-wires using a patented external connector device that theoretically offers robust stability and early mobilization [46]. Miyamoto et al. report favorable results at 15-month follow-up with mean QuickDASH of 6.36, grip strength 96% of the contralateral side, and 100% union [46].

Arthrodesis

In select cases, when significantly comminuted CMC fracture-dislocations occur, primary arthrodesis may also be performed as the initial treatment [25]. This approach is thought to be better tolerated in fracture-dislocations involving the central column due to the rigidity of the second and third CMC joints at baseline. At the time of index fracture fixation, however, it is impossible to predict those fracture injuries that will go on to develop symptomatic arthritis or those that a patient cannot compensate or modify their activity to overcome. Therefore, unless the fracture is completely unamenable to fixation, we would reserve arthrodesis as a salvage option.

Salvage

Even when prompt and effective treatment of CMC fracture injuries is performed, patients can develop symptomatic posttraumatic osteoarthritis. In these instances, the most reliable and reproducible salvage operation for a painful and arthritic CMC joint is a CMC joint arthrodesis [25]. In their series of 20 patients with CMC fracture-dislocations, two patients had a salvage arthrodesis, one at 4 months and another at 10 months, after a dorsal second and third CMC fracture-dislocation failed closed reduction and immobilization. One patient had full grip strength and was immediately able to return to work, albeit with significant pain, while the other had 59% grip strength compared to the contralateral side and was unable to return to work due to disabling pain. Both patients underwent second and third CMC joint arthrodesis with the former having a subsequently excellent outcome, while the latter only achieved a satisfactory result [25].

Clendenin and Smith report their experience with fifth metacarpal/hamate arthrodesis using iliac crest bone graft for symptomatic posttraumatic osteoarthritis secondary to prior CMC fracture-dislocation in seven patients with average 2-year follow-up [11]. Fusion was performed in 20–30° of flexion with the graft press fit into a dorsally created slot and sometimes supplemented with pins. These authors found marked to complete pain relief and return to pre-injury occupation in all patients with full flexion-extension and an improvement in grip strength by 48% [11]. Further, they described using a pre-surgical diagnostic injection of local anesthetic into the fifth CMC joint to isolate the source of pain and reject the idea of additionally needing to fuse the fourth CMC joint if not a pain generator. Once fused, it is important to note that the normal mobility of the transverse carpal arch is permanently altered and metacarpal motion occurs through the hamate-triquetral articulation [47]. Importantly, given load transference to this adjacent joint, there is a risk of future secondary arthritis at this articulation in addition to the standard risks of delayed union, nonunion, and infection associated with any fusion surgery [48].

To provide an alternative to arthrodesis surgery and its inherent risks, Green and Kilgore performed three cases of fifth metacarpal resection and hemiarthroplasty using a stemmed Silastic toe prosthesis [47]. The major benefit of this approach is maintenance of motion. Final follow-up occurred 9 months to 2 years after surgery and all patients were without pain, had 15° to full arc of CMC motion, and good grip strength [47]. Alternatively, Gainor et al. reported on ten cases of base of the fifth metacarpal excisional arthroplasty with interposition of a rolled palmaris longus tendon autograft spacer [48]. At a mean follow-up of 5 years, they reported good to excellent functional and cosmetic results and maintained hand motion and power grip without the loss of metacarpal height, malalignment, or malrotation [48]. The Dubert procedure or "stabilization arthroplasty of the fifth ray" described in 1994 is another non-fusion salvage option [49]. This procedure involves resection of the fifth metacarpal base with fusion of the residual proximal fifth metacarpal to the fourth metacarpal. Using a variation of this technique on five patients with posttraumatic osteoarthritis of the small finger, Bain et al. report low pain and high visual analogue satisfaction scores in addition to preserved motion and grip strength [50].

While these resections, tissue interpositions, and silicone arthroplasties have been reported, long-term results and their reliability, in addition to their role in CMC joints outside of the small finger, are unknown.

Hamatometacarpal Base Fracture-Dislocation

CMC fracture-dislocations involving a fracture of the distal carpal row are even more rare than those involving the metacarpal base (Fig. 11.5). These unique injuries are thought to represent 26% of all CMC fracture-dislocations [24]. First classified by Cain et al. in 1987, hamatometacarpal fracture-dislocations are the most common carpometacarpal fracture-dislocation involving a carpal fracture [24, 27]. The mechanism of injury is similar to fracture-dislocations involving a metacarpal fracture. Instead, the fracture location and type of fracture line are likely dependent on the degree of palmar flexion of the digit at the time of injury [27]. Further, Cain et al. suggest that load transmission at the time of injury is always initiated through the fourth metacarpal first, therefore always involving a fourth metacarpal base fracture [27]. Once the fourth metacarpal is shortened, then the load is transferred to the more mobile fifth CMC joint through the strong intermetacarpal ligaments. Based on the degree of palmar flexion of the digit at the time of injury, various patterns of metacarpal base and/or hamate fractures may occur. These authors report that closed reduction and immobilization is typically sufficient for Type I fractures if the joint is stable, with pinning and open reduction and internal fixation reserved for Type Ia and Type Ib fractures, respectively (Table 11.1). Type II and III fractures necessitated open reduction and fixation to restore a congruent joint surface. As previously mentioned, Lee et al. expanded upon the Cain classification system using CT imaging to characterize the amount of hamate involvement and to be more inclusive of a variety of metacarpal base fractures (Table 11.1) [30]. When treating patients according to the fracture type, as defined by the fracture line of the hamate and percentage of the hamate involved, these authors reported good to excellent results in 35 of 37 patients treated. As such, they advocated closed reduction and percutaneous pinning for Type I fractures (with stable hamate fractures), and open reduction with internal fixation of all Type II and Type III fractures with unstable hamate fractures [30].

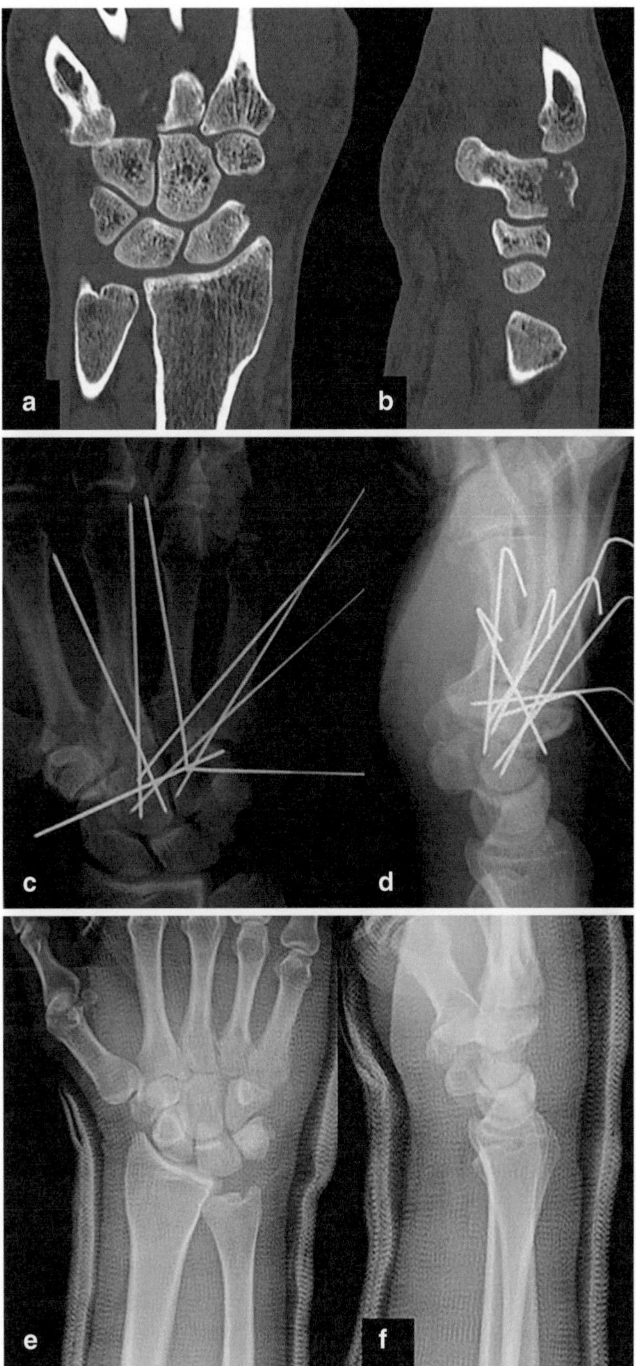

Fig. 11.5 Coronal (**a**) and sagittal (**b**) CT scan sections of right wrist demonstrating third through fifth CMC dislocations with comminuted fracture of the dorsal hamate. AP (**c**) and lateral (**d**) views of the wrist after open reduction and percutaneous pinning were performed 5 days after injury. Pins were removed at 7 weeks, and a short arm cast was applied (**e** and **f**)

Other Distal Carpal Row Fracture-Dislocation

Other fracture-dislocations affecting the carpal bones of the central column (e.g. trapezoid and capitate) may also occur. Mechanism of injury is again no different. Early recognition and expeditious reduction of trapezoid or capitate fracture-dislocations is highly recommended. Unlike unstable hamatometacarpal injuries, dorsally displaced metacarpals of the central column indirectly cause narrowing of the nearby carpal canal and may lead to the development of median nerve compression or entrapment. Garcia-Elias et al. found three cases of acute carpal tunnel syndrome among five patients who had a diagnostic delay in the presence of a CMC fracture-dislocation while there were no cases of carpal tunnel syndrome in the eight patients who had immediate recognition and treatment [24]. Garcia-Elias et al. found predictably good results in their series of second and third CMC fracture-dislocations involving the trapezoid and capitate as long as they were treated without delay [24].

Complications

Some of the more common complications associated with both nonoperative and operative treatment of metacarpal base and CMC fracture-dislocations include diminished grip strength and range of motion, continued pain, and a prominent carpal boss [25]. As previously mentioned, arthrodesis is a viable salvage option to effectively address symptoms of continued pain. As an alternative, some authors advocate for corrective osteotomy and capsulectomy for painful malunions with the rationale that correction of the deformity has the potential to improve hand function and dexterity enough to allow a patient to return to their functional needs [51]. Freeland and Lily suggested two possible strategies when considering metacarpal osteotomy for this indication [51]. The first is to act early with an osteotomy performed within 10 weeks of malunion in order to maximize early recovery of motion and to prevent the formation of scar, adhesions, or contractures that may alter hand and finger mechanics; the second strategy involves intervening later and after allowing patients to reach maximum clinical improvement despite the malunion. In the later strategy, they suggest repeating a clinical and physical examination at 3 months or later to see if the patient has adequately compensated or would still benefit from a corrective osteotomy [51].

Black et al. described CMC joint resection arthroplasty for 13 cases of isolated fifth metacarpal malunion and three cases of fourth and fifth metacarpal malunions treated without surgery [52]. At mean of 28-months of follow-up, they reported ten patients as being completely asymptomatic, all patients returned to full work, full grip strength, and retained motion of 25° and 15° of motion at the CMC joints for the small and ring fingers, respectively. Three patients had continued pain and underwent revision surgery, one with CMC joint arthrodesis and two with revision resection arthroplasty [52].

The deep motor branch of the ulnar nerve is at risk both during initial fracture injury and during the surgical treatment of metacarpal base and CMC fracture-dislocation injuries [25, 40, 53–55]. Peterson et al. reported the case of a fifth metacarpal base fracture associated with an ulnar motor branch neuropraxia after a closed reduction and casting was performed [55]. The neuropraxia was identified as intrinsic weakness and wasting 4 weeks after injury once the cast was removed, and it completely resolved by 4 months postoperatively. The authors are unclear if the nerve symptoms were due to the space-occupying effect of the fracture fragment and hematoma or due to the cast application and molding. Murphy et al. described a missed fifth metacarpal base fracture with volar dislocation of the metacarpal shaft that presented 8 weeks after injury with persistent weakness, aching in the hypothenar eminence, and wasting of the intrinsic musculature. The authors performed an ORIF with K-wires as well as exploration of the Guyon's canal and ulnar nerve neurolysis. By 4 months postoperatively, the patient had almost fully recovered [54]. Saing et al. reported on three cases after CRPP of fourth and fifth CMC fracture-dislocations presenting 3–4 weeks postoperatively with a claw hand and weak intrinsics [40]. All patients were treated with pin removal and ulnar nerve neurolysis with full recovery noted 16 weeks to 9 months postoperatively.

Psychological Influence on Outcomes

In their systematic review, Chaves et al. offer a unique perspective on patients who typically sustain a metacarpal base or CMC fracture-dislocation injury [6]. Their perception is, given the most common mechanism associated with these injuries is a fist strike—secondary to a fight, assault, or self-mutilation—this patient population has a unique and consistent psychological profile and set of personality traits that impacts treatment and outcomes on multiple levels [6]. The example these authors use for comparison is patients who sustain a fifth metacarpal neck fracture or "boxer's fracture." Mercan et al. specifically compared the psychopathology and personality features of patients with boxer's fractures to a healthy control group of other patients who sustained an alternative upper extremity fracture. These authors found significantly higher rates of anxiety and maladaptive personality traits present in patients with boxer's fractures [56]. If these findings could be extrapolated to metacarpal base and CMC fracture-dislocations based on mechanism alone, it would provide some explanation for other findings seen in this population, namely poor follow-up rates and long delays prior seeking treatment [6].

Summary

Metacarpal base and CMC fracture-dislocations are uncommon hand injuries that require prompt recognition and treatment to avoid debilitating sequelae. While some series report reasonably good results with nonoperative treatment, the vast majority are indicated for surgery. Closed reduction and percutaneous pinning may be appropriate when an anatomic reduction can be obtained. Failing that, an open reduction may be necessary. The goal of surgery is to restore strength and dexterity while avoiding complications of persistent pain, nonunion, malunion, and posttraumatic osteoarthritis. If addressed early, results can be good to excellent. Although several creative salvage alternatives have been described, chronic metacarpal base and CMC fracture-dislocations or those that have gone on to develop posttraumatic arthritis are most reliably treated with CMC joint arthrodesis. Social and situational factors may influence outcomes so one should be reminded that it is more important to treat the individual patient and not just the injury.

References

1. Bushnell BD, Draeger RW, Crosby CG, Bynum DK. Management of intra-articular metacarpal base fractures of the second through fifth metacarpals. J Hand Surg. 2008;33(4):573–83.
2. Cassell O, Vidal P. An unreported cause of rupture of the extensor pollicis longus tendon. J Hand Surg. 1996;21(5):640–1.
3. Cobbs KF, Owens WS, Berg EE. Extensor carpi radialis brevis avulsion fracture of the long finger metacarpal: a case report. J Hand Surg. 1996;21(4):684–6.
4. Sadr B, Lalehzarian M. Traumatic avulsion of the tendon of extensor carpi radialis longus. J Hand Surg. 1987;12(6):1035–7.
5. Treble N, Arif S. Avulsion fracture of the index metacarpal. J Hand Surg. 1987;12(1):1–2.
6. Chaves C, Dubert T. Ulnar-sided carpometacarpal fractures and fractures-dislocations. A systematic review and publication guidelines. Orthop Traumatol Surg Res. 2020;106(8):1637–43.
7. Bora FWA Jr, Didizian NH. The treatment of injuries to the carpometacarpal joint of the little finger. JBJS. 1974;56(7):1459–63.
8. Mueller JJ. Carpometacarpal dislocations: report of five cases and review of the literature. J Hand Surg. 1986;11(2):184–8.
9. Nakamura K, Patterson RM, Viegas SF. The ligament and skeletal anatomy of the second through fifth carpometacarpal joints and adjacent structures. J Hand Surg. 2001;26(6):1016–29.
10. El-shennawy M, Nakamura K, Patterson RM, Viegas SF. Three-dimensional kinematic analysis of the second through fifth carpometacarpal joints. J Hand Surg. 2001;26(6):1030–5.
11. Clendenin MB, Smith RJ. Fifth metacarpal/hamate arthrodesis for posttraumatic osteoarthritis. J Hand Surg. 1984;9(3):374–8.
12. Dukas AG, Wolf JM. Management of complications of periarticular fractures of the distal interphalangeal, proximal interphalangeal, metacarpophalangeal, and carpometacarpal joints. Hand Clin. 2015;31(2):179–92.
13. Petrie PW, Lamb DW. Fracture-subluxation of base of fifth metacarpal. Hand. 1974;6(1):82–6.
14. Thomas WO, Gottliebson W, D'Amore T, Harris C, Parry S. Isolated palmar displaced fracture of the base of the index metacarpal: a case report. J Hand Surg. 1994;19(3):455–6.
15. Kuschner SH, Shepard L, Stephens S, Gellman H. Fracture of the index metacarpal base with subluxation of the trapeziometacarpal joint. A case report. Clin Orthop Relat Res. 1991;264:197–9.
16. Takami H, Takahashi S, Ando M. Isolated volar displaced fracture of the ulnar condyle at the base of the index metacarpal: a case report. J Hand Surg. 1997;22(6):1064–6.
17. Rotman MB, Pruitt DL. Avulsion fracture of the extensor carpi radialis brevis insertion. J Hand Surg. 1993;18(3):511–3.
18. Tsiridis E, Kohls-Gatzoulis J, Schizas C. Avulsion fracture of the extensor carpi radialis brevis insertion. J Hand Surg Br. 2001;26(6):596–8.

19. Boles SD, Durbin RA. Simultaneous ipsilateral avulsion of the extensor carpi radialis longus and brevis tendon insertions: case report and review of the literature. J Hand Surg. 1999;24(4):845–9.
20. Viegas SF, Patterson RM, Hokanson JA, Davis J. Wrist anatomy: incidence, distribution, and correlation of anatomic variations, tears, and arthrosis. J Hand Surg. 1993;18(3):463–75.
21. Tay S, Leow M, Tan E. Use of dorsal buttress plate fixation for ulnar carpometacarpal joint fracture dislocations for early mobilization: outcomes of 11 cases. Musculoskelet Surg. 2019;103(1):77–82.
22. Root M. Biomechanical examination of the foot. J Am Podiatry Assoc. 1973;63(1):28–9.
23. Yoshida R, Shah MA, Patterson RM, Buford WL Jr, Knighten J, Viegas SF. Anatomy and pathomechanics of ring and small finger carpometacarpal joint injuries. J Hand Surg. 2003;28(6):1035–43.
24. Garcia-Elias M, Bishop A, Dobyns J, Cooney W, Linscheid R. Transcarpal carpometacarpal dislocations, excluding the thumb. J Hand Surg. 1990;15(4):531–40.
25. Lawlis J III, Gunther S. Carpometacarpal dislocations. Long-term follow-up. JBJS Am. 1991;73(1):52–9.
26. Gilula L. Carpal injuries: analytic approach and case exercises. Am J Roentgenol. 1979;133(3):503–17.
27. Cain JE Jr, Shepler TR, Wilson MR. Hamatometacarpal fracture-dislocation: classification and treatment. J Hand Surg. 1987;12(5):762–7.
28. McDonald LS, Shupe PG, Hammel N, Kroonen LT. The intermetacarpal angle screening test for ulnar-sided carpometacarpal fracture-dislocations. J Hand Surg. 2012;37(9):1839–44.
29. Kim JK, Shin SJ. A novel hamatometacarpal fracture–dislocation classification system based on CT scan. Injury. 2012;43(7):1112–7.
30. Lee S-U, Park I-J, Kim H-M, Jeong C, Oh J-R. Fourth and fifth carpometacarpal fracture and dislocation of the hand: new classification and treatment. Eur J Orthop Surg Traumatol. 2012;22(7):571–8.
31. Kjaer-Petersen K, Jurik A, Petersen L. Intra-articular fractures at the base of the fifth metacarpal: a clinical and radiographical study of 64 cases. J Hand Surg. 1992;17(2):144–7.
32. Lundeen JM, Shin AY. Clinical results of intraarticular fractures of the base of the fifth metacarpal treated by closed reduction and case immobilization. J Hand Surg Br. 2000;25(3):258–61.
33. Niechajev I. Dislocated intra-articular fracture of the base of the fifth metacarpal: a clinical study of 23 patients. Plast Reconstr Surg. 1985;75(3):406–10.
34. Schortinghuis J, Klasen H. Open reduction and internal fixation of combined fourth and fifth carpometacarpal (fracture) dislocations. J Trauma Acute Care Surg. 1997;42(6):1052–5.
35. Gehrmann S, Kaufmann R, Grassmann J, Lögters T, Schädel-Höpfner M, Hakimi M, et al. Fracture-dislocations of the carpometacarpal joints of the ring and little finger. J Hand Surg Eur Vol. 2015;40(1):84–7.
36. Crichlow T, Hoskinson J. Avulsion fracture of the index metacarpal base: three case report. J Hand Surg. 1988;13(2):212–4.
37. Jessa KK, Hodge JC. Avulsion fracture of tendon of extensor carpi radialis longus: unknown mechanism. J Emerg Med. 1997;15(2):201–7.
38. Goedkoop A, van Onselen E, Karim R, Hage J. The 'mirrored' Bennett fracture of the base of the fifth metacarpal. Arch Orthop Trauma Surg. 2000;120(10):592–3.
39. Mozaffarian K, Vosoughi AR, Hedjazi A, Zarenezhad M, Nazmi MK. The safest direction of percutaneous pinning for achieving firm fixing of the fifth carpometacarpal joint. J Orthop Sci. 2012;17(6):757–62.
40. Saing MH, Lee SY, Raphael JS. Percutaneous pinning of fifth carpal–metacarpal fracture–dislocations: an alternative pin trajectory. Hand. 2008;3(3):251–6.
41. Tan ES, Chao TS. Dorsal buttress plate fixation of ulnar carpometacarpal joint fracture dislocations. THUES. 2016;20(2):77–82.
42. Iwata N, Komura S, Hirakawa A, Kanamori S, Masuda T, Ito Y, et al. Dorsal buttress plate fixation for the treatment of fracture–dislocation of the fifth carpometacarpal joint with avulsion fracture of the hamate: a case report. Arch Orthop Trauma Surg. 2019;139(1):135–9.

43. Voigt C. Osseous rupture of the attachment of the tendon of the extensor carpi radialis brevis muscle. Handchir Mikrochir Plast Chir. 1989;21(6):331–3.
44. Höcker K, Spitz H. Osseous avulsion injury of the extensor carpi radialis brevis tendon from the base of the 3rd metacarpal bone. Handchir Mikrochir Plast Chir. 2000;32(2):112–4.
45. Johnson AE, Puttler EG. Avulsion of the extensor carpi radialis brevis insertion: a case report and review of the literature. Mil Med. 2006;171(2):136–8.
46. Miyamoto H, Adi M, Taleb C, Zemirline A, Bodin F, Gay A, et al. Fifth carpometacarpal fracture dislocations fixed with Meta-HUS®: a series of 31 cases. Eur J Orthop Surg Traumatol. 2015;25(3):477–82.
47. Green WL, Kilgore ES. Treatment of fifth digit carpometacarpal arthritis with Silastic prosthesis. J Hand Surg. 1981;6(5):510–4.
48. Gainor BJ, Stark HH, Ashworth CR, Zemel NP, Rickard TA. Tendon arthroplasty of the fifth carpometacarpal joint for treatment of posttraumatic arthritis. J Hand Surg. 1991;16(3):520–4.
49. Dubert T. Stabilized arthroplasty of the 5th metacarpal bone. A therapeutic proposal for the treatment of old fractures-luxations of the 5th metacarpal bone. Ann Hand Upper Limb Surg. 1994;13(5):363–5.
50. Bain GI, Unni PR, Mehta JA, Eames MH. Arthrodesis of ring finger and little finger metacarpal bases for little finger carpometacarpal joint arthritis. J Hand Surg. 2004;29(5):449–52.
51. Freeland AE, Lindley SG. Malunions of the finger metacarpals and phalanges. Hand Clin. 2006;22(3):341–55.
52. Black DM, Watson HK, Vender MI. Arthroplasty of the ulnar carpometacarpal joints. J Hand Surg. 1987;12(6):1071–4.
53. Dahlin L, Palffy L, Widerberg A. Injury to the deep branch of the ulnar nerve in association with dislocated fractures of metacarpals II–IV. Scand J Plast Reconstruc Surg Hand Surg. 2004;38(4):250–2.
54. Murphy TP, Parkhill WS. Fracture-dislocation of the base of the fifth metacarpal with an ulnar motor nerve lesion: case report. JOT. 1990;30(12):1585–7.
55. Peterson P, Sacks S. Fracture-dislocation of the base of the fifth metacarpal associated with injury to the deep motor branch of the ulnar nerve: a case report. J Hand Surg. 1986;11(4):525–8.
56. Mercan S, Uzun M, Ertugrul A, Ozturk I, Demir B, Sulun T. Psychopathology and personality features in orthopedic patients with boxer's fractures. Gen Hosp Psychiatry. 2005;27(1):13–7.

Adult Metacarpal Shaft Fractures

12

R. Christopher Chadderdon and Alexander A. Hysong

Introduction

In the USA, metacarpal fractures are some of the most common upper-extremity injuries. They account for up to 18% of all below elbow fractures and up to 44% of all hand fractures [1–3]. Metacarpal fractures most commonly afflict male patients in their second and third decades of life following a fall or direct contact with a solid object [3]. Eighty-eight percent of these fractures occur in non-thumb metacarpals with the fifth metacarpal being most common [2].

Appropriate locomotor function of the human hand depends on the balanced function of the intrinsic muscles of the fingers and the extrinsic finger flexors and extensors. The longitudinal bones of the hand play a critical role in maintaining this balance. Fractures of the metacarpals lead to disruption of this delicate system and can result in mechanical dysfunction [4]. The degree of dysfunction varies substantially depending on patient characteristics, the mechanism of injury, and fracture morphology. Thus, "ideal" management of metacarpal fractures requires consideration of each of these unique factors.

Regardless of the fracture in question, the primary goals of treatment remain the same: restoration of skeletal stability while maintaining hand function. These two goals, however, are often in conflict with one another [5]. Restoring anatomic bony alignment helps avoid biomechanical consequences of malunion. However, prolonged immobilization during healing can result in joint contractures, tendon adhesion, and scarring, leading to permanent loss of range of motion and stiffness [6].

R. C. Chadderdon (✉)
Orthocarolina Hand Center, OrthoCarolina, Charlotte, NC, USA

Atrium Health, Department of Orthopaedic Surgery, Charlotte, NC, USA
e-mail: Christopher.Chadderdon@orthocarolina.com

A. A. Hysong
Orthopaedic Residency, Atrium Health Carolinas Medical Center, Charlotte, NC, USA
e-mail: Alexander.hysong@atriumhealth.org

Similarly, operatively treated metacarpal fractures can result in stiffness via scar/adhesion formation secondary to iatrogenic soft tissue injury. As the body's most dynamic appendage, the hand is particularly susceptible to the sequalae of stiffness [6]. Despite advances in technology, the majority of metacarpal shaft fractures still can, and should, be managed nonoperatively.

This chapter will serve as a review of the evaluation and management of metacarpal shaft fractures.

Anatomy/Pathoanatomy of the Non-thumb Metacarpals

Appropriate management of metacarpal shaft fractures begins with an understanding of the anatomy and biomechanics of the uninjured hand.

Osteology

The four non-thumb metacarpals all exhibit similar osseous morphology. Each metacarpal is comprised of a quadrilateral base that tapers in to a tubular and concave shaft, all terminating in a cam-shaped head [7, 8]. Despite these similarities, each of the metacarpals does exhibit unique characteristics. For example, the index metacarpal has the longest length and widest diameter, the ring finger metacarpal has the smallest diameter, and the small finger metacarpal is the shortest [9].

Together, through the stability provided by their articulations and their stout intermetacarpal ligaments, the concave metacarpals form the longitudinal and transverse arches of the hand [1, 8]. These arches provide support for the hand and aid with grasp.

Of particular relevance to the management of metacarpal shaft fractures are the carpometacarpal articulations. Each metacarpal exhibits a unique articulation with one or more of the distal carpal bones. The relative motion permitted by each of these articulations has implications on both the native function of each digit and degree of deformity that is tolerated following a fracture [1, 9]. The second metacarpal, which articulates with the trapezoid and trapezium, and the third metacarpal, which articulates with the capitate, are relatively fixed at their carpometacarpal (CMC) joints, thus permitting very little motion. Functionally, this helps with precise grip and power pinch. In contrast, fourth metacarpal, which articulates with the capitate and hamate, and the fifth metacarpal, which articulates with the hamate, allow for roughly 15° and 25° of sagittal plane motion at their CMC joints, respectively [8]. Functionally, this allows the hand to more easily accommodate different shaped objects and assist with power grasp [9] (Fig. 12.1).

In the setting of trauma, the mobility of the more ulnar CMC articulations puts them at higher risk of dislocation. Following a metacarpal shaft fracture, however, this motion also allows the ring and small fingers to compensate for a greater degree of sagittal plane angulation of the metacarpal before clinically significant

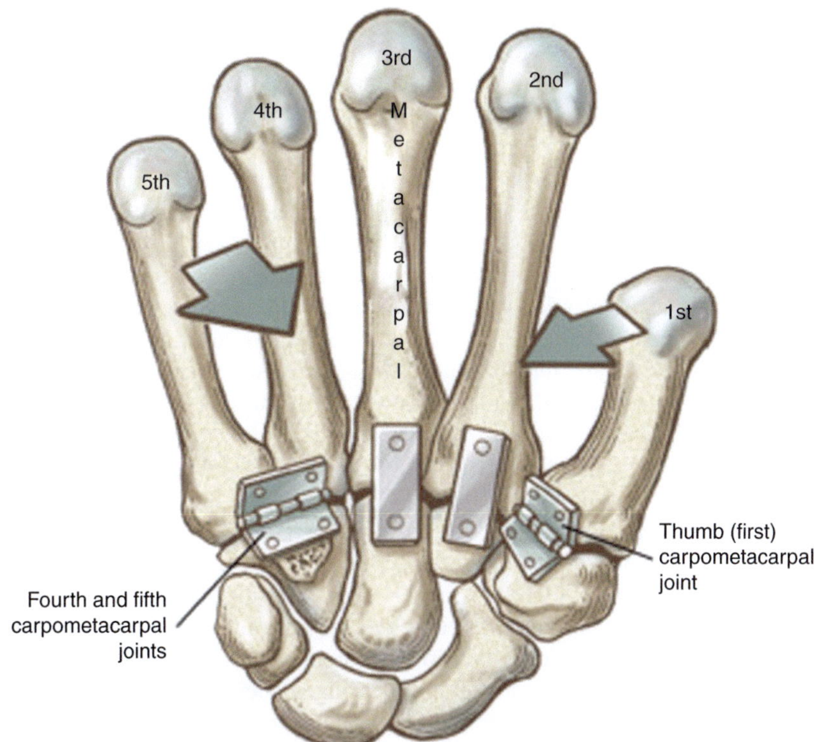

Fig. 12.1 Palmar view of the right hand showing a schematic representation of the relative mobility across the five carpometacarpal (CMC) joints. The first, fourth, and fifth CMC joints are relatively mobile, whereas the second and third CMC joints have much more limited motion. The motion of each CMC joint has implications as it relates to tolerance for angulation of fractures of their respective metacarpals. (**Source:** With permissions from: Donald A. Neumann. (2009). *Kinesiology of the Musculoskeletal System* (2nd ed.). Mosby/Elsevier. Page 250)

dysfunction is noted [7–9]. As a general rule, the hand can accommodate 10–15° of apex dorsal angulation of the metacarpal more than the available CMC motion of the involved digit.

Distally, each metacarpal articulates with a single proximal phalanx at the metacarpophalangeal joint (MCPJ). Each MCPJ is a multiaxial condyloid joint that permits flexion and extension and variable degrees of radial and ulnar deviation, contingent upon the position of the joint in space. When the MCPJ is fully extended, it tolerates a substantial radial and ulnar deviation of the finger. This is because the distal articular surface of the metacarpal head is relatively narrow, allowing the collateral ligaments to relax. In full flexion, the proximal phalanx articulates with the volar aspect of the metacarpal head which is wider and more prominent than the tip of the metacarpal. These features tighten the collateral ligaments in flexion, resulting in increased stability, and decreased radial and ulnar motion [7–9].

Muscular/Ligamentous Anatomy

In addition to osseous anatomy, there are a number of muscular and ligamentous structures relevant to the evaluation and treatment of metacarpal shaft fractures (some of which are alluded to previously).

Within the palm, the interossei and lumbricals muscles arise from metacarpals and flexor digitorum profundus tendons, respectively, and their tendons travel volar to the central axis of rotation of the MCPJ. These structures coalesce distally to form the lateral bands and insert dorsally onto the proximal phalanx and extensor expansion. This anatomic relationship is the primary driving force behind flexion at the MCPJ [7, 8]. Additionally, the extrinsic flexor and extensor tendons cross into the hand and insert distally into the phalanges and extensor expansion, respectively. The base of each metacarpal, with the exception of the ring finger, serves as an insertion point for a wrist flexor and/or extensor. The flexor carpi radialis (FCR) and extensor carpi radialis longus (ECRL) insert on the base of the index-finger metacarpal, the extensor carpi radialis brevis (ECRB) inserts on the base of the middle-finger metacarpal, and the extensor carpi ulnaris (ECU) and the flexor carpi ulnaris (FCU) insert on the base of the fifth metacarpal [1]. Together, these structures act as important deforming forces following metacarpal shaft fractures.

Proximally and distally, there are important ligamentous structures that act as static stabilizers for the metacarpals. The metacarpal bases are constrained by dense capsular tissue and numerous dorsal and volar ligaments that traverse among the metacarpals and the distal carpal bones [10]. Distally, the proper and accessory collateral ligaments originate from collateral recesses of the metacarpal head and insert distally into the proximal phalanx and volar plate, respectively [7, 8]. The collateral recess serves as an important anatomic landmark for operative fixation of metacarpal fractures (this will be addressed later in the chapter).

In addition to being an insertion for the accessory collateral ligament, the volar plate functions primarily as a dense fibrocartilaginous restraint to hyperextension at the MCPJ. While the volar plate itself does not provide any inherent stability to the metacarpal shaft, the volar plates of the non-thumb metacarpals are interconnected by the deep transverse intermetacarpal ligament. This stout structure is the primary stabilizer of the distal arch of the palm and helps prevent proximal migration of the metacarpal head and neck following shaft fractures [1, 7, 9].

Pathoanatomy/Mechanism/Clinical Relevance

Metacarpal fractures are classified in the same manner as other long bones in the body: Intraarticular, open/closed, transverse, short oblique, spiral, and all with varying degrees of comminution (Fig. 12.2) [1, 7, 11]. For the purposes of this chapter, we will focus predominantly on fractures involving the metacarpal shaft.

The specific fracture pattern that is observed depends upon the causative mechanism of injury. Transverse fractures are often caused by a direct blow to the dorsum of the hand with higher energy mechanisms creating comminution. Spiral shaft

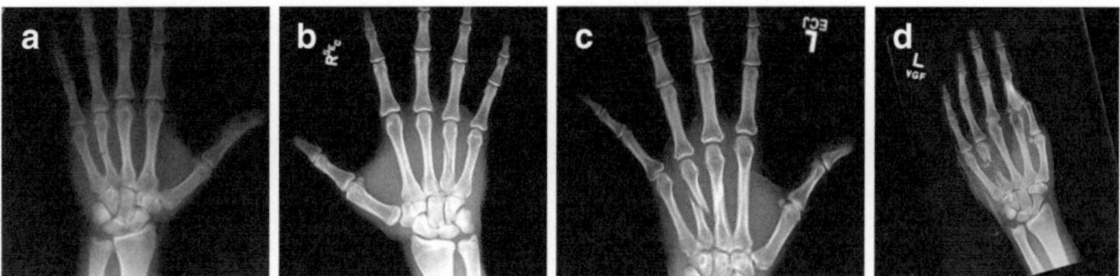

Fig. 12.2 There are several common metacarpal shaft fracture patterns, each with a different typical mechanism of injury, and each poses different considerations as it relates to treatment options. (**a**) Transverse fracture (of fourth metacarpal). (**b**) Long spiral oblique fracture (of fourth metacarpal). (**c**) Short oblique of third and fourth metacarpal. (**d**) Comminuted/ballistic (of fourth metacarpal). (**Source:** Authors' clinical X-rays)

fractures are most frequently the result of a twisting mechanism of the finger. A comminuted shaft fracture with a bending wedge fragment is typically caused by a bending mechanism with associated axial compression. A short oblique fracture is the result of a twisting mechanism with concurrent axial load [11]. Alternatively, ballistic and blast injuries can lead to unpredictable fracture patterns, which often involve significant comminution, soft tissue injury, and occasionally bone loss [12].

Following most metacarpal shaft fractures, the pull of the intrinsic hand musculature creates an apex dorsal deformity. As mentioned prior, the tendons of the intrinsics traverse volar to the axis of rotation of the metacarpal head before inserting into the extensor hood. Thus, when they contract they lever metacarpal head volarly and the fracture site protrudes dorsally [1, 7, 11]. Excessive angulation of the metacarpal can result in compensatory hyperextension that the MCPJ and extensor lag at the PIP and DIPJs. This phenomenon is referred to as "pseudoclawing" and can impair a patient's ability to grip. The amount of angulation that is tolerated by each metacarpal is directly related to the amount of motion that is present within each respective CMC joint and the proximity of the fracture to the metacarpal neck. In the ring and small fingers, hyperextension through the CMC joint can allow for patients to compensate for a greater amount of apex dorsal angulation through the metacarpal. In fact, literature suggests that patients can tolerate anywhere from 30 to 70+ degrees of apex dorsal angulation of the fourth and fifth metacarpal necks with little functional deficit [13, 14]. Additionally, angular deformities are poorly tolerated as the fracture lines occur closer to the isthmus of the metacarpal shaft. Tolerated angulation for metacarpal shaft fractures is as follows: 10–20° for the index and middle fingers and 20–25° for the ring and small fingers [1, 8, 9, 11].

In addition to angulation, metacarpal shortening is another important deformity that should be considered in length-unstable fracture patterns (spiral, oblique, comminuted, etc.). In isolated metacarpal fractures, shortening tends to be more common in the border digits (index and small fingers). This is because the transverse intermetacarpal ligaments act to suspend the central metacarpals. In most cases, the deep transverse intermetacarpal ligament prevents shortening more than 3–4 mm in the long and ring fingers [1, 15, 16]. Cosmetically, fracture shortening alone can be quite subtle, presenting as a loss of knuckle contour [1, 7, 9, 15]. Functionally,

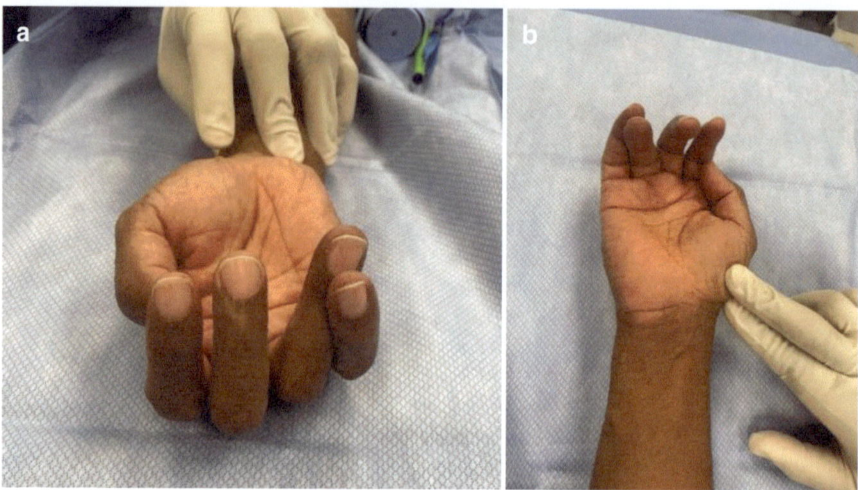

Fig. 12.3 Example of a malrotated fracture of the right fourth metacarpal. Dorsal (**a**) and palmar (**b**) views of the crossover, or "scissoring" of the ring finger beneath the adjacent small finger. (**Source:** Author's Clinical photos)

however, excessive shortening can have important consequences. As the metacarpal shortens, there is relative lengthening or laxity of the extrinsic finger extensors and flexors, thus altering the native length-tension relationship in these muscles. While clinical evidence is limited, cadaveric studies have shown that for every 2 mm of metacarpal shortening there is a corresponding 7° extensor lag at the MCPJ [15]. Additionally, cadaveric studies estimate that for every 2 mm of shortening there is an 8% loss in interosseous muscle power [17]. These findings, in addition to the fact the MCPJs exhibit a natural 20° of hyperextension, explain why several studies suggest that 3–6 mm is considered an acceptable amount of shortening with tolerated functional loss [1, 15, 18, 19].

The third and final way that metacarpal fractures can deform is via malrotation. Malrotation is often the least well tolerated deformity of metacarpal fractures as even small degrees of rotation tend to be an indication for intervention (Fig. 12.3). As little as 1° of metacarpal shaft rotation can lead to 5° of digital rotation. On average 5° of digital rotation can cause 1.5 cm of digital overlap/scissoring while attempting to make a fist [1, 16, 18, 20]. Scissoring deformities can significantly impair hand function.

Treatment Indications/Options

Like any other fracture in the body, metacarpal fractures can be managed both operatively and nonoperatively. The decision of whether to pursue surgery for a metacarpal shaft fracture depends largely on the specific fracture pattern, associated injuries, and patient characteristics/desires. Both options have relative indications and associated benefits and risks that should be considered.

Table 12.1 List of the commonly accepted apex dorsal shaft angulation, shortening, and apex dorsal neck angulation of metacarpal shaft fractures [1, 2, 7, 8]

	Shaft angulation (°)	Shaft shortening (mm)	Neck angulation (°)
Second and third metacarpal	10	4–6	15
Fourth metacarpal	20–30	4–6	30–40
Fifth metacarpal	30–40	4–6	50–70+

Nonoperative

Nonoperative management is the most common treatment modality for metacarpal shaft fractures and often yields excellent results [21]. The success of nonoperative management reflects the hand's remarkable versatility and its capacity for functional compensation. Moreover, small functional deficits from malunion are often preferable to the risk of surgical sequalae and/or complications [1, 18].

However, nonoperative treatment modalities are vast, each with differing indications and respective treatment algorithms. In general, the "acceptable" parameters of deformity following an extraarticular fracture are listed in Table 12.1 [1, 14, 22, 23]. If a fracture deformity is within these parameters and the fracture is stable, many advocate for minimally protective splinting without manipulation and early range of motion. Outside of these parameters the recommendation is often for reduction and immobilization [2, 18]. However, it is important to note that many of these ranges are derived from cadaveric and anatomic studies, which do not always correlate with clinical significance [24].

Angulation, Shortening, and Reduction

Of the three possible metacarpal fracture deformities (angulation, shortening, rotation), angulation is the best controlled by nonoperative modalities. As previously described, the respective sagittal plane angular deformity tolerated by each metacarpal increases as we progress from radial to ulnar and from midshaft to metacarpal neck. This greater tolerance for angular deformity of the more ulnar digits relates directly to the amount of compensatory motion that is available at the respective CMC joints [1, 8]. In metacarpal fractures with significant angulation, reduction to an acceptable parameter is often recommended prior to immobilizing. The most commonly cited technique for reduction was described by Jahss in 1938 (coined the "Jahss maneuver"). It involves full flexion at the MCP joint with subsequent dorsally directed pressure through the axis of the proximal phalanx of the same digit (Fig. 12.4). This technique serves to both relax the pull of the intrinsic musculature and counter the apex dorsal deformity that is present in most metacarpal fractures [25, 26]. Once restored to a more "appropriate" alignment the fractures are then immobilized and allowed to heal.

While the concepts of "reduction" and "immobilization" may appear quite mundane, there has been a considerable amount of research dedicated to determining the best practices for conservatively treating metacarpal fractures. Many of these studies explore the two conflicting goals of hand fracture management: fracture stability and hand mobility. For example, some studies recommend against reduction and rigid immobilization altogether following certain fracture types. Specifically, Van

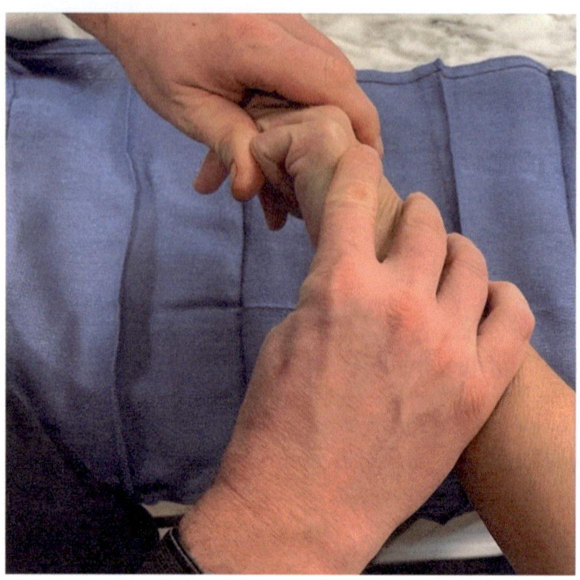

Fig. 12.4 Maneuver for reduction of apex-dorsally angulated metacarpal neck and shaft fractures, known as the Jahss Maneuver (1938). The MCP joint is flexed to 90°, then using one's contralateral hand, a volarly directed force is applied to the metacarpal just proximal to the fracture, and a dorsally directed force is applied to the distal fracture fragment by axially loading the proximal phalanx. (**Source:** Author's clinical photos)

Aaeken et al. conducted a prospective randomized control trial comparing closed reduction and casting versus only soft dressing and buddy taping for angulated fifth MC shaft fractures. At 4 months, there were no differences found in either group's pain, qDASH scores, function, or strength even with fractures displaying 70° of initial apex dorsal angulation. Furthermore, the soft dressing group missed significantly less days of work than the reduction and casting group, with the major downside of no reduction being permanent loss of knuckle contour [24]. In fact, some studies go as far as to suggest that closed reduction and casting is an unreliable method for maintaining anatomic alignment, and that if stability is the primary objective, then operative intervention should be pursued instead [27].

Finally, there is evidence that the clinical impact of metacarpal shortening may not be quite as impactful as previously thought. As mentioned prior, cadaveric studies have demonstrated that there is a 7° extensor lag with every 2 mm of MC shortening [15]. One case series reported the outcomes of 42 patients with length-unstable long oblique metacarpal fractures (that did not require reduction) treated with a simple volar wrist splint and immediate mobilization. As expected, the fractures did shorten, but all healed with otherwise acceptable radiographic parameters. Though patients did exhibit an initial extensor lag of the injured finger (mean 26°) this lag completely resolved in all patients by 9-month follow-up. The injured hand did, however, exhibit some diminished strength compared to the contralateral side at 1 year follow-up possibly related to the impact of shortening on intrinsic muscle function [17, 28].

While these findings are not universally applicable, they do exemplify that conventional wisdom may not always correlate with clinical outcomes. The same is true for the different forms of immobilization that are used for metacarpal fractures (Fig. 12.5).

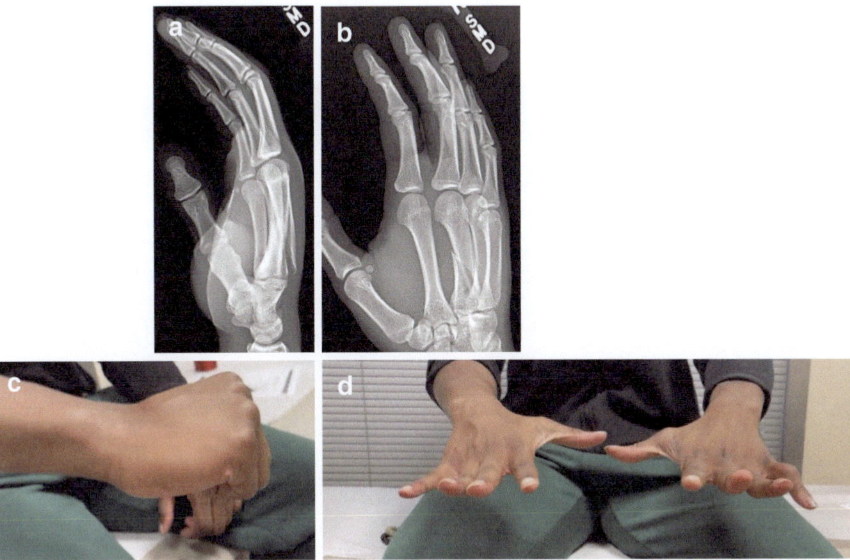

Fig. 12.5 Clinical example of a long oblique third metacarpal fracture (**a**—acute X-rays) treated conservatively with a volar splint. The fracture has healed in a foreshortened position with slight angulation (**b**). Despite the dorsal hump noted while the patient makes a fist (**c**), there is no clinical malrotation or extensor lag noted at 4 months after injury (**c** and **d**). (**Source:** Author's clinical photos)

Immobilization

When electing to perform reduction and cast immobilization of metacarpal fractures, there are two primary goals: maintenance of reduction and prevention of long-term stiffness. Over time, there have been many iterations of hand/upper-extremity casts attempting to strike this balance [29].

For example, in 1938 Jahss, along with his reduction technique, described a casting technique which held the MPCJ and digit in flexion [26]. Additional cast types include the Goldberg "cast and vice," the Galveston brace, Konradsen's "functional cast," the specifics of which are all beyond the scope of this chapter [28]. An important concept of hand immobilization, however, was described by Professor James at the University of Edinburgh in the 1960s. He described the functional position of the hand, since termed the "Edinburgh" or "intrinsic plus" position [30]. The "ideal" intrinsic plus position is described as the wrist in 30° of extension, MCPJ in 90° of flexion, and the interphalangeal joints in 0° of extension (Fig. 12.6) [26]. Theoretically, this position has multiple beneficial effects. It places the MCPJ collateral ligaments on maximum tension due to the cam shape of the metacarpal head. Full extension of the interphalangeal tensions the collateral ligaments of the PIP and DIP joints, and it also relaxes the deforming forces of the intrinsic musculature [22, 26]. Thus, it was believed that casting in this position would limit post-cast stiffness by reducing the risk of soft tissue contractures.

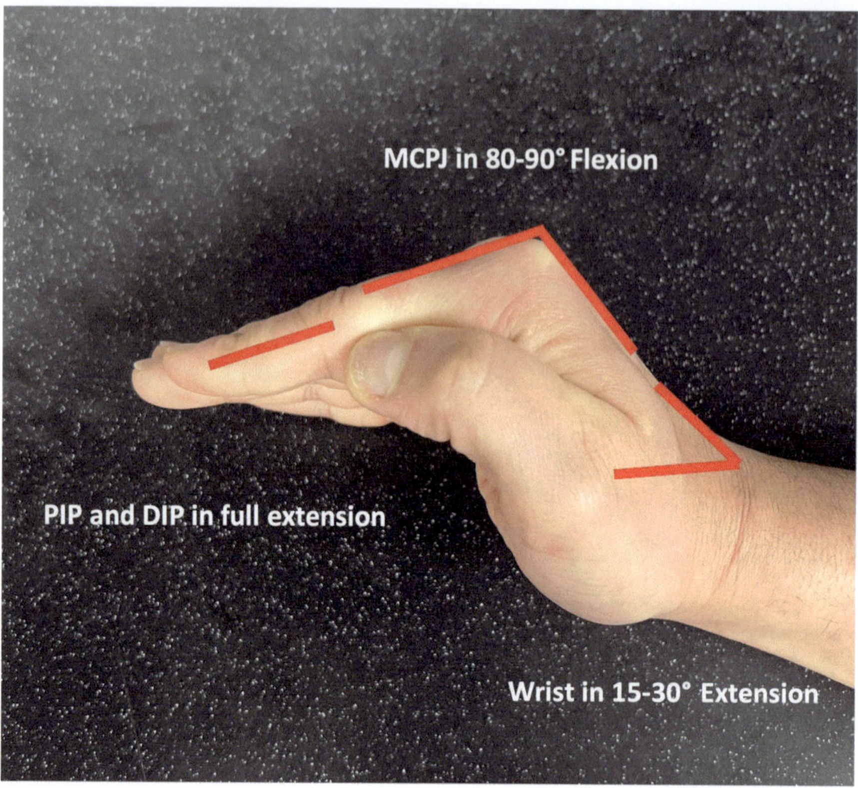

Fig. 12.6 The "Edinburgh" or "intrinsic plus" position of immobilization. The wrist is in 30° of extension, MCPJs in 90° of flexion, and the interphalangeal joints in full extension. (**Source:** Author's clinical photos)

This concept motivated the use of "radial gutter" and "ulnar gutter" casts (or close variations) (Fig. 12.7) in the immobilization of metacarpal neck and shaft fractures. For decades to follow, intrinsic plus positioning has been the standard of care for conservative management of metacarpal fractures, and the results of these casts have been excellent [22, 28].

However, appropriately applying these casts often requires a skilled technician, they can be quite cumbersome for patients, and extensive immobilization can render the rest of the patient's hand unusable. For this reason, several authors have challenged this convention, to see if the intrinsic plus position has any major impact on functional outcomes. Tavassoli et al. compared three different forms of immobilization for fifth metacarpal fractures: MCPJ in flexion with full interphalangeal motion permitted, MCPJ in flexion and interphalangeal joints fixed in extension, and MCPJ in extension and full interphalangeal joint permitted. When they assessed patient's radiographic alignment, strength, and range of motion at 9 weeks post injury, there was no difference in among groups [22]. Three years later Hofmeister et al. performed a randomized control trial comparing fifth metacarpal fractures

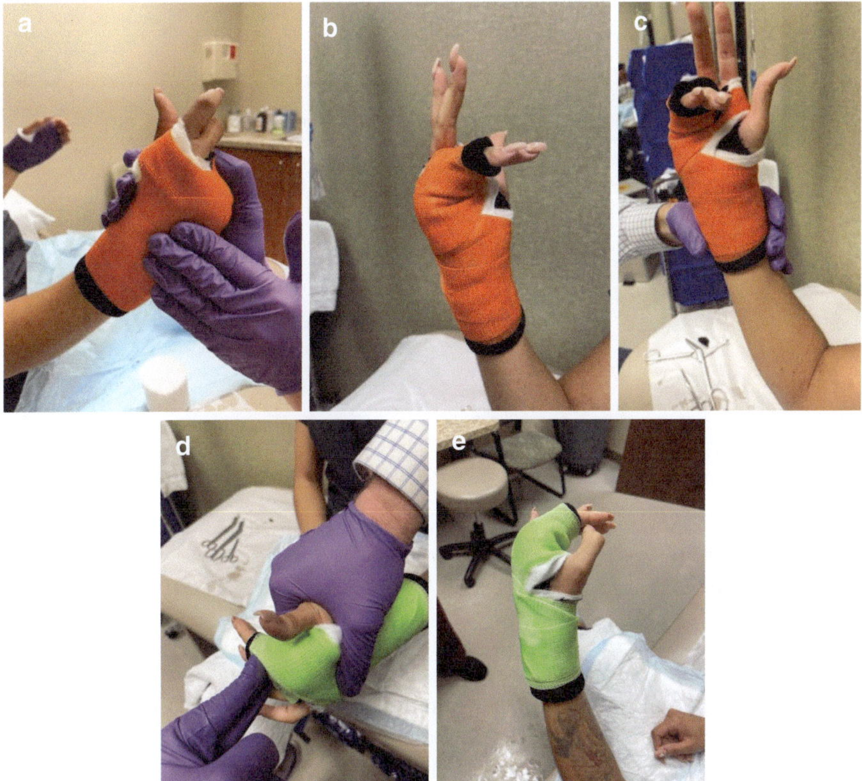

Fig. 12.7 Examples of an ulnar gutter cast (**a–c**) and radial gutter cast (**d, e**). Application the cast (**a, d**), placing 2 of the patient's fingers in an "intrinsic plus" position while concurrently correcting apex dorsal angulation with a dorsal mold. (**Source:** Author's clinical photos)

immobilized with the MCPJ in flexion with interphalangeal joints fixed in extension versus MCPJ in extension with interphalangeal joint motion permitted. They also found no functional or radiographic differences between the two groups. These findings suggest that functional positioning of the hand may not be as important as previously perceived, and that ease of application and maintaining hand function may be more important.

For fractures of the metacarpal shaft in particular, several authors advocate for hand-based splints and casts that do not immobilize any joints at all. In 1984 Barton et al. described a "shorthand cast" which utilizes a hand-based 3-point mold to maintain metacarpal reduction (Fig. 12.8). Studies like the one published by Debnath et al. in 2004 revealed excellent maintenance of reduction (average 40 at injury to 8° of apex dorsal deformity at final follow-up) [29]. This cast type provides the added benefit of full digital and wrist range of motion, which permits much more use of the hand when compared to more extensive forms of immobilization.

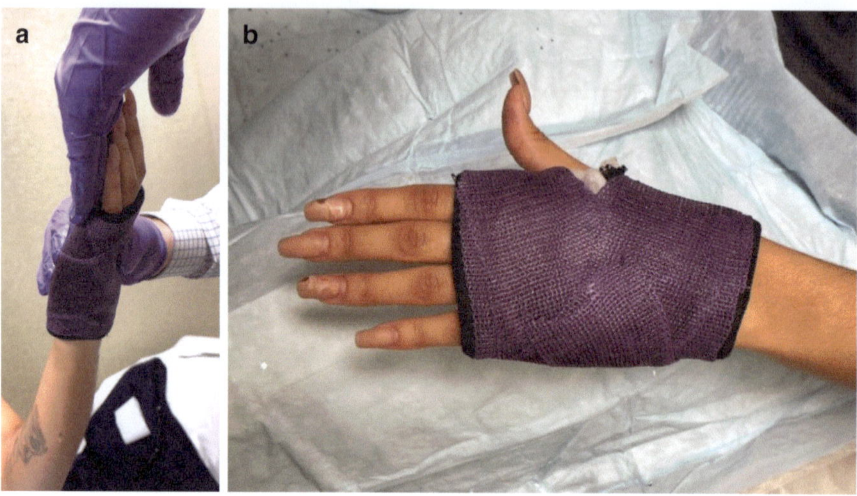

Fig. 12.8 Example of a hand-based cast. Application of a "shorthand cast" which utilizes a hand-based 3-point mold (**a**) to maintain metacarpal reduction, and the final appearance of the cast (**b**) which allows near-normal range of motion of the wrist and MCPJs. (**Source:** Author's clinical images)

In terms of duration, most publications advocate for 4–6 weeks of immobilization prior to cast removal and progression of hand use [1, 7, 9]. At this point casts should be removed and patients should be assessed for tenderness at their fracture site. A painless fracture is suggestive of clinical healing and often precedes obvious evidence of radiographic union [7].

With all of the conflicting information about conservative management of metacarpals, it is difficult to make any strong recommendations about the ideal technique. In general, however, it is important to remember that most metacarpal fractures can be treated effectively without surgical intervention. Additionally, when using a cast to maintain a reduction, techniques that maintain joint mobility and optimize patient comfort may be equally as effective as the more extensive casting techniques that were traditionally used.

Operative

Indications

There are very few, if any, hard operative indications for metacarpal shaft fractures. For isolated metacarpal shaft fractures one of the strongest indications for initial operative management is significant malrotation of the metacarpal (causing scissoring of the digits). As mentioned above, malrotation is both very poorly tolerated by patients and poorly controlled by any reduction or immobilization. A second common indication for surgery is failure to maintain a reduction via conservative measures, though as we can see the hand can tolerate quite a bit of malunion with little functional deficit.

Further relative indications for surgery include open fractures, polytraumatized patients (to help with early weightbearing and mobility), multiple metacarpal shaft fractures in the same hand, and patient preference [1]. Importantly, a patient's profession and/or desire to return to normal activity often plays a significant role in deciding whether or not to operate on a metacarpal fracture. For example, a professional athlete may elect to have surgery in order to return to weightbearing and competition more quickly [9]. Additionally, a profession that requires precise finger function, such as a concert pianist, may elect to have surgery in order to avoid functional deficits that a malunion may cause.

Techniques

There are numerous techniques available to the surgeon, including pin/k-wire fixation, interfragmentary screw fixation, wiring techniques, dorsal plate and screw fixation, and intramedullary stabilization. There are multiple factors that determine the choice of technique including patient factors, surgeon preference, and fracture pattern. Due to the large variation in fracture patterns, mechanism of injury, biologic factors, and other variables, there is an absence of well-performed level I or II evidence comparing different surgical approaches. Thus the literature remains unclear as to providing the surgeon with specific guidance as to the optimum choice of fracture fixation for specific metacarpal fractures. Perhaps more important in the hand than elsewhere, the surgeon should bear in mind the need to obtain adequate skeletal stability while performing as little soft tissue dissection as possible.

Plate and Screw Fixation

Plate fixation of the metacarpal shaft is typically performed with a direct dorsal surgical approach to the hand, with radial or ulnar retraction of the overlying extrinsic extensor tendons (Fig. 12.9). Relative indications for plate and screw fixation

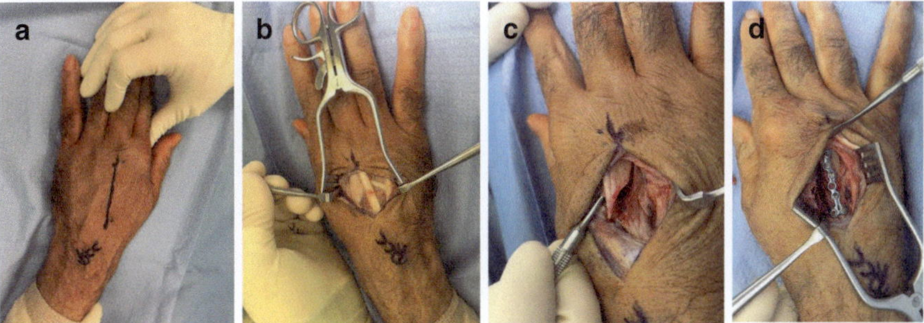

Fig. 12.9 Plate fixation of the metacarpal shaft is typically performed with a direct dorsal surgical approach to the hand (**a**). Exposure of the overlying extrinsic extensor tendon (**b**), blunt retraction of the extensor tendon and fracture exposure (**c**) and plate/screw osteosynthesis (**d**). (**Source:** Author's clinical photos)

include: Displaced transverse or oblique fracture patterns, and comminuted fractures for which the plate is utilized in part as a bridging fixation device. Displaced fractures of all patterns may require extraction of interposed soft tissue, such as interosseous muscle and periosteum. For oblique fracture patterns, in particular, it is important to visualize the proximal and distal apices in order to ensure the absence of interposed soft tissue and confirm restoration of length and alignment. An open approach thus allows for direct visualization and reduction of the fracture. Obtaining an anatomic reduction with most fracture patterns is typically achieved, often with the assistance of reduction tools such as dental picks and small bone reduction clamps.

The surgeon must be cognizant of restoring appropriate length of the fractured metacarpal, especially in regard to fracture patterns at risk for foreshortening (i.e. spiral, oblique, and comminuted fractures). Although no well-performed correlative in vivo studies have been performed (and as referenced previously), cadaveric studies have predicted that for every 2 mm of shortening of the metacarpal, there is a correlative 7° of extension lag at the metacarpophalangeal and 8% loss of grip power [15, 17]. With all fracture patterns, ensuring appropriate rotation is paramount, as only a few degrees of malrotation may result in the overlap of digits with fist formation [18, 20]. Intraoperative assessment of rotation is imperative for all forms of fracture fixation and will be discussed later in the chapter.

There are many implant options available for dorsal plate and screw fixation. Most are comprised of either stainless steel or titanium. Additionally, there are different of choices of plate design, length, shape, thickness, and screw size. Generally speaking, implant sizes range between 1.3 and 2.7 mm in width, and the choice of size is determined by diameter of the bone. Relatively thicker plate is indicated when bridging across a comminuted segment. As with many areas of orthopedics, newer generations of plates have a lower profile, thus offering a lower potential for soft tissue irritation and adhesions (Fig. 12.10).

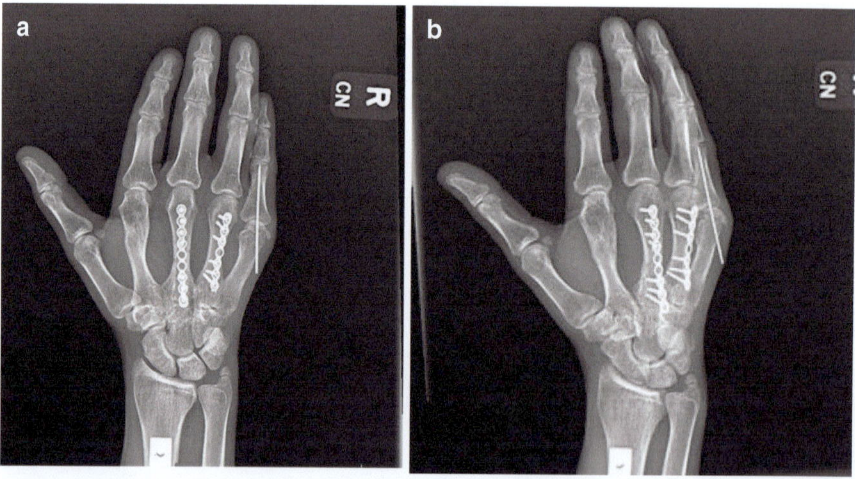

Fig. 12.10 Postoperative radiographs of healed right third and fourth right metacarpal fractures after low-profile plate and screw fixation. (**a**) AP view of hand, and (**b**) oblique view of hand. (**Source:** Author's clinical photos)

Conventional teaching is that six cortices should be achieved on either side of the fracture. However with locking plate/screw technology, Barr et al. demonstrated in a biomechanical study that two bicortical locking screws on each side of the fracture may be equivalent to three bicortical nonlocking screws on each side of the fracture [31]. It is thus possible that locked plates may allow for less dissection and soft tissue disruption. Moreover, some proximal and distal shaft fracture patterns do not allow for three holes of plate fixation on both sides of the fracture.

Some advocate for plating on surfaces other than the dorsum of the metacarpal. Chiu et al. explored this technique and demonstrated in a biomechanical study that lateral metacarpal plate fixation confers less mechanical strength than k-wire fixation [32]. The major benefit of this technique is the lower potential for extensor tendon adhesion.

In most cases, the stability of a dorsal plate and screw construct permits early range of motion and therapy; however, there is appropriate concern about the potential for loss of motion due to adhesion of extensor tendons to the plate's surface and due to the increased scarification caused by the surgical dissection necessary fracture exposure and plate application. Complication rates following plate and screw fixation of the metacarpal are variable, but overall quite high ranging from 32% to 36% [33, 34]. In a 1998 study examining 66 MC fractures, stiffness was one of the more commonly reported complications with a total arc of motion (TAM) less than 220° at final follow-up, variable amounts of extensor lag, and contractures [1]. In a 2002 study examining 105 MC fractures the most common complication was poor healing with 7.5% of patients developing malunion and 7.5% developing nonunion. Stiffness was a close second at 10% [34]. However, the rate of adhesions of the overlying extrinsic extensor tendons after plate fixation of the metacarpal shaft is relatively low compared to fixation of phalangeal fractures, due to less anatomic intimacy between bone and tendon at this level (extensor tendon Zone VI). This is, in part, reflected by the better outcomes after plate fixation of metacarpals compared to phalanges. Using TAM as a primary outcome, Page and Stern reported that 76% of metacarpal fractures fixated with plates and screws achieved a TAM >220°, compared to 11% in plate-fixated phalangeal fractures [33].

Stable plate fixation of metacarpal fractures allows for relatively early mobilization and therapy, which may mitigate some of the increased risk of adhesions and stiffness conferred by the open surgical technique. Time to radiographic union varies, but the surgeon should be aware that time to consolidation may be longer with a transverse fracture pattern as opposed to oblique, likely due to the larger bony interface with more oblique patterns [35].

Percutaneous and Wire Fixation

Intramedullary fixation of displaced metacarpal fractures with k-wires was first described in 30 patients by Lord in 1957, and he reported that this technique resulted in earlier return to work with no infections or refractures [36]. This technique, predominantly performed in a percutaneous manner with smooth wires, has evolved

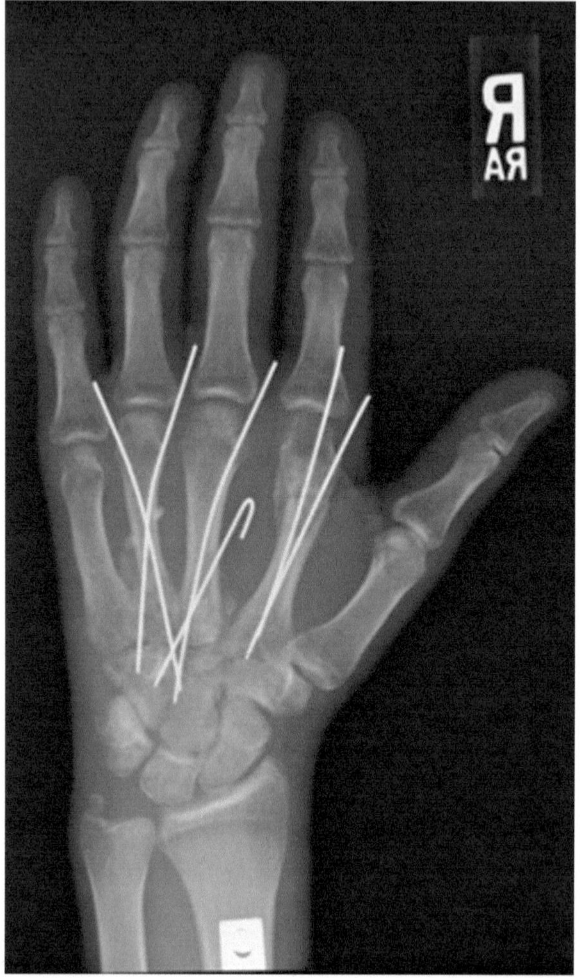

Fig. 12.11 Case example of multiple metacarpal fractures fixed with multiple k-wires. The second (distal shaft) and fourth (proximal shaft) fractures are each stabilized with 2 sized 0.045 in. longitudinal K-wires. (**Source:** Author's clinical photos)

vis-à-vis wire size, entry points, number of wires, and wire construct. Many metacarpal fractures can be reduced in a closed fashion under fluoroscopic guidance, allowing percutaneous placement of k-wires. The fracture patterns most amenable to longitudinal k-wire fixation include transverse and short oblique fracture patterns, although long oblique fractures can also be addressed with longitudinal k-wires as long as the surgeon is watchful that foreshortening through the fracture does not occur (Fig. 12.11).

The most common k-wiring technique for metacarpal shaft fractures is closed reduction and percutaneous pinning (CRPP) utilizing retrograde intramedullary fixation, with an entrance point in the ulnar or radial aspect of the metacarpal head or collateral recesses. Utilizing a wire driver, the k-wire can be passed longitudinally across the fracture, coming to rest in the subchondral bone at the base of the metacarpal (Fig. 12.12). At least two k-wires should be utilized to stabilize most

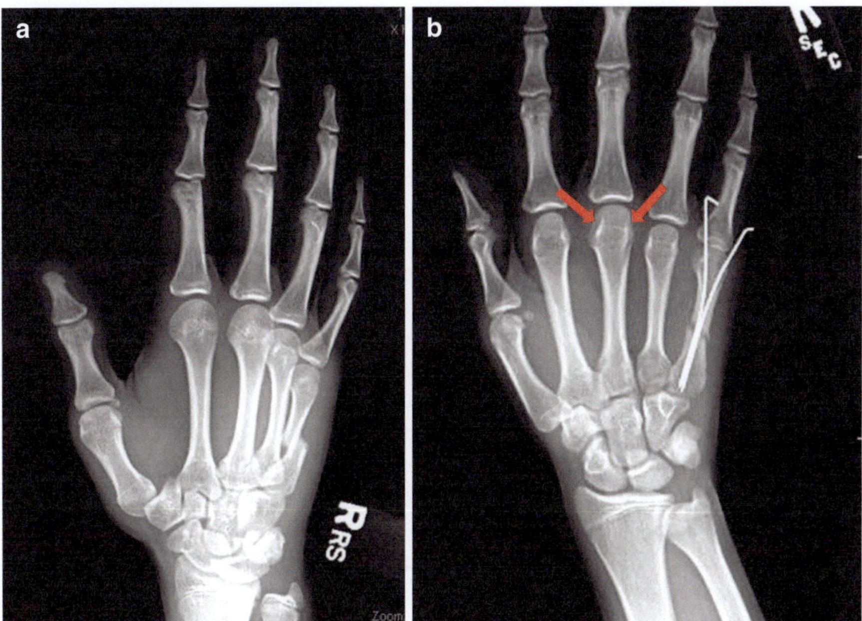

Fig. 12.12 Preoperative (**a**) and postoperative (**b**) X-rays of a right transverse fifth metacarpal shaft fracture stabilized by 2 sized 0.045 in. longitudinal k-wires. The entrance points for these percutaneous k-wires are the radial and ulnar collateral recesses. Red arrows pointing to the collateral recesses of the third Metacarpal. The proximal tip of the k-wires is resting in the subchondral bone at the base of the metacarpal. (**Source:** Author's clinical photos)

metacarpal shaft fractures, and the majority of adult metacarpal medullary canals will support two 0.045 in. k-wires. The use of this size k-wire also allows the surgeon to "bounce" the k-wire off the inner cortex with an oscillation or a firm-push drill technique. Although a less common approach, antegrade k-wire fixation has been reported by van Bussel et al. to have 100% union (in 34 fractures) and excellent clinical outcomes [37].

As with all k-wire techniques, a decision must be made whether to cut the wire deep to the skin, or the leave the wire prominent. The benefit of exposed (non-buried) k-wires is ease of in-office removal, but with the obvious concern of accidental early removal (i.e. with bandage changes, therapy, etc.). Terndrup et al. demonstrated an increased need for a surgical procedure to remove buried k-wires (17%) that were not deemed accessible in an office-based setting [38]. Another common concern with percutaneous wire fixation is the potential risk of pin-tract irritation/infection and osteomyelitis as sequelae. However literature supports that there is no significant increased relative risk of infection with exposed (non-buried) k-wires compared to buried [39]. Conversely, an additional concern with retrograde passage of k-wires is tethering of the extensor mechanism at the metacarpophalangeal joint (either sagittal band or tendon proper), which may limit excursion of the tendons and lead to adhesions [37, 40]. The extensor mechanism effectively envelops the dorsal and lateral aspects of the metacarpo-phalangeal joint and metacarpal neck, resulting in this risk of tethering from penetrating k-wires. Also, the extensor mechanism at this level is comparatively intimate with the bony and capsuloligamentous structures, rendering this anatomy more prone to adhesions.

Given the aforementioned concerns, several studies have explored the complication profile of IM k-wire fixation. The complication rate ranges from 15% to 20% with one of the more commonly reported complications being pin-tract infection and osteomyelitis. Additionally, there are reports of tendon injury, nerve injury, mal-union/nonunion, and pin migration though all of these are relatively less common (<3% each) [41–43]. One of the more frequent arguments against k-wire fixation is the need for delayed rehabilitation given the relative flexibility of the fixation construct. Dreyfuss et al. compared intramedullary pinning to plate fixation for 39 metacarpal shaft fractures and found significantly improved outcomes range of motion, grip strength, rotational alignment, and DASH score in the plated group [44]. The authors concluded that plate fixation should be used instead of smooth pin fixation of metacarpal fractures.

Despite findings like these, intramedullary k-wires remain an excellent option for fixation of metacarpal shaft fractures. The decision to use k-wires depends on a number of factures including fracture configuration, resource availability, surgeon preference, etc.

Isolated Screw Fixation

Isolated lag screw fixation is another commonly employed technique for metacarpal shaft fractures. They are indicated in long oblique shaft fractures that meet operative criteria (angulation, rotation, and/or shortening). It is recommended that isolated lag screws be used in fractures that are at least two times longer than the diameter of the metacarpal shaft [45]. Fractures of this length and configuration allow the screws to capture cortices of both fragments at multiple levels, which would otherwise be very difficult in short oblique or transverse fractures. When used appropriately, interfragmentary lag screws provide the benefit of anatomic cortical apposition with interfragmentary compression. This technique has been shown to be biomechanically more stable than k-wire fixation for oblique metacarpal fracture [46]. Theoretically, this promotes primary bone healing and provides stability for early range of motion following surgery [7, 9, 45].

With regard to technique, most surgeons advocate for an open or mini-open approach to the dorsum of the metacarpal. Through direct visualization and fluoroscopic imaging, the fracture is reduced. Often, the proximal and distal apices provide an excellent read for accurate reduction. Once reduced, the fracture is then held with a pointed reduction clamp and or a smooth wire [45]. Next, two to three bicortical screws are placed across the fracture site (orthogonal to the metacarpal and orthogonal to the fracture line) [7, 9, 18, 45, 47]. Additionally, it is recommended that the screws be at least two screw diameters away from the fracture apices to

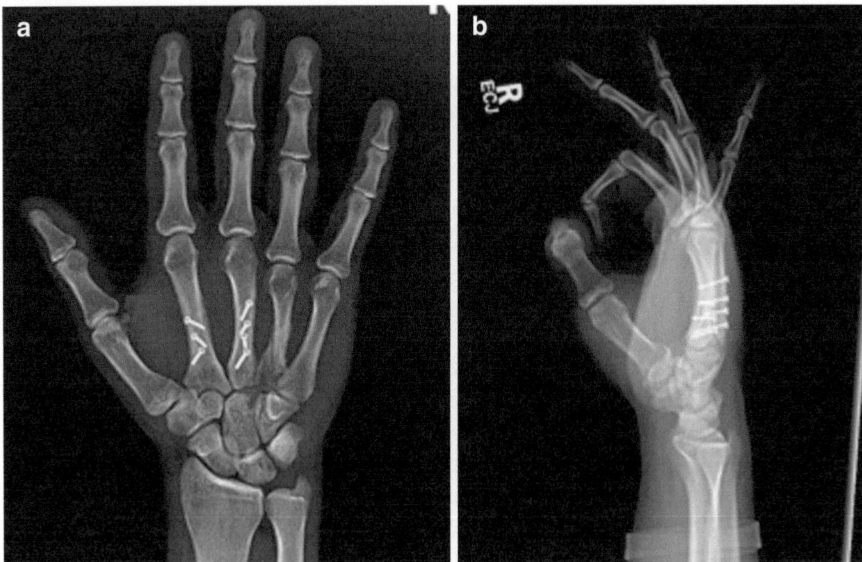

Fig. 12.13 Case example of right second and third oblique metacarpal shaft fracture treated with multiple lag screws. Anteroposterior (**a**) and lateral (**b**) X-rays of healed fractures, demonstrating three sized 2.0 mm cortical screws in the second metacarpal and four sized 2.0 mm screws in the third metacarpal. (**Source:** Author's Clinical Photos)

avoid fragmentation of the fracture spikes [45]. When placed appropriately, the screw trajectories are often divergent in the axial plane which is also visualized on X-ray imaging (Fig. 12.13).

When placing the screws, classic lag screw technique states that the near cortex should be over drilled with a drill bit that equals the thread diameter of the planned screw and the far cortex should be drilled with a drill bit matching the core diameter of the screw. This allows for a fully threaded screw to compress the near fragment to the far fragment, theoretically improving cortical contact [48]. However, both clinical and biomechanical studies have shown that simply using positional, bicortical self-tapping screws is equally as effective as lag screws when treating these fractures [48, 49]. Proponents of the "bicortical screw" technique state that it is less technically demanding and may decrease the risk of fracture propagation since only one, core diameter, sized drill bit is used [50].

Finally, there is a lack of consensus in literature regarding the number and size of screws that should be used for this technique. Authors report using 1.5–2.7 mm interfragmentary screws to fix long oblique fractures, and they differ on whether 2 or 3 screws should be used [45, 48–50]. Cheah et al. displayed that 3, 1.5 mm screws and 2, 2.0 mm screws were biomechanically similar with the 2.0 mm group showing slightly less loosening [51]. A more recent biomechanical study by white et al. in 2021 compared 1.2, 1.5 mm, 2.0 mm, and 2.3 mm, 2 screw fixation construction in a 3D printed metacarpal. They found no significant differences in peak load to failure in any of the cohorts. Importantly, they did find a higher rate of drill bit deformation and fracture in the 1.2 mm screw group and a higher rate of fracture propagation in the 2.3 mm screw group. They concluded that either 1.5 mm or 2.0 mm, 2 screw techniques should be used for this technique [49].

In summary, isolated screw techniques are an effective way to treat long oblique metacarpal shaft fractures. When used appropriately, they may help minimize the complications of plate and screw fixation while affording the benefit of early range of motion to avoid stiffness.

IM Screw Fixation

Over the past decade and a half, intramedullary screw (IM screw) fixation has been introduced as a hybrid solution for the fixation of metacarpal shaft fractures. In theory, IM screws combine the rigid fracture stability of open reduction and plate/ screw fixation with the soft tissue preservation of percutaneous k-wire fixation [52]. Thus, when used appropriately, IM screws can allow for early motion, rapid rehabilitation, and decreased postoperative stiffness.

Brief History of IM Screws

Intramedullary fixation of metacarpal fractures is not a new concept; however, the technique for IM fixation has undergone several iterations over the past 50+ years. One of the earliest reports of IM fixation was in 1971 when Milford et al. reported using medullary pegs of bone to treat malunions of the metacarpal [53]. The use of intramedullary "screws" was not reported until 1978, when Tamai and Irigaray reported using IM screws during digital replantation surgery [54]. In subsequent years, extraarticular intramedullary k-wire fixation was developed with excellent results. However, this technique required an open approach to the fracture site and the absence of any fixation between the k-wire and the bone allowed for pin migration [53]. Ultimately, in 2010 Boulton et al. published the first case report of using a retrograde, trans-articular intramedullary headless compression screw to fix a metacarpal fracture. Specifically, he used a 3.0 mm screw to fix a displaced, comminuted, subcapital fifth MC neck fracture. The patient was allowed to perform range of motion as tolerated on postoperative day 5. The patient achieved functional range of motion at 6 weeks postoperatively and the fracture united without complication or deformity [52]. Since their conception, the application and advancement of IM metacarpal screws has taken off in the realm of hand surgery.

Implants

While there are many manufacturers that produce headless metacarpal screws, there are two major screw designs that are currently offered [55]. The older and more commonly used (at least in literature) is that of a classic headless compression screw

Fig. 12.14 There are two primary intramedullary screw designs. (**a**) Headless screws with a smooth shaft and threaded ends. All distal threads must be past the fracture to obtain adequate fixation. (**b**) A conical and fully threaded screw, with either variable thread pitch or constant thread pitch providing either uniform or no compression, respectively. Not all threads need to cross the fracture to obtain purchase. (**Source:** Author's clinical photos)

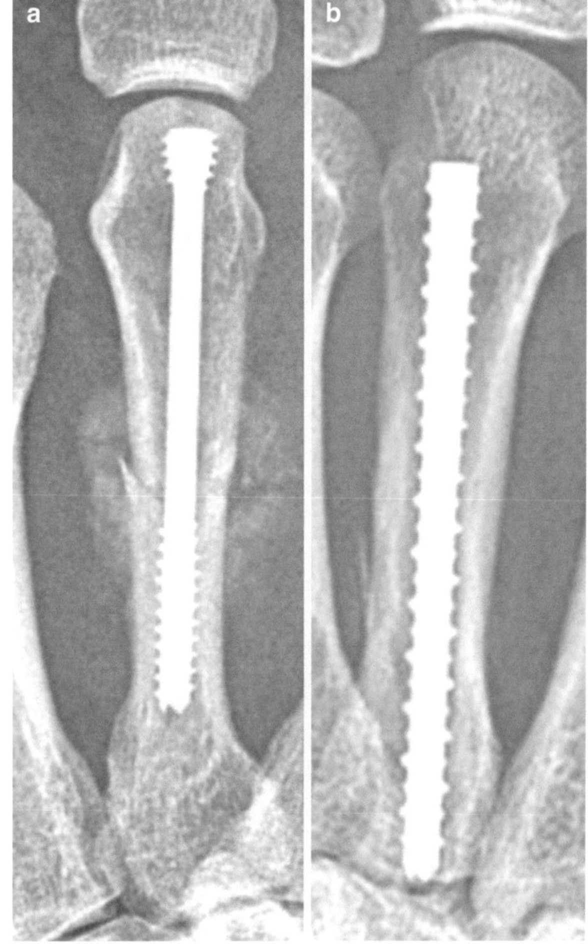

design. These screws have a smooth shaft and threaded ends. These screws come in a wide variety of sizes, they provide compression at the fracture, and all distal threads must be past the fracture to obtain adequate fixation. The second, newer, design is a conical and fully threaded screw. These screws are designed with either variable thread pitch or constant thread pitch providing either uniform or no compression, respectively. Importantly, not all threads need to cross the fracture to obtain purchase (Fig. 12.14).

Though it is beyond the scope of this chapter, "canal-screw mismatch" is a concern when using IM screws for metacarpal fixation. The wide range of metacarpal lengths and endosteal diameters can make it difficult to pass a screw or lead to poor fracture purchase if an inappropriate screw size is selected. Several authors have sought to address this concern by comparing radiographic analysis of metacarpals to the different screws available on the market [56–58].

Techniques/Articular Considerations

The most common technique described is retrograde placement of the screw through the metacarpal head [55, 59, 60]. In short, a small longitudinal incision is typically made over the metacarpal head and a small longitudinal split in the extensor tendon and a limited dorsal arthrotomy. The tendon is retracted and protected, while the surgeon obtains the appropriate start point for the screw. Clinical and radiographic studies have shown that the ideal start point is at the dorsal central third of the metacarpal head, which is in-line with the canal [55]. Alternatively, some advocate for a completely percutaneous technique without any tendon visualization or retraction. While cadaveric studies have shown that there is less risk of tendon damage with the mini-open approach, the difference may not be clinically relevant [61–63]. Currently, there is no clinical evidence supporting one approach over the other.

Next, the fracture is reduced, the guidewire is advanced to the metacarpal base, and a measurement is made. Finally, the guidewire is over drilled and the appropriately sized screw is placed with the proximal threads buried beneath the articular cartilage (Fig. 12.15) [52, 55, 64, 65].

One of the more commonly cited concerns of this technique is the fact that it requires penetration of the joint surface. Berg et al. performed a quantitative 3-dimensional analysis to determine the extent of this articular injury. They found that with a 3.0 mm screw there was very minimal articular injury and a maximum of 12% overlap with the base of the proximal phalanx. This overlap only occurred with hyperextension of the MCPJ [55, 64] (Fig. 12.16). Despite this lack of overlap, there is still concern that the articular injury itself may result in later development of arthritis. Early and midterm results following this technique have not shown any evidence of early arthritis; however, long-term data is still pending [26, 55, 60, 64].

Antegrade intramedullary screw fixation of metacarpals has been proposed as a potential solution to the risk of MCPJ and extensor tendon injury. Hoang et al. described a technique of retrograde guidewire passage starting at the MC head and advancing to the base of the MC. No incision is formally made over the MCPJ. Rather, an incision is made at the base of the MC and the soft tissues are retracted as the guidewire is advanced out of the MC base. Next, the guidewire is over drilled antegrade and a headless screw is placed [66–68]. Currently, there are no clinical outcomes for this technique.

Indications/Applications

Early in their conception, IM screws were reserved predominantly for length-stable metacarpal neck and shaft fractures. As we can see in (Fig. 12.17), IM headless compression screws provide both a strong load-sharing construct and compression through a length-stable fracture [69, 70].

However, in highly comminuted, length-unstable fractures, the use of an IM screw was initially deemed to be contraindicated, resulting in the preferential use crossing k-wire or plate and screw fixation [69]. The rationale was that the use of

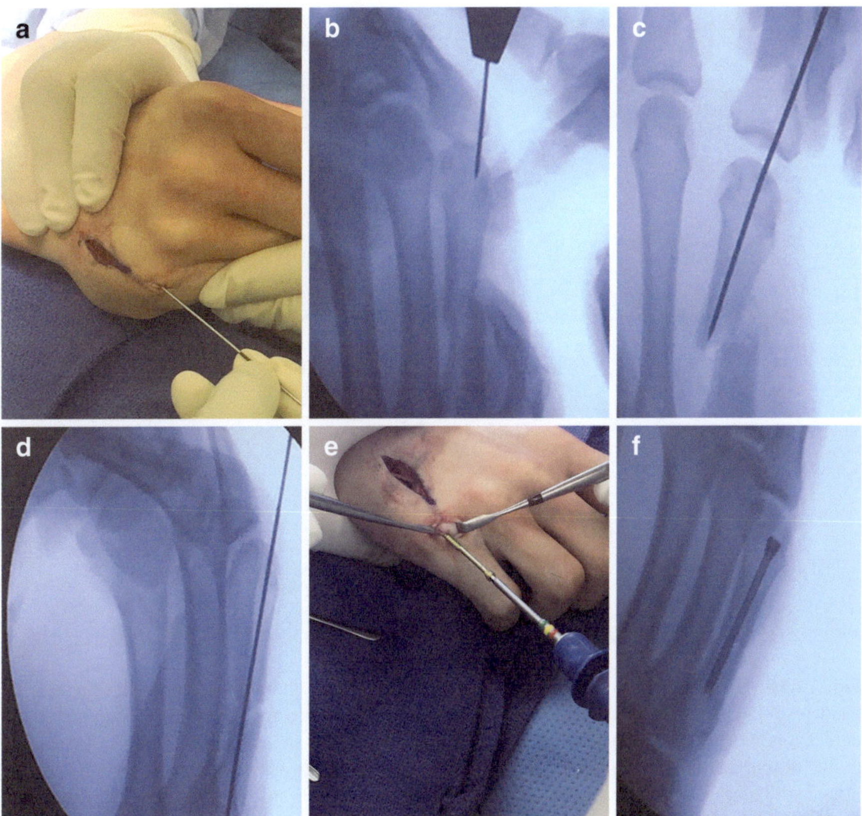

Fig. 12.15 Case example, demonstrating surgical steps for placement of an intramedullary screw for fixation of a transverse fifth metacarpal shaft fracture. (**a**) After a mini-open approach to this subacute fracture to perform osteoclasis, a guidewire for a cannulated headless screw is placed percutaneously into the dorsal central 1/3 of the metacarpal head. (**b**) Confirmation of appropriate starting point with intraoperative fluoroscopy, and (**c**) passage of the guidewire to the fracture site. (**d**) The fracture is reduced, and the guidewire is passed across the fracture. (**e**) After a small incision is made surrounding the entry point of the guidewire, the small extensor tendon-splitting approach to the metacarpal head is made to expose the dorsal central aspect of the meta-carpal head, and the headless screw is passed over the guidewire. (**f**) Final intraoperative fluoroscopy after final placement of the screw and removal of the guidewire. (**Source:** Author's Clinical Photos)

single compression screw along the length of a comminuted metacarpal would result in shortening through the fracture site.

To address this concern, Piñal et al. published a case series in 2015 of more complex screw configurations that can be used to provide stability in length-unstable fractures. For example, they described a technique of "Y-struting" where the endosteal friction fit of two divergent IM screws is used to maintain length in an otherwise length-unstable metacarpal fracture. While no definitive conclusions could be drawn, outcomes of such techniques appeared to be favorable [69].

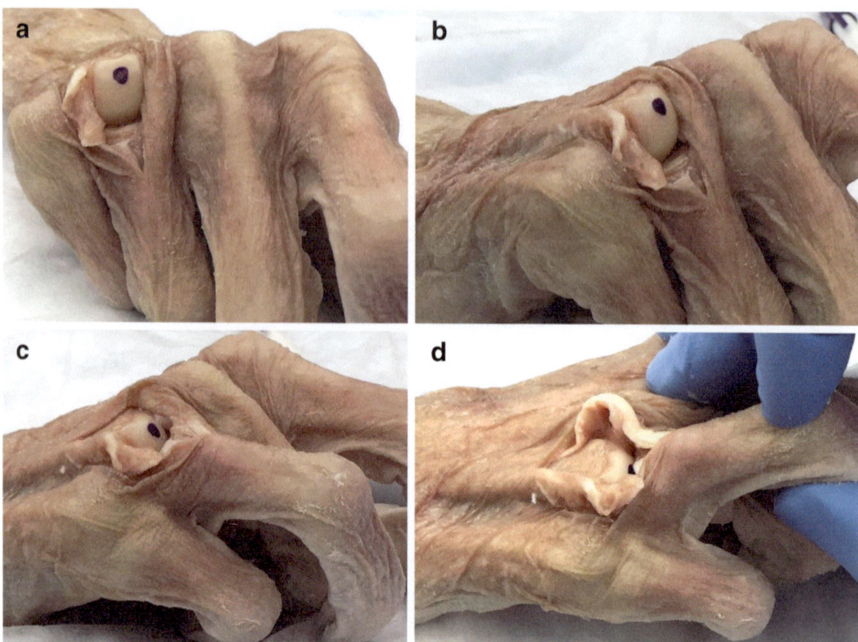

Fig. 12.16 Cadaveric demonstration of location of a typical chondral defect in the metacarpal head resulting from placing a retrograde intramedullary metacarpal screw/nail. The size of the defect is represented by an ink dot with the MCPJ flexed to 90° (**a** and **b**), at 20° of flexion (**c**) and in 20° of hyperextension (**d**). This demonstrates that the metacarpal head defect only engages the dorsal articular base of the proximal phalanx with the MCPJ in positions of hyperextension. (**Source:** Author's cadaveric photos)

More recently, however, the development of fully threaded, conical metacarpal screws has broadened the indications for IM screw fixation. These screws are specifically designed to be non-compressive and thread purchase throughout the length of the endosteum. In theory, these screws can be used in comminuted and long oblique fractures with a decreased risk of fracture shortening (Fig. 12.18). While clinical data is limited, the application of these conical screws at this authors' institution has been effective.

Fig. 12.17 Case example. Preoperative (**a**) and postoperative (**b**) X-ray of a transverse right fifth metacarpal fracture fixed with an intramedullary screw. (**Source:** Author's clinical photos)

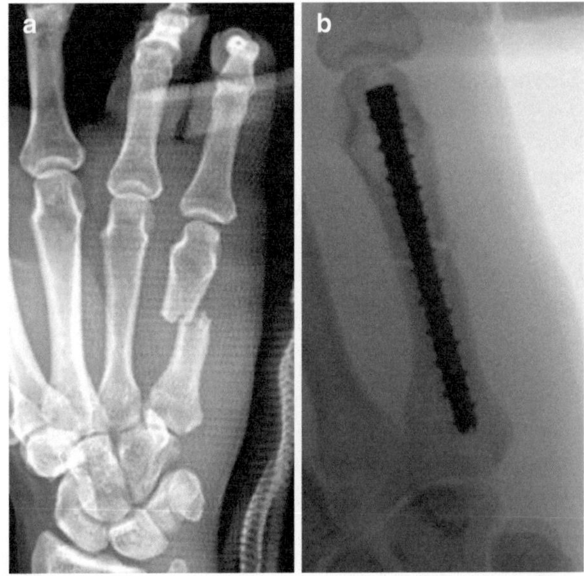

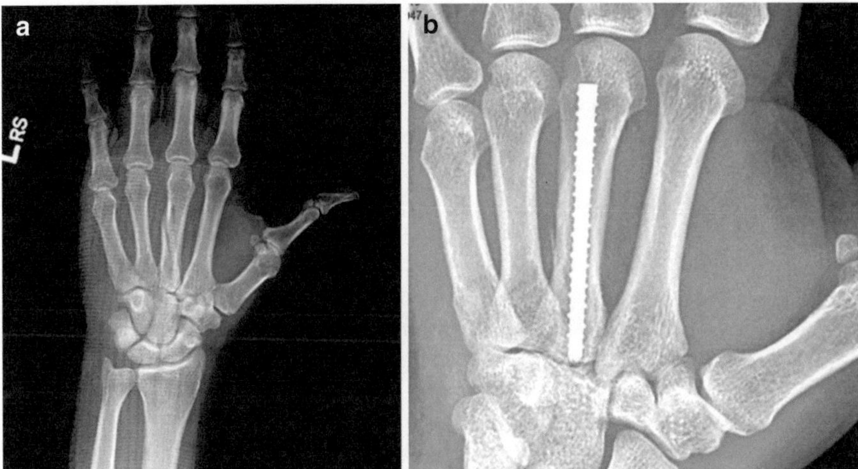

Fig. 12.18 Case example. Preoperative (**a**) and postoperative (**b**) X-ray of a long oblique left third metacarpal fractur fixed with an intramedullary headless conical screw. Despite the oblique fracture pattern, the non-compressive screw design allows preservation of length of the metacarpal. (**Source:** Author's Clinical Photos)

Outcomes (Biomechanical/Clinical)/Complications

Biomechanical Outcomes

Much like an intramedullary femoral nail, the intramedullary metacarpal screw functions as a load-sharing device. Theoretically, this allows for earlier weightbearing and mobilization [71]. Additionally, micromotion at the fracture site encourages rapid healing through secondary bone healing and callus formation. However, if being used to permit early active hand motion, it is important to know if metacarpal nails can actually withstand the forces that they are subject to in the early postoperative period.

To date, there have been several biomechanical studies comparing metacarpal screws to other forms of fracture fixation. In 2021, Dyrna et al. performed 3-point bend testing of lag screws, dorsal plates, and IM headless compression screws. They found that IM screws had the highest peak load to failure of all three modalities [46]. Also in 2021, Galbraith et al. compared IM screws to k-wires and dorsal metacarpal plates. Overall, they found that plating provided the most stability (with IM screws close behind), and that both IM screws and plates provided stability far in excess of what was required in the early hand rehabilitation period [72]. Finally, Melamed et al. compared IM screws to both locked and unlocked dorsal plates and found that IM screws provided the least stability. It is important to note, however, that only short 2.4 mm headless compression screws were used in this study [73]. Three more studies have been performed, all of which corroborate the previous findings that the intramedullary screws are stiffer than k-wire fixation but either as stiff or less stiff than plate and screw fixation [74].

Based on the available results, it appears that intramedullary screws can provide stability that is comparable to other commonly used metacarpal fixation strategies. Its biomechanical profile may actually be ideal in that it provides enough stability to permit early range of motion, but is not too rigid as to prevent secondary bone healing and callus formation [74]. Nonetheless, in order to improve fracture stability, IM screws should be appropriately sized to achieve adequate endosteal purchase.

Clinical Outcomes/Cost/Complications

Currently, long-term data and comparative studies on the outcomes of IM screw fixation are limited. However, the available literature is overall very positive. In 2021, Hug et al. published a systematic review of 2 prospective and 16 retrospective studies, reporting the outcomes of IM screw fixation for both metacarpal and phalangeal fractures. In total, 630 metacarpal fractures were included for analysis with an average follow-up of 18 months. The study revealed a 100% union rate with an average time to union of 5.7 weeks. Functionally, the total active range of motion at final follow-up was 240°, and grip strength was 97.5% of the contralateral (uninjured) side. They reported an overall complication rate of 2.5% which included: 0.3% loss of reduction, 0% infection, 1.7% restricted range of motion, 0.5% screw protrusion. Notably, there were nine refractures in the metacarpal cohort. In two of these cases a bent screw was left in place, in the seven other cases the screw was removed and plate fixation was performed [75].

Of note, the longest reported follow-up for IM screw fixation is by Pogetti et al. [76]. They reported 4-year outcomes following both IM fixation of MC and phalanx fractures. Functional and radiographic outcomes are excellent like those reported by Hug et al. [75]. Importantly, they reported no radiographic signs of osteoarthritis in any of their 173 patients, despite retrograde placement of the screw via a transarticular approach.

Finally, one of the common arguments against use of IM screws is the concern for implant associated costs. Recently, a study out of the UK compared the cost of uncomplicated IM screw fixation to k-wire fixation of metacarpal and phalangeal fractures. The study demonstrated no significant difference in total associated costs (including return to surgery for implant removal, and complications such as infection). In fact, when complications were excluded and when compared to k-wire fixation with buried wires, IM screws were found to be significantly cheaper overall [77].

When used appropriately, IM screws for metacarpal fractures are a promising new technique with excellent short- and midterm outcomes and growing applications. The major benefit of IM screws is that they avoid stiffness by permitting early range of motion with minimal soft tissue disruption. For this reason, they may be the only available operative modality that bolsters both stability and functionality following metacarpal fractures.

Other Techniques/Combination Techniques

In addition, to the aforementioned techniques, there are other, less common, metacarpal fixation strategies that have been described in literature with favorable results.

The first is cerclage wire fixation of the long oblique metacarpal fractures. It was first described by Gropper et al. in 1984 and in their publication they recommended "scoring" the bone to prevent migration of the cerclage wire along the metacarpal shaft [78]. This technique was later modified in 2016 by Al-Qattan et al. who described using dental wire (either true cerclage or interosseous loops for proximal and distal oblique fractures). They reported a case series of 19 patients who received cerclage wiring with full functional recovery and excellent radiographic outcomes and no complications [79]. Other clinical studies on this technique are quite limited.

Another technique is external fixation of metacarpal fractures. The proponents of external fixation explain that it combines the minimal invasiveness of k-wires and the stability of open reduction and plate fixation (similar to IM screw fixation). Despite studies that report excellent outcomes (like the one by Margić et al. in 2006), external fixation is not regularly used in practice [80]. This is likely due to the fact that external fixators (even with the most subtle designs) are cumbersome, unsightly, can be difficult for patients to manage, and other internal fixation techniques are equally as successful. Thus, they are typically reserved for injuries with significant soft tissue damage and/or active infections.

Finally, any of the techniques that have been presented can be used in combination with one another to achieve appropriate fracture reduction and stability. For example, surgeons can combine lag screw and plate fixation or cerclage wire and k-wire fixation if the fracture necessitates. If a hand surgeon is familiar with the available techniques and their respective advantages and pitfalls, it will help him/her choose the appropriate fixation construct for the specific fracture that he/she is addressing.

Rotational Assessment

Following all forms of surgical intervention, it is critical to assess clinical rotation. There are techniques for assessing rotation that can be used intraoperatively (immediately following fixation). First, clinicians can assess for the collinearity of the nail plates with the fingers in extension. Second, the wrist can be taken through passive flexion and extension to assess rotation during tenodesis of the digits. When the digits are fully extended, there should be a normal cascade from index to small finger. In passive flexion, all the digits should be pointed generally toward the distal pole of the scaphoid and distal aspect of the carpal tunnel without crossover (Fig. 12.19). Additionally, in recent years, WALANT (wide awake local anesthesia no tourniquet) surgery has become more common in hand surgery even for metacarpal fracture fixation. In this setting, digital rotation can be assessed as the patient actively flexes and extends their fingers in the operating room [81]. More details on this topic will be covered in the chapter on WALANT hand surgery.

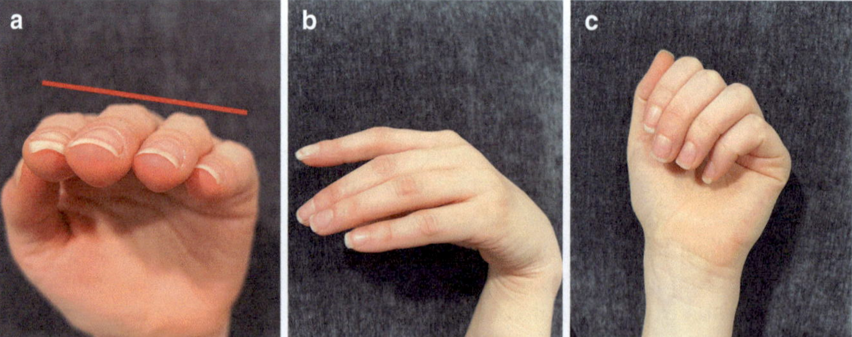

Fig. 12.19 Assessment of correct rotational alignment of the fingers. All nail plates should be collinear when the fingers are in extension (**a**). Also, the wrist can be taken through passive flexion and extension to assess rotation during tenodesis of the digits. When the digits are fully extended (i.e. with wrist in flexion), there should be a normal cascade from index to small finger (**b**). When the digits are flexed (i.e. with wrist in extension), all the digits should be pointed generally toward the distal pole of the scaphoid and distal aspect of the carpal tunnel without crossover (**c**). (**Source:** Author's clinical photos)

Conclusion

Successful metacarpal fracture management (like all hand fractures) requires a delicate balance of bony fixation to avoid the biomechanical consequences of malunion and early mobilization to avoid stiffness. Nonoperative management should typically be considered for most fractures. However, when operative management is preferred surgeons must select the fixation technique that most appropriately addresses the individual fracture with the best chance of permitting early active hand and finger motion. Over the past decade, intramedullary screw fixation has demonstrated excellent outcomes with expanding indications. Surgeons should strive to be comfortable with the pros/cons of the various fixation techniques so that they can offer the best treatment for each individual patient based upon fracture/patient parameters.

References

1. Kollitz KM, Hammert WC, Vedder NB, Huang JI. Metacarpal fractures: treatment and complications. Hand. 2014;9(1):16–23. https://doi.org/10.1007/s11552-013-9562-1.
2. Henry MH. Fractures of the proximal phalanx and metacarpals in the hand: preferred methods of stabilization. J Am Acad Orthop Surg. 2008;16(10):586–95. https://doi.org/10.5435/00124635-200810000-00004.
3. Nakashian MN, Pointer L, Owens BD, Wolf JM. Incidence of metacarpal fractures in the US population. Hand (N Y). 2012;7(4):426–30. https://doi.org/10.1007/S11552-012-9442-0.
4. Smith R. Intrinsic muscles of the fingers: function, dysfunction, and surgical reconstruction. Instr Course Lect. 1975;24
5. Taghinia AH, Talbot SG. Phalangeal and metacarpal fractures. Clin Plast Surg. 2019;46(3):415–23. https://doi.org/10.1016/J.CPS.2019.02.011.
6. Brand PW. Mechanical factors in joint stiffness and tissue growth. J Hand Ther. 1995;8(2):91–6. https://doi.org/10.1016/S0894-1130(12)80305-X.
7. Chin SH, Vedder NB. MOC-PSSM CME article: metacarpal fractures. Plast Reconstr Surg. 2008;121(1 Suppl):1. https://doi.org/10.1097/01.PRS.0000294704.48126.8C.
8. Panchal-Kildare S, Malone K. Skeletal anatomy of the hand. Hand Clin. 2013;29(4):459–71. https://doi.org/10.1016/J.HCL.2013.08.001.
9. Wahl EP, Richard MJ. Management of metacarpal and phalangeal fractures in the athlete. Clin Sports Med. 2020;39(2):401–22. https://doi.org/10.1016/J.CSM.2019.12.002.
10. Nakamura K, Patterson RM, Viegas SF. The ligament and skeletal anatomy of the second through fifth carpometacarpal joints and adjacent structures. J Hand Surg Am. 2001;26(6):1016–29. https://doi.org/10.1053/JHSU.2001.26329.
11. Kozin SH, Thoder JJ, Lieberman G. Operative treatment of metacarpal and phalangeal shaft fractures. J Am Acad Orthop Surg. 2000;8(2):111–21. https://doi.org/10.5435/00124635-200003000-00005.
12. Ghareeb PA, Daly C, Liao A, Payne D. Current trends in the management of ballistic fractures of the hand and wrist: experiences of a high-volume level I trauma center. Hand (N Y). 2018;13(2):176–80. https://doi.org/10.1177/1558944717697432.
13. Strub B, Schindele S, Sonderegger J, Sproedt J, Von Campe A, Gruenert JG. Intramedullary splinting or conservative treatment for displaced fractures of the little finger metacarpal neck? A prospective study. J Hand Surg Eur Vol. 2010;35(9):725–9. https://doi.org/10.1177/1753193410377845.
14. Theeuwen GAJM, Lemmens JAM, van Niekerk JLM. Conservative treatment of boxer's fracture: a retrospective analysis. Injury. 1991;22(5):394–6. https://doi.org/10.1016/0020-1383(91)90103-L.

15. Strauch RJ, Rosenwasser MP, Lunt JG. Metacarpal shaft fractures: the effect of shortening on the extensor tendon mechanism. J Hand Surg Am. 1998;23(3):519–23. https://doi.org/10.1016/S0363-5023(05)80471-X.
16. Eglseder WA Jr, Juliano PJ, Roure R. Fractures of the fourth metacarpal. J Orthop Trauma. 1997;11(6):441–5. https://doi.org/10.1097/00005131-199708000-00014.
17. Meunier MJ, Hentzen E, Ryan M, Shin AY, Lieber RL. Predicted effects of metacarpal shortening on interosseous muscle function. J Hand Surg Am. 2004;29(4):689–93. https://doi.org/10.1016/j.jhsa.2004.03.002.
18. Freeland AE, Orbay JL. Extraarticular hand fractures in adults: a review of new developments. Clin Orthop Relat Res. 2006;445:133–45. https://doi.org/10.1097/01.BLO.0000205888.04200.C5.
19. Christoforetti JJ, Krupp RJ, Singleton SB, Kissenberth MJ, Cook C, Hawkins RJ. Arthroscopic suture bridge transosseous equivalent fixation of rotator cuff tendon preserves intratendinous blood flow at the time of initial fixation. J Shoulder Elb Surg. 2012;21(4):523–30. https://doi.org/10.1016/J.JSE.2011.02.012.
20. Royle SG. Rotational deformity following metacarpal fracture. J Hand Surg Br. 1990;15(1):124–5. https://doi.org/10.1016/0266-7681_90_90068-F.
21. Poolman RW, Goslings JC, Lee J, Statius Muller M, Steller EP, Struijs PAA. Conservative treatment for closed fifth (small finger) metacarpal neck fractures. Cochrane Database Syst Rev. 2005;2005(3):CD003210. https://doi.org/10.1002/14651858.CD003210.PUB3.
22. Tavassoli J, Ruland RT, Hogan CJ, Cannon DL. Three cast techniques for the treatment of extra-articular metacarpal fractures. Comparison of short-term outcomes and final fracture alignments. J Bone Joint Surg Am. 2005;87(10):2196–201. https://doi.org/10.2106/JBJS.D.03038.
23. Soong M, Chase S, George Kasparyan N. Metacarpal fractures in the athlete. Curr Rev Musculoskelet Med. 2017;10(1):23–7. https://doi.org/10.1007/s12178-017-9380-0.
24. van Aaken J, Fusetti C, Luchina S, et al. Fifth metacarpal neck fractures treated with soft wrap/buddy taping compared to reduction and casting: results of a prospective, multicenter, randomized trial. Arch Orthop Trauma Surg. 2016;136(1):135–42. https://doi.org/10.1007/S00402-015-2361-0.
25. Jahss S. Fractures of the metacarpals: a new method of reduction and immobilization. J Bone Joint Surg. 1938;20(1):178–86.
26. Carreño A, Ansari MT, Malhotra R. Management of metacarpal fractures. J Clin Orthop Trauma. 2020;11(4):554–61. https://doi.org/10.1016/J.JCOT.2020.05.043.
27. Pace GI, Gendelberg D, Taylor KF. The effect of closed reduction of small finger metacarpal neck fractures on the ultimate angular deformity. J Hand Surg Am. 2015;40(8):1582. https://doi.org/10.1016/j.jhsa.2015.05.013.
28. Al-Qattan MM. Outcome of conservative management of spiral/long oblique fractures of the metacarpal shaft of the fingers using a palmar wrist splint and immediate mobilisation of the fingers. J Hand Surg Eur Vol. 2008;33(6):723–7. https://doi.org/10.1177/1753193408093559.
29. Debnath UK, Nassab RS, Oni JA, Davis TRC. A prospective study of the treatment of fractures of the little finger metacarpal shaft with a short hand cast. J Hand Surg Am. 2004;29 B(3):214–7. https://doi.org/10.1016/j.jhsb.2004.02.020.
30. Iqbal A, Cattell AE, Dhillon S. A simple technique to ensure adequate moulding of a cast into the Edinburgh position. Ann R Coll Surg Engl. 2012;94(2):133. https://doi.org/10.1308/rcsann.2012.94.2.134.
31. Barr C, Behn AW, Yao J. Plating of metacarpal fractures with locked or nonlocked screws, a biomechanical study: how many cortices are really necessary? Hand. 2013;8(4):454. https://doi.org/10.1007/s11552-013-9544-3.
32. Chiu YC, Hsu CE, Ho TY, Ting YN, Tsai MT, Hsu JT. Bone plate fixation ability on the dorsal and lateral sides of a metacarpal shaft transverse fracture. J Orthop Surg Res. 2021;16(1):441. https://doi.org/10.1186/s13018-021-02575-3.
33. Page SM, Stern PJ. Complications and range of motion following plate fixation of metacarpal and phalangeal fractures. J Hand Surg Am. 1998;23(5):827–32. https://doi.org/10.1016/S0363-5023(98)80157-3.

34. Fusetti C, Meyer H, Borisch N, Stern R, Santa DD, Papaloïzos M. Complications of plate fixation in metacarpal fractures. J Trauma. 2002;52(3):535. https://doi.org/10.1097/00005373-200203000-00019.
35. Fusetti C, Della Santa DR. Influence of fracture pattern on consolidation after metacarpal plate fixation. Chir Main. 2004;23(1):32. https://doi.org/10.1016/j.main.2003.12.002.
36. Alhujayri AK, Alohaideb NS, Alarfaj SF, Alhodaib NI. Intra-medullary, at fracture site introduction of K-wires for metacarpal fracture fixation (in-site technique). A new fixation technique and a case series. Int J Surg Case Rep. 2020;73:218. https://doi.org/10.1016/j.ijscr.2020.07.032.
37. van Bussel EM, Houwert RM, Kootstra TJM, et al. Antegrade intramedullary Kirschner-wire fixation of displaced metacarpal shaft fractures. Eur J Trauma Emerg Surg. 2019;45(1):65. https://doi.org/10.1007/s00068-017-0836-0.
38. Terndrup M, Jensen T, Kring S, Lindberg-Larsen M. Should we bury K-wires after metacarpal and phalangeal fracture osteosynthesis? Injury. 2018;49(6):1126. https://doi.org/10.1016/j.injury.2018.02.027.
39. Khan H, Adil A, Ul Ain N, Qureshi BA, Chishti UF, Malik TS. Outcome of buried versus exposed Kirchner wires in terms of infection in fractures of phalanges and metacarpal bones of hand. Cureus. 2022;14:e22515. https://doi.org/10.7759/cureus.22515.
40. Kim JK, Kim DJ. Antegrade intramedullary pinning versus retrograde intramedullary pinning for displaced fifth metacarpal neck fractures. Clin Orthop Relat Res. 2015;473(5):1747. https://doi.org/10.1007/s11999-014-4079-7.
41. Ozer K, Gillani S, Williams A, Peterson SL, Morgan S. Comparison of intramedullary nailing versus plate-screw fixation of extra-articular metacarpal fractures. J Hand Surg Am. 2008;33(10):1724–31. https://doi.org/10.1016/j.jhsa.2008.07.011.
42. Hsu LP, Schwartz EG, Kalainov DM, Chen F, Makowiec RL. Complications of K-wire fixation in procedures involving the hand and wrist. J Hand Surg Am. 2011;36(4):610–6. https://doi.org/10.1016/j.jhsa.2011.01.023.
43. Botte MJ, Davis JLW, Rose BA, et al. Complications of smooth pin fixation of fractures and dislocations in the hand and wrist. Clin Orthop Relat Res. 1992;276:194–201. https://doi.org/10.1097/00003086-199203000-00025.
44. Dreyfuss D, Allon R, Izacson N, Hutt D. A comparison of locking plates and intramedullary pinning for fixation of metacarpal shaft fractures. Hand. 2019;14(1):27. https://doi.org/10.1177/1558944718798854.
45. Jones NF, Jupiter JB, Lalonde DH. Common fractures and dislocations of the hand. Plast Reconstr Surg. 2012;130(5):722e. https://doi.org/10.1097/PRS.0b013e318267d67a.
46. Dyrna FGE, Avery DM, Yoshida R, et al. Metacarpal shaft fixation: a biomechanical comparison of dorsal plating, lag screws, and headless compression screws. BMC Musculoskelet Disord. 2021;22(1):1–8. https://doi.org/10.1186/s12891-021-04200-0.
47. Souza JM, Cheesborough JE, Ko JH, Cho MS, Kuiken TA, Dumanian GA. Targeted muscle reinnervation: a novel approach to postamputation neuroma pain. Clin Orthop Relat Res. 2014;472(10):2984–90. https://doi.org/10.1007/S11999-014-3528-7.
48. Roth JJ, Auerbach DM. Fixation of hand fractures with bicortical screws. J Hand Surg Am. 2005;30(1):151. https://doi.org/10.1016/j.jhsa.2004.07.016.
49. White MJ, Parr WCH, Wang T, Schick BF, Walsh WR. Effect of bicortical interfragmentary screw size on the fixation of metacarpal shaft fractures: a 3-dimensional-printed biomechanical study. J Hand Surg Glob Online. 2021;3(3):154. https://doi.org/10.1016/j.jhsg.2021.01.003.
50. Liporace FA, Kinchelow T, Gupta S, Kubiak EN, McDonnell M. Minifragment screw fixation of oblique metacarpal fractures: a biomechanical analysis of screw types and techniques. Hand. 2008;3(4):311. https://doi.org/10.1007/s11552-008-9108-0.
51. Eu-Jin Cheah A, Behn AW, Comer G, Yao J. A biomechanical analysis of 2 constructs for metacarpal spiral fracture fixation in a cadaver model: 2 large screws versus 3 small screws. J Hand Surg Am. 2017;42(12):1033.e1. https://doi.org/10.1016/j.jhsa.2017.07.018.

52. Boulton CL, Salzler M, Mudgal CS. Intramedullary cannulated headless screw fixation of a comminuted subcapital metacarpal fracture: case report. J Hand Surg Am. 2010;35(8):1260–3. https://doi.org/10.1016/j.jhsa.2010.04.032.

53. Grundberg AB. Intramedullary fixation for fractures of the hand. J Hand Surg Am. 1981;6(6):568–73. https://doi.org/10.1016/S0363-5023(81)80134-7.

54. Irigaray A. New fixing screw for completely amputated fingers. J Hand Surg Am. 1980;5(4):381. https://doi.org/10.1016/S0363-5023(80)80181-X.

55. Ten Berg PWL, Mudgal CS, Leibman MI, Belsky MR, Ruchelsman DE. Quantitative 3-dimensional CT analyses of intramedullary headless screw fixation for metacarpal neck fractures. J Hand Surg Am. 2013;38(2):322–30.e2. https://doi.org/10.1016/j.jhsa.2012.09.029.

56. Dunleavy ML, Candela X, Darowish M. Morphological analysis of metacarpal shafts with respect to retrograde intramedullary headless screw fixation. Hand. 2020;17:602. https://doi.org/10.1177/1558944720937362.

57. Okoli M, Chatterji R, Ilyas A, Kirkpatrick W, Abboudi J, Jones CM. Intramedullary headless screw fixation of metacarpal fractures: a radiographic analysis for optimal screw choice. Hand. 2020;17:245. https://doi.org/10.1177/1558944720919897.

58. Douglass N, Yao J. Nuts and bolts: dimensions of commonly utilized screws in upper extremity surgery. J Hand Surg Am. 2015;40(2):368. https://doi.org/10.1016/j.jhsa.2014.11.012.

59. Ruchelsman DE, Puri S, Feinberg-Zadek N, Leibman MI, Belsky MR. Clinical outcomes of limited-open retrograde intramedullary headless screw fixation of metacarpal fractures. J Hand Surg Am. 2014;39(12):2390–5. https://doi.org/10.1016/j.jhsa.2014.08.016.

60. Eisenberg G, Clain JB, Feinberg-Zadek N, Leibman M, Belsky M, Ruchelsman DE. Clinical outcomes of limited open intramedullary headless screw fixation of metacarpal fractures in 91 consecutive patients. Hand. 2020;15(6):793–7. https://doi.org/10.1177/1558944719836235.

61. Urbanschitz L, Dreu M, Wagner J, Kaufmann R, Jeserschek JM, Borbas P. Cartilage and extensor tendon defects after headless compression screw fixation of phalangeal and metacarpal fractures. J Hand Surg Eur Vol. 2020;45(6):601. https://doi.org/10.1177/1753193420919060.

62. Colzani G, Tos P, Battiston B, Merolla G, Porcellini G, Artiaco S. Traumatic extensor tendon injuries to the hand: clinical anatomy, biomechanics, and surgical procedure review. J Hand Microsurg. 2016;08(01):2. https://doi.org/10.1055/s-0036-1572534.

63. Mahylis JM, Burwell AK, Bonneau L, Marshall LM, Mirarchi AJ. Drill penetration injury to extensor tendons: a biomechanical analysis. Hand. 2017;12(3):301. https://doi.org/10.1177/1558944716668824.

64. Esteban-Feliu I, Gallardo-Calero I, Barrera-Ochoa S, Lluch-Bergadà A, Alabau-Rodriguez S, Mir-Bulló X. Analysis of 3 different operative techniques for extra-articular fractures of the phalanges and metacarpals. Hand. 2021;16(5):595. https://doi.org/10.1177/1558944719873144.

65. Beck CM, Horesh E, Taub PJ. Intramedullary screw fixation of metacarpal fractures results in excellent functional outcomes: a literature review. Plast Reconstr Surg. 2019;143(4):1111–8. https://doi.org/10.1097/PRS.0000000000005478.

66. Hoang D, Vu CL, Jackson M, Huang JI. An anatomical study of metacarpal morphology utilizing CT scans: evaluating parameters for antegrade intramedullary compression screw fixation of metacarpal fractures. J Hand Surg Am. 2021;46(2):149.e1. https://doi.org/10.1016/j.jhsa.2020.08.007.

67. Hoang D, Huang J. Antegrade intramedullary screw fixation: a novel approach to metacarpal fractures. J Hand Surg Glob Online. 2019;1(4):229. https://doi.org/10.1016/j.jhsg.2019.07.002.

68. Hoang D, Vu CL, Huang JI. Evaluation of antegrade intramedullary compression screw fixation of metacarpal shaft fractures in a cadaver model. J Hand Surg Am. 2021;46(5):428.e1. https://doi.org/10.1016/j.jhsa.2020.10.026.

69. Del Piñal F, Moraleda E, Rúas JS, De Piero GH, Cerezal L. Minimally invasive fixation of fractures of the phalanges and metacarpals with intramedullary cannulated headless compression screws. J Hand Surg Am. 2015;40(4):692. https://doi.org/10.1016/j.jhsa.2014.11.023.

70. Guidi M, Frueh FS, Besmens I, Calcagni M. Intramedullary compression screw fixation of metacarpal and phalangeal fractures. EFORT Open Rev. 2020;5(10):624–9. https://doi.org/10.1302/2058-5241.5.190068.

71. Bong MR, Kummer FJ, Koval KJ, Egol KA. Intramedullary nailing of the lower extremity: biomechanics and biology. J Am Acad Orthop Surg. 2007;15(2):97–106. https://doi.org/10.5435/00124635-200702000-00004.
72. Galbraith JG, Huntington LS, Borbas P, Ackland DC, Tham SK, Ek ET. Biomechanical comparison of intramedullary screw fixation, dorsal plating and K-wire fixation for stable metacarpal shaft fractures. J Hand Surg Eur Vol. 2022;47(2):172. https://doi.org/10.1177/17531934211017705.
73. Melamed E, Hinds RM, Gottschalk MB, Kennedy OD, Capo JT. Comparison of dorsal plate fixation versus intramedullary headless screw fixation of unstable metacarpal shaft fractures: a biomechanical study. Hand. 2016;11(4):421. https://doi.org/10.1177/1558944716628485.
74. Morway GR, Rider T, Jones CM. Retrograde intramedullary screw fixation for metacarpal fractures: a systematic review. Hand. 2021;18:67. https://doi.org/10.1177/1558944720988073.
75. Hug U, Fiumedinisi F, Pallaver A, et al. Intramedullary screw fixation of metacarpal and phalangeal fractures—a systematic review of 837 patients. Hand Surg Rehabil. 2021;40(5):622–30. https://doi.org/10.1016/J.HANSUR.2021.04.009.
76. Poggetti A, Fagetti A, Lauri G, Cherubino M, Borelli PP, Pfanner S. Outcomes of 173 metacarpal and phalangeal fractures treated by intramedullary headless screw fixation with a 4-year follow-up. J Hand Surg Eur Vol. 2021;46(5):466–70. https://doi.org/10.1177/1753193420980324.
77. Brewer CF, Young-Sing Q, Sierakowski A. Cost comparison of Kirschner wire versus intramedullary screw fixation of metacarpal and phalangeal fractures. Hand (N Y). 2021; https://doi.org/10.1177/15589447211030690.
78. Gropper PT, Bowen V. Cerclage wiring of metacarpal fractures. Clin Orthop Relat Res. 1984;188:203. https://doi.org/10.1097/00003086-198409000-00028.
79. Al-Qattan MM, Al-Lazzam A. Long oblique/spiral mid-shaft metacarpal fractures of the fingers: treatment with cerclage wire fixation and immediate post-operative finger mobilisation in a wrist splint. J Hand Surg Eur Vol. 2007;32(6):637–40. https://doi.org/10.1016/J.JHSE.2007.05.016.
80. Margić K. External fixation of closed metacarpal and phalangeal fractures of digits. A prospective study of one hundred consecutive patients. J Hand Surg Am. 2006;31(1):30. https://doi.org/10.1016/j.jhsb.2005.09.013.
81. Lalonde DH. Latest advances in wide awake hand surgery. Hand Clin. 2019;35(1):1–6. https://doi.org/10.1016/J.HCL.2018.08.002.

Metacarpal Head and Neck Fractures

13

Richard J. Tosti

Epidemiology and Mechanism

Metacarpal head and neck fractures are commonly encountered by treated physicians representing 18% of all fractures below the elbow and up to 44% of all hand fractures [1, 2]. The highest risk demographic is young adults; males represent 76% of those identified with a metacarpal fracture. The most common mechanism that results in head and neck fractures is an axial compression usually from a clenched fist impacting a solid object. However, solid objects impacting the hand or falls are also not uncommonly recorded in the history. Avulsion fractures are uncommon at the metacarpophalangeal (MP) joints of the fingers but may occur when excessive radial or ulnar deviation is impressed upon the fingers such as "jamming" a finger while playing sports.

Classification

Although no classification is widely used, fractures can be described by location and morphology. Intra-articular fractures of the head of the metacarpal may be partial or complete articular, simple or comminuted, or in the coronal or sagittal planes. Metacarpal neck fractures occur at the metaphyseal region and usually deform in apex dorsal angulation. These fractures may present as transverse, oblique, or spiral and may be simple or comminuted. It is not uncommon for these fractures to rupture through the dorsal skin as result of the relative subcutaneous position of the bone.

R. J. Tosti (✉)
Rothman Orthopaedic Institute, Thomas Jefferson University, Philadelphia, PA, USA

Avulsion fractures of the metacarpal head may have displaced or nondisplaced fragments from their respective condyles and may be considered stable or unstable with respect to the MP joint.

Physical Exam

Open fractures are usually obvious upon inspection in apex dorsal fractures, but volar lacerations may be hidden from vision beneath the fingers. The knuckle prominence may be shortened. Swelling and joint effusion are often present. A dorsal "bump" deformity may present over an angulated neck fracture. Range of motion is often reduced due to pain and guarding. Intra-articular fractures may have a block to motion and could additionally be assessed with an intra-articular injection of local anesthesia. Neck fractures should be critically examined for rotatory deformities, which is performed best with the patient making a composite fist. If the patient is guarding, placing the wrist into extension and allowing the fingers to flex by tenodesis effect can be helpful to make an assessment of rotational alignment. Rotational orientation of the digits can be viewed by the cascade, the orientation of the nail plates, or overlapping of the digits. Additionally angulated neck fractures should be checked for the ability to extend the MP joint using the contralateral hand as a reference. Avulsion fractures should be tested for joint stability. The patient should be able to complete a smooth arc of motion and should be stable to varus/valgus forces in extension and at 30° of flexion. Usually varus or valgus deviation of 15° greater than the opposite side or 30° total indicates an unstable joint.

Imaging

Suspected fractures of the hand are first evaluated with orthogonal radiographs. A Brewerton view may be helpful in assessing metacarpal head fractures; the plate is placed against the dorsum of patient's fingers with the wrist in neutral. The patient then flexes the MP joints to 65° and the beam is directed ulnar to radial at 15°. A computed tomography scan may be of utility for complex intra-articular fractures to assessment displacement, loose bodies, or for presurgical planning. Magnetic resonance imaging is useful for identifying occult fractures or pure ligamentous injuries.

Treatment

The goal of treatment in metacarpal head fractures is to ensure a congruent articulation to prevent post-traumatic arthrosis and promote unimpeded motion. Most surgeons would agree that large (>25%) or displaced (>1 mm) intra-articular fragments would be indicated for surgery. Also fragments that may block motion due to loose body formation or incongruity should also be treated operatively.

Metacarpal neck fractures are more controversial. Traditionally, acceptable angulation is often defined as 10°, 20°, 30°, 40° for the index, middle, ring, and small, respectively. However, a recent study that surveyed 250 surgeons of the ASSH had shown wide variation in their preferred treatment method based on small finger angulation with some surgeons accepting up to 70° of deformity [3]. Sagittal plane deformity is most often apex dorsal angulation due to the forces of the intrinsic and extrinsic flexors. Angular deformity and shortening may result in an extensor lag of the digit, which would impede the ability to open the hand to acquire large objects. In a cadaveric study by Strauch et al. it was estimated that every 2 mm of shortening resulted in 7° of extensor lag [4]. Additionally, a severe malunion may cause pain and weakness with grasp as the metacarpal head experiences increased contact pressures and the flexor digit minimi is placed in a disadvantaged position [5, 6]. Fractures with a rotatory deformity result in overlapping or "scissoring" of the digits when forming a composite fist, thus are usually treated surgically.

Avulsion fractures may be considered for operative treatment if largely displaced, comprise a large portion of the articular surface, or associated with joint instability.

Nonoperative Management

For metacarpal head fractures, immobilization in a hand based orthosis for 4–6 weeks is appropriate for nondisplaced fractures without a block to motion. The MP joint is usually positioned in flexion or "safety position" to maintain tension on the collateral ligaments and prevent an extension contracture. Active and passive motion exercises are initiated once clinical union is perceived by the surgeon and strength and weight bearing begin after radiographic union.

Metacarpal neck fractures have a variety of described treatment methods and none has been shown to be superior. One perspective is to immobilize the hand in "safety position" to protect the MP joints against extension contracture. However, this method is sometimes criticized as immobilization in flexion will further deform an apex dorsal fracture. Another strategy is to immobilize the MP in extension as this imparts a corrective force of the distal fragment and may be better tolerated [7]. Although this strategy may be criticized for its risk of extension contracture, a study by Hofmeister et al. had noted no differences in range of motion or deformity between immobilizing the MP joint in flexion or extension [7]. A third option is to buddy strap the injured digit to the adjacent digit. A study by Catalan et al. noted that immobilization was not superior to buddy strapping with immediate motion for fractures with less than 70° of angulation [8].

It should be noted that prior to immobilizing the fracture, an attempt at closed reduction could be made under local anesthesia. This is best performed within the first few days after the injury. For an apex dorsal fracture, the surgeon places a dorsally directed force on the distal fragment. Alternatively, the Jahss maneuver may also be performed whereby the surgeon will flex the MP joint and use the base of the proximal phalanx to direct a dorsal force on the head of the metacarpal [9].

Avulsion fractures of the fingers are usually treated nonoperatively by buddy strapping the finger to the finger adjacent to the fracture. Early range of motion exercises are performed. A short period of immobilization may be considered in cases with severe pain or swelling.

Operative Management

Metacarpal head fractures are usually approached dorsally through an extensor tendon splitting or release of the sagittal band. The dorsal capsule is incised to expose the fragments. A volar approach may be necessary in the case of coronal shear injury. The A1 flexor pulley is released and the flexor tendons are retracted. The volar plate is incised to expose the joint. In either case, a joint debridement and lavage will remove loose bodies and large fragments are reduced and provisionally secured with K wires. Most often small (1.3–1.5 mm) headed or headless screws are placed in a retrograde orientation. Headed screws will need to be counter sunk beneath the chondral surface to avoid impingement.

Severely damaged metacarpal head fractures may also be treated with a spanning bridge plate if adequate bone stock is still present. The bridge plate is removed at 6–12 weeks postoperatively and is concomitantly performed with a tenolysis and arthrolysis. For those without adequate bone stock a resection arthroplasty or implant arthroplasty may be a salvage option (Fig. 13.1).

Metacarpal neck fractures may be secured by a variety of techniques. Internal fixation with a plate and screw construct may be necessary for comminuted fractures or those with bone loss. A direct dorsal incision with retraction of the extensor

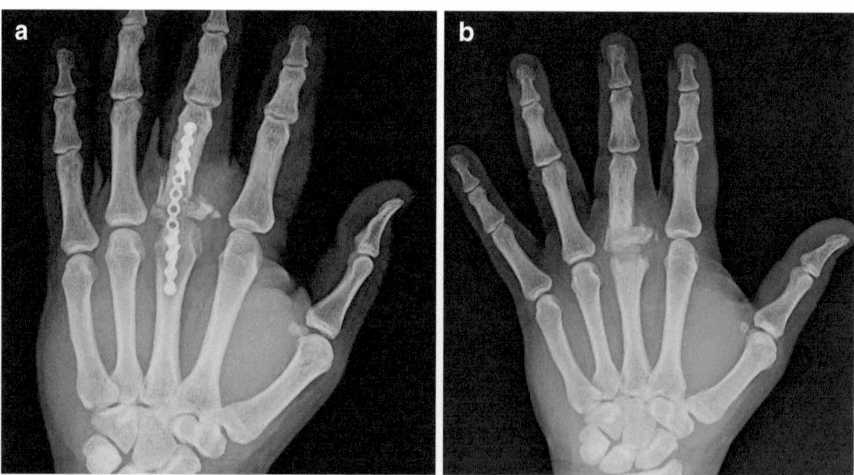

Fig. 13.1 (a) Bridge plate construct over comminuted proximal phalanx and metacarpal head fracture resulting from a gunshot. (b) This was later removed and replaced with a silastic joint

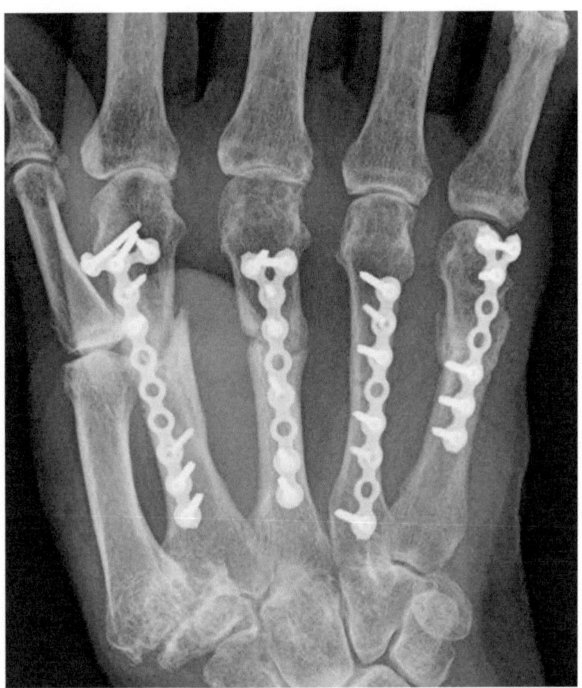

Fig. 13.2 Plate a screw constructs for metacarpal neck and shaft fractures in an open avulsion injury

tendon will place surgeon directly on the fracture. Screws are often unicortical locking screws in the metacarpal head (Fig. 13.2).

A less invasive internal fixation option is placing retrograde headless intramedullary screw. This can be done percutaneous or through a small extensor splitting approach of the MP joint. The screw diameter is templated by placing the screw over the metacarpal isthmus on live fluoroscopy. The ring finger metacarpal has the thinnest diameter [10]. The fracture is reduced using a dorsal applied force and guide wire is started between the dorsal third and the midpoint of the metacarpal head. It is then advanced retrograde across the fracture and into the base of the metacarpal. A cannulated drill is used to puncture the metacarpal head, and the headless screw is advanced to a subchondral position (Fig. 13.3).

Immediate motion is usually started with internal fixation techniques; these constructs are usually strong enough to support normal physiological forces and the early motion reduces stiffness.

K wires are also preferred by some surgeons. Two crossing retrograde K wires may be placed across the fracture site (Fig. 13.4). Several antegrade K wires (bouquet pinning) may be placed from the metacarpal base and into the head to serve as an internal stent. Alternatively, K wires may be placed transversely across adjacent metacarpal heads. The wires remain in place for 4–6 weeks and are usually removed in the office. They may be buried beneath the skin or exposed. Early motion is possible with K wires but is more difficult than internal fixation.

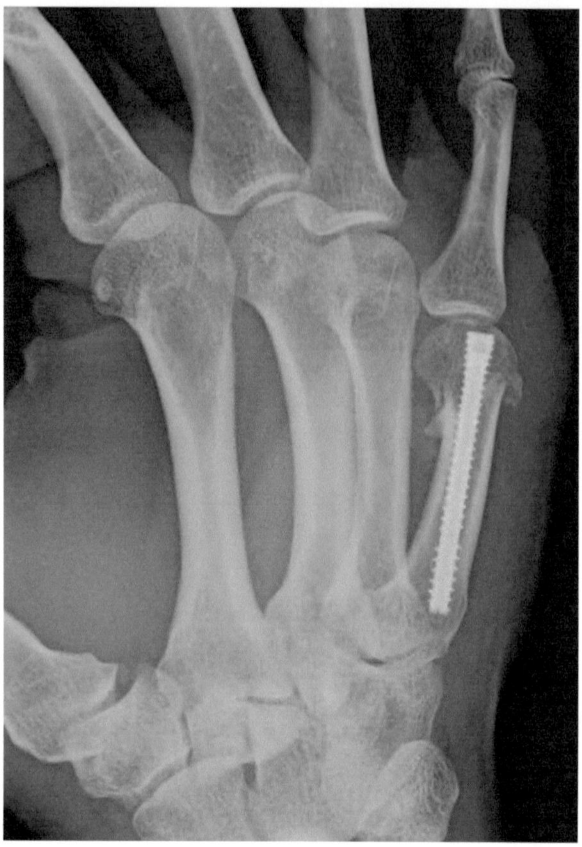

Fig. 13.3 Intramedullary screw fixation for metacarpal neck fracture

Avulsion fractures are also treated through a dorsal approach. Large fragments can be secured with a screw or a small threaded pin cut on the cortical surface. Small fragments can be secured with a tension band or a bone anchor. The tension band is placed by drilling an anterior to posterior bone tunnel in the metacarpal shaft. A wire or suture is passed into the bone tunnel, crossed, and then transversely pierces the Sharpey fibers of the fragment. The free ends are either tied or twisted depending on the material suture or wire, respectively. A bone anchor can also be placed into the fracture site and the limbs of the suture can grasp the ligamentous portion of the avulsed fragment or may be passed directly through two small bone tunnels in the fragment.

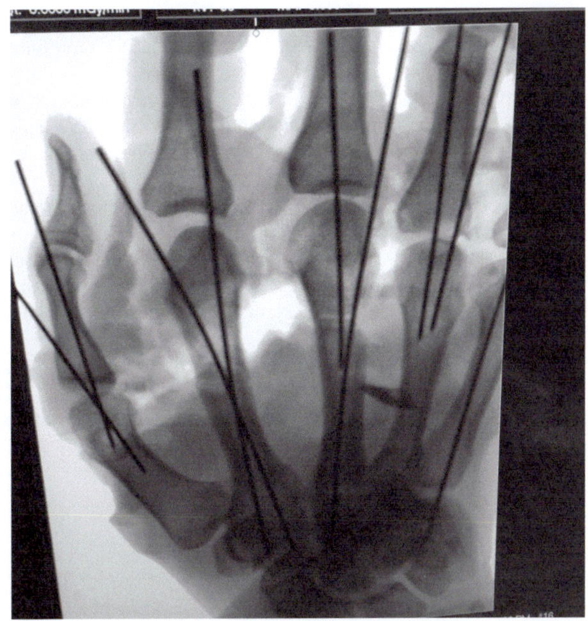

Fig. 13.4 Retrograde intramedullary cross pinning of a metacarpal fracture in a hand during replantation surgery

Outcomes

Overall outcomes for surgical treatment of metacarpal head fractures are generally favorable but dependent on the severity of injury and the state of the overlying soft tissue. Stiffness is a common complication especially with more complex fractures or with those that require more dissection [11, 12]. Infection is a rare complication but may reach as high as 11% with open fractures [13].

References

1. Chung KC, Spilson SV. The frequency and epidemiology of hand and fore-arm fractures in the United States. J Hand Surg Am. 2001;26:908–15.
2. Kollitz KM, Hammert WC, Vedder NB, Huang JI. Metacarpal fractures: treatment and complications. Hand (N Y). 2014;9(1):16–23.
3. Tosti R, Ilyas AM, Mellema JJ, Guitton TG, Ring D, Science of Variation Group. Interobserver variability in the treatment of little finger metacarpal neck fractures. J Hand Surg Am. 2014;39(9):1722–7.
4. Strauch RJ, Rosenwasser MP, Lunt JG. Metacarpal shaft fractures: the effect of shortening on the extensor tendon mechanism. J Hand Surg Am. 1998;23(3):519–23.
5. Birndorf MS, Daley R, Greenwald DP. Metacarpal fracture angulation decreases flexor mechanical efficiency in human hands. Plast Reconstr Surg. 1997;99:1079–83.
6. Ali A, Hamman J, Mass DP. The biomechanical effects of angulated boxer's fractures. J Hand Surg. 1999;24A:835–44.

 7. Hofmeister EP, Kim J, Shin AY. Comparison of 2 methods of immobilization of fifth metacarpal neck fractures: a prospective randomized study. J Hand Surg [Am]. 2008;33:1362–8.
 8. Martínez-Catalán N, Pajares S, Llanos L, Mahillo I, Calvo E. A prospective randomized trial comparing the functional results of buddy taping versus closed reduction and cast immobilization in patients with fifth metacarpal neck fractures. J Hand Surg Am. 2020;45(12):1134–40.
 9. Jahss SA. Fractures of the metacarpals: a new method of reduction and immobilization. J Bone Joint Surg. 1938;20:178–86.
10. Okoli M, Lutsky K, Rivlin M, Katt B, Beredjiklian P. Metacarpal bony dimensions related to headless compression screw sizes. J Hand Microsurg. 2020;12(Suppl 1):S39–44.
11. Fusetti C, Meyer H, Borisch N, et al. Complications of plate fixation in metacarpal fractures. J Trauma. 2002;52:535–9.
12. Page SM, Stern PJ. Complications and range of motion following plate fixation of metacarpal and phalangeal fractures. J Hand Surg [Am]. 1998;23:827–32.
13. McLain RF, Steyers C, Stoddard M. Infections in open fractures of the hand. J Hand Surg [Am]. 1991;16:108–12.

Adult Thumb Metacarpal Fractures

14

Virgenal Owens, Julia Mastracci, and R. Glenn Gaston

Epidemiology

First metacarpal fractures are common orthopedic injuries, comprising about 4% of fractures of the hand. Roughly 80% involve the metacarpal base, and 20% of these involve the articular surface of the first carpometacarpal joint [1, 2].

Mechanism of Injury and Biomechanics

First metacarpal fractures typically result from an axial load, while the thumb is in a flexed position. This mechanism occurs with falls, a solid object striking the hand, as well as a clenched fist striking a solid object. Fractures of the metacarpal base are most common and can be associated with first carpometacarpal joint subluxation or dislocation, as well as trapezial fractures. Deforming muscular forces include the pull of the adductor pollicis, which adducts and supinates the distal fragment, the abductor pollicis longus, which shortens and causes apex-dorsal angulation of the proximal fragment, and the extensor pollicis longus, which contributes to metacarpophalangeal joint hyperextension. These forces can lead to metacarpal height loss, first webspace narrowing, and loss of up to 40% of hand function [3, 4].

V. Owens · J. Mastracci
Department of Orthopaedic Surgery, Atrium Health Musculoskeletal Institute, Charlotte, NC, USA

R. G. Gaston (✉)
OrthoCarolina Hand Center, Charlotte, NC, USA
e-mail: Glenn.Gaston@orthocarolina.com

Classification

First metacarpal fractures can be classified as extra-articular or intra-articular injuries. Extra-articular injuries include metacarpal shaft and epi-basal fractures. Intra-articular fractures include Bennett or Rolando type fractures.

First metacarpal head fractures can also occur but are rare due to the traumatic forces dissipating through the metaphysis.

Shaft fractures are typically transverse or oblique in nature and include epi-basal fractures, which are the most common type of shaft fracture. Epi-basal fractures typically occur at the proximal metaphyseal–diaphyseal junction.

Bennett fractures involve a variable-sized volar-ulnar intra-articular fragment that is held by the volar oblique ligament. The volar oblique ligament (also known as the beak ligament) originates on the palmar tubercle of the trapezium and inserts on the first metacarpal base fracture fragment [5]. The remaining metacarpal shaft displaces proximally, radially, and dorsally due to the deforming forces of the abductor pollicis longus and adductor pollicis. These deforming forces can often lead to joint subluxation or dislocation. Bennett fractures represent 30% of metacarpal fractures and are four times more common than Rolando fractures [3].

Rolando fractures are complete articular fractures at the base of the thumb metacarpal. These fractures involve at least three separate fragments and result from a higher amount of force than Bennett fractures.

Fracture patterns in all groups can include transverse, oblique, or spiral patterns.

Physical Exam

Examination should begin with inspection, assessing for swelling, ecchymosis, and open injury. Clinical signs of deformity include dorsal prominence of the metacarpal base, metacarpophalangeal joint hyperextension, and first webspace narrowing. Range of motion at the carpometacarpal (CMC) joint may be limited with flexion, extension, adduction, and/or abduction, and there may be associated instability.

Imaging

Radiographic evaluation of the hand for suspected fractures should begin with orthogonal radiographs. For the thumb, Robert's view, obtained by hyper-pronating the thumb to rest on the cassette, provides a true AP of the CMC joint. Bett's view is a lateral radiograph of the first metacarpal, which involves placing the hand flat on the cassette, pronating the hand 15–35° while aiming the beam 15° distal to proximal. Robert's and Bett's views allow for evaluation of the first carpometacarpal joint, in addition to the trapezoid and scaphoid [6]. Computed tomography can be helpful to evaluate complex intra-articular fractures, loose bodies, and for preoperative planning. Magnetic resonance imaging can be helpful if there is concern for ligamentous injury or occult fracture.

Treatment

Non-operative Management

The majority of extra-articular first metacarpal fractures can be treated with closed reduction and casting. In the first metacarpal shaft, up to 30° of angulation is acceptable for non-operative management [7]. Closed reduction is performed via longitudinal traction, volar pressure on the apex of the fracture, and pronation of the distal fracture fragment. If non-operative management is performed, radiographs in cast should be taken frequently to ensure that the reduction is maintained during the 4–6 weeks of immobilization.

There remains some debate on whether Bennett fractures without joint subluxation are best managed with non-operative versus operative intervention. Several studies have demonstrated good outcomes, including little to no pain and preserved thumb function, following non-operative management of Bennett fractures [8, 9]. Other literature reports higher incidence of symptomatic arthritis, decreased strength, and decreased thumb mobility following non-operative management of Bennet fractures [10, 11]. Overall, Bennett fractures with less than 2 mm of intra-articular displacement and without joint subluxation have better outcomes following non-operative management, which includes closed reduction and immobilization in thumb spica cast for 4–6 weeks.

Operative Management

While metacarpal head fractures are uncommon, displaced intra-articular metacarpal head fractures are ideally managed with closed reduction and percutaneous pinning (CRPP) or open reduction internal fixation (ORIF) to achieve and maintain anatomic alignment.

Unstable extra-articular first metacarpal shaft fractures require CRPP if reduction cannot be achieved and maintained with casting (Figs. 14.1 and 14.2). Open or extremely comminuted first metacarpal shaft fractures occasionally require external fixation (Fig. 14.3) [12].

Bennett fractures with greater than 2 mm of intra-articular displacement or joint subluxation are best managed with operative intervention. Reduction and fixation can be achieved through CRPP or ORIF, with literature demonstrating no difference in clinical outcomes between the two [13, 14]. Percutaneous pinning can be performed with obliquely placed Kirschner wires (k-wires) removed at 4–6 weeks post-operatively (Fig. 14.4). If the volar-ulnar fragment is too small to allow for fixation, pinning can be performed between the larger metacarpal base and the trapezium. Some surgeons advocate for k-wire fixation between the first and second metacarpals [15]. Irreducible fractures are generally best managed with open reduction through a Wagner volar approach at the radial aspect of the thenar muscles, curving ulnarly to the distal wrist flexion crease. The thenar muscles are retracted distally and the first carpal-metacarpal joint capsule is

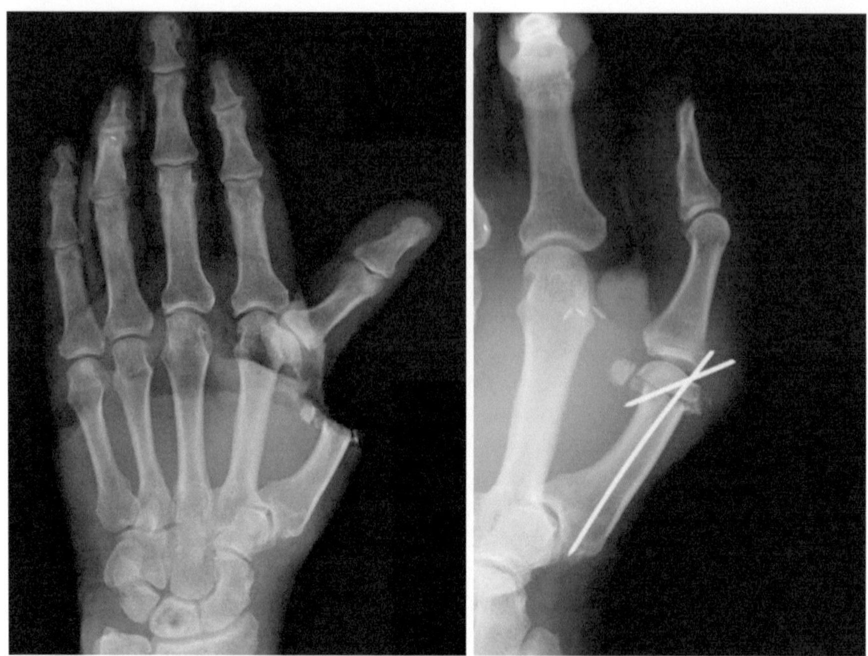

Fig. 14.1 Fixation of unstable thumb metacarpal shaft fracture with k-wires

Fig. 14.2 Percutaneous pinning of extra-articular thumb metacarpal fracture

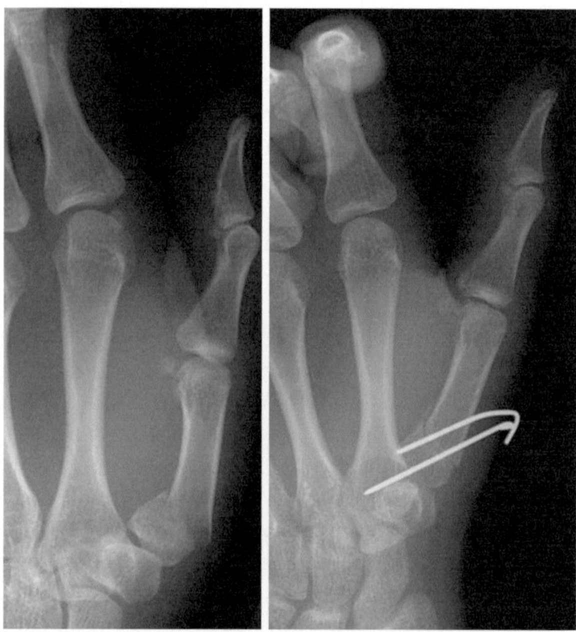

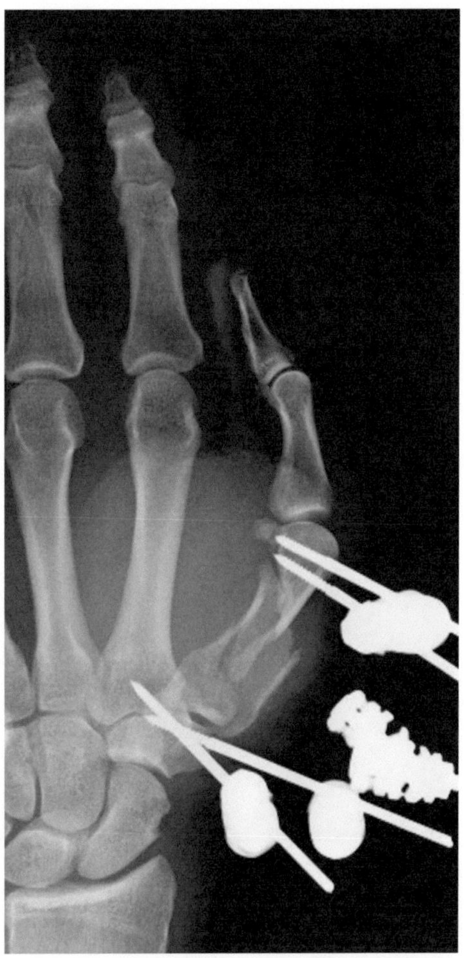

Fig. 14.3 External fixation of comminuted first metacarpal shaft fracture

incised. Options for internal fixation include pinning, independent screw fixation through the volar-ulnar fragment and metacarpal or plate and screw fixation (Fig. 14.5).

Rolando fractures are best treated with operative fixation. CRPP may be utilized in select clinical scenarios; however, CRPP may not provide adequate fixation given the comminuted nature of Rolando fractures. ORIF can be performed with k-wires or plate fixation (Fig. 14.6). A Wagner approach to the first metacarpal base can be used, as described above. Uludag et al. reported excellent results in Rolando fractures treated with locked plate and screw constructs [16]. In the setting of severely comminuted or open fractures, this fracture pattern may be best treated with an external fixation device [17–19]. If significant bone loss exists, bone allograft or autograft can be used.

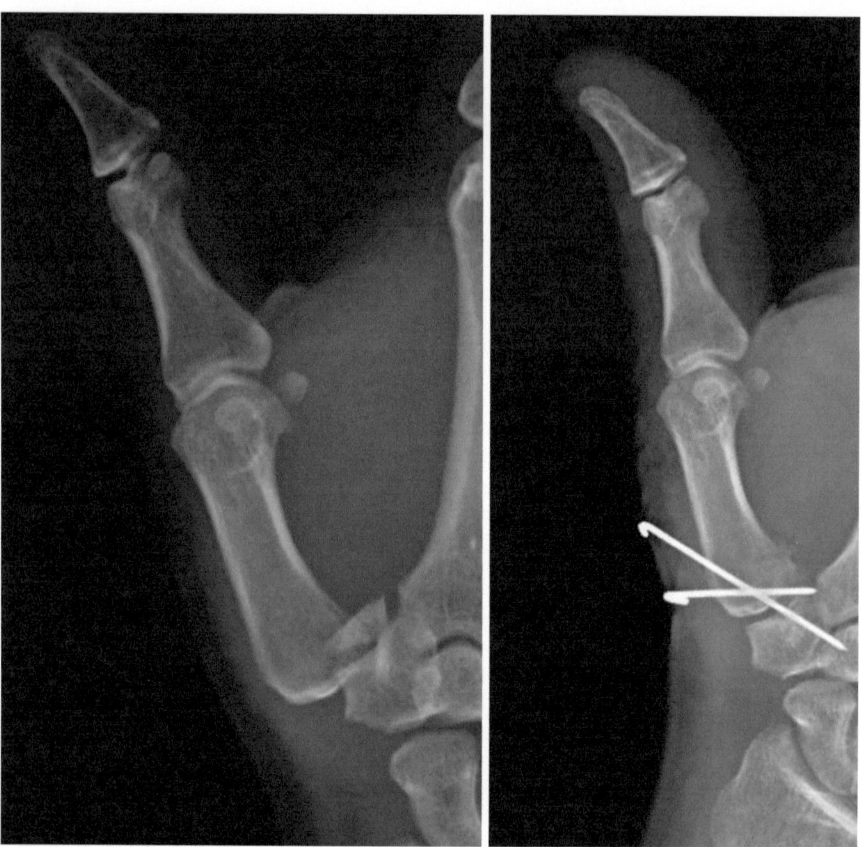

Fig. 14.4 Percutaneous pinning of thumb Bennett fracture

Fig. 14.5 Screw fixation
of thumb Bennett fracture

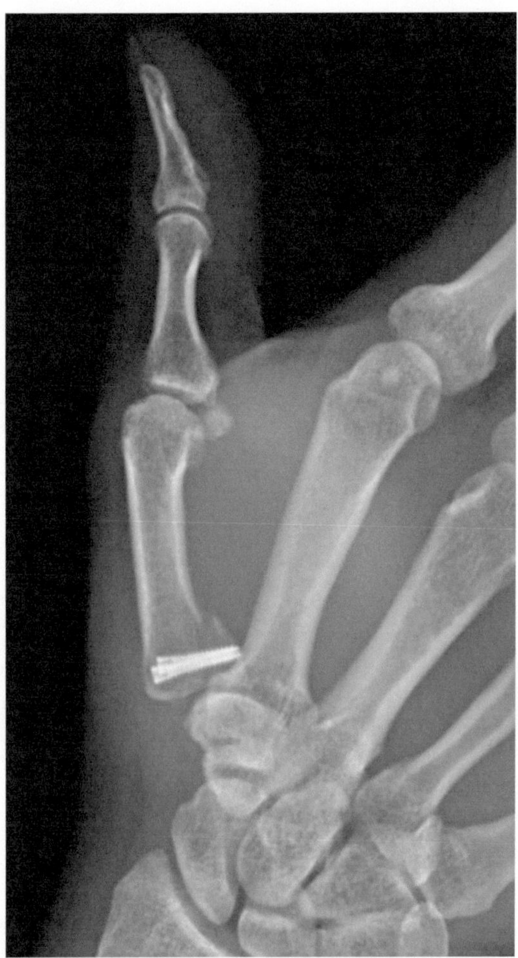

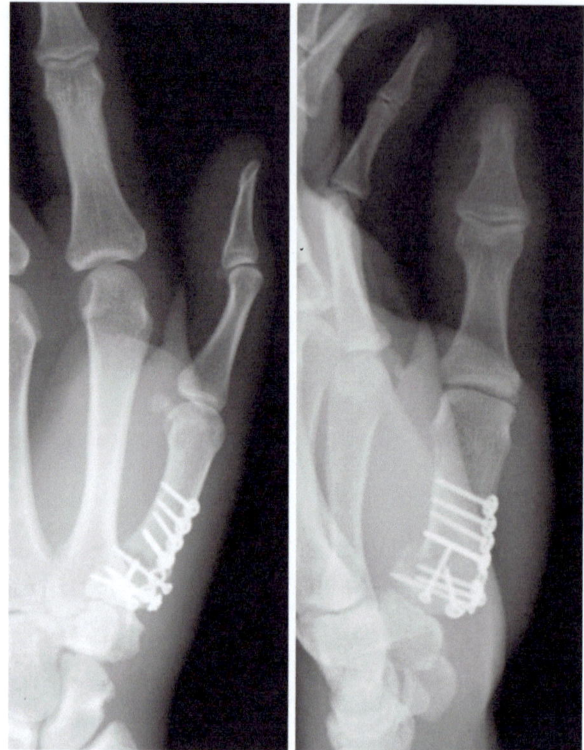

Fig. 14.6 Plate and screw fixation of thumb Rolando fracture

Outcomes

First metacarpal treatment outcomes are good overall but depend on the severity of the injury, quality of the soft tissues, and prompt identification and management. Extra-articular thumb metacarpal fractures typically have good outcomes with reduction followed by splinting or casting. Displaced, intra-articular metacarpal base fractures fare better with operative treatment, as studies have shown that conservative treatment is associated with increased varus angulation, trapeziometacarpal joint subluxation, decreased range of motion, and loss of grip strength [20, 21]. Surgical outcomes and functional scores are excellent regardless of the fixation method [22, 23]. Stiffness is a common complication that is worse with more complex fractures [21].

References

1. Stanton JS, Dias JJ, Burke FD. Fractures of the tubular bones of the hand. J Hand Surg Eur Vol. 2007;32(6):626–36. https://doi.org/10.1016/j.jhse.2007.06.017.
2. Wang W, Zeng M, Yang J, Wang L, Xie J, Hu Y. Clinical efficacy of closed reduction and percutaneous parallel K-wire interlocking fixation of first metacarpal base fracture. J Orthop Surg Res. 2021;16(1):454. https://doi.org/10.1186/s13018-021-02600-5.

3. Brown MT, Rust PA. Fractures of the thumb metacarpal base. Injury. 2020;51(11):2421–8. https://doi.org/10.1016/J.INJURY.2020.07.053.
4. Fischborn T, Beckenbauer D, Held M, Daigeler A, Medved F. Analysis of operative techniques of fractures of the first metacarpal base. Ann Plast Surg. 2018;80(5):507–14. https://doi.org/10.1097/SAP.0000000000001293.
5. McCann MR, Rust PA, Wallace R. The stabilising effect of the anterior oblique ligament to prevent directional subluxation at the trapeziometacarpal joint of the thumb: a biomechanical cadaveric study. Arch Bone Jt Surg. 2018;6(2):105. Accessed 10 Sept 2022. /pmc/articles/PMC5867353/.
6. Carlsen BT, Moran SL. Thumb trauma: Bennett fractures, Rolando fractures, and ulnar collateral ligament injuries. J Hand Surg. 2009;34(5):945–52. https://doi.org/10.1016/j.jhsa.2009.03.017.
7. Day C. Green's operative hand surgery. In: Wolfe S, Hotchkiss R, Pederson W, Kozin S, Cohen M, editors. Green's operative hand surgery. 7th ed. Elsevier; 2017.
8. Cannon SR, Dowd GSE, Williams DH, Scott JM. A long-term study following Bennett's fracture. J Hand Surg Br. 1986;11(3):426–31. https://doi.org/10.1016/0266-7681(86)90172-5.
9. Milogević I, Sudjić V, Bumbasirević V, Lesić A, Damjanović G, Bumbasirević M. [Nonoperative treatment of fractures of the base of the first metacarpal bone—Bennett fracture]. Acta Chir Iugosl. 2005;52(2):67–71. https://doi.org/10.2298/ACI0502067M.
10. Kjær-Petersen K, Langhoff O, Andersen K. Bennett's fracture. J Hand Surg Br. 1990;15(1):58–61. https://doi.org/10.1016/0266-7681(90)90049-A.
11. Livesley PJ. The conservative management of Bennett's fracture-dislocation: a 26-year follow-up. J Hand Surg Br. 1990;15(3):291–4. https://doi.org/10.1016/0266-7681(90)90006-P.
12. Dailiana Z, Agorastakis D, Varitimidis S, Bargiotas K, Roidis N, Malizos KN. Use of a mini-external fixator for the treatment of hand fractures. J Hand Surg Am. 2009;34(4):630–6. https://doi.org/10.1016/J.JHSA.2008.12.017.
13. Timmenga EJF, Blokhuis TJ, Maas M, Raaijmakers ELFB. Long-term evaluation of Bennett's fracture. A comparison between open and closed reduction. J Hand Surg Br. 1994;19(3):373–7. https://doi.org/10.1016/0266-7681(94)90093-0.
14. Lutz M, Sailer R, Zimmermann R, Gabl M, Ulmer H, Pechlaner S. Closed reduction transarticular Kirschner wire fixation versus open reduction internal fixation in the treatment of Bennett's fracture dislocation. J Hand Surg Br. 2003;28(2):142–7. https://doi.org/10.1016/S0266-7681(02)00307-8.
15. van Niekerk JLM, Ouwens R. Fractures of the base of the first metacarpal bone: results of surgical treatment. Injury. 1989;20(6):359–62. https://doi.org/10.1016/0020-1383(89)90014-4.
16. Uludag S, Ataker Y, Seyahi A, Tetik O, Gudemez E. Early rehabilitation after stable osteosynthesis of intra-articular fractures of the metacarpal base of the thumb. J Hand Surg Eur Vol. 2015;40(4):370–3. https://doi.org/10.1177/1753193413494035.
17. Buchler U, McCollam SM, Oppikofer C. Comminuted fractures of the basilar joint of the thumb: combined treatment by external fixation, limited internal fixation, and bone grafting. J Hand Surg Am. 1991;16(3):556–60. https://doi.org/10.1016/0363-5023(91)90032-7.
18. El-Sharkawy AA, El-Mofty AO, Moharram AN, Abou Elatta MM, Asal F. Management of Rolando fracture by modified dynamic external fixation: a new technique. Tech Hand Up Extrem Surg. 2009;13(1):11–5. https://doi.org/10.1097/BTH.0B013E3181847652.
19. Houshian S, Jing SS. Treatment of Rolando fracture by capsuloligamentotaxis using mini external fixator: a report of 16 cases. Hand Surg. 2013;18(1):73–8. https://doi.org/10.1142/S0218810413500147.
20. Abid H, Shimi M, el Ibrahimi A, el Mrini A. Articular fracture of the base of the thumb metacarpal: comparative study between direct open fixation and extrafocal pinning. Chir Main. 2015;34(3):122–5. https://doi.org/10.1016/J.MAIN.2015.01.008.
21. Liverneaux PA, Ichihara S, Hendriks S, Facca S, Bodin F. Fractures and dislocation of the base of the thumb metacarpal. J Hand Surg Eur Vol. 2015;40(1):42–50. https://doi.org/10.1177/1753193414554357.

22. Kollitz KM, Hammert WC, Vedder NB, Huang JI. Metacarpal fractures: treatment and complications. Hand. 2014;9(1):16–23. https://doi.org/10.1007/s11552-013-9562-1.
23. Wong VW, Higgins JP. Evidence-based medicine: management of metacarpal fractures. Plast Reconstr Surg. 2017;140(1):140e–151. https://doi.org/10.1097/PRS.0000000000003470.

Adult Phalangeal Base Fractures: Pilons, Avulsions, PIPJ Fracture-Dislocations

15

Keith T. Aziz, Daniel A. London, and Peter J. Stern

Introduction

Fractures of the phalanges are among the most common upper extremity injuries encountered. One study of several statewide emergency department and inpatient databases demonstrated that phalangeal fractures occur with more regularity than metacarpal fractures (at a rate of 12.5 compared to 8.4 per 10,000 persons annually) [1, 2]. In a review of all phalangeal and metacarpal fractures that presented to a single institution, Stanton et al. found that approximately 70% of digital fractures occurred in patients between the ages of 11 and 45 and 54% of these fractures involved the phalanges [3]. Stanton et al. additionally noted that the base was the most injured part of both the proximal and middle phalanges and that it was roughly equivalent to the tuft in terms of the most injured part of the distal phalanx [3]. Further, they noted that only 10% of intra-articular fractures were non-displaced and 19% of extra-articular fractures were non-displaced [3].

There are several different management options for the treatment of phalangeal base fractures, ranging from buddy taping with early mobilization to operative treatment with surgical fixation. The most optimal management requires careful consideration of patient demographics, rehabilitative potential, fracture morphology and stability, and awareness of the relevant anatomy. The goal of any treatment should be the preservation of pain-free stability and range of motion.

K. T. Aziz (✉)
Department of Orthopaedic Surgery, Mayo Clinic Jacksonville, Jacksonville, FL, USA

D. A. London
Department of Orthopaedic Surgery, University of Missouri, Columbia, MO, USA

P. J. Stern
Department of Orthopaedic Surgery, University of Cincinnati College of Medicine, Cincinnati, OH, USA
e-mail: pstern@handsurg.com

J. M. Abzug et al. (eds.), *Pediatric and Adult Hand Fractures*,
https://doi.org/10.1007/978-3-031-32072-9_15

Anatomy of the Metacarpophalangeal Joint

The metacarpophalangeal (MP) joint is a diarthrodial joint formed by the articulation of the metacarpal head with the base of the proximal phalanx. The metacarpal head has a complex geometry with asymmetry in the coronal and sagittal planes but is primarily convex [4]. The base of the proximal phalanx is concave, and the combined bony morphology allows for the MP joint to demonstrate motion in flexion, extension, abduction, adduction, and rotation [5]. The MP joint has a broader arc of motion than the proximal and distal interphalangeal joints [5]. The plurality of the planes of motion of the MP joint affords the opportunity for the digits to be positioned in several configurations and allows optimal interaction with the environment; however, this range of motion is possible because of a lack of inherent bony constraint. Because of this, the soft tissue stabilizers, notably the proper collateral ligaments, accessory collateral ligaments, palmar plate, and capsule play a significant role in MP joint stability and function.

In a cadaveric study, Minami et al. found that the collateral ligaments were the primary stabilizers in distraction, dorso-volar dislocation, abduction–adduction, and pronation–supination [6]. The metacarpal head has a radial and ulnar depression that is dorsal to the axis of rotation (about one-third of the distance dorsal to volar) and serves as the origin (footprint) of the proper collateral ligaments (Fig. 15.1a–c) [7]. The proper collateral ligaments then insert on the volar aspect of the proximal phalanx (about one-fourth of the distance from volar to dorsal), causing the proper collateral ligaments to be tighter in flexion than extension. Additionally, the cam shape of the metacarpal head causes the phalangeal base to move in a palmar direction with flexion—further tightening the collateral ligaments [6, 7]. The accessory collateral ligaments contribute mostly to stability with adduction and abduction and originate volar to the proper collateral ligament while inserting into the volar plate [7]. As a result of the origin and insertion of the accessory collateral ligaments, they are tight in extension. The volar plate only has a significant role in preventing dorsal dislocation when the MP joint is in extension [6]. The volar plate is a fibrocartilaginous structure with thick attachments distally at the volar aspect of the proximal phalanx and a loose membranous insertion proximal to the metacarpal head. The insertion proximal to the metacarpal head creates a retrocondylar space and the loose insertion allows for some hyperextension [5, 6]. Finally, the dorsal capsule provides some additional stability to the MP joint and provides stability to distraction as well as pronation and supination of the joint [6].

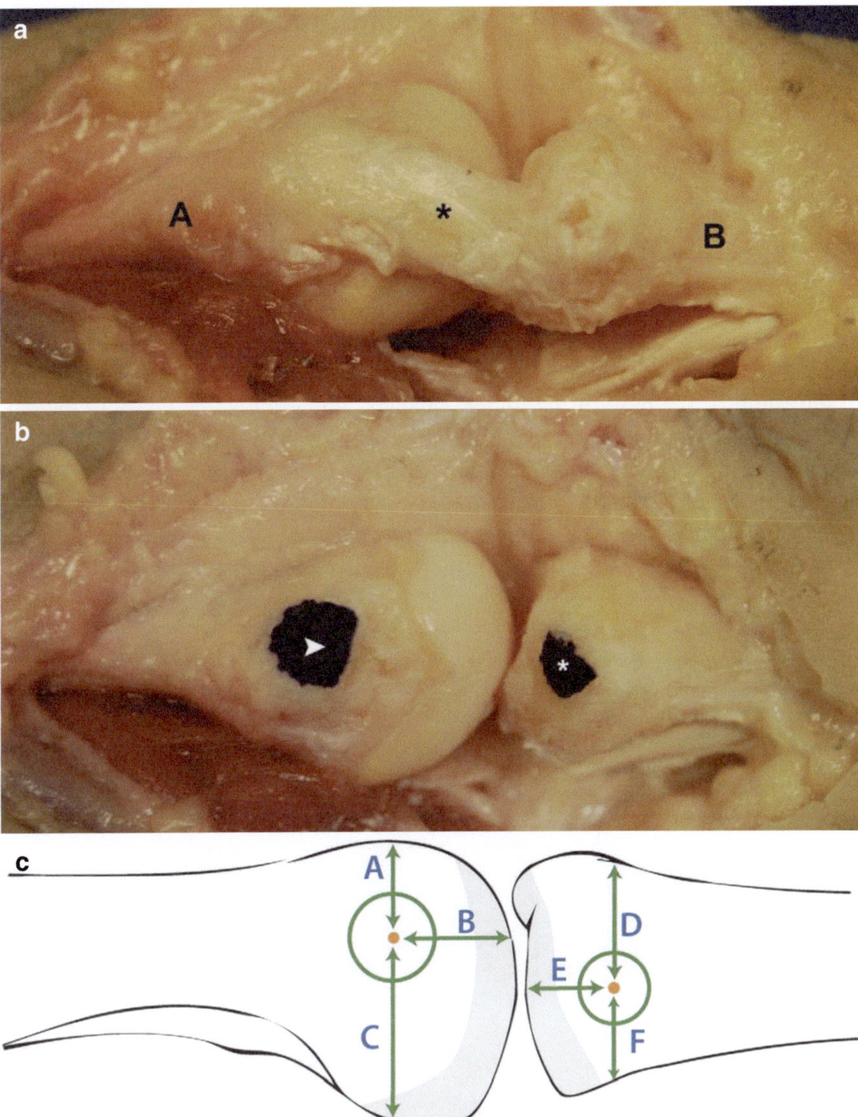

Fig. 15.1 (**a**) Cadaveric dissection showing the gross anatomy of the proper radial collateral ligament (*) of the MP joint, with demonstration of the dorsal origin on the metacarpal (A) and the insertion on the proximal phalanx (B). (From Dy et al. [7]). (**b**) Cadaveric dissection after removal of the proper radial collateral ligament, showing the origin on the metacarpal head (arrow) and insertion on the proximal phalanx base (*). (From Dy et al. [7]). (**c**) Diagrammatic representation of the origin of the proper collateral ligament on the metacarpal head, demonstrating the distances from the dorsal surface of the metacarpal head (A), the articular surface of the metacarpal head (B), and the volar surface of the metacarpal head (C)—as well as the distance from the dorsal surface of the proximal phalanx (D), articular surface of the proximal phalanx base (E), and the volar surface of the proximal phalanx base (F). (From Dy et al. [7])

Anatomy of the Proximal Interphalangeal Joint

The proximal interphalangeal (PIP) joint is a hinged diarthrodial joint with motion primarily in the sagittal plane, allowing flexion and extension. The head of the middle phalanx has a central intercondylar depression and the base of the middle phalanx has a sagittal beak that corresponds to the intercondylar depression and forms a specific joint cavity between the articulations on each condyle of the proximal phalanx head (Fig. 15.2) [8]. The intercondylar depression and corresponding beaking of the base of the middle phalanx impart some inherent stability in the coronal plane, and Minamikawa et al. found that only 50% of the collateral ligaments needed to remain intact to allow for adequate joint stability [8, 9]. In the sagittal plane, the radius of curvature of the proximal phalanx head is smaller than the radius of curvature of the base of the middle phalanx, imparting some laxity to the PIP joint that has led some to describe the joint as a "sloppy" hinge (Fig. 15.3) [8]. Caravaggi et al. have demonstrated that in addition to soft tissue releases, disruption of the volar lip of the middle phalanx is necessary to impart considerable instability to the joint, which supports the higher degree of bony constraint seen in the PIP joint [10]. The range of motion of the PIP joint required for normal function is greater

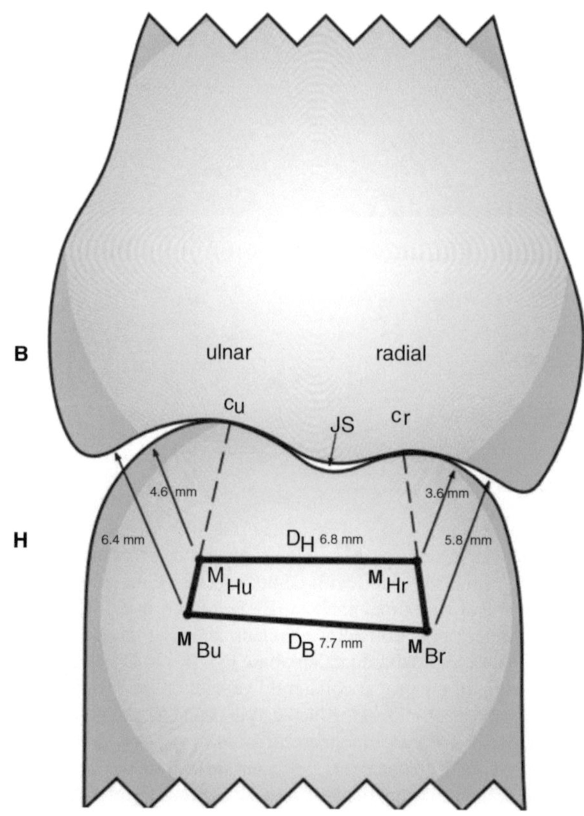

Fig. 15.2 Demonstration of a transverse cross section of the PIP joint, showing the articulating surfaces of the condyles of the proximal phalanx (H) and the base of the middle phalanx (B) with two contact points. The ulnar radii are larger than the radial ones, and in the middle of the joint, there is a small central cavity (JS). *Cr* contact radial, *Cu* contact ulnar, *DB* distance between both centers of the base of the middle phalanx, *DH* distance between both condyle centers, *JS* joint space, *MBr* curvature center of the proximal end of the middle phalanx, radial, *MBu* curvature center of the proximal end of the middle phalanx, ulnar, *MHr* curvature center radial condyle, *MHu* curvature center ulnar condyle. (From Dumont et al. [8])

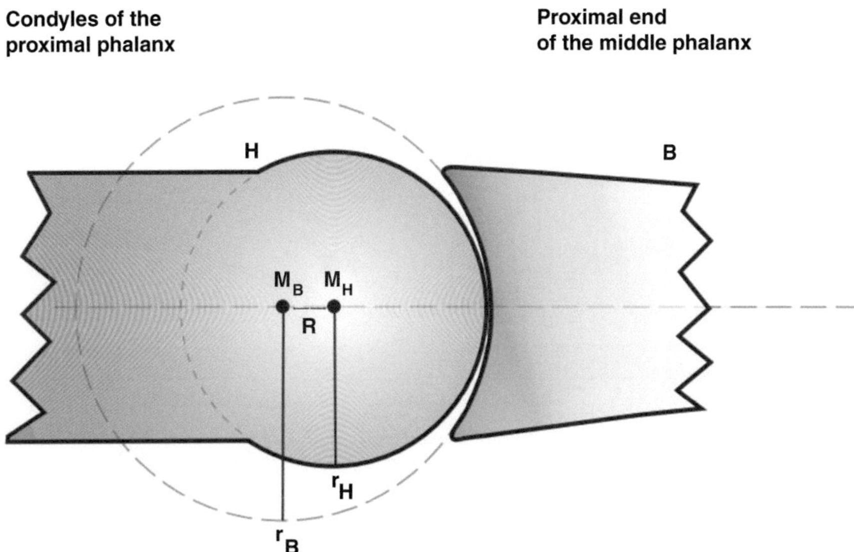

Fig. 15.3 The radii of curvatures of the base of the middle phalanx (rB) and the head of the proximal phalanx (rH) as well as the distance between the centers of rotation (R) are demonstrated. *B* base of the middle phalanx, *H* head of the proximal phalanx, *MB* curvature center of the base of the middle phalanx, *MH* curvature center of the head of the proximal phalanx. (From Dumont et al. [8])

than the functional range of motion of both the MP and distal interphalangeal (DIP) joints [5]. Stiffness is a common complication after managing dislocations of the PIP joint, and awareness of the soft tissue stabilizers is critical in the management of joint contractures following injury.

The collateral ligaments of the PIP joint are the primary stabilizers to radial and ulnar stress. The PIP joint has both proper and accessory collateral ligaments, with the proper collateral ligaments originating from concavities at about the center of rotation of the PIP joint on either side of the head of the proximal phalanx (Fig. 15.4a, b) [11]. The insertion of the proper collateral ligament is very broad and inserts on both the volar plate and the volar aspect of the base of the middle phalanx [11–13]. Because the proper collateral ligament originates from almost the center of rotation of the proximal phalanx head, and the radius of curvature of the proximal phalanx head is relatively constant, the tension in the proper collateral ligaments is fairly constant throughout the flexion and extension arc. The accessory collateral ligaments of the PIP joints originate proximally and volarly to the center of rotation and insert on the volar plate and the dorsal aspect of the flexor sheath [11, 13]. As a result, the accessory collateral ligaments are tight in extension, but relaxed in flexion—which is why the accessory collateral ligaments are prone to contracture if the PIP joint is placed or held in flexion [11]. Compounding the risk of accessory ligament contractures is the fact that swelling, trauma, or hemorrhage affecting the joint often results in flexion of the PIP joint to about 40°, which allows for maximum

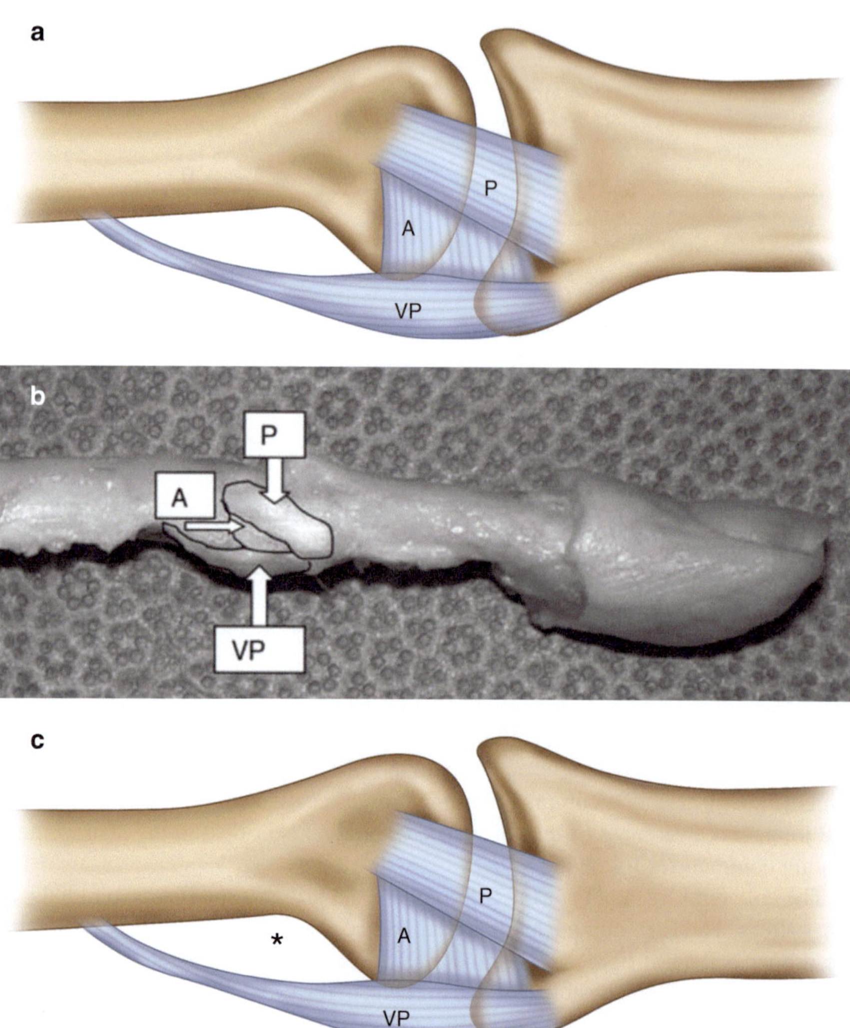

Fig. 15.4 (**a**) Diagrammatic representation of the soft tissue attachments of the PIP joint, showing the origin and insertion of the proper collateral ligament (P), accessory collateral ligament (A), and volar plate (VP). (**b**) Cadaveric dissection demonstrating the soft tissue attachments around the PIP joint, showing the origin and insertion of the proper collateral ligament (P), accessory collateral ligament (A), and volar plate (VP). (From Hogan et al. [11]). (**c**) Diagrammatic representation of the soft tissue attachments of the PIP joint, showing Drucker's space (*) as well as the proper collateral ligament (P), accessory collateral ligament (A), and volar plate (VP)

capsular volume but then places the accessory collateral ligaments in a position where they are prone to contracture. The volar plate of the PIP joint is similar to the volar plate of the MP joint in that it is a fibrocartilaginous structure that has a robust distal insertion at the base of the middle phalanx. Proximally, the volar plate originates well proximal to the head of the proximal phalanx by membranous checkrein ligaments (see Fig. 15.5a, b), creating the retrocondylar space of Drucker (see asterisk in Fig. 15.4c). Drucker's space provides a potential space for the volar plate to be accommodated during flexion, and the formation of scar tissue in this space limits flexion.

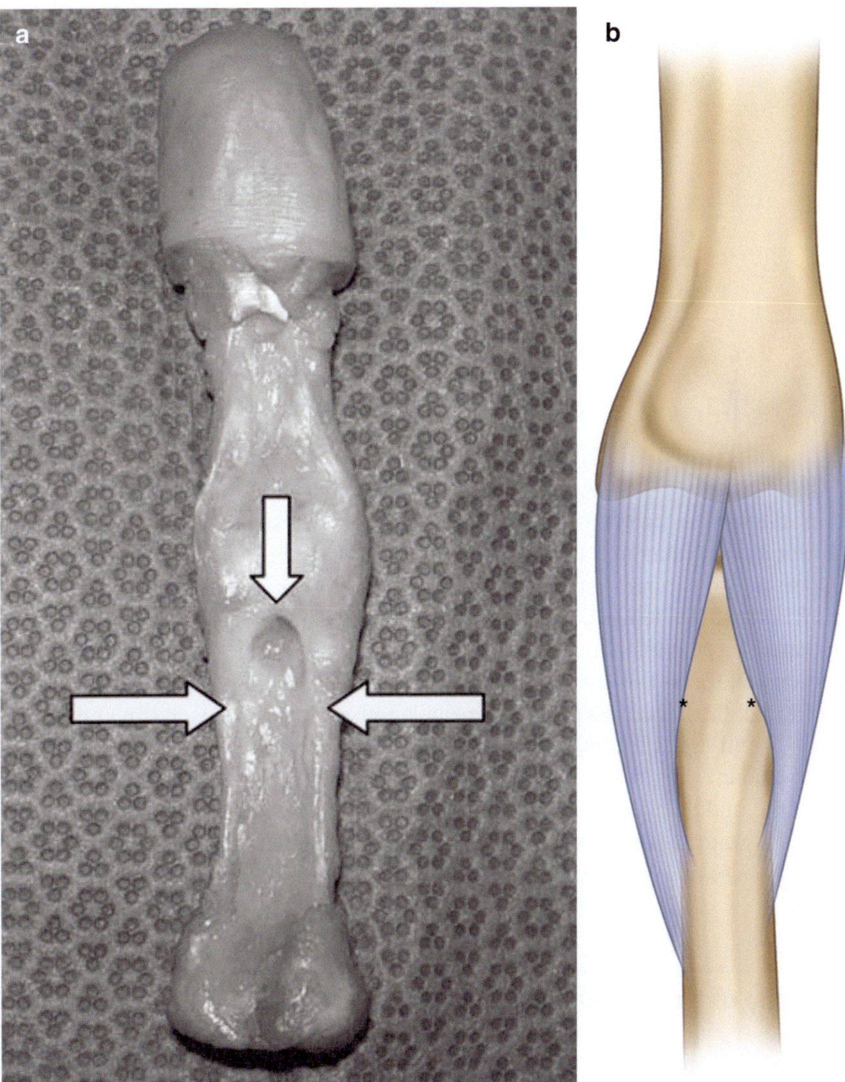

Fig. 15.5 (a) Cadaveric dissection showing the checkrein ligaments (horizontal white arrows) and membranous portion of the volar plate (vertical white arrow), as well as diagrammatic representation (b) of the checkrein ligaments (black asterisk) ((a) from Hogan et al. [11], (b) is personal figure)

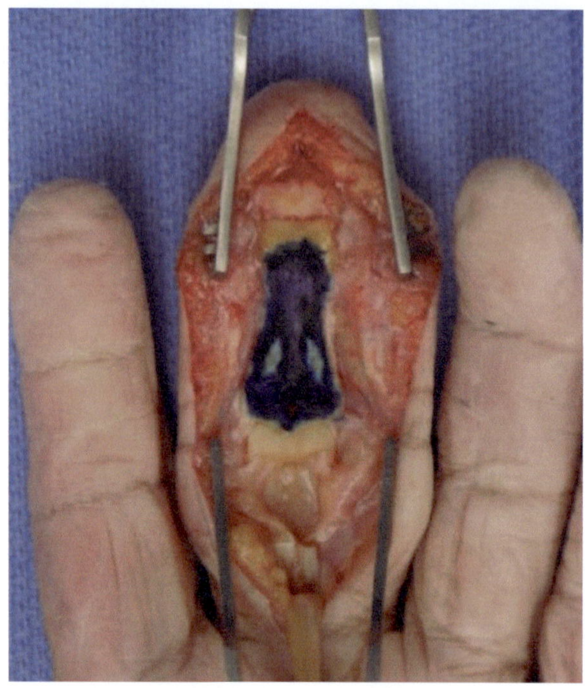

Fig. 15.6 Cadaveric dissection after removal of the FDS insertion, with methylene blue staining demonstrating the entirety of the FDS insertion. (From Nicholson et al. [14])

In addition to ligamentous and fibrocartilaginous stabilizers, the flexor and extensor tendons that help stabilize the joint. The tendons that help stabilize the PIP joint include the central slip of the extrinsic extensors and the flexor digitorum superficialis (FDS) tendon. The FDS tendon has a broad insertion. Nicholson et al. performed a cadaveric study investigating the characteristics of the FDS tendon insertion and found that the proximal aspect began an average of 3.22 mm distal to the PIP joint flexion crease [14]. The mean length and width of each slip of the FDS was 5.15 mm and 1.9 mm, respectively, and spans a considerable amount of the middle phalanx (Fig. 15.6) [14]. The central slip inserts on the dorsal aspect of the base of the middle phalanx and prevents volar subluxation or dislocation of the PIP joint [15]. Scarring or contracture of the dorsal apparatus can cause a swan neck posture, whereas laxity or disruption of the central slip can result in a boutonniere posture.

Anatomy of the Distal Interphalangeal Joint

The osseous anatomy of the DIP joint is very similar to that of the PIP joint, in that the head of the middle phalanx has prominent radial and ulnar condyles with an intercondylar groove [16]. The base of the distal phalanx has some slight differences in that the concavities in the base of the distal phalanx are asymmetric with the ulnar side of the distal phalanx base having a greater radius of curvature [16].

There still are both radial and ulnar convexities in the base of the head of the middle phalanx, with a central ridge—which itself confers some additional stability in the coronal plane [16]. The DIP joint has the lowest functional arc of motion and lowest total range of motion of all joints in the finger [5, 8]. The DIP joint is stabilized in the coronal plane by both accessory and collateral ligaments, with the proper collateral ligaments originating just dorsal to the center of rotation of the head of the middle phalanx and inserting on the lateral aspect of the base of the distal phalanx [17]. Its proper collateral ligaments are taught in flexion and relaxed in extension [17]. The accessory collateral ligaments originate on the radial and ulnar epicondyles and then insert on the volar plate and are taught in extension and relaxed in flexion [17]. The volar plate is different from the volar plate of the PIP joint in that there are no checkrein ligaments and is weakly attached to the distal margin of the FDS insertion by membranous fibers [18]. Distally, the volar plate has strong attachments to the volar lip of the distal phalanx base [18]. The terminal tendon and the flexor digitorum profundus (FDP) also provide stability. Chepla et al. performed a cadaveric study to characterize the FDP insertional anatomy and found that the proximal aspect of the FDP insertion on average was 1.2 mm from the volar aspect of the distal phalangeal base [19]. The average length of the FDP insertion is 6.2 mm and the average width is 7.9 mm [19]. The distance from the dorsal aspect of the distal phalangeal base to the insertion of the terminal tendon inserts directly onto the dorsal aspect of the distal phalanx base, and the distal aspect of the terminal tendon insertion is only 1.2 mm proximal to the germinal matrix [19–21]. Managing distal phalangeal base fractures is challenging because of the close proximity of these structures, and it is not uncommon to consider salvage procedures especially when significant articular damage has been sustained.

Assessment

History and Mechanism

A thorough history and physical examination is paramount in order to formulate an appropriate treatment plan. The mechanism of injury should be identified, as associated pathologies that may have been missed on initial evaluation. Additionally, the resulting fracture pattern is usually dependent on mechanism of injury—e.g. a direct axial blow will cause a different fracture pattern than a torsional or hyperextension injury.

Clinical Findings and Physical Examination

On inspection, often there is considerable swelling and tenderness of the affected digit. The dorsal skin creases overlaying the interphalangeal and MP joints are often obscured secondary to swelling. Clinical malrotation or angulation will have considerable impact on treatment. To identify malrotation, ask the patient to actively make a fist, which can demonstrate any crossover or scissoring. If the patient is in considerable pain and has difficulty performing active range of motion, a digital block should be administered after performing a baseline sensory and vascular exam. While injection of a local anesthetic can provide adequate analgesia to allow for assessment of active motion, if this is administered in an asymmetric fashion it can give the appearance of subtle angulation or rotation (or mask existing deformity).

Imaging: Radiographs

Dedicated anteroposterior (AP) and lateral radiographs of the affected digit should always be obtained. Hand radiographs are not appropriate for assessing digital pathology distal to the MP joint (Fig. 15.7a). If an intra-articular or juxta-articular fracture is suspected, the beam should be coned over the affected joint. While oblique radiographs are not routinely obtained, they can be useful in identifying certain fracture patterns or recognizing the extent and direction of rotational deformity. Subtle injuries are often missed, and it is important to be vigilant and not rely exclusively on a radiologist's interpretation (Fig. 15.7a, b). There are a number of features that are important to consider when assessing radiographs of the finger. In the extended finger, the dorsal cortices of the proximal, middle, and distal phalanges are collinear (Fig. 15.8a). Unrecognized volar or dorsal subluxation may considerably compromise final range of motion. Additionally, the head of the proximal and middle phalanges are coplanar on the lateral view, and any rotational difference must be carefully

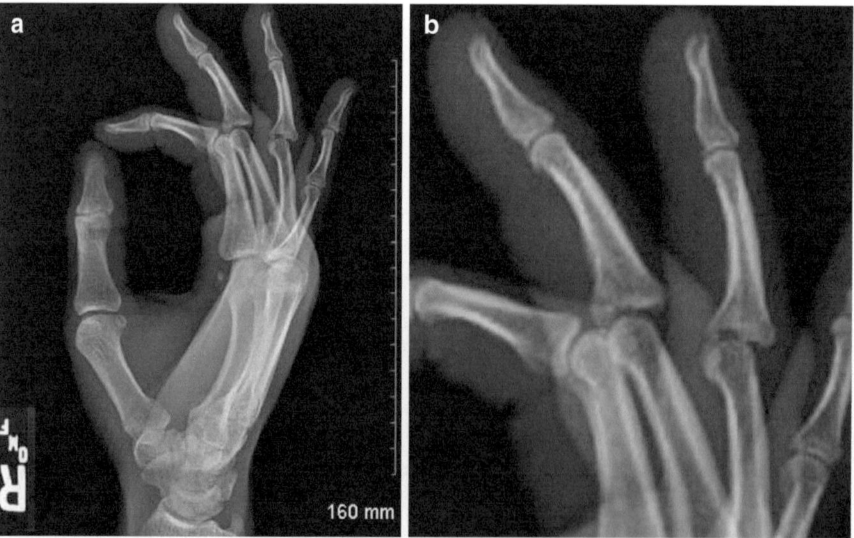

Fig. 15.7 (a) Lateral radiograph of the right hand obtained by the Emergency Department for suspected injuries to the long and ring finger. Unfortunately not appropriate for evaluation and read as normal by the radiologist. (b) Enhanced zoom demonstrating that the proximal and middle phalanx dorsal cortices are not coplanar. The volar articular impaction upon referral to our practice

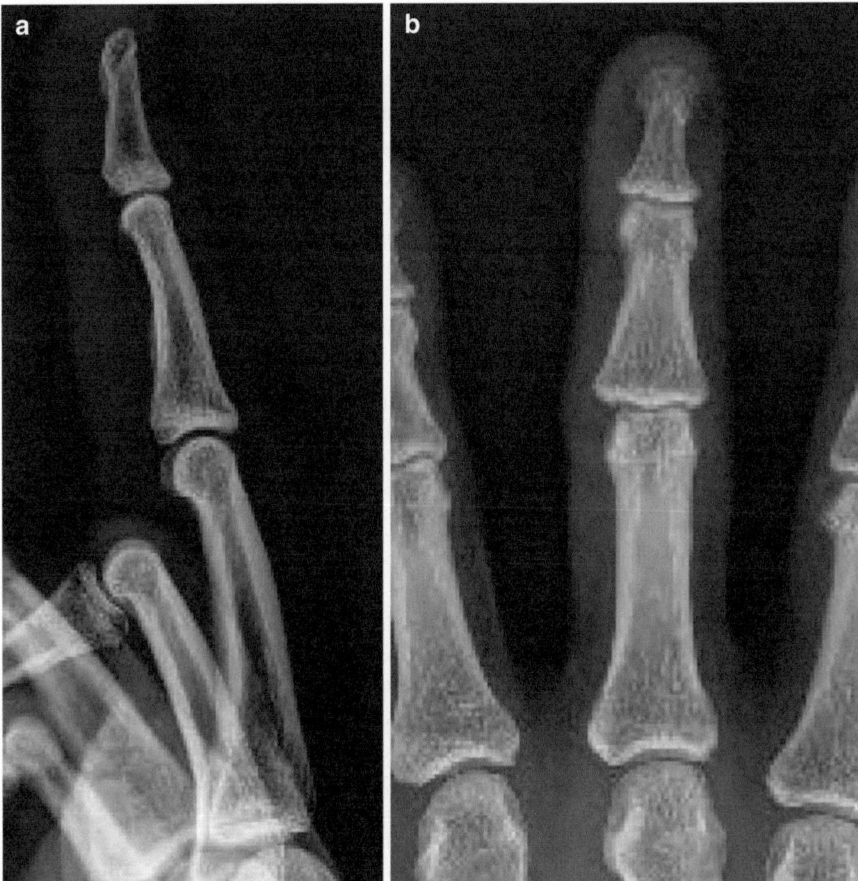

Fig. 15.8 (**a**) Lateral radiograph of the right long finger demonstrating that the middle and proximal phalangeal heads are coplanar, and that the dorsal profile of all three phalanges is parallel. (**b**) AP radiograph of the right long finger demonstrates that the condyles of the middle and proximal phalanges are colinear

assessed on clinical examination (Fig. 15.8a). On the AP radiograph, the condyles of the middle and proximal phalanges are collinear (Fig. 15.8b). Frequently the combination of a thorough clinical exam and plain radiographs is adequate to diagnose acute pathology; however, if it is necessary to further characterize phalangeal base fractures, computed tomography (CT) can prove to be quite useful.

Imaging: Computed Tomography (CT)

Certain fracture patterns are difficult to assess with plain radiographs, and the literature has shown that it is not possible to use the number of fracture fragments to predict the extent of phalangeal base articular involvement [22]. Lateral and even oblique radiographs of the MP joint can mask fractures because of overlap of adjacent joints. If intra-articular fracture is suspected, CT is a reasonable consideration to establish a definitive diagnosis [23]. Further, some phalangeal base fractures are impaction fractures—and identifying the extent of articular impaction can be helpful in preoperative planning [24]. Faccioli et al. compared the use of cone-beam CT with multi-slice CT in characterizing phalangeal base fracture morphology and found that cone-beam CT was able to characterize articular involvement equally well with significantly lower radiation exposure [25].

Imaging: Magnetic Resonance Imaging (MRI)

MRI is rarely necessary to evaluate isolated phalangeal base fractures. Several prior studies have shown exceptional sensitivity and specificity in evaluating volar plate, collateral ligament, and tendon injuries about the MP, PIP, or DIP joints [26–29].

Imaging: Ultrasound

Ultrasound is another modality that can be used in the evaluation of injuries of the fingers. It is highly operator dependent [30–32]. Advantages include low cost, ability to deploy at the bedside in clinic, and potential for dynamic evaluation of digital injuries. Ultrasonography has been used to successfully diagnose collateral ligament, volar plate, and tendon injuries—and recently there has been some effort to deploy ultrasound to assess bony pathology and fractures [33, 34].

Classification

Fractures and fracture-dislocations of the PIP joint have been extensively studied and many of the principles that are used to assess and treat PIP joint injuries can be applied to the MP and DIP joints. Additionally, another chapter in this textbook will focus on DIP phalangeal base fractures (Chap. 18). PIP joint fracture-dislocations and middle phalangeal base fractures can be classified by stability, and if unstable the direction of instability.

Stable Versus Unstable

Stable and pain-free range of motion of the PIP joint is the goal of treatment. Instability must be recognized. Eaton speculated that articular involvement may predispose to instability, and he postulated that a "critical corner" of the middle phalangeal base was involved in instability of the PIP joint [35]. Subsequent studies by Hastings and Krakauer supported the notion that stability of the PIP joint could be predicted by extent of middle phalangeal base articular involvement [36–38].

Biomechanical studies showed that if >50% of the volar base of the middle phalanx base was involved, then the joint would be unstable [36–38]. If <30% of the middle phalangeal base was involved, the PIP joint is usually stable, and involvement of 30–50% of the middle phalangeal base could be tenuous (Table 15.1 and Fig. 15.9) [36–38].

Dorsal PIP Fracture-Dislocation

Dorsal PIP fracture-dislocations occur as a result of detachment of the volar plate from the base of the middle phalanx with or without fracture of the volar lip of the middle phalanx. An intact volar plate serves as a checkrein to PIP joint hyperextension and when detached with or without fracture dorsal subluxation of the middle phalanx can occur (Fig. 15.10a). The dorsal subluxation of the middle phalanx causes a space between the head of the proximal phalanx and the base of the middle

Table 15.1 Stability based classification of PIP joint fracture-dislocations (from Kiefhaber et al. [38])

Palmar lip fracture
Stable (<30% articular surface, reduced in extension)
No PIP hyperextension
Hyperextensible PIP (swan neck)
Tenuous (30–50% articular surface and reduction maintained with <30° flexion)
Unstable (>50% articular surface or 30–50% requiring >30° of flexion to maintain reduction)
Dorsal lip fracture
Stable (in extension)
Unstable (palmar translation of middle phalanx)
Pilon fracture

PIP proximal interphalangeal

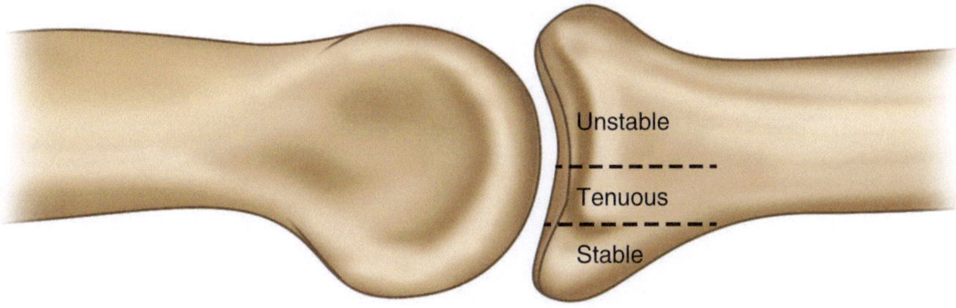

Fig. 15.9 Palmar lip fracture classification. Stable fractures involve less than 30% of the articular surface and demonstrate no tendency to subluxate, even when the proximal interphalangeal (PIP) joint is fully extended. Tenuous fractures involve 30–50% of the middle phalangeal articular surface but remain reduced when the joint is flexed to less than 30°. All PIP joint fractures involving greater than 50% of the joint surface are categorized as unstable. Fractures involving 30–50% of the middle phalangeal base that require more than 30° of flexion to maintain reduction are also classified as unstable. (From Kiefhaber et al. [38])

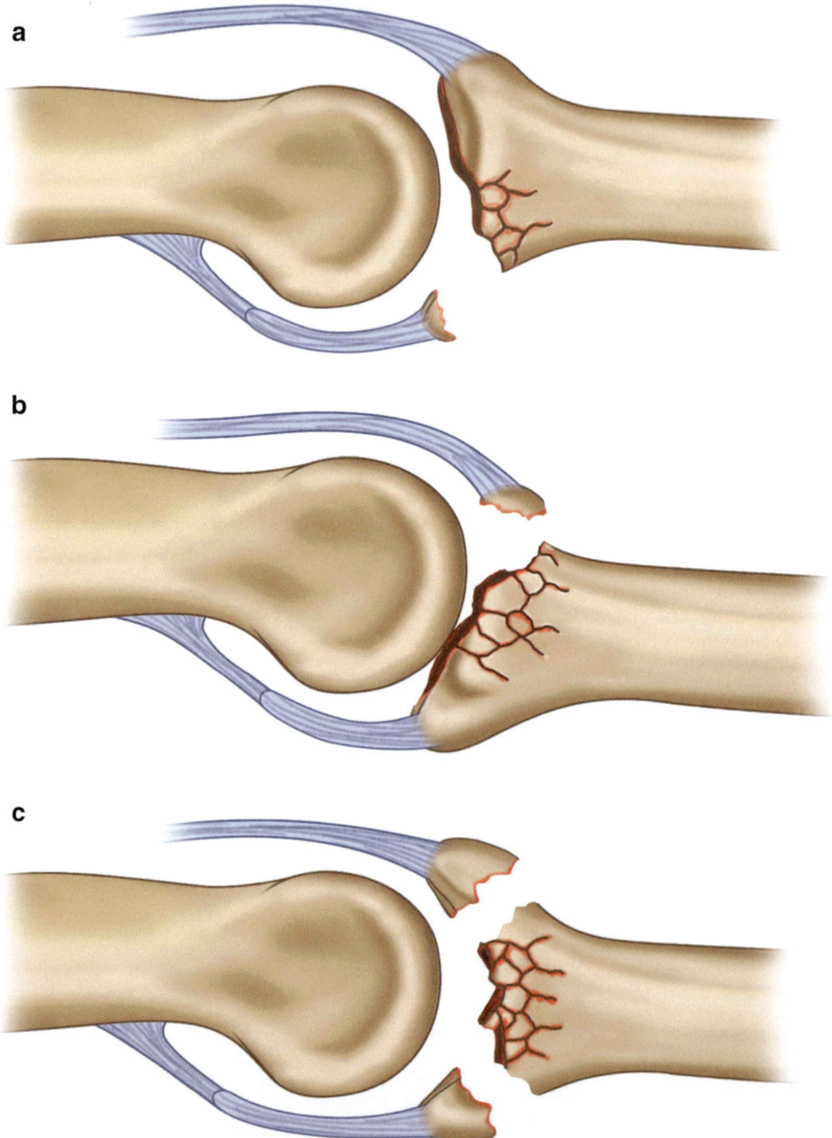

Fig. 15.10 Proximal interphalangeal joint fracture dislocation patterns. (**a**) Palmar lip fracture with dorsal subluxation. Palmar lip fractures can be of the avulsion or impaction shear type. In the impaction shear injury depicted here, the palmar 50% of the articular surface is damaged. The palmar plate remains attached to the anterior lip of the middle phalanx and there is impaction of articular cartilage into the underlying metaphyseal bone. Subtle dorsal subluxation is appreciated by observing a V-shaped gap between the articular surfaces of the head of the proximal phalanx and the undamaged portion of the middle phalanx base. (**b**) Dorsal lip fracture with palmar subluxation. Dorsal lip fractures can be of the avulsion or impaction shear type. Loss of middle phalangeal articular surface contour, as depicted in this impaction shear injury, accentuates palmar translation of the middle phalanx. (**c**) Pilon fracture. By definition, pilon fractures include disruption of both the dorsal and palmar cortical margins. The central articular fragments are often comminuted and impacted into the underlying metaphyseal bone. (From Kiefhaber et al. [38])

phalanx that is highlighted by the "V" sign (Fig. 15.10a). Dorsal fracture-dislocations can occur either by hyperextension of the PIP joint, where the robust insertion of the volar plate fails in tension, or from an impaction and shearing secondary to axial force applied to a flexed PIP joint [39, 40].

Volar PIP Fracture-Dislocation

Volar PIP fracture-dislocations are uncommon and occur as a result of central tendon insufficiency with or without a fracture of the dorsal lip of the middle phalangeal base [41]. The PIP joint loses a dorsal buttress and the joint subluxates volarly (Fig. 15.10b). Volar fracture-dislocations can either occur by hyperflexion, where the dorsal lip fails in tension, or by impaction and shearing in an extended joint [39, 40, 42]. In addition to losing the dorsal buttress, there is unopposed pull of the flexor digitorum sublimis (FDS) on the PIP as a result of loss of the extensor tendon pull.

Pilon Type Fracture-Dislocation

Pilon type fracture-dislocations of the PIP joint are also uncommon and were first described by Stern et al. [43]. Pilon PIP joint fracture-dislocations require involvement of both the dorsal and volar margins of the middle phalangeal articular surface and also involve extensive central depression, comminution, and splay (Fig. 15.10c). Pilon type injuries occur as a result of axial force being applied to the PIP joint. This injury can be difficult to manage; in the study by Stern et al., no patients regained full motion [43].

Treatment

The goal of treating phalangeal base fractures is to achieve a pain-free, stable joint with restoration of range of motion. During treatment, serial radiographs are important to ensure that the joint is anatomically reduced. Interestingly, the articular reduction has not been shown to reliably correlate to range of motion or development of arthrosis—suggesting that it is reasonable to accept some degree of articular step-off as long as the joint is concentrically reduced [44–46].

Non-operative Treatment

Buddy Taping

In a stable dorsal PIP joint fracture-dislocation the lateral radiograph of the affected digit should demonstrate a reduced joint, with coplanar middle and proximal phalangeal heads, and absence of the V-sign. Phair et al. noted in a study on conservative treatment that immobilization caused increased morbidity, specifically stiffness of the interphalangeal joints [47]. Immobilization is not recommended, and it is important to counsel patients on the importance of early motion [47]. If a dorsal fracture-dislocation of the PIP joint is stable, non-operative treatment by anchoring the affected digit to the neighboring digit by neighbor strapping (buddy taping) with tape or Velcro straps [47, 48]. The size of the volar articular fragment does not predict outcome, but Lee et al. found that greater displacement or rotation of the fracture fragments and presence of subluxation or dislocation of the fragment was associated with the failure of conservative treatment (Fig. 15.11) [48, 49]. While a

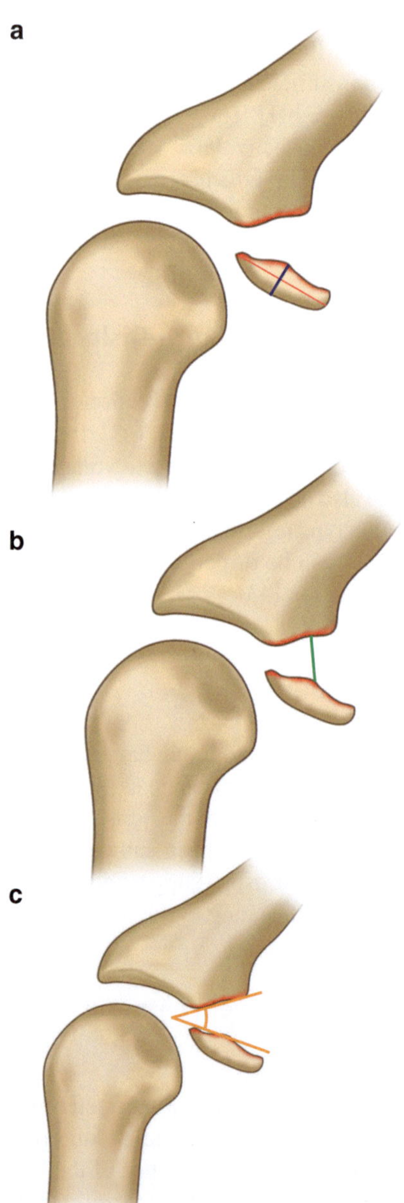

Fig. 15.11 (a) On the lateral radiograph, the longest proximal-distal length was defined as the height and the longest anteroposterior line perpendicular to it, as the width. The fragment size was evaluated as the area by multiplying the width (indicated in red) by the height (indicated in blue). (b) The distance between the bisector at the volar fracture surface of the middle phalangeal base and the bisector at the fracture fragment was measured to assess the extent of displacement (green). (c) The angle created between the volar fracture surface of the middle phalangeal base and the surface of the fracture fragment was measured to assess the extent of rotation (orange)

majority of patients can have an excellent or good outcome following early mobilization with buddy taping, presentation more than 3 weeks after injury is associated with poor prognosis [49].

Extension Block Splint

In dorsal PIP fracture-dislocations that have tenuous stability, such that there is involvement of 30–50% of the articular surface, they may be treated with figure of eight extension block splinting, provided that adequate reduction of the PIP joint can be maintained (Fig. 15.12) [50]. When stability is tenuous, the joint often has to be flexed to achieve reduction—but if >30° of flexion is required to maintain joint reduction there is increased risk of stiffness and poor functional outcome (Fig. 15.13a) [50, 51]. Additionally, it is critical that the PIP joint does not hinge during flexion—as this is a contraindication to treatment with extension block splinting (Fig. 15.13b). While some series have noted that it is acceptable to immobilize the PIP joint in up to 60° of flexion for a short time, most experience with extension block splinting has found that cases that require increased immobilization or increased flexion are better treated with operative intervention [38, 39, 50].

Dorsal AlumaFoam Splint

Non-operative management of *volar* PIP joint fracture-dislocations can be achieved with dorsal AlumaFoam splinting, with the PIP joint immobilized in full extension. Because of the rarity of volar PIP joint fracture-dislocations, there is limited literature to support closed management. With such injuries, there is loss of the extensor mechanism through disruption of the insertion of the central slip. Kang and Stern have suggested that adequate restoration of central slip function may be achieved as long as the avulsed fracture fragment is displaced less than 2 mm [39]. The PIP joint is immobilized for 3–4 weeks, and the DIP and MP joints are left free and mobilization is encouraged [39, 42]. If there is enough displacement to cause extensor lag, then surgical intervention should be considered [39, 42].

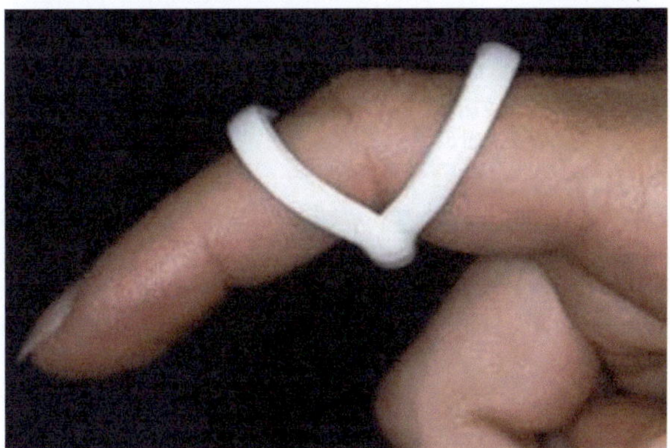

Fig. 15.12 Demonstration of a figure of eight splint for immobilization of stable phalangeal base fracture-dislocations. (Accessed from https://emedicine.medscape.com/article/1287715-treatment on 9/6/2021)

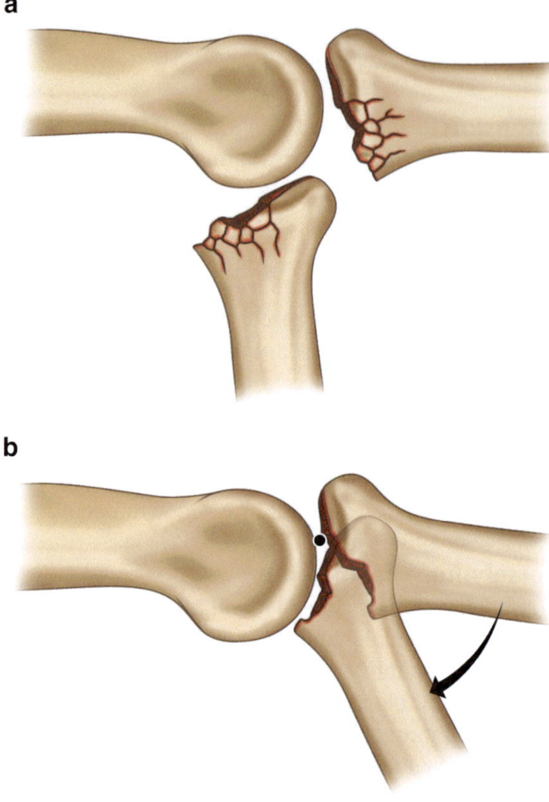

Fig. 15.13 Proximal interphalangeal flexion/glide versus hinging. (**a**) Restoration of the normal glide of the middle phalanx around the head of the proximal phalanx requires complete elimination of middle phalangeal dorsal subluxation. (**b**) Hinging of the middle phalanx (depicted here) portends an unacceptable clinical result. (From Kiefhaber et al. [38])

Operative Treatment

Extension Block Pinning

In unstable dorsal PIP fracture-dislocations, operative intervention is indicated. Extension block pinning is minimally invasive. The PIP joint is flexed to achieve concentric reduction and a trans-articular Kirschner wire (K-wire) is inserted into the head of the proximal phalanx to prevent dorsal subluxation of the middle phalanx [52]. The ability to actively flex the PIP joint is maintained. The K-wire is removed at 3 weeks, and an extension block splint is used for another 2 weeks [52, 53]. Newington et al. reported their °experience with extension block pinning in ten patients, noting that at 16 years the mean PIP arc of motion was 85° and that there was a mean flexion contracture of 8° [53]. It is important to avoid pinning in excessive flexion (greater than 15–20°) to avoid a PIP joint flexion contracture [38].

Closed Reduction and Percutaneous Pinning

In PIP fracture-dislocations with large fracture fragments, it may be possible to perform closed reduction and percutaneous pinning (CRPP). Often it is necessary to perform trans-articular pinning or extension block pinning in addition to fixation of

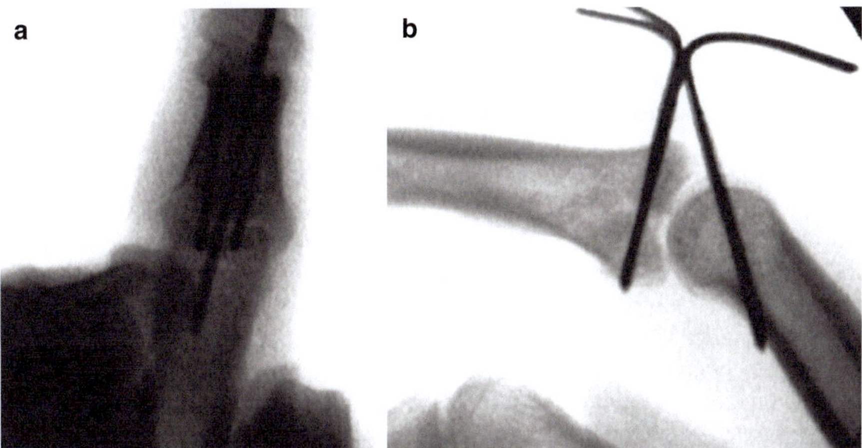

Fig. 15.14 AP (**a**) and lateral (**b**) intraoperative fluoroscopy demonstrating closed reduction and percutaneous pinning with extension block pinning. (From Vitale et al. [54])

the fracture fragments to provide enough construct stability to ensure adequate healing (Fig. 15.14a, b) [54]. CRPP can be performed in either dorsal or volar PIP joint fracture-dislocations. Vitale et al. reported six patients with CRPP and extension block pinning for unstable dorsal PIP joint fracture-dislocations [54]. K-wires were left in place for 3.5–4 weeks and then removed in clinic [54]. Following removal, under digital block, passive manipulation was recommended to break up tendon adhesions [54]. The mean arc of motion was 89° with a 4° flexion contracture [54]. The authors reported excellent VAS and DASH scores and noted excellent range of motion of the DIP joint [54]. In another small series, comparison of CRPP with open reduction and internal fixation (ORIF) demonstrated comparable outcomes in arc or motion and flexion contracture [55].

Open Reduction and Internal Fixation

Open reduction and internal fixation of PIP joint fracture-dislocations is technically demanding but can produce excellent outcomes in the appropriate patient population [24]. ORIF can be accomplished with screws, plates, or cerclage wiring. ORIF is best equipped to treat fracture-dislocations large fracture fragments or if there is a need for metaphyseal bone grafting with associated articular impaction. While excellent outcomes have been reported in ORIF, there is also the potential for complications and loss of function [43, 55]. ORIF is technically demanding, and there is potential for soft tissue scaring and adhesions.

Hamilton et al. reported nine patients who underwent ORIF for unstable dorsal fracture-dislocations with an average follow-up of 3.5 years [56]. In their series, the average final arc of motion of the PIP joint was 70°, with an average flexion contracture of 14°, though seven of nine patients had painless range of motion and the remaining two patients only had pain with heavy activity [56]. Grant et al. reported 14 patients who underwent ORIF for unstable fracture-dislocations of the PIP joint with an average follow up of 3 years [57]. In their series, the final arc of motion was highly dependent on acute intervention—with patients who were treated within 14 days of injury having an average of 100° final arc of motion compared to 86° in patients who presented more than 2 weeks after injury [57].

Static and Dynamic External Fixator

If PIP fracture-dislocations are unstable not amenable to CRPP or ORIF, then external fixation can be utilized. External fixation depends on indirect reduction using the soft tissues and ligamentotaxis to achieve appropriate alignment of the fracture fragments. External fixation can be either static or dynamic [58, 59]. There are several configurations for dynamic external fixators (Fig. 15.15) [59–62]. The goal is to unload the PIP articular surface, allow early motion, and promote healing with minimal additional soft tissue trauma. In order to allow for appropriate motion with a dynamic external fixator, it is critical to place a K-wire through the center of rotation of the head of the proximal phalanx (Fig. 15.16c). Ellis et al. reported eight patients

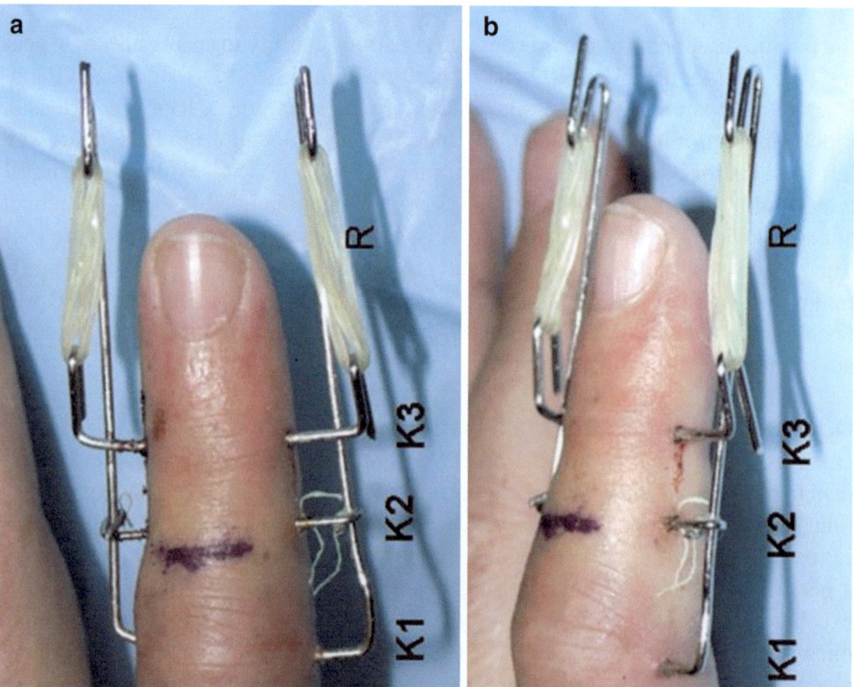

Fig. 15.15 Intraoperative photographs taken after placement of external fixator (patient 1). Proximal (K1), middle or "translational stability" (K2), and distal (K3) K-wires seen along with rubber bands (R) on both anteroposterior (**a**) and lateral (**b**) views. (From Ellis et al. [59])

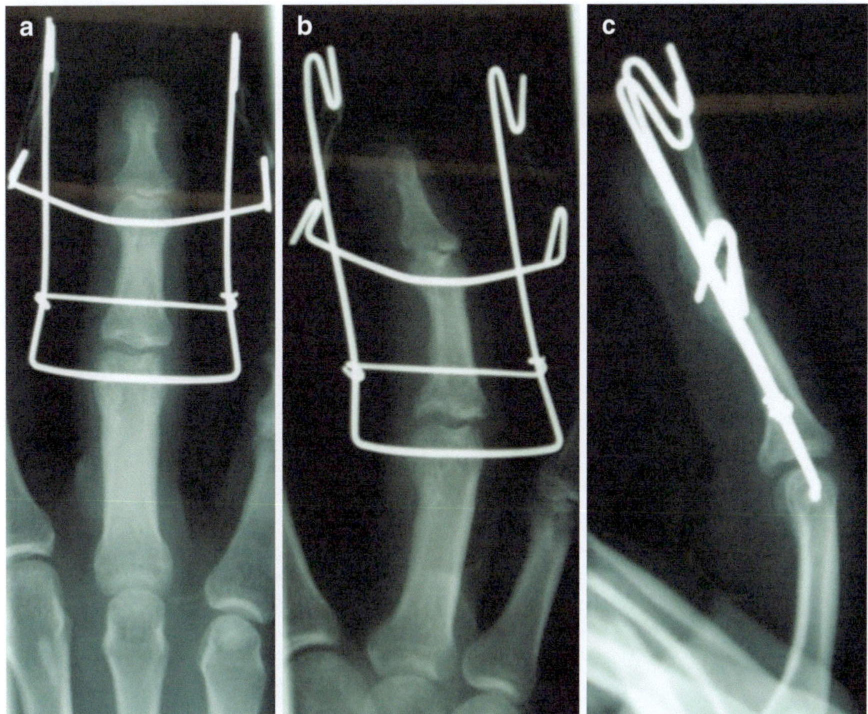

Fig. 15.16 Radiographs after placement of external fixator (patient 2). Anteroposterior (**a**), oblique (**b**), and lateral (**c**) demonstrating concentrically reduced PIP joint. Three pins well fixed: (1) center of rotation proximal phalangeal condyles, (2) proximal shaft of middle phalanx, (3) distal condyles of middle phalanx. (From Ellis et al. [59])

treated with dynamic external fixation at an average follow-up of 26 months. The average arc of motion of the PIP joint was 88° with minimal pain and 92% grip strength compared to the contralateral hand [59]. Importantly, Ellis et al. noted that final radiographic follow-up demonstrated a concentric reduction in all PIP joints, with evidence of early arthrosis or articular step-off in 5 of 8 patients [59].

Volar Plate Arthroplasty

Historically, dorsal PIP joint fracture-dislocations were managed with volar plate arthroplasty [63]. The initial rationale for volar plate arthroplasty was to restore the volar buttress and prevent dorsal subluxation of the middle phalanx, which is performed by advancing the volar plate into the osseous defect on the volar aspect of the base of the middle phalanx (Fig. 15.17) [63]. While volar plate arthroplasty today is less commonly performed, Dionysian and Eaton reported 17 patients with an average follow-up of 11.5 years [64]. The average range of motion of the PIP joint was 85° in patients who had surgery within 4 weeks of injury and remodeling

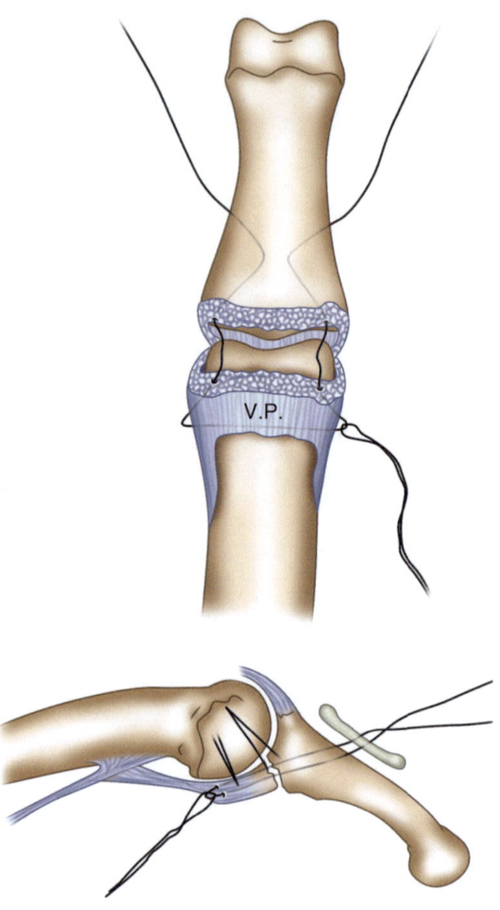

Fig. 15.17 Diagrammatic representation of the technique for volar plate advancement arthroplasty, showing volar and lateral appearance. (From Eaton et al. [63])

of the articular surface of the base of the middle phalanx was noted [63, 64]. Consistent with other series, if surgery was done more than 4 weeks following injury, the range of motion was comparatively reduced at an average of 61° [64].

Bridge Plating

Recently another treatment option has recently been proposed for unstable PIP joint fracture-dislocations that are not amenable to open reduction and internal fixation that avoids the need for percutaneous pins. Ozer introduced bridge plating (Figs. 15.18 and 15.19) [65]. Small stab incisions are made in the dorsal apparatus, and the bridge plate is left in place for 4–6 weeks [65]. During plate removal, tenolysis is recommended. Ozer reported his experience with one patient, who maintained 90% of PIP motion at final follow-up but also lost significant DIP joint range of motion [65]. In a case report, Selverian and Jones also described a similar outcome with PIP and DIP joint range of motion [66].

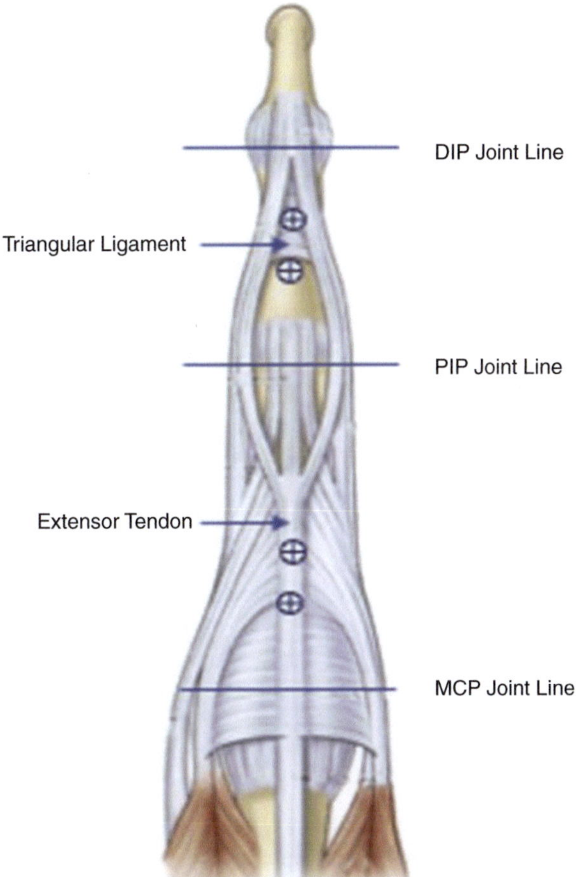

Fig. 15.18 Placement of proximal and distal screws is shown on the extensor surface of the digit. Two small stab incisions are made to split the extensor tendon and the triangular ligament to place screws as shown. (From Ozer [65])

Salvage Options

Hemi-hamate Arthroplasty

Hastings et al. first introduced hemi-hamate arthroplasty after extensive cadaveric and biomechanical research [67]. In hemi-hamate arthroplasty, the volar middle phalangeal base is replaced with a size-matched osteo-articular autograft from the hamate [67]. The central ridge of the hamate, which divides the fourth and fifth carpometacarpal (CMC) joints, serves as an excellent replacement for the sagittal ridge at the base of the middle phalanx (Fig. 15.20) [68]. When placing the hamate autograft, it is important to recall that the cartilage thickness of the hamate differs from the cartilage thickness of the base of the middle phalanx—so radiographs may give the appearance of a step-off when one does not exist (Fig. 15.21a–c) [68, 69]. Also assess for coronal plane angulation—as it can be subtle and when not addressed, it can adversely impact patient outcomes. Capo et al. did a cadaveric study assessing

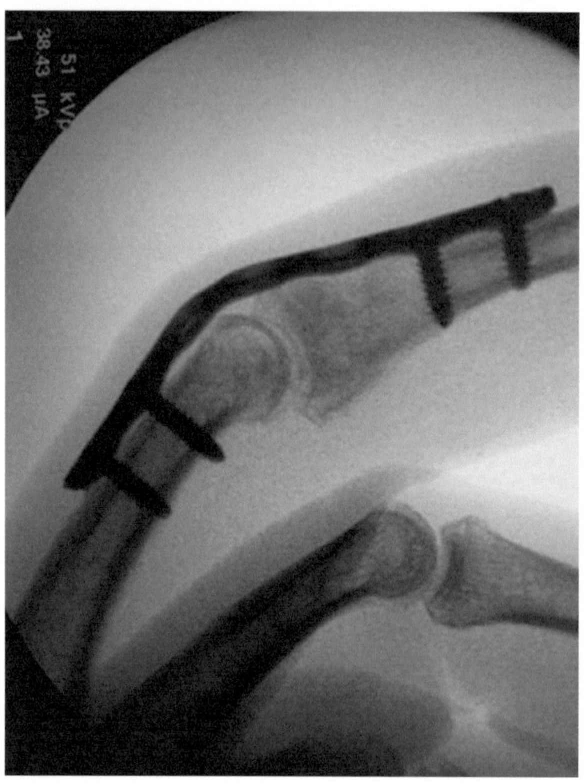

Fig. 15.19 Fluoroscopic image in the lateral plane shows satisfactory alignment of the joint and the fracture after bone grafting. (From Ozer [65])

CMC joint stability after harvesting the hamate and found that the removal of the central portion of the hamate did not cause obvious clinical instability or dislocation [70]. Williams et al. reported 13 patients treated with hemi-hamate arthroplasty with an average follow-up of 16 months and found a mean PIP arc of motion of 85° with minimal pain and an average 82% grip strength of the contralateral hand [70]. Calfee et al. reported outcomes for hemi-hamate arthroplasty used to treat 33 patients with acute or chronic PIP fracture-dislocations [71]. At an average of 4.5 years after the initial injury, they found an average arc of PIP motion of 69° with an average pain score of 2.5 and good grip strength [71].

Implant Arthroplasty

Implant arthroplasty is a salvage procedure and is rarely indicated. Both silicone and pyrocarbon implants have been described [72, 73]. Henry reported a pyrocarbon hemiarthroplasty 18 months after surgery with a PIP joint arc of motion was 95° . Criner and Ilyas reported on silicone arthroplasty for chronic PIP fracture-dislocations, and in four patients the average PIP joint arc of motion was 76° at 20 months with minimal pain [73].

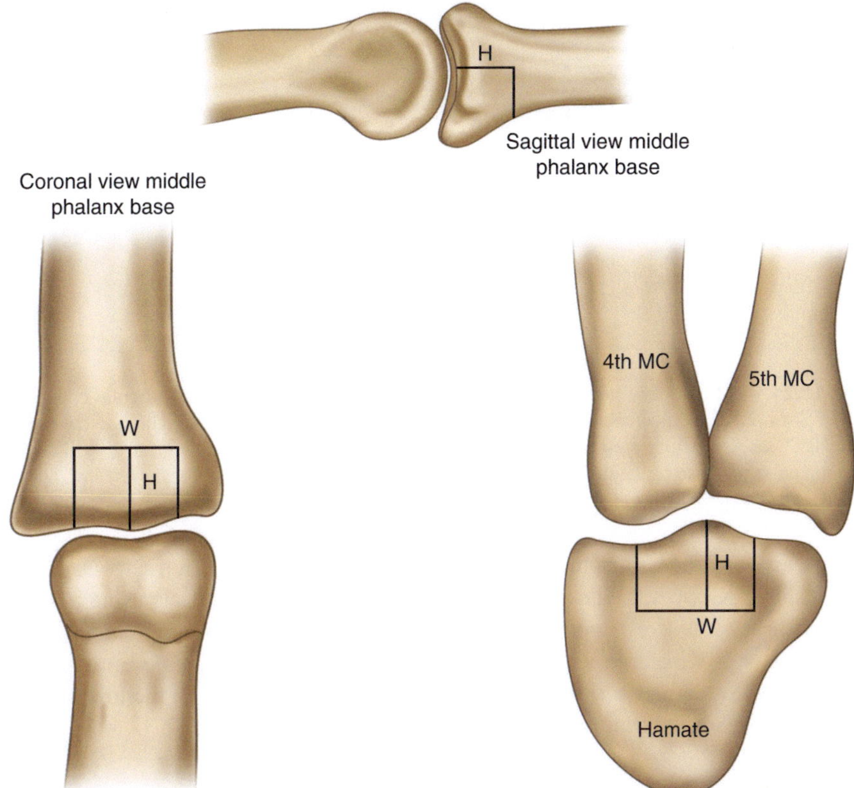

Fig. 15.20 Graft dimensions: Use the central articular ridge of the middle phalangeal base to establish the center of the graft. Measure the amount of missing articular surface radial and ulnar to this midline ridge and determine the needed width of the graft (W). Transfer the measurements of the missing articular surface to the hamate centering the proposed graft on the articular ridge between the articulations of the fourth and fifth metacarpals. The graft should be harvested slightly larger than the measurements to accommodate for the thickness of the saw blade. Once harvested, the graft can be further tailored to the exact size and shape needed

Arthrodesis

Occasionally there is no motion sparing option available for salvage of the PIP joint. In such cases, arthrodesis is a reliable procedure for achieving pain-free stability [74]. Stern et al. reported on their experience of 203 patients who underwent 290 tension band fusions of the MP and PIP joints and found a 97% rate of union with excellent pain relief [75]. Nine percent of cases required hardware removal. In a more recent series, Hussain et al. reported on 415 patients who underwent PIP joint fusion with a tension band construct and an average of 1.3 years of follow-up. In their series, there was a 10% nonunion rate and a 15% reoperation rate [76].

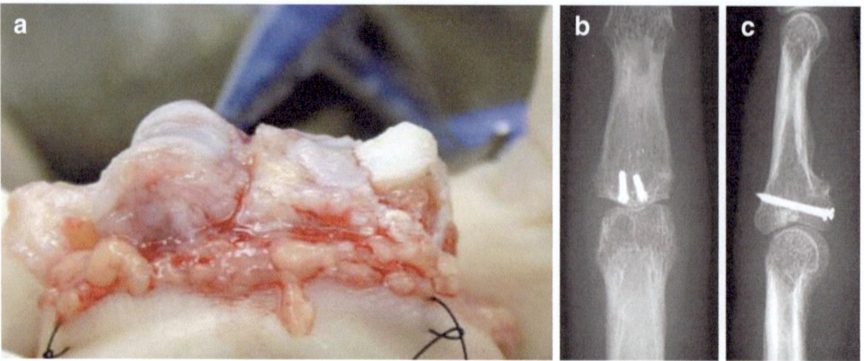

Fig. 15.21 (**a**) Intraoperative lateral view of inset graft with reconstitution of articular concavity and volar lip. (**b**) AP postoperative radiograph. (**c**) Lateral postoperative radiograph. Note radiographic "false" articular step-off created by thicker articular cartilage present at distal hamate compared to the base of the middle phalanx. No step-off is noted on the clinical view intraoperatively (**a**). (From Williams et al. [68])

Alternative arthrodesis techniques can employ headless compression screws, plates, staples, and K-wires. Leibovic and Strickland compared arthrodesis using a headless compression screw with other techniques—and found that the nonunion rate was 21% with Kirschner wires, 4.5% with tension band wires, and no nonunions occurred with Herbert screws [77]. Additionally, the etiology with the lowest nonunion rate was acute traumatic fusion and post-traumatic salvage [77].

Summary

Phalangeal base fractures and PIP joint fracture-dislocations are challenging injuries. Often, the initial evaluation following injury to be done by a physician that lacks expertise in hand and upper extremity surgery and delays in care or missed diagnoses can adversely impact patient outcomes. The goals of managing these injuries are to restore stable, functional, and pain-free range of motion. There are a host of therapeutic options for treatment. It is incumbent upon the surgeon to consider both patient and fracture patterns and selecting the best treatment option.

References

1. Karl JW, Olson PR, Rosenwasser MP. The epidemiology of upper extremity fractures in the United States, 2009. J Orthop Trauma. 2015;29(8):e242–4.
2. Ootes D, Lambers KT, Ring DC. The epidemiology of upper extremity injuries presenting to the emergency department in the United States. Hand (N Y). 2012;7(1):18–22.
3. Stanton JS, Dias JJ, Burke FD. Fractures of the tubular bones of the hand. J Hand Surg Eur Vol. 2007;32(6):626–36.

4. Hoang D, Vu CL, Jackson M, Huang JI. An anatomical study of metacarpal morphology utilizing CT scans: evaluating parameters for antegrade intramedullary compression screw fixation of metacarpal fractures. J Hand Surg Am. 2021;46(2):149.e1–8.

5. Bain GI, Polites N, Higgs BG, Heptinstall RJ, McGrath AM. The functional range of motion of the finger joints. J Hand Surg Eur Vol. 2015;40(4):406–11.

6. Minami A, An KN, Cooney WP, Linscheid RL, Chao EY. Ligament stability of the metacarpophalangeal joint: a biomechanical study. J Hand Surg Am. 1985;10(2):255–60.

7. Dy CJ, Tucker SM, Kok PL, Hearns KA, Carlson MG. Anatomy of the radial collateral ligament of the index metacarpophalangeal joint. J Hand Surg Am. 2013;38(1):124–8.

8. Dumont C, Albus G, Kubein-Meesenburg D, Fanghänel J, Stürmer KM, Nägerl H. Morphology of the interphalangeal joint surface and its functional relevance. J Hand Surg Am. 2008;33(1):9–18.

9. Minamikawa Y, Horii E, Amadio PC, Cooney WP, Linscheid RL, An KN. Stability and constraint of the proximal interphalangeal joint. J Hand Surg Am. 1993;18(2):198–204.

10. Caravaggi P, Shamian B, Uko L, Chen L, Melamed E, Capo JT. In vitro kinematics of the proximal interphalangeal joint in the finger after progressive disruption of the main supporting structures. Hand (N Y). 2015;10(3):425–32.

11. Hogan CJ, Nunley JA. Posttraumatic proximal interphalangeal joint flexion contractures. J Am Acad Orthop Surg. 2006;14(9):524–33.

12. Bogumill GP. A morphologic study of the relationship of collateral ligaments to growth plates in the digits. J Hand Surg Am. 1983;8(1):74–9.

13. Leibovic SJ, Bowers WH. Anatomy of the proximal interphalangeal joint. Hand Clin. 1994;10(2):169–78.

14. Nicholson LT, Hill JR, McKnight B, Heckmann N, Stevanovic M, Ghiassi A. Redefining zone ii: anatomy of the flexor digitorum superficialis insertion. Hand (N Y). 2019;14(3):377–80.

15. Clavero JA, Alomar X, Monill JM, et al. MR imaging of ligament and tendon injuries of the fingers. Radiographics. 2002;22(2):237–56.

16. Graham KS, Goitz RJ, Kaufmann RA. Curvatures of the DIP joints of the hand. Hand (N Y). 2014;9(4):522–8.

17. Shrewsbury MM, Johnson RK. Ligaments of the distal interphalangeal joint and the mallet position. J Hand Surg Am. 1980;5(3):214–6.

18. Craig SM. Anatomy of the joints of the fingers. Hand Clin. 1992;8(4):693–700.

19. Chepla KJ, Goitz RJ, Fowler JR. Anatomy of the flexor digitorum profundus insertion. J Hand Surg Am. 2015;40(2):240–4.

20. Schweitzer TP, Rayan GM. The terminal tendon of the digital extensor mechanism: part II, kinematic study. J Hand Surg Am. 2004;29(5):903–8.

21. Shum C, Bruno RJ, Ristic S, Rosenwasser MP, Strauch RJ. Examination of the anatomic relationship of the proximal germinal nail matrix to the extensor tendon insertion. J Hand Surg Am. 2000;25(6):1114–7.

22. Janssen SJ, Ter Meulen DP, Hageman MGJS, Earp BE, Ring D. Quantitative 3-dimensional CT analyses of fractures of the middle phalanx base. Hand (N Y). 2015;10(2):210–4.

23. Chitnis SS, Chitnis SL. Indication for CT following index finger metacarpophalangeal joint dislocation—a case report. Trauma Case Rep. 2018;18:31–6.

24. Wolfe SW, Katz LD. Intra-articular impaction fractures of the phalanges. J Hand Surg Am. 1995;20(2):327–33.

25. Faccioli N, Foti G, Barillari M, Atzei A, Mucelli RP. Finger fractures imaging: accuracy of cone-beam computed tomography and multislice computed tomography. Skelet Radiol. 2010;39(11):1087–95.

26. Rubin DA, Kneeland JB, Kitay GS, Naranja RJ. Flexor tendon tears in the hand: use of MR imaging to diagnose degree of injury in a cadaver model. AJR Am J Roentgenol. 1996;166(3):615–20.

27. Drapé JL, Silbermann-Hoffman O, Houvet P, et al. Complications of flexor tendon repair in the hand: MR imaging assessment. Radiology. 1996;198(1):219–24.

28. Drapé JL, Dubert T, Silbermann O, Thelen P, Thivet A, Benacerraf R. Acute trauma of the extensor hood of the metacarpophalangeal joint: MR imaging evaluation. Radiology. 1994;192(2):469–76.
29. Hinke DH, Erickson SJ, Chamoy L, Timins ME. Ulnar collateral ligament of the thumb: MR findings in cadavers, volunteers, and patients with ligamentous injury (Gamekeeper's thumb). AJR Am J Roentgenol. 1994;163(6):1431–4.
30. Read JW, Conolly WB, Lanzetta M, Spielman S, Snodgrass D, Korber JS. Diagnostic ultrasound of the hand and wrist. J Hand Surg Am. 1996;21(6):1004–10.
31. Allen GM, Drakonaki EE, Tan MLH, Dhillon M, Rajaratnam V. High-resolution ultrasound in the diagnosis of upper limb disorders: a tertiary referral centre experience. Ann Plast Surg. 2008;61(3):259–64.
32. Bajaj S, Pattamapaspong N, Middleton W, Teefey S. Ultrasound of the hand and wrist. J Hand Surg Am. 2009;34(4):759–60.
33. Lee SA, Kim BH, Kim S-J, Kim JN, Park S-Y, Choi K. Current status of ultrasonography of the finger. Ultrasonography. 2016;35(2):110–23.
34. Champagne N, Eadie L, Regan L, Wilson P. The effectiveness of ultrasound in the detection of fractures in adults with suspected upper or lower limb injury: a systematic review and subgroup meta-analysis. BMC Emerg Med. 2019;19(1):17.
35. Eaton RG. Joint injuries of the hand. Springfield, IL: Charles C. Thomas; 1971. p. 9–34.
36. Hastings H, Carroll C. Treatment of closed articular fractures of the metacarpophalangeal and proximal interphalangeal joints. Hand Clin. 1988;4(3):503–27.
37. Krakauer JD, Stern PJ. Hinged device for fractures involving the proximal interphalangeal joint. Clin Orthop Relat Res. 1996;327:29–37.
38. Kiefhaber TR, Stern PJ. Fracture dislocations of the proximal interphalangeal joint. J Hand Surg Am. 1998;23(3):368–80.
39. Kang R, Stern PJ. Fracture dislocations of the proximal interphalangeal joint. J Am Soc Surg Hand. 2002;2(2):47–59.
40. Akagi T, Hashizume H, Inoue H, Ogura T, Nagayama N. Computer simulation analysis of fracture dislocation of the proximal interphalangeal joint using the finite element method. Acta Med Okayama. 1994;48(5):263–70.
41. Thompson JS, Eaton RG. Volar dislocation of the proximal interphalangeal joint. J Hand Surg. 1977;2:232.
42. Caggiano NM, Harper CM, Rozental TD. Management of proximal interphalangeal joint fracture dislocations. Hand Clin. 2018;34(2):149–65.
43. Stern PJ, Roman RJ, Kiefhaber TR, McDonough JJ. Pilon fractures of the proximal interphalangeal joint. J Hand Surg Am. 1991;16(5):844–50.
44. Salter RB. The physiologic basis of continuous passive motion for articular cartilage healing and regeneration. Hand Clin. 1994;10(2):211–9.
45. Morgan JP, Gordon DA, Klug MS, Perry PE, Barre PS. Dynamic digital traction for unstable comminuted intra-articular fracture-dislocations of the proximal interphalangeal joint. J Hand Surg Am. 1995;20(4):565–73.
46. Calfee RP, Sommerkamp TG. Fracture-dislocation about the finger joints. J Hand Surg Am. 2009;34(6):1140–7.
47. Phair IC, Quinton DN, Allen MJ. The conservative management of volar avulsion fractures of the P.I.P. joint. J Hand Surg Br. 1989;14(2):168–70.
48. Lee S, Jang SJ, Jeon SH. Factors related to failure of conservative treatment in volar plate avulsion fractures of the proximal interphalangeal joint. Clin Orthop Surg. 2020;12(3):379–85.
49. Gaine WJ, Beardsmore J, Fahmy N. Early active mobilisation of volar plate avulsion fractures. Injury. 1998;29(8):589–91.
50. McElfresh EC, Dobyns JH, O'Brien ET. Management of fracture-dislocation of the proximal interphalangeal joints by extension-block splinting. J Bone Joint Surg Am. 1972;54(8):1705–11.
51. Kuczynski K. The proximal interphalangeal joint. Anatomy and causes of stiffness in the fingers. J Bone Joint Surg Br. 1968;50(3):656–63.

52. Viegas SF. Extension block pinning for proximal interphalangeal joint fracture dislocations: preliminary report of a new technique. J Hand Surg Am. 1992;17(5):896–901.
53. Newington DP, Davis TR, Barton NJ. The treatment of dorsal fracture-dislocation of the proximal interphalangeal joint by closed reduction and Kirschner wire fixation: a 16-year follow up. J Hand Surg Br. 2001;26(6):537–40.
54. Vitale MA, White NJ, Strauch RJ. A percutaneous technique to treat unstable dorsal fracture-dislocations of the proximal interphalangeal joint. J Hand Surg Am. 2011;36(9):1453–9.
55. Aladin A, Davis TRC. Dorsal fracture-dislocation of the proximal interphalangeal joint: a comparative study of percutaneous Kirschner wire fixation versus open reduction and internal fixation. J Hand Surg Br. 2005;30(2):120–8.
56. Hamilton SC, Stern PJ, Fassler PR, Kiefhaber TR. Mini-screw fixation for the treatment of proximal interphalangeal joint dorsal fracture-dislocations. J Hand Surg Am. 2006;31(8):1349–54.
57. Grant I, Berger AC, Tham SKY. Internal fixation of unstable fracture dislocations of the proximal interphalangeal joint. J Hand Surg Br. 2005;30(5):492–8.
58. Yousaf O, Yousaf IS, Giladi AM, Katz RD. Syringe external fixator: an inexpensive static-to-dynamic treatment for comminuted intra-articular phalangeal fractures. Tech Hand Up Extrem Surg. 2020;24(3):126–30.
59. Ellis SJ, Cheng R, Prokopis P, et al. Treatment of proximal interphalangeal dorsal fracture-dislocation injuries with dynamic external fixation: a pins and rubber band system. J Hand Surg Am. 2007;32(8):1242–50.
60. Kastenberger T, Kaiser P, Keller M, Schmidle G, Gabl M, Arora R. Clinical and radiological midterm outcome after treatment of pilonidal fracture dislocations of the proximal interphalangeal joint with a parabolic dynamic external fixator. Arch Orthop Trauma Surg. 2020;140(1):43–50.
61. Kodama A, Sunagawa T, Nakashima Y, et al. Joint distraction and early mobilization using a new dynamic external finger fixator for the treatment of fracture-dislocations of the proximal interphalangeal joint. J Orthop Sci. 2018;23(6):959–66.
62. Deshmukh SC, Kumar D, Mathur K, Thomas B. Complex fracture-dislocation of the proximal interphalangeal joint of the hand. Results of a modified pins and rubbers traction system. J Bone Joint Surg Br. 2004;86(3):406–12.
63. Eaton RG, Malerich MM. Volar plate arthroplasty of the proximal interphalangeal joint: a review of ten years' experience. J Hand Surg Am. 1980;5(3):260–8.
64. Dionysian E, Eaton RG. The long-term outcome of volar plate arthroplasty of the proximal interphalangeal joint. J Hand Surg Am. 2000;25(3):429–37.
65. Ozer K. Temporary bridge plate fixation of pilon fractures of the proximal interphalangeal joint. J Hand Surg Am. 2019;44(6):524.e1–6.
66. Selverian S, Jones CM. Case report: bridge plating for unstable pip fracture dislocation. Arch Bone Jt Surg. 2020;8(6):739–43.
67. Hastings H, Capo J, Steinberg B, Stern P. Hemicondylar hamate replacement arthroplasty for proximal interphalangeal joint fracture/dislocations. Presented at the 54th Annual Meeting of the American Society for Surgery of the Hand; Boston, MA, 2–4 Sept, 199.
68. Williams RMM, Hastings H, Kiefhaber TR. Pip fracture/dislocation treatment technique: use of a hemi-hamate resurfacing arthroplasty. Tech Hand Up Extrem Surg. 2002;6(4):185–92.
69. Podolsky DJ, Mainprize J, McMillan C, Binhammer P. Suitability of using the hamate for reconstruction of the finger middle phalanx base: an assessment of cartilage thickness. Plast Surg (Oakv). 2019;27(3):211–6.
70. Capo JT, Hastings H, Choung E, Kinchelow T, Rossy W, Steinberg B. Hemicondylar hamate replacement arthroplasty for proximal interphalangeal joint fracture dislocations: an assessment of graft suitability. J Hand Surg Am. 2008;33(5):733–9.
71. Calfee RP, Kiefhaber TR, Sommerkamp TG, Stern PJ. Hemi-hamate arthroplasty provides functional reconstruction of acute and chronic proximal interphalangeal fracture-dislocations. J Hand Surg Am. 2009;34(7):1232–41.
72. Henry M. Prosthetic hemi-arthroplasty for post-traumatic articular cartilage loss in the proximal interphalangeal joint. Hand (N Y). 2011;6(1):93–7.

73. Criner KT, Ilyas AM. Silicone arthroplasty for chronic proximal interphalangeal joint dislocations. Tech Hand Up Extrem Surg. 2011;15(4):209–14.
74. Jones BF, Stern PJ. Interphalangeal joint arthrodesis. Hand Clin. 1994;10(2):267–75.
75. Stern PJ, Gates NT, Jones TB. Tension band arthrodesis of small joints in the hand. J Hand Surg Am. 1993;18(2):194–7.
76. Hussain HM, Roth AL, Sultan AA, Anis HK, Stern PJ. Nonunion and reoperation following proximal interphalangeal joint arthrodesis and associated patient factors. Hand (N Y). 2022;17(3):566–71. Published online 8 Aug 2020.
77. Leibovic SJ, Strickland JW. Arthrodesis of the proximal interphalangeal joint of the finger: comparison of the use of the Herbert screw with other fixation methods. J Hand Surg Am. 1994;19(2):181–8.

Adult Phalangeal Shaft Fractures

16

Jesse B. Jupiter

Introduction

The diaphyseal skeleton of the proximal and middle phalanges' anatomic design in the hand is consistent with that found in other short and long bones in the human skeleton. Yet they differ substantially due to their inherent relationship to the complexity of the gliding structures which envelope the bones. Furthermore, the overall length of these tubular bones represents a perfect example of the universal formula of a logarithmic formula found throughout nature as described by Fibonacci in the thirteenth century [1]. This formula puts the proximal interphalangeal joint of the digit exactly at the center of a spiral which does not change its shape as it grows and maintains the balance of digital arc of motion. The overriding goal in the management of fractures of the diaphyseal segments of the phalanges is to preserve the structural length and alignment along with restoration of the normal arc of digital motion, thus restoring the prehensile function unique to the human hand.

Fracture Assessment

Every phalangeal diaphyseal fracture will have its own "personality." The fracture pattern may be simple versus complex and comminuted; stable or unstable; displaced or nondisplaced; or open versus closed (Table 16.1).

Strickland et al. and several other authors have identified a number of patients related and fracture related factors that will contribute to an unsatisfactory outcome on digital function [2–6]. These include patient age, comorbidities, associated

J. B. Jupiter (✉)
Department of Orthopaedic Surgery, Massachusetts General Hospital, Boston, MA, USA
e-mail: jjupiter1@partners.org

Table 16.1 The assessment of the fracture personality

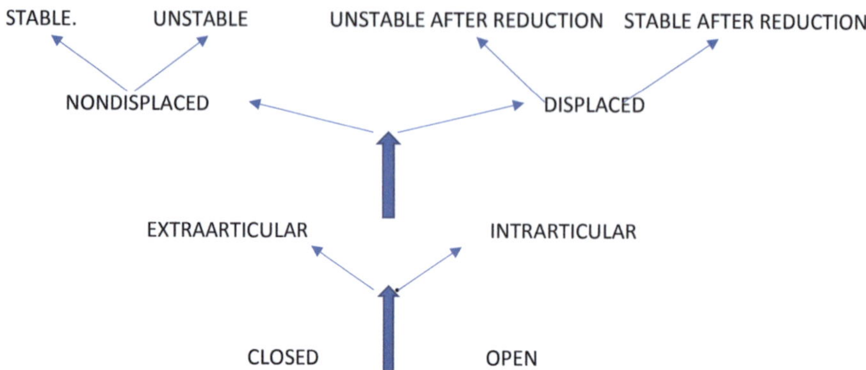

osteoarthritis, and motivation and compliance, while injury characteristics include soft issue disruption, associated tendon and/or nerve injury, articular involvement, bone loss, or multiple injuries.

Diaphyseal fractures may be transverse, oblique, spiral, or comminuted. Spiral or oblique fractures will more commonly be seen in closed fractures of the proximal phalanx, while transverse fractures tend to be more common involving the diaphysis of the middle phalanx. Oblique and/or spiral fractures, when displaced, will present with rotational deformity as well as digital shortening. Transverse fractures of the proximal phalanx tend to produce apex-volar angulatory deformity with the proximal segment flexed due to the insertion of the interosseous muscles, while the distal fragment extends due to the pull of the common extensor apparatus.

Fracture stability may be difficult to accurately assess from radiologic views alone and is best evaluated clinically by having the patient fully flex and extend the involved digit. This may require a temporary digital block anesthetic. Open and/or comminuted fractures will be unstable and may angulate and shorten or rotate [1, 7, 8].

Treatment

Nondisplaced Fractures

After assessment of clinical alignment and assurance that the fracture is stable and nondisplaced even with digital motion, immobilization with either a splint or cast should maintain the metacarpal phalangeal joints in 70° of flexion, interphalangeal joints in extension, and wrist slightly extended. Immobilization should not extend beyond 3 weeks. In the setting of a compliant patient, the involved digit can be "buddy strapped" to the adjacent digit(s). In either case, an X-ray at 1 week post-injury will be needed to confirm that the fracture remains stable.

Stable Fracture After Closed Reduction

Transverse fractures in particular are often stable after a closed fracture reduction as long as appropriate splint or cast is applied with the hand and wrist joints in the safe position. Clinical assurance must be taken after reduction to assess rotational and angular realignment. Control radiographs should be taken weekly until immobilization is removed at 3 weeks post-injury.

Alternatively, "extension block" immobilization with transverse proximal phalanx diaphyseal fractures with the cast or splint holding the metacarpophalangeal joint at 70° of flexion and extending over the proximal interphalangeal joint will permit digital flexion helping the overlying muscles to provide a dynamic flexion force while preventing an extension deformity and the fracture site. In general, no more than 10° of angular deformity in the coronal or sagittal plane is acceptable (Fig. 16.1).

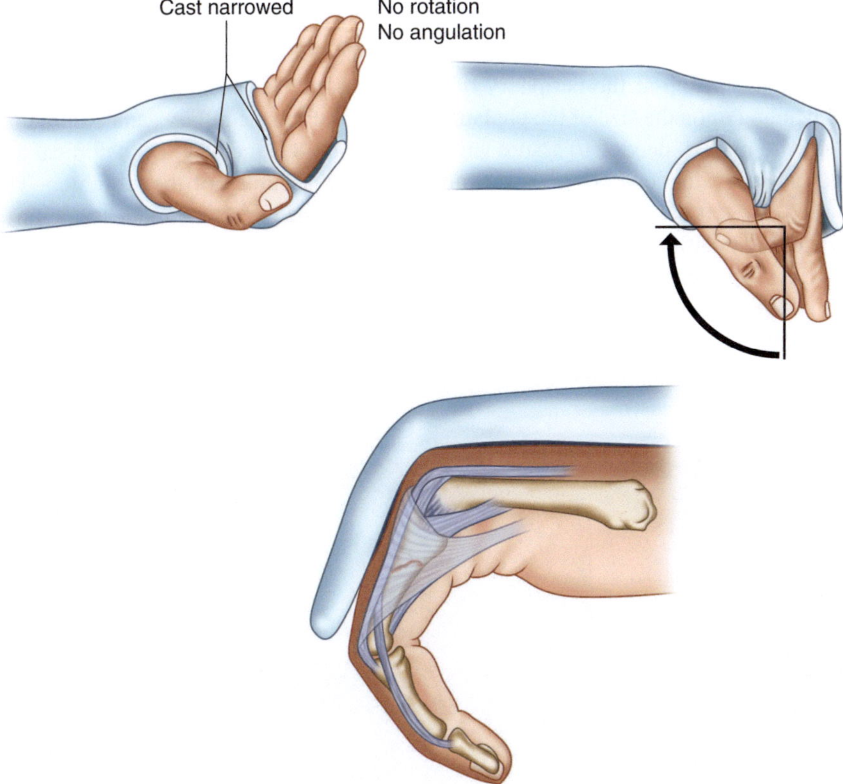

Fig. 16.1 The extension block cast maintains the metacarpophalangeal joint in about 70° of flexion but allows active flexion at the proximal interphalangeal joints allowing there to be dynamic forces to help maintain the reduction. (Adapted from Jupiter JB, Belsky MR. Fractures and dislocations in the hand. In Browner BD, Jupiter JB, Levine A et al. co-editors. Skeletal Trauma ed. 1. Philadelphia 1992, WB Saunders pp. 925–1024)

If attempting to reduce and hold a displaced spiral or oblique fracture, a word of caution is required as rotational correction may actually not occur at the fracture site but may occur through the metacarpophalangeal joint. This may be appreciated only at the point when immobilization is ended at 3 weeks and the rotational deformity at the healing fracture site now apparent.

Unstable Fracture After Closed Reduction Percutaneous Kirschner Wire Fixation

Transverse Fracture of the Proximal Phalanx

After satisfactory anesthesia has been achieved, the reduction technique is equivalent to that described above. Using fluoroscopic control, an antegrade placement of a 0.035 in. or 0.045 in. smooth Kirschner wire can be directed through the metacarpal head or placed on either side of the head and extended down the medullary cavity of the proximal phalanx. Alternatively, the Kirschner wire can be placed antegrade starting at the periphery of the articular base of the proximal phalanx. Depending upon the size of the phalanx and width of the medullary canal, more than one wire may be needed to assure angular and rotational control. Both clinical and radiologic evaluations are necessary to ensure the accuracy of the reduction. The wire(s) are left out of the skin and protected with gauze dressing and a cast applied in the safe position as noted above [9] (Fig. 16.2a, b).

Unstable transverse fractures of the middle phalanx can be stabilized after reduction with crossed Kirschner wires with care to avoid the wires crossing at the fracture site which may result in distraction of the fracture and delay in healing. Follow-up radiographs weekly for 3 weeks is advisable prior to pin removal in 3–4 weeks.

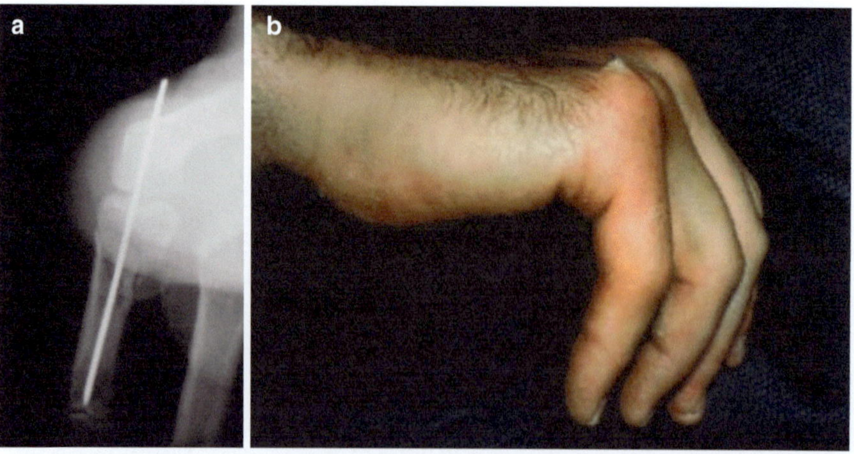

Fig. 16.2 (**a** and **b**) A transverse proximal phalanx fracture treated with closed reduction and percutaneous pinning

Closed Reduction and Percutaneous Kirschner Wire Fixation of Unstable Spiral or Oblique Diaphyseal Fractures

Unstable spiral and oblique fractures prove more difficult to both achieve an anatomic reduction as well as successfully stabilize with percutaneous Kirschner wires. Provisional reduction requires longitudinal traction and the use of a pointed reduction clamp to help realign the fracture and maintain the reduction while 2 or 3 0.035 in. Kirschner wires are placed perpendicular to the bone and pass through both cortices. Ideally the use of an oscillating drill will help to minimize injury to the overlying extensor mechanism. Fluoroscopic control followed by a careful assessment of the rotational and angular alignment must be done before further immobilization applied. If satisfactory, the pins are left outside of the skin and digit immobilized for 3 weeks at which time the pins are removed and active motion begun. Postoperatively, the digit should be X-rayed weekly for 3 weeks. At most 3 mm of shortening and 15° of angulation are acceptable (Fig. 16.3a–d, Table 16.2).

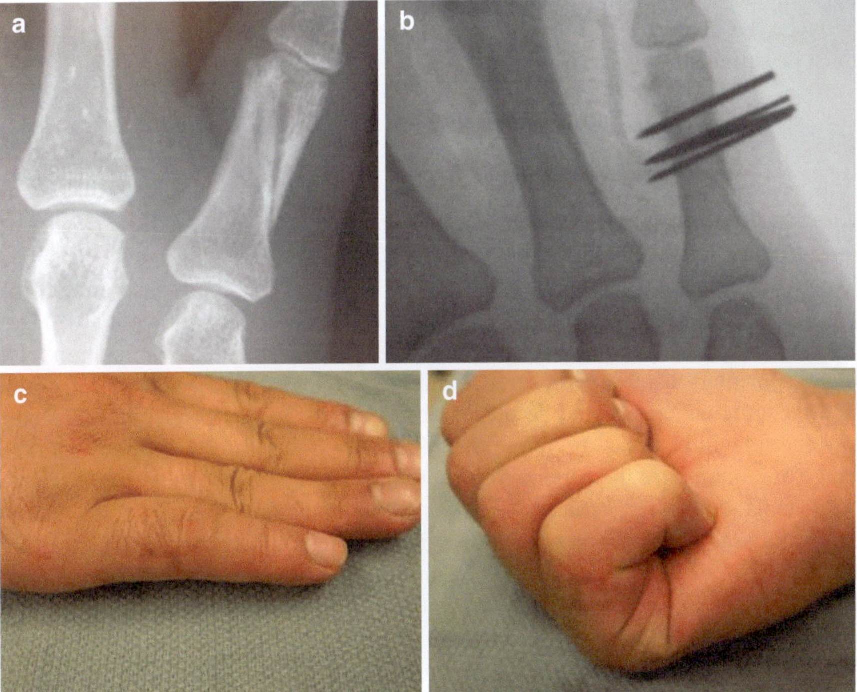

Fig. 16.3 (**a**) A displaced long oblique fracture of the proximal phalanx of the right little finger. (**b**) The reduced fracture is stabilized with multiple percutaneous Kirschner wires. (**c** and **d**) Nearly full extension and flexion were achieved following fracture healing

Table 16.2 Percutaneous Kirschner wire fixation

Indications
Unstable fractures
Advantages
Technique and equipment simple
Maintains intact soft tissue envelope
Disadvantages
Pin track infection
Joint stiffness

Open Reduction and Internal Fixation

The need for open reduction and stable internal fixation increases with associated injuries including open fractures, combined injuries involving two or more associated structures in the digit, or fractures unable to be reduced by traction and manipulation.

Surgical exposure can be either midaxial or dorsal with the interval in the proximal phalanx developed between the lateral band and central extensor tendon. If needed, one lateral band can be excised to facilitate exposure and limit adhesions between the hardware and this portion of the extensor mechanism. The exposure must be sufficient to visualize the entire extent of the fracture lines.

Fracture Fixation

Kirschner wire fixation as described above can effectively be applied in most of these fractures with the exception of those comminuted or with associated bone loss. To enhance the stability, a thin stainless steel wire can be looped around the points of the pins and brought over the dorsal surface as a figure of eight [10, 11].

Some long oblique and spiral fractures will be amenable to stable fixation with interfragmentary compression screw fixation. Usually 1.3 or 1.5 mm sized screws will be sufficient and should be placed perpendicular to the fracture line. At least two screws will be necessary to provide rotational stability and allow postoperative range of motion once the patient is comfortable (Fig. 16.4a–d) (Table 16.3).

Plate fixation is best indicated for those comminuted fractures, those with extensive soft tissue injury or some fractures with bone loss. Plates can be applied either on the dorsal or lateral side of the phalanx depending upon the soft tissue injury (Fig. 16.5a, b). Plates often have to be removed after fracture healing due to the bulk of the implant [12–15] (Table 16.4).

External Skeletal Fixation

Highly comminuted open or contaminated fractures as well as fracture with bone or soft tissue loss may be stabilized effectively with external fixation [16] (Table 16.5).

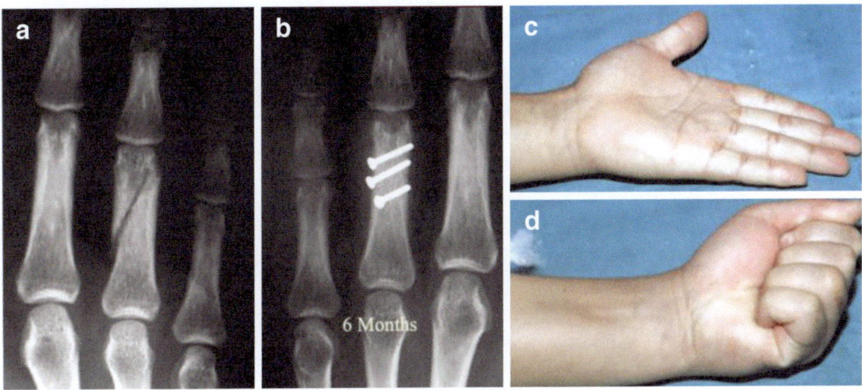

Fig. 16.4 (**a**) A displaced long oblique fracture of the ring finger proximal phalanx. (**b**) Stable fixation with three interfragmentary screws. (**c** and **d**) Full range of motion and full fracture healing after 3 weeks

Table 16.3 Interfragmentary screw fixation

Indications
Displaced spiral or long oblique fractures
Advantages
Stable fracture fixation for functional rehabilitation
Predictable union when properly applied
Low profile implant
Disadvantages
Technically demanding
Requires operative exposure

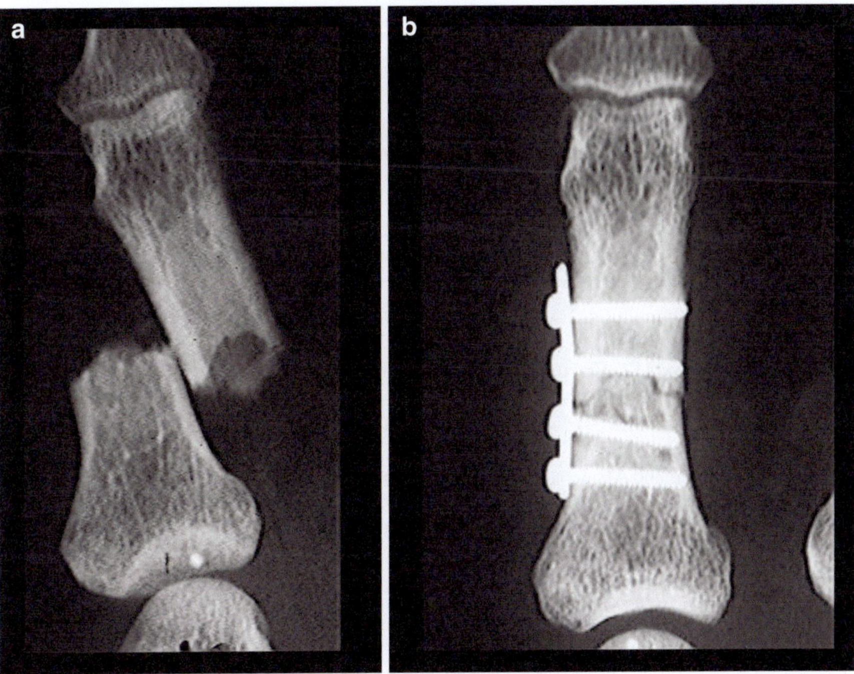

Fig. 16.5 (**a** and **b**) Lateral plate fixation of a displaced transverse proximal phalanx fracture

Table 16.4 Plate fixation

Indications
    Comminuted fractures
    Fractures with bone loss
Advantages
    Stable fixation
    Maintains or restores length and alignment
Disadvantages
    Technically more difficult
    Little room for error
    Bulk of implant

Table 16.5 Indications for external fixation

Indications
    Highly comminuted fractures
    Fractures with bone loss
    Infected fractures
Advantages
    Avoids operative manipulation of fracture fragments
    Maintains length and alignment with traction without crossing joints
    Ease of access to soft tissue injury
    May be placed percutaneously
Disadvantages
    Complex frame applications
    Pins can injure overlying tendons
    Pin infection
    May delay healing

Complications

Diaphyseal fractures of the hand phalanges range widely from simple, nondisplaced to those with extensive soft tissue and complex fracture patterns. Delayed or non-healing, deformity, articular stiffness, infection, loss of overall motion and strength are among the well recognized complications and care must always be taken to minimize these from occurring.

References

1. Jupiter JB, Belsky MR. Fractures and dislocations of the hand. In: Browner BD, Jupiter JB, Levine A, et al., editors. Skeletal trauma. Philadelphia: WB Saunders; 1992. p. 925–1024.
2. Strickland JW, Steichen JB, Kleinman WB, et al. Phalangeal fractures: factors influencing digital performance. Orthop Rev. 1982;11:39–50.
3. Duncan RW, Freeland AE, Jabaley ME, et al. Open hand fractures: an analysis of active motion and complications. J Hand Surg Am. 1993;18:387–94.
4. Huffaker WH, Wray RC Jr, Weeks PM. Factors influencing final range of motion in the fingers after fractures of the hand. Plast Reconst Surg. 1979;63:82–7.
5. Ip WY, Ng KH, Chow SP. A prospective study of 924 digital fractures of the hand. Injury. 1996;27:279–85.

6. Pun WK, Chow SP, So YC, et al. A prospective study on 284 digital fractures of the hand. J Hand Surg Am. 1989;14:474–81.
7. Stern PJ. Management of fractures of the hand over the last 25 years. J Hand Surg Am. 2000;25:817–23.
8. Reyes FA, Latta LL. Conservative management of difficult hand fractures. Clin Orthop Res Res. 1987;214:23–30.
9. Belsky MR, Eaton RG, Lane LB. Closed reduction and internal fixation of proximal phalangeal fractures. J Hand Surg Am. 1984;9:725–9.
10. Petilivan O, Kiral A, Solakoglu C, et al. Tension band wiring of unstable fractures of the proximal and middle phalanges of the hand. J Hand Surg Br. 2004;29:130–4.
11. Lister G. Intraosseous wiring of the digital skeleton. J Hand Surg Am. 1978;3:427–35.
12. Swanson TV, Szablo RM, Anderson DD. Open hand fractures: prognosis and classification. J Hand Surg Am. 1991;16:101–7.
13. Ouellette EA, Dennis JJ, Latta LL, et al. The role of soft tissues in plate fixation of proximal phalanx fractures. Clin Orthop Relat Res. 2004;418:213–8.
14. Nunley JA, Kleon P. Biomechanical analysis and functional testing of plate fixation devices for proximal phalangeal fractures. J Hand Surg Am. 1991;32:270–5.
15. Page SM, Stern PJ. Complications and range of motion following plate fixation of metacarpal and phalangeal fractures. J Hand Surg Am. 1998;23:827–32.
16. Ashmead D IV, Rothkopf DM, Walton RL, et al. Treatment of hand injuries by external fixation. J Hand Surg Am. 1992;17:956–64.

Adult Phalangeal Condyle Fractures

17

Anna Luan and Jeffrey Yao

Anatomy and Pathophysiology

Phalangeal condyle fractures, or phalangeal head fractures, can be challenging injuries to treat. The phalangeal head consists of two condyles that fit closely in a tongue-in-groove fashion with the base of the more distal phalanx to form the interphalangeal joint. Because phalangeal condyle fractures involve the interphalangeal joint articular surface, appropriate treatment is critical to reestablishing range of motion and the ultimate function of the joint. While these joints are not high load-bearing joints, outcomes are dependent on stability and alignment [1]. The interphalangeal joint is stabilized by multiple important soft tissue structures. The proper and accessory collateral ligaments along the radial and ulnar aspects of the joint prevent lateral deviation in the coronal plane. The volar plate at the palmar surface of the joint limits hyperextension. Secondary stabilizers include the central slip, lateral bands, and flexor tendons [2].

Phalangeal condyle fractures are common injuries among athletes and young adults. They may occur from axial loading of the digit or a lateral force resulting in avulsion through the collateral ligament [3]. These fractures are commonly sustained as sports injuries, such as from contact sports or from the force of a ball between two outstretched and flexed digits [4, 5], or from fighting and assault. The mechanism of injury may contribute to the pattern of fracture observed. Axial loading or a lateral force can cause a tilting force at the joint, leading to a shearing stress at the condyle, which is less likely to lead to comminution [3]. However, high energy axial loading directed centrally can cause comminuted bicondylar "pilon"-type fractures, with compression of the subchondral bone and buckling of the articular surface [3]. While there does not appear to be any overall differential incidence

A. Luan · J. Yao (✉)
Department of Orthopaedic Surgery, Robert A. Chase Hand and Upper Limb Center, Stanford University Medical Center, Palo Alto, CA, USA
e-mail: aluan@stanford.edu; jyao@stanford.edu

J. M. Abzug et al. (eds.), *Pediatric and Adult Hand Fractures*,
https://doi.org/10.1007/978-3-031-32072-9_17

between radial or ulnar condylar involvement [5], the fractured condyle tends to be more frequently toward the midline of the hand when there is a distraction mechanism causing a tension load [4].

Principles of Management

Preoperative evaluation should include a focused examination and radiographs. The digit should be evaluated for angulation or malrotation. Unicondylar fractures can be easily missed or misdiagnosed as a sprain, as the patient may maintain good flexion and extension of the digit [1]. Radiographs should be obtained in the standard anteroposterior and lateral views, as well as the oblique view of the finger in question [1]. Articular step-offs and lateral displacement can often be visualized on the anteroposterior radiograph, while articular incongruity and palmar displacement can be diagnosed on a lateral view. The oblique view should be included to fully assess fracture geometry and orientation. Misdiagnosis can result in subsequent displacement, malunion, and dissatisfaction.

Condylar fractures follow a classification system introduced by London et al. [6] (Fig. 17.1). Type I condylar fractures are stable without displacement, type II fractures are unicondylar and unstable, and type III fractures are bicondylar and/or comminuted.

Type I condylar fractures may be treated nonoperatively. However, many fractures are unstable even when nondisplaced at presentation, and therefore, patients managed nonoperatively must be followed extremely closely with weekly radiographs to monitor for subsequent displacement. Unfortunately, nonoperative treatment has less success in adults compared to children, potentially due to thinner periosteum and therefore less stabilization by the surrounding soft tissues [3]. If there is any question of instability or displacement, operative intervention should be pursued.

Type II condylar fractures are inherently unstable, often due to shearing forces. These fractures require operative treatment with reduction and fixation. Weiss and Hastings further classified type II unicondylar fractures of the proximal phalanx (Fig. 17.2), describing unicondylar fractures by their fracture pattern: oblique volar

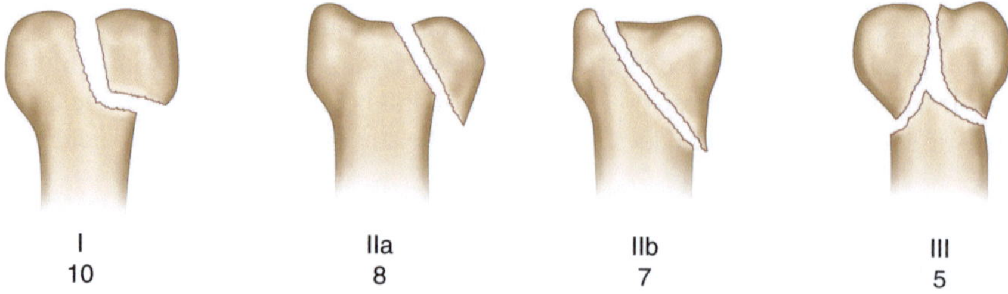

Fig. 17.1 Types of phalangeal condyle fractures. (From London PS. Sprains and Fractures Involving the Interphalangeal Joints. Hand. 1971 Apr;3(2):155–8)

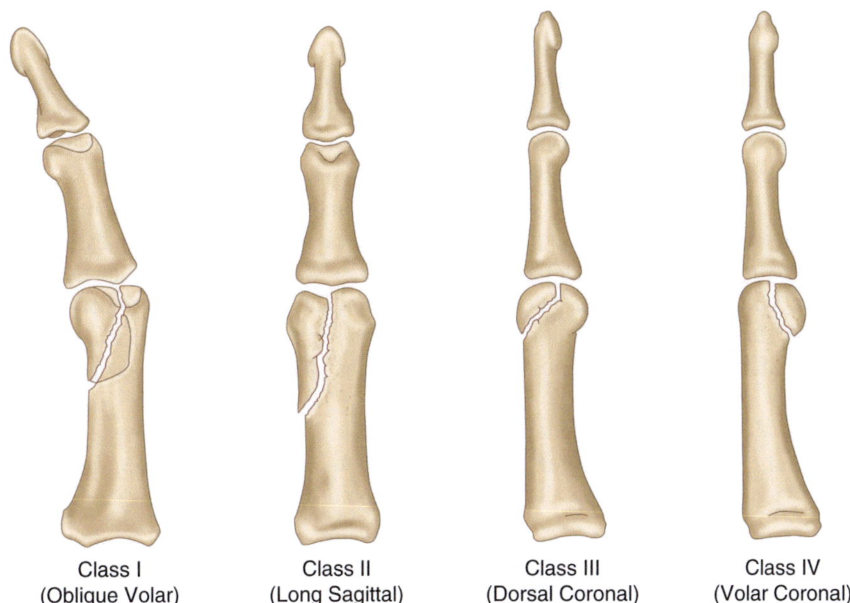

Fig. 17.2 Patterns of unicondylar phalangeal head fractures. (From Weiss A-PC, Hastings H. Distal unicondylar fractures of the proximal phalanx. The Journal of Hand Surgery. 1993 Jul;18(4):594–9)

(class I), long sagittal (class II), dorsal coronal (class III), or volar coronal (class IV) [4]. Class I unicondylar fractures extend from the proximal metaphyseal flare of the phalanx to the intracondylar depression at the articular surface, with the distal fracture fragment lying volar to the phalangeal shaft. Class II fractures lie in a sagittal plane, while class I fractures are neither in a sagittal nor coronal plane. Class III fractures involve a small distal fragment that lies dorsal, and class IV fractures involve a small distal fragment that lies volar.

Finally, type III condylar fractures are bicondylar and/or comminuted and almost universally require operative treatment. These fractures typically require an open approach to reduce the fracture and restore the articular surface. In bicondylar fractures with a compressed and buckled articular surface, reduction can be challenging to achieve. It may not be possible to fully reestablish the articular surface in severely comminuted fractures.

Appropriate management of a phalangeal condylar fracture requires accurate assessment of the stability of a fracture. Condylar fractures are often inherently unstable, even when initially nondisplaced [3]. The presence of comminution and small articular fragments can often make it difficult to achieve and maintain reduction. Malunion can result in pain, deformity, loss of motion, and articular incongruity [3, 7]. While articular remodeling is commonly observed, leading to low rates of symptomatic osteoarthritis [1], deformity and lateral deviation are still likely to occur, and therefore reestablishment of alignment is still necessary. Greater displacement is often an indicator of increased instability due to greater disruption of the periosteum and soft tissues.

Chronicity of a condylar fracture may also determine approach to management. Condylar fractures may be treated on a semi-elective basis, as there has been no difference demonstrated in outcomes with fixation at 2 weeks when compared to more urgent fixation [3]. However, in some fractures, treatment within 5–7 days following injury may enable closed reduction and percutaneous fixation. While reduction and fixation of condylar fractures can be performed even up to 8 weeks after the initial injury [3], the reduction may be less stable over time as the interdigitations of the fractured ends become less pronounced. Overall, fixation particularly at more than 5 weeks post-injury has been shown to result in more residual stiffness of the affected joint [3], and fixation should be attempted within a few weeks of injury.

Overall, the goals of treatment are to maximize function and minimize pain and deformity. Therefore, management should strive to restore articular congruency and to provide stable fixation to allow for early range of motion.

Nonoperative Management

Nonoperative management is reserved for type I condylar fractures, which are stable and nondisplaced. Patients must be monitored closely during nonoperative treatment, as even initially nondisplaced fractures may frequently be unstable and become displaced over time. The digit should be immobilized with a digital splint in extension, and then protected mobilization begun after 4 weeks [3, 7]. After beginning mobilization, buddy strapping or buddy taping should be continued for another 3 weeks [3]. One should closely monitor with weekly radiographs for the first 3 weeks to check for displacement and maintain a low threshold for operative intervention [7]. Many initially nondisplaced fractures will become displaced over this timeframe and require operative fixation.

Operative Management

Indications for operative management of phalangeal condyle fractures are broad and include any condylar fracture that is unstable and/or displaced.

Some fractures may be amenable to closed reduction and percutaneous fixation, typically within the first week following the injury. Longitudinal traction is applied to facilitate reduction, and a finger trap may be used to assist in providing traction. Reduction may be held by one or two bone reduction clamps to help apply compression. A Kirschner wire (K-wire) may be placed into the fracture fragment and used as a joystick to manipulate fracture fragments to achieve reduction. A small incision at the fracture may be utilized to help facilitate reduction using a dental pick [8]. Once reduction is confirmed with fluoroscopy, two or three 0.028-in. or 0.035-in. K-wires can then be used to percutaneously fix the fracture. Percutaneous fixation may also be achieved with small cannulated screws [9]. An additional derotational K-wire may be placed in addition to the percutaneous screw. In oblique fractures, K-wires or lag screws should be placed perpendicular to the fracture line. Due to lack of direct visualization, adequate reduction after fixation must be carefully confirmed with radiographs.

Open reduction and fixation is recommended for type III condylar fractures and other displaced fractures that cannot be adequately reduced through a closed approach. Several approaches to the condyle have been previously described [10].

Dorsal approaches address the extensor mechanism using varying techniques. A longitudinal incision is made either in the dorsal midline, a curvilinear or lazy S fashion, or radially or ulnarly on the side of the fracture [10]. Dorsal veins that are encountered should be preserved if possible. The incision may be carried down to enter the joint through the interval between the central slip and the lateral band of the extensor apparatus [1], or the extensor tendon may be split longitudinally [11]. Alternatively, the central slip may be divided to provide greater exposure of the joint, although the tendon must then be repaired afterward. The Chamay approach involves the division of the central tendon at the junction of the proximal and middle third of the proximal phalanx by creating a distally based triangular tendon flap, reflecting the tendon distally with the distal central slip insertion left intact. The cut central slip is then repaired at the conclusion of the fixation. Care should be taken to restore the original tension of the central tendon. The central slip may be detached at its insertion instead but must then be reattached at the base of the middle phalanx using sutures or suture anchors to prevent the development of an extensor lag and/or boutonniere deformity.

The lateral approach involves a mid-axial incision and requires a bilateral approach for bicondylar fractures [3]. In the lateral approach, an incision is made in the vertical retinacular fibers and the collateral ligament exposed and preserved. The neurovascular bundle is protected volarly. Careful preservation of the collateral ligament attachments helps to decrease the risk of avascular necrosis by maintaining the vascular supply to the condyles [8]. If the proper collateral ligament is released for increased exposure of the joint, it must be repaired after fixation is completed. The periosteum is then incised at the lateral border of the volar plate, and the structures are elevated in a single layer along with the extensor mechanism. Advocates of the lateral approach argue that this minimizes adhesions between the extensors and periosteum and therefore decreases subsequent stiffness of the digit. The condyle can then be visualized and flipped into the wound [3]. Following fixation, the vertical retinacular fibers and periosteum are repaired with absorbable suture.

Finally, in the volar approach, a Bruner, zigzag, or Bruner-midlateral hybrid incision is made at the skin, with the base of the flap designed on the more involved side of the joint [10]. The flexor tendon sheath and neurovascular bundles are visualized, and the flexor tendon sheath is incised between the A2 and A4 pulleys [12]. The flexor tendons are retracted either to one side or the two slips of the flexor digitorum superficialis split and retracted to either side, and one or both of the accessory collateral ligaments are incised sharply. Next, the volar plate is detached either distally or proximally and the articular surface visualized. Alternatively, two incisions may be made in the flexor tendon sheath and accessory collateral ligaments on either side of the volar plate, and the flexor sheath and volar plate mobilized en bloc [13]. The volar plate must be repaired in this approach, and the collateral ligaments and flexor tendon sheath may also be repaired.

After exposure of the fracture site, the fracture surfaces are cleaned of hematoma, and the fracture reduced under direct visualization. The condylar fragment should be exposed, but care taken to preserve the attachment of the collateral ligament(s). Detachment may result in instability and also devascularization of the joint [1]. Visual confirmation of adequate reduction and restoration of the articular surface should be obtained. Reduction may be assisted with the use of K-wires, a dental pick, or bone reducing clamps. A 0.028-in. K-wire may be used to provide provisional fixation. In type III bicondylar fractures, it is suggested that the condyles are first fixed to each other with either a K-wire or screw, followed by fixation of the condylar head construct to the remainder of the phalanx.

Fixation may be achieved with a number of different techniques, including K-wire fixation, percutaneous screw fixation, a low-profile plate, or external fixation. Biomechanical stability has been shown to be relatively equivalent among fixation methods in a proximal phalanx unicondylar fracture model [14]. At least two 0.028-in. or 0.035-in. K-wires are driven from the fragment into the intact phalangeal shaft, or in the opposite direction from the intact phalanx to the fragment, depending on fracture geometry (Fig. 17.3). K-wire placement should avoid the collateral ligaments, which if impinged could decrease ligament excursion [4]. Percutaneous K-wire fixation provides the advantage of avoiding disruption of the blood supply. However, multiple K-wires are typically necessary to prevent rotation and loosening [4]. A single K-wire is inadequate to provide fixation and can lead to loss of reduction [4, 15, 16]. Furthermore, care must be taken as repeated attempts at placement may contribute to greater comminution of the fragment [8]. Finally, as K-wires do not compress across the fracture site and also splint the overlying soft

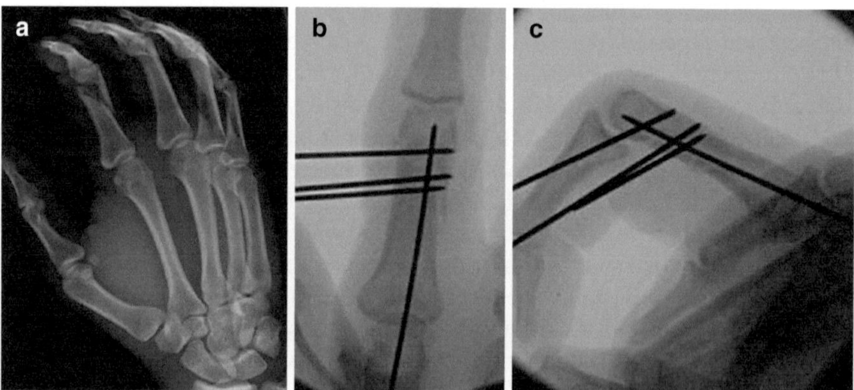

Fig. 17.3 Percutaneous fixation with K-wires of a condylar fracture of the proximal phalanx, with an additional intramedullary K-wire for longitudinal stability. (**a**) Oblique proximal phalangeal fracture of the index finger. (**b**) AP radiograph following K-wire fixation of the index proximal phalanx fracture. (**c**) Lateral radiograph following K-wire fixation of the index proximal phalanx fracture. (From Cotterell IH, Richard MJ. Metacarpal and Phalangeal Fractures in Athletes. Clinics in Sports Medicine. 2015 Jan;34(1):69–98)

tissues, K-wire fixation may prohibit early mobilization. Despite these limitations, some suggest that fixation with multiple K-wires may provide the best final range of motion among techniques [1].

Percutaneous screw fixation may be achieved with either headless compression screws [9], bicortical screws [17], or lag screws [3, 18]. The collateral ligament may need to be elevated slightly to provide enough exposure for screw placement. The condylar fragment is examined to determine appropriate screw diameter. The fracture fragment should be 2.5–3 times the external diameter of the screw to prevent further comminution of the fragment [1]. Common hardware options range from a 1.2 to 1.5 mm lag screw [1, 3, 15, 19] or a 1.5 mm headless compression screw. Proponents of small headless cannulated screws argue that they minimize irritation of the collateral ligament and adhesions associated with scarring [20, 21]. Shewring advocated for fixation with a single 1.2 or 1.4 mm self-tapping lag screw, which provides compression across the fracture and allows for early mobilization (Fig. 17.4) [3]. Other authors use a minimum of two screws to prevent loss of

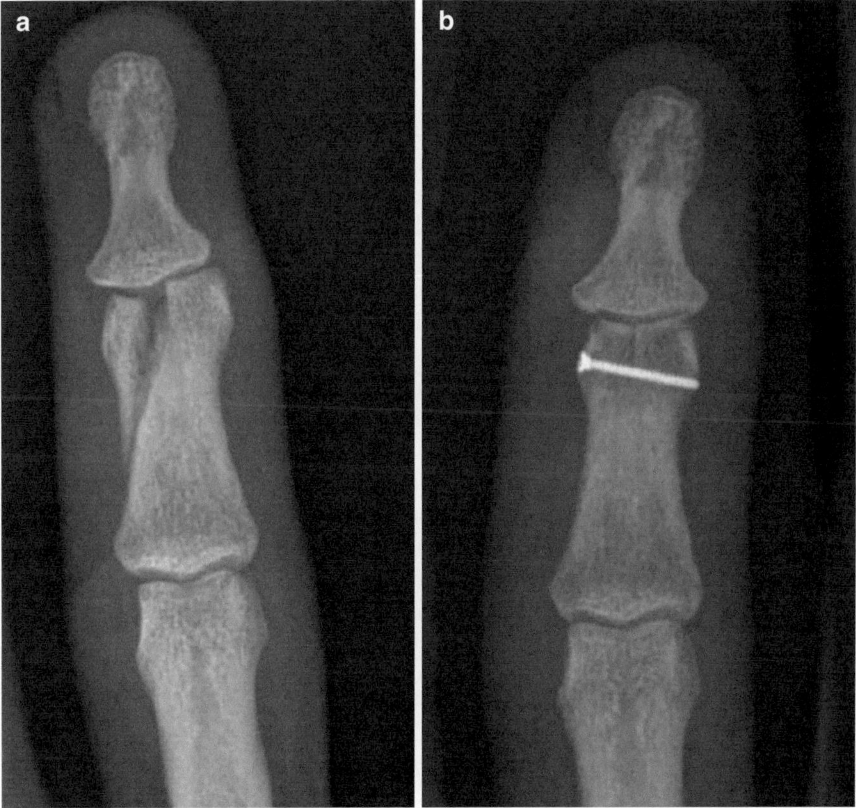

Fig. 17.4 Fixation of an unstable unicondylar phalangeal fracture with a single screw. (**a**) Intracondylar fracture of the middle phalanx. (**b**) Screw fixation of the intracondylar fracture of the middle phalanx. (From Shewring DJ, Miller AC, Ghandour A. Condylar fractures of the proximal and middle phalanges. J Hand Surg Eur Vol. 2015 Jan;40(1):51–8)

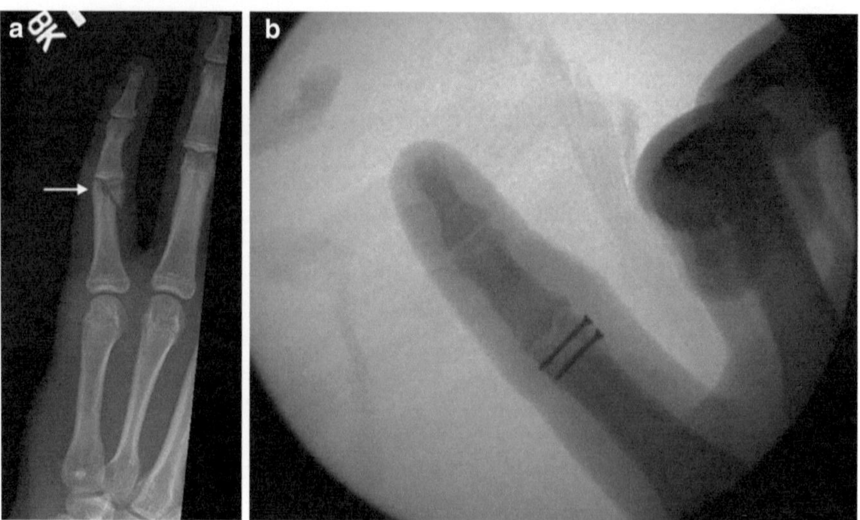

Fig. 17.5 A unicondylar proximal phalangeal fracture (**a**) with open reduction and internal fixation with two 1.2 mm screws (**b**). (From Ganesh Kumar N, Chung KC. An Evidence-Based Guide for Managing Phalangeal Fractures. Plastic & Reconstructive Surgery. 2021 May;147(5):846e–61e)

reduction from rotation or loosening [1]. Use of either a derotational K-wire or a second screw may provide additional rotational stability (Fig. 17.5), particularly if the interdigitations of the fracture surface have become less pronounced due to delayed presentation after injury. Screws should be placed just dorsal and proximal to the origin of the collateral ligament to preserve its insertion and avoid transfixing the ligament. If the collateral ligament was elevated for screw placement, it is then replaced over the screw. Countersinking is important to embed the head of the screw and minimize interference with the collateral ligament.

A low-profile 1.5 or 2 mm minicondylar blade plate may be used if the fracture extends into the metaphysis or diaphysis, or for bicondylar or comminuted fractures (Fig. 17.6) [8, 22, 23]. The minicondylar plate provides stable fixation of periarticular fragments and allows for early active range of motion. The 1.5 mm plate is typically utilized, although the 2 mm plate may also be suitable for the proximal phalanx. The plate can be placed laterally or dorsally, with lateral placement recommended due to decreased risk of potential friction on the extensor tendon and subsequent impingement of gliding. Locking screws can be helpful to enhance stability when bony deficiency is present or when comorbidities pose risk of poor healing [24]. Challenges of using the minicondylar plate for phalangeal condyle fractures include the small fragments, the implant's bulky size relative to the phalanx and lack of forgiveness of plate application, limited surrounding soft tissue to accommodate the implant, need for more extensive dissection, and risk of adhesions. Small fragments may be further comminuted or split with screw placement. Extensive soft tissue damage may preclude the use of a plate due to lack of soft tissue coverage.

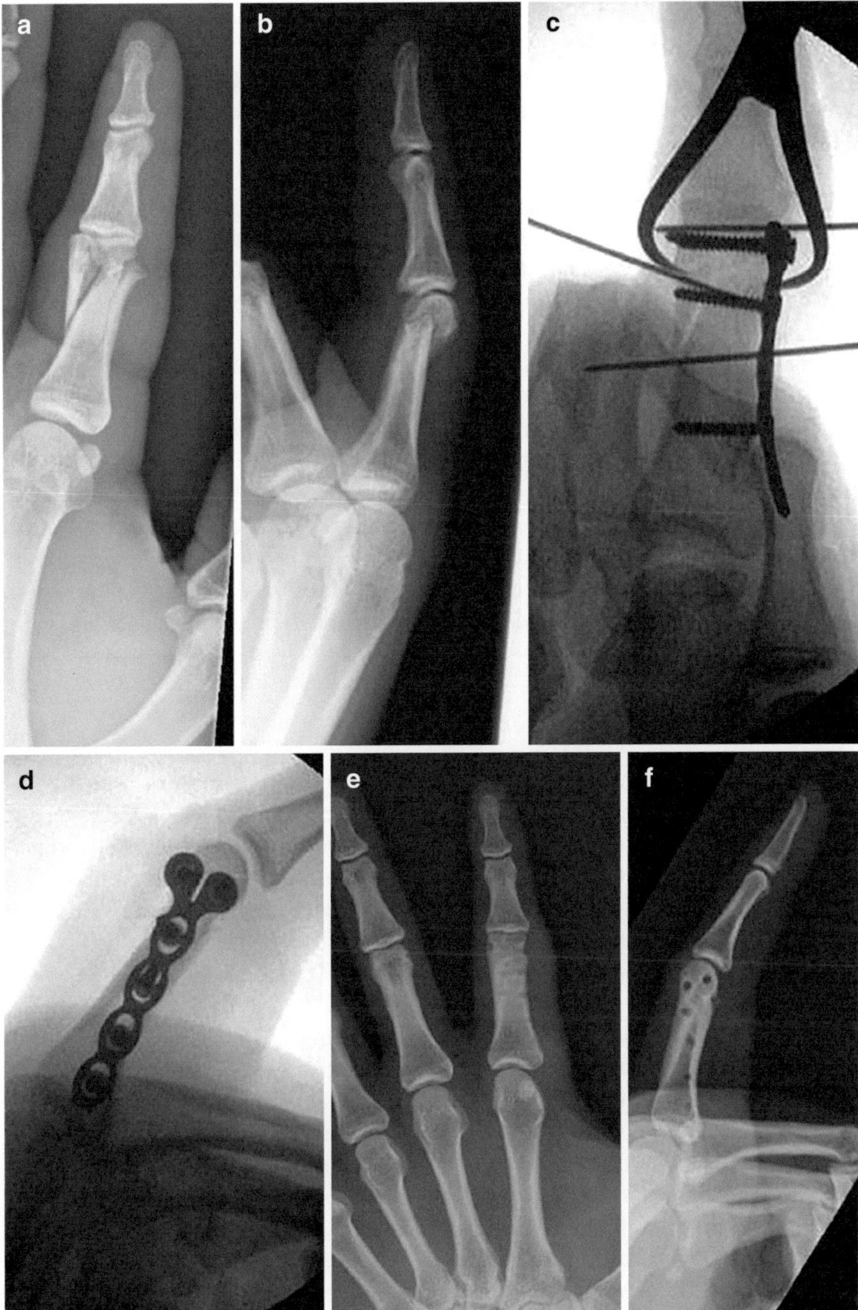

Fig. 17.6 Open reduction and fixation of a comminuted condylar fracture of the proximal phalanx (**a, b**) utilizing a fixed-angle locking plate (**c, d**). The patient subsequently underwent plate removal and tenolysis 8 months later (**e, f**). (From Cotterell IH, Richard MJ. Metacarpal and Phalangeal Fractures in Athletes. Clinics in Sports Medicine. 2015 Jan;34(1):69–98)

Other techniques of fixation have also been described. Sammut and Evans have reported on the use of a bone tie for fixation of condylar fractures [25]. In this technique, a bone tie provides compression between fragments. However, the bulkiness of the device may cause impingement on the collateral ligament and can also require significant stripping of the soft tissues [3]. Interosseous wiring can also provide compression and fixation [26], but is technically difficult due to the passing of wires through multiple drill holes, often requiring extensive soft tissue dissection.

Finally, dynamic external fixation can be applied for 4 weeks if there is significant comminution present and the fragments are too small for fixation [27–29]. Techniques utilize the principles of distraction and ligamentotaxis to reduce the fragments. Early motion prevents stiffness and adhesions, reduces swelling, and promotes articular remodeling [29, 30]. In severely comminuted fractures, the articular surface may not be able to be fully restored. There will be some articular remodeling with dynamic external fixation, but patients should be cautioned that residual stiffness will occur. Regardless, primary arthrodesis should be avoided if possible.

Restoration of congruity of the articular surfaces should be confirmed on a lateral view, which should demonstrate superimposition of the condyles. The periosteum and any other divided structures are repaired with absorbable suture. A splint should be applied with the interphalangeal joint in extension to prevent extensor lag.

Post-operative Care

Patients are seen within the first post-operative week. Radiographs in the anteroposterior, lateral, and oblique views are taken to confirm maintenance of reduction and fixation. If stable fixation is confirmed, early mobilization is recommended to prevent stiffness. If percutaneous K-wire fixation was used, K-wires are removed at 3–4 weeks post-operatively. Screws and plates are not routinely removed unless there is a need for capsulotomy or if there are significant adhesions.

Patients are referred to hand therapy to begin supervised mobilization [31]. With stable fixation, active range of motion is initiated at 5–7 days post-operatively. Efforts should be made to reduce pain and swelling, which if unaddressed will encourage the patient to bring the joint into a flexed position. Mobilization is limited only by patient discomfort and can minimize residual stiffness. The joint should be splinted in full extension initially post-operatively as well as rested in extension in between exercises, as the most common complication is extensor lag with loss of full extension. Short-arc active range of motion is conducted hourly. Continued passive motion with rigid internal fixation can prevent adhesions and stiffness, reduce edema, and promote articular remodeling [30]. Range of motion should take place within 3 weeks. If the central slip was incised and repaired, full joint flexion should be avoided for 3 weeks to allow for the sutured tendon to heal [31].

Complications

The most common complication is stiffness, which typically presents as extensor lag or a flexion joint contracture. Extensor lag ranging between 5° and 35° is common regardless of dorsal, lateral, or volar approach [3, 10]. Interestingly, approaches that avoid the central slip may frequently still develop extensor lag, potentially due to adhesions or the role of the lateral bands in achieving full extension. Soft tissue adhesions may occur in the planes of dissection around the extensor apparatus, particularly with rigid fixation. Treatment may include tenolysis, hardware removal, and/or capsulotomies. Extensor lag can often be at least partially corrected with dynamic extension splinting [1]. Serial casting may be necessary for longstanding or severe flexion contractures greater than 45° [2]. Attempts should be made to prevent stiffness by establishing stable fixation to limit immobilization and by reducing pain and edema to improve patient participation in therapy [2].

Improper bony healing may result in delayed union, nonunion, or malunion. Delayed union and nonunion may be treated with cancellous bone grafting. Malunion can result in pain, deformity, loss of motion, and articular incongruity (Fig. 17.7) [3, 7]. If articular incongruity is not restored, posttraumatic arthritis may

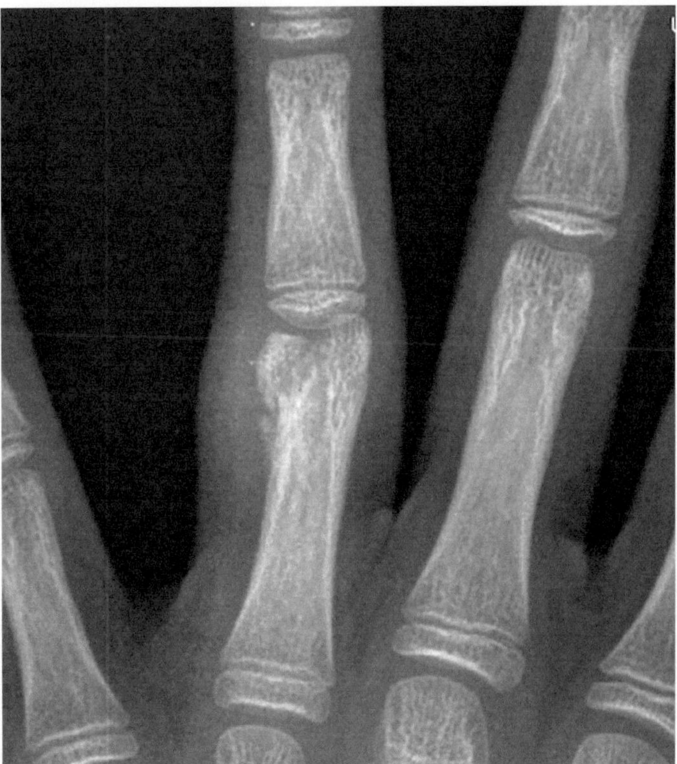

Fig. 17.7 Malunion of a phalangeal condyle fracture resulting in articular incongruity and angular deformity. (From Shewring DJ, Miller AC, Ghandour A. Condylar fractures of the proximal and middle phalanges. J Hand Surg Eur Vol. 2015 Jan;40(1):51–8)

occur. Malunion may require a corrective intercondylar osteotomy to treat, either through the healed fracture site or a longitudinal condylar advancement osteotomy [32]. Avascular necrosis of condylar fracture fragments is less common, but risk can be minimized by careful limited dissection and preservation of the collateral ligament attachments. Loss of fixation may ultimately require arthrodesis of the joint.

Other hardware complications include pin migration and breakage and screw loosening. Patients may have discomfort due to presence of hardware requiring subsequent hardware removal. Prominent screw heads or plates may cause irritation and friction on surrounding structures, with a risk of tendon rupture if placed beneath the extensor tendon. Wound healing complications may lead to hardware exposure, particularly in cases of significant soft tissue injury. Overall complications have been shown to increase with greater soft tissue injury and in open fractures [23, 33]. Infection can occur in the setting of hardware and may ultimately require hardware removal and loss of fixation. Acutely, presence of percutaneous wires may provide a site for pin tract infections. If left untreated, chronic infections may lead to osteomyelitis.

References

1. Wolfe SW, Pederson WC, Kozin SH, Cohen MS. Green's operative hand surgery, vol. 1. 7th ed. Philadelphia, PA: Elsevier; 2017. 978 p.
2. Kamnerdnakta S, Huetteman HE, Chung KC. Complications of proximal interphalangeal joint injuries: prevention and treatment. Hand Clin. 2018;34(2):267–88.
3. Shewring DJ, Miller AC, Ghandour A. Condylar fractures of the proximal and middle phalanges. J Hand Surg Eur Vol. 2015;40(1):51–8.
4. Weiss A-PC, Hastings H. Distal unicondylar fractures of the proximal phalanx. J Hand Surg Am. 1993;18(4):594–9.
5. McCue FC, Honner R, Johnson MC, Gieck JH. Athletic injuries of the proximal interphalangeal joint requiring surgical treatment. J Bone Joint Surg Am. 1970;52(5):937–56.
6. London PS. Sprains and fractures involving the interphalangeal joints. Hand. 1971;3(2):155–8.
7. Carpenter S, Rohde RS. Treatment of phalangeal fractures. Hand Clin. 2013;29(4):519–34.
8. Cotterell IH, Richard MJ. Metacarpal and phalangeal fractures in athletes. Clin Sports Med. 2015;34(1):69–98.
9. Gaston RG, Chadderdon C. Phalangeal fractures. Hand Clin. 2012;28(3):395–401.
10. Cheah AE-J, Yao J. Surgical approaches to the proximal interphalangeal joint. J Hand Surg Am. 2016;41(2):294–305.
11. Swanson AB, Maupin BK, Gajjar NV, Swanson GD. Flexible implant arthroplasty in the proximal interphalangeal joint of the hand. J Hand Surg Am. 1985 Nov;10(6 Pt 1):796–805.
12. Lin HH, Wyrick JD, Stern PJ. Proximal interphalangeal joint silicone replacement arthroplasty: clinical results using an anterior approach. J Hand Surg Am. 1995;20(1):123–32.
13. Herren DB, Simmen BR. Palmar approach in flexible implant arthroplasty of the proximal interphalangeal joint. Clin Orthop Relat Res. 2000;(371):131–5.
14. Sirota MA, Parks BG, Higgins JP, Means KR. Stability of fixation of proximal phalanx unicondylar fractures of the hand: a biomechanical cadaver study. J Hand Surg Am. 2013;38(1):77–81.
15. Hastings H, Carroll C. Treatment of closed articular fractures of the metacarpophalangeal and proximal interphalangeal joints. Hand Clin. 1988;4(3):503–27.
16. James JIP. Fractures of the proximal and middle phalanges of the fingers. Acta Orthop Scand. 1962;32(1–4):401–12.

17. Roth JJ, Auerbach DM. Fixation of hand fractures with bicortical screws. J Hand Surg Am. 2005;30(1):151–3.
18. Ford D, Elhadidi S, Lunn P, Burke F. Fractures of the phalanges: results of internal fixation using 1.5mm and 2mm A. O. screws. J Hand Surg Br. 1987;12(1):28–33.
19. Ganesh Kumar N, Chung KC. An evidence-based guide for managing phalangeal fractures. Plast Reconstr Surg. 2021;147(5):846e–1.
20. Geissler WB. Operative fixation of metacarpal and phalangeal fractures in athletes. Hand Clin. 2009;25(3):409–21.
21. Geissler WB. Cannulated percutaneous fixation of intra-articular hand fractures. Hand Clin. 2006;22(3):297–305.
22. Büchler U, Fischer T. Use of a minicondylar plate for metacarpal and phalangeal periarticular injuries. Clin Orthop Relat Res. 1987;(214):53–58.
23. Ouellette EA, Freeland AE. Use of the minicondylar plate in metacarpal and phalangeal fractures. Clin Orthop Relat Res. 1996;(327):38–46.
24. Lögters TT, Lee HH, Gehrmann S, Windolf J, Kaufmann RA. Proximal phalanx fracture management. Hand (N Y). 2018;13(4):376–83.
25. Sammut D, Evans D. The bone tie: a new device for interfragmentary fixation. J Hand Surg. 1999;24(1):64–9.
26. Rayhack JM, Bottke CA. Intraosseous compression wiring of displaced articular condylar fractures. J Hand Surg Am. 1990;15(2):370–3.
27. Fahmy NRM, Harvey RA. The "S" Quattro in the management of fractures in the hand. J Hand Surg. 1992;17(3):321–31.
28. Khan W, Fahmy N. The S-Quattro in the management of acute intraarticular phalangeal fractures of the hand. J Hand Surg. 2006;31(1):79–92.
29. Schenck RR. Dynamic traction and early passive movement for fractures of the proximal interphalangeal joint. J Hand Surg Am. 1986;11(6):850–8.
30. Salter RB. The physiologic basis of continuous passive motion for articular cartilage healing and regeneration. Hand Clin. 1994;10(2):211–9.
31. Hardy MA. Principles of metacarpal and phalangeal fracture management: a review of rehabilitation concepts. J Orthop Sports Phys Ther. 2004;34(12):781–99.
32. Teoh LC, Yong FC, Chong KC. Condylar advancement osteotomy for correcting condylar malunion of the finger. J Hand Surg Br. 2002;27(1):31–5.
33. Chow SP, Pun WK, So YC, Luk KDK, Chiu KY, Ng KH, et al. A prospective study of 245 open digital fractures of the hand. J Hand Surg. 1991;16(2):137–40.

Adult Bony Mallet Fractures

18

Andrew J. Miller and Philip M. Petrucelli

Introduction

Mallet finger is a term used to characterize an injury to the distal phalangeal (DIP) joint of the finger that results in a discontinuity to the terminal extensor tendon and its bony insertion. This results in an extensor lag deformity at the DIP joint. Secondarily, disruption of the extensor mechanism of the DIP joint may lead to an imbalance between the intrinsic and extrinsic extension mechanism that gradually results in hyperextension at the proximal interphalangeal (PIP) joint and the characteristic swan neck deformity. Mallet finger has also been described as a "drop" finger or "baseball" finger. Mallet finger can be purely ligamentous, bony, or a combination of the two. The focus of this chapter will be on the bony mallet injury of an adult [1, 2].

Presentation

Mallet injuries are most commonly seen in young, adult males. Peak incidence among females is around middle age, where incidence among males and females begins to steadily decline as they reach older age [3]. The long, ring, and small fingers of the dominant hand are most commonly affected [4]. The injuries are typically sustained while participating in sports or work-related activity. Lower energy mechanisms are less common but may occur where the digit is caught in an article of clothing [5]. The most common mechanism is sudden and forceful flexion of an extending DIP joint. Less commonly, it can be caused by hyperextension of the DIP

A. J. Miller (✉)
Philadelphia Hand to Shoulder Center, Thomas Jefferson University, Philadelphia, PA, USA

P. M. Petrucelli
Thomas Jefferson University, Philadelphia, PA, USA

joint, resulting in a large fracture at the base of the distal phalanx [1]. Sharp lacerations across zone 1 or zone 2 of the extensor tendon may also result in a mallet deformity as well.

Classification

The two most commonly used classification systems are Wehbe and Schneider as well as the Doyle classifications. Wehbe and Schneider, specifically designed for bony mallet injuries, is divided into three types based on the degree of DIP joint subluxation or the presence of epiphyseal or physeal injuries. Each type is then divided into three subtypes based on the degree of articular surface involvement [6] (Fig. 18.1).

The Doyle classification accounts for both soft tissue and bony mallet injuries. Type I is a closed injury with or without a small, dorsal avulsion fracture. Type II is an open injury due to laceration. Type III is an open injury due to deep abrasion involving skin and tendon. Type IV is a fracture, subdivided into three types. Type A is a distal phalanx physeal injury. Type B is a fracture fragment involving 20–50% of the articular surface. Type C is a fracture fragment involving greater than 50% of the articular surface (Fig. 18.2) [1]. Patel et al. defined acute injuries as those presenting within 4 weeks from injury, and chronic injuries as those presenting greater than 4 weeks from injury [7].

Fig. 18.1 Wehbe and Schneider classification. (Adapted from Wehbe MA, Schneider LH. Mallet Fractures. The Journal of Bone and Joint Surgery. 1984;66(5): 658–669)

	Description
Type	
I	No DIP joint subluxation
II	DIP joint subluxation
III	Epiphyseal and physeal injuries
Subtype	
A	< 1/3 articular surface
B	1/3 to 2/3 articular surface
C	>2/3 articular surface

Type I	Closed injury, with or without small dorsal avulsion fracture
Type II	Open injury, laceration of tendon
Type III	Open injury with loss of skin, subcutancous cover, and tendon substance
Type IV	Mallet fracture
A	Transepiphyscal plate fracture in children
B	Hyperflexion injury with fracture of articular surface of 20% to 50%
C	Hyperextension injury with fracture of the articular surface>50% and with early or late volar subluxation of distal phalanx

Fig. 18.2 Doyle classification. (From Doyle JR: Extensor tendons: acute injuries. In Green D, editor: Green's operative hand surgery, ed 4, New York, 1999, Churchill Livingstone, pp 195–198)

Evaluation

The evaluation of a suspected mallet injury should begin with a thorough history and physical examination. The history should focus on the mechanism and timing from injury. The physical exam should focus on range of motion, specifically at the DIP joint. Generally, patients will have loss of active extension of the DIP joint, but maintenance of active flexion and passive extension at the DIP joint. Range of motion at the PIP joint and deformity (such as swan neck) should be examined. Radiographs of the affected digit should be obtained to assess for any fracture or joint incongruity, taking into consideration the size of the fracture fragment as well the amount of displacement (Fig. 18.3) [2]. The presence of arthritis should be noted as well. In cases of a mallet injury, CT or MRI is rarely beneficial.

Moradi et al. were able to identify factors associated with DIP joint subluxation based on the size of the articular fragment and amount of displacement. Subluxation was observed when the fragment size involved more than 39% of the articular surface. For every 1% increase in articular surface involvement, they found a 4% increase in risk of subluxation [8].

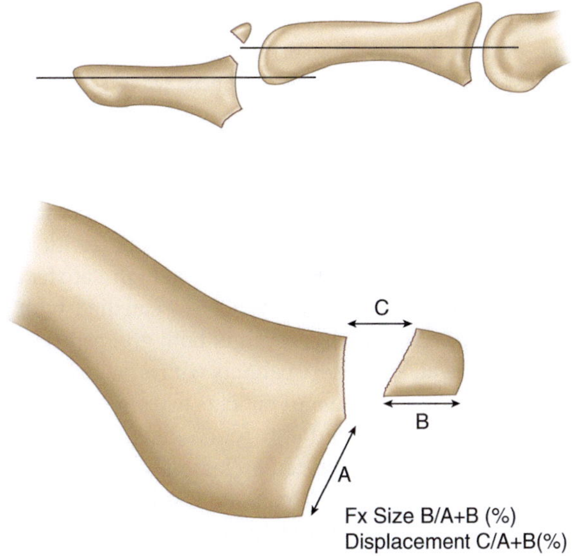

Fig. 18.3 Assessment of distal interphalangeal joint subluxation, fracture size, and fracture displacement. (Adapted from Wehbe MA, Schneider LH. Mallet Fractures. The Journal of Bone and Joint Surgery. 1984;66(5): 658–669)

Treatment

Nonoperative Treatment

The most common treatment method for acute, closed bony mallet injuries is non-operative management in the form of splinting. The goal of the use of a splint is to maintain the DIP joint in slight hyperextension without blanching the skin. The splint may extend proximally to provide a dorsal block at the PIP joint if a swan neck deformity is present. The splint should be worn at all times for the initial 8 weeks, even during skin hygiene. The patient can then be re-evaluated in the office and if upon removal of the splint, the DIP joint rests back in flexion, the splint should be worn at all times for an additional 6–8 weeks. If there is no residual deformity, the splint should be maintained at nighttime for an additional 2–4 weeks before discontinuing as part of a weaning process. Buddy tape can be used for an additional 6–8 weeks for use during athletic activities. Elastic therapeutic tape may also be placed longitudinally from the volar fingertip to the dorsal middle phalangeal region to provide an extension support. There are many variations of splints such as the Mexican hat splint, Kleinert modified, stack splint, aluminum foam, Abouna splint, and perforated thermoplastic splint [1].

In a study by Kalainov et al, 22 closed, bony mallet injuries involving more than one-third of the articular surface were treated with a thermoplastic DIP joint extension splint. Average delay to treatment was 21 days, and average length of treatment was 5.5 weeks. There were split into two treatment groups, where the first showed no evidence of DIP joint subluxation (9 cases), while the second group showed radiographic evidence of DIP joint palmar subluxation (13 cases). At final follow-up, there was no significant difference in outcomes between the two groups. All patients reported minimal difficulties with activities of daily living while wearing the splint. Patients reported relatively high satisfaction with finger function and treatment outcome. Patients were less satisfied with final finger appearance. The DIP joint extensor lag improved in both groups [9].

Okafor et al. studied 31 patients with a mallet injury treated with a thermoplastic splint. Thirty-five percent of patients had an intra-articular fracture. Average follow-up time was 5 years, and they found that 90% of patients were satisfied with their final result and 68% reported no loss of ability to perform precision tasks [10].

Trickett et al. also showed good results with nonoperative management of bony mallet injuries regardless of fragment size or articular subluxation. A total of 218 mallet fractures were treated using a custom-made thermoplastic splint. Average length of follow-up was 4 years. The joint was incongruent in 50 of the 218 cases, and the majority of fractures involved between 1/3 and 2/3 of the articular surface. There were no significant differences in range of motion, extensor lag, or patient evaluation measure associated with DIP joint subluxation or the articular fragment size. Superficial skin irritation and temporary swan neck deformity were the most common complications, which were treated with splint modification and all resolved [11].

Gaberman reported on 75 patients comparing early versus delayed splinting, which included 13 bony mallet injuries that involved less than 1/3 of the articular surface. In the delayed group, treatment was initiated on average 8 weeks after injury compared to 4 days in the early treatment group. The splint was worn continuously for 7 weeks. They found successful outcomes even in the delayed group with no significant difference between early versus delayed treatment in regard to extensor lag or treatment success [12].

When comparing different types of splints, in a blinded, prospective, randomized study, Pike et al. compared volar, dorsal, and custom thermoplastic splints. Eighty-seven patients were randomized to each group. All patients had Doyle Type I fractures. There was no significant difference between the groups in regard to extensor lag. However, there was a trend towards superiority in the custom thermoplastic group. There was only one major complication, which involved a full-thickness ulceration over the dorsum of the DIP joint that required antibiotics. This occurred with the dorsal thermoplastic splint [13].

In another prospective, randomized controlled trial, O'Brien compared the use of an aluminum splint, custom thermoplastic splint, and stack splint for mallet injuries. There were 64 subjects, of which 28 sustained a bony injury. There was no difference in residual extensor lag among the three splints. However, the custom thermoplastic splint was found to result in higher compliance rates and less likely to result in treatment failure [14].

Warren compared the use of the stack splint versus the Abouna splint (rubber coated wire splint) in a study of 116 randomized patients. There was bony involvement in 31.9% of cases. The outcomes were similar between the two groups. However, the Abouna splint was associated with more skin complications and lower patient satisfaction [15].

Operative Treatment

Operative intervention is generally recommended if the fracture involves more than 30% of the articular surface or if there is volar subluxation of the distal phalanx. There are many different surgical treatment options for bony mallet injuries, which have been described in the literature. These include the use of Kirschner (K) wires, screws, suture, or hook plate (Figs. 18.4, 18.5, and 18.6) [16–29]. Classically, percutaneous pinning is the mainstay of treatment. This can usually be accomplished by closed techniques where an extension blocking K-wire is placed in the middle phalanx to reduce the fracture fragment, followed by an additional K-wire across the DIP joint to hold the reduction in place. The use of screws, hook plates, tension bands, or pull-through sutures require an open technique.

Hofmeister reported on 24 bony mallet fractures that involved 40% of the articular surface treated with extension block pinning. The average time to fracture union was 35 days, average extension loss was 4°, and average DIP flexion was 77° at final follow-up. There were five minor complications, which included three superficial

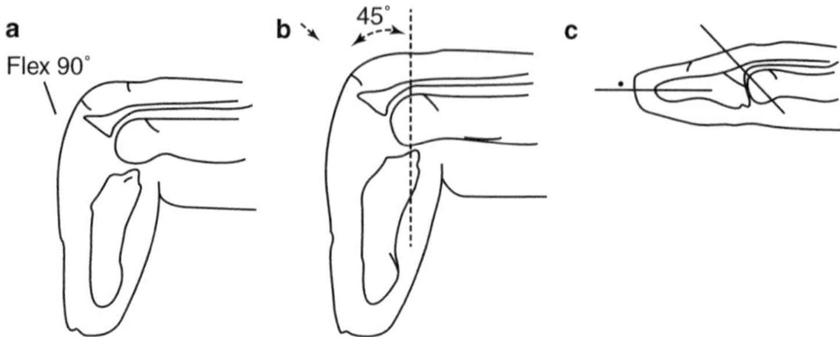

Fig. 18.4 Example of extension block pinning. (**a**) The DIP joint is flex 90 degrees. (**b**) The exension block pin is inserted just proximal to the mallet fragment at a 45 degree angle into the articular surface of P2. (**c**) The distal phalanx is extended to neutral and a transarticular pin is placed in retrograde fashion while the mallet fragment is reduced (From Hofmeister EP, Mazurek MT, Shin AY. Extension Block pinning for Large Mallet Fractures. The Journal of Hand Surgery. 2003; 28(3):453–459)

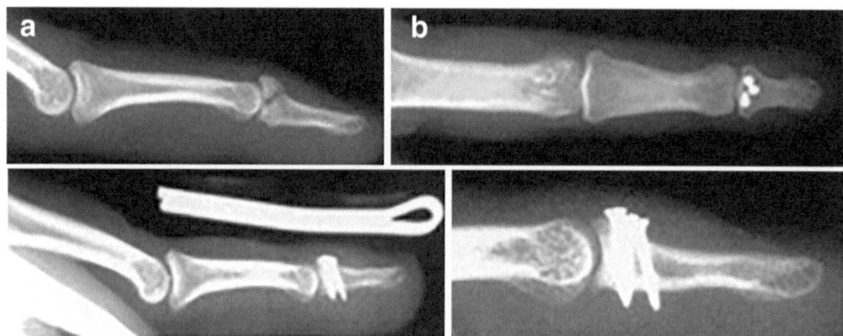

Fig. 18.5 Example of open reduction and screw fixation. (**a**) A large reducible bony mallet fragment. (**b**) AP of a bony mallet fragment fixed with 3 cortical screws. (**c**) Lateral of the bony mallet screw fixation. (**d**) Magnified lateral view of the bony mallet ORIF (From Kronlage SC, Faust D. Open Reduction and Screw Fixation of Mallet Fractures. Journal of Hand Surgery (European Volume). 2004;29(2):135–138)

pin site infections that resolved with oral antibiotics and two cases of mild displacement of the reduction (<2 mm). There were no non-unions or malunions [16].

Lubahn reported on 31 patients with bony mallet injuries treated with either a splint or by open reduction internal fixation with a Kirschner wire. In the closed treatment group, there was 20–30° of extension lag with an average range of motion (ROM) of 35° compared to 0–20° of extension lag in the open treatment group with average ROM of 55° [30].

In a recent randomized clinical trial, Thillemann et al. compared extension block pinning versus splinting in 32 patients with bony mallet fractures involving at least

Fig. 18.6 Example of hook plate construct. (**a**) Lateral of a hook plate reducing the bony mallet fragment. (**b**) AP of a hook plate reducing the bony mallet fragment (From Teoh LC, Lee JYL. Mallet Fractures: A Novel Approach to Internal Fixation Using a Hook Plate. Journal of Hand Surgery (European Volume). 2007;32(1):24–30)

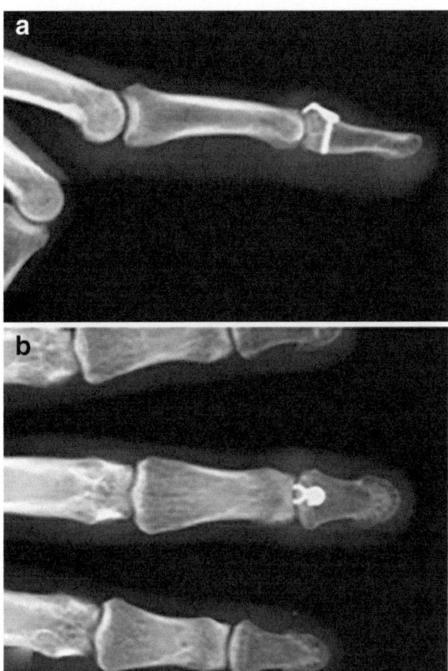

one-third of the articular surface. There was no significant difference among final extension lag or patient reported outcomes. Flexion and active range of motion at the DIP joint was better in the splinting group. However, three patients developed secondary subluxation at the DIP joint [31].

Auchincloss compared splinting to internal fixation in a prospective, randomized controlled trial. Out of 41 cases treated with either a splint or percutaneous fixation with a K-wire, the results were similar between the two groups based on subjective and objective standards if they were treated within the first week from injury. The study also showed that those treated in a delayed fashion may benefit more from internal fixation [32].

Yoon et al. compared nonoperative treatment to extension block pinning in 49 patients with a bony mallet fracture involving more than one-third of the articular surface. They found no significant difference among the average extension lag, flexion of the DIP joint, and pain scores between the two groups. All of the fractures in both groups healed by 3 months [33].

One study compared extension block pinning or open reduction and hook plate fixation among 22 patients with a bony mallet fracture that involved at least 25% of the articular surface. There was no significant difference in pain scores, mean extensor lag, and functional outcomes. Extension block pinning was found to be more cost-effective when compared to hook plate fixation [17].

Kronlage and Faust showed that open reduction and screw fixation can lead to satisfactory outcomes in patients with bony mallet injuries. They treated twelve patients with mallet fractures that involved more than one-third of the articular surface. At final follow-up, average range of motion was from 6° to 70° and loss of reduction occurred in one patient. Ten of the twelve patient showed no evidence of degenerative changes at the DIP joint, and there were no infections or nail deformities in the entire group [20].

Damron et al. performed a retrospective review of 19 patients with irreducible mallet finger fractures that failed splinting. All patients were treated with open reduction and a tension band technique. The average follow-up time was 8.2 years. Results showed 89% had no residual deformity, significant pain, or major disability. DIP joint range of motion averaged from 1 degree of hyperextension to 69° of flexion [29].

Complications

Stern and Kastrup compared complications from splinting versus surgical treatment among 123 mallet injuries, which included 82 bony injuries [34]. Surgery had a 53% complication rate, of which 76% were considered long-term. Only one mallet injury in the splint group had a long-term complication, which was a minor nail deformity. The most common complication in the surgery group was infection, followed by permanent nail deformity, joint incongruity, pin failure, and radial or ulnar prominence or deviation.

Similarly, Kang et al. found a 41% complication rate in mallet injuries that were treated surgically with open reduction and trans-articular fixation across the DIP joint with K-wire. The most common complication was marginal skin necrosis, followed by recurrent mallet deformity, pin tract infection, and nail deformity. Despite these complications, all 59 cases in this study went on to successful union [35].

Discussion

Mallet injuries are common injuries in the young adult male population. Mechanisms are usually forceful flexion of an extending DIP joint but can also less commonly result from a hyperextension of the DIP joint. The characteristic finding on examination is an extensor lag of the DIP joint. Bony mallet injuries that involve greater than 1/3 of the articular surface or with joint subluxation are often treated surgically. There is insufficient evidence to support operative treatment over nonoperative treatment when there is no joint subluxation present. There is also no significant difference in outcomes among the different types of surgical techniques [36, 37]. We recommend nonoperative treatment in the form of a custom thermoplastic stack splint for 8 weeks for bony mallet injuries without joint subluxation and that involve less than 1/3 of the articular surface. We recommend operative management for bony mallet injuries with joint subluxation, involvement of greater than 1/3 articular disruption, or open mallet injuries. Complications are higher with operative treatment, with infection and skin necrosis most commonly seen.

References

1. Doyle JR. Extensor tendons: acute injuries. In: Green DP, Pederson CW, Hotchkiss RN, editors. Green's operative hand surgery. 4th ed. New York: Churchill Livingstone; 1999. p. 195–8.
2. Lamaris GA, Matthew MK. The diagnosis and management of mallet finger injuries. Hand (N Y). 2017;12(3):223–8.
3. Clayton RAE, Court-Brown CM. The epidemiology of musculoskeletal tendinous and ligamentous injuries. Injury. 2008;39(12):1338–44.
4. Stark HH, Boyes JH, Wilson JN. Mallet finger. J Bone Joint Surg Am. 1962;44(6):1061–8.
5. Robb WA. The results of treatment of mallet finger. J Bone Joint Surg Br Vol. 1959;41(3):546–9.
6. Wehbe MA, Schneider LH. Mallet fractures. J Bone Joint Surg. 1984;66(5):658–69.
7. Patel MR, Desai SS, Bassini-Lipson L. Conservative management of chronic mallet finger. J Hand Surg. 1986;11(4):570–3.
8. Moradi A, Braun Y, Oflazoglu K, Meijs T, Ring D, Chen N. Factors associated with subluxation in mallet fracture. J Hand Surg Eur Vol. 2017;42(2):176–81.
9. Kalainov DM, Hoepfner PE, Hartigan BJ, Carroll C, Genuario J. Nonsurgical treatment of closed mallet finger fractures. J Hand Surg. 2005;30(3):580–6.
10. Okafor B, Mbubaegbu C, Munshi I, et al. Mallet deformity of the finger: five year follow-up of conservative treatment. J Bone Joint Surg Br Vol. 1997;79(4):544–7.
11. Trickett RW, Brock J, Shewring DJ. The non-operative management of bony mallet injuries. J Hand Surg Eur Vol. 2021;46(5):460–5.
12. Gaberman SF, Diao E, Peimer CA. Mallet finger: results of early versus delayed closed treatment. J Hand Surg. 1994;19(5):850–2.
13. Pike J, Mulpuri K, Metzger M, et al. Blinded, prospective, randomized clinical trial comparing volar, dorsal, and custom thermoplastic splinting in treatment of acute mallet finger. J Hand Surg. 2010;35(4):580–8.
14. O'Brien LJ, Bailey MJ. Single blind, prospective, randomized controlled trial comparing dorsal aluminum and custom thermoplastic splints to stack splint for acute mallet finger. Arch Phys Med Rehabil. 2011;92(2):191–8.
15. Warren RA, Norris SH, Ferguson DG. Mallet finger: a trial of two splints. J Hand Surg Br. 1988;66(5):658–9.
16. Hofmeister EP, Mazurek MT, Shin AY. Extension block pinning for large mallet fractures. J Hand Surg. 2003;28(3):453–9.
17. Toker S, Türkmen F, Pekince O, Korucu İ, Karalezli N. Extension block pinning versus hook plate fixation for treatment of mallet fractures. J Hand Surg. 2015;40(8):1591–6.
18. Takami H, Takahashi S, Ando M. Operative treatment of mallet finger due to intra-articular fracture of the distal phalanx. Arch Orthop Trauma Surg. 2000;120:9–13.
19. Bauze A, Bain GI. Internal suture for mallet finger fracture. J Hand Surg Br Eur Vol. 1999;24(6):688–92.
20. Kronlage SC, Faust D. Open reduction and screw fixation of mallet fractures. J Hand Surg Eur Vol. 2004;29(2):135–8.
21. Tetik C, Gudemez E. Modification of the extension block Kirschner wire technique for mallet fractures. Clin Orthop Relat Res. 2002;404:284–90.
22. Yamanaka K, Sasaki T. Treatment of mallet fractures using compression fixation pins. J Hand Surg Br Eur Vol. 1999;24(3):358–60.
23. Ulusoy MG, Karalezli N, Kocer U. Pull-in suture technique for the treatment of mallet finger. Plast Reconstr Surg. 2006;118(3):696–702.

24. Teoh LC, Lee JYL. Mallet fractures: a novel approach to internal fixation using a hook plate. J Hand Surg Eur Vol. 2007;32(1):24–30.
25. Lee YH, Kim JY, Chung MS. Two extension block Kirschner wire technique for mallet finger fractures. J Bone Joint Surg. 2009;91(11):1478–81.
26. Fritz D, Lutz M, Arora R, et al. Delayed Kirschner wire compression technique for mallet fracture. J Hand Surg Eur Vol. 2005;30(2):180–4.
27. Rocchi L, Genitiempo M. Percutaneous fixation of mallet fractures by the "umbrella handle" technique. J Hand Surg Eur Vol. 2006;31(4):407–12.
28. Badia A, Riano F. A simple fixation method for unstable bony mallet finger. J Hand Surg. 2004;29(6):1051–5.
29. Damron TA, Engber WD. Surgical treatment of mallet finger fractures by tension band technique. Clin Orthop Relat Res. 1994;300:133–40.
30. Lubahn JD. Mallet finger fractures: a comparison of open and closed technique. J Hand Surg Am. 1989;14(2 Pt 2):394–6.
31. Thillemann JK, Thillemann TM. Splinting versus extension-block pinning of bony mallet finger: a randomized clinic trial. J Hand Surg Eur Vol. 2020;45(6):574–81.
32. Auchincloss JM. Mallet-finger injuries: a prospective, controlled trial of internal and external splintage. Hand. 1982;14(2):168–73.
33. Yoon JO, Baek H, Kim JK. The outcomes of extension block pinning and nonsurgical management for mallet fracture. J Hand Surg. 2017;42(5):387.e1–7.
34. Stern PJ, Kastrup JJ. Complications and prognosis of treatment of mallet finger. J Hand Surg. 1988;13(3):329–34.
35. Kang HJ, Shin SJ, Kang ES. Complications of operative treatment for mallet fractures of the distal phalanx. J Hand Surg Br. 2001;26(1):28–31.
36. Handoll HHG, Vaghela MV. Interventions for treating mallet finger injuries. Cochrane Database Syst Rev. 2004;(3):CD004574.
37. Lin JS, Samora JB. Surgical and nonsurgical management of mallet finger: a systematic review. J Hand Surg. 2018;43(2):146–63.

Fingertip Injuries

19

Shruthi Deivasigamani, Benjamin Gundlach, and Adam Strohl

Section I: Anatomy

Nail Complex

The **nail**, or nail plate, itself is a rigid structure overlying the distal dorsal aspect of the finger pulp (Fig. 19.1). The nail is comprised of layers of stratum corneum cells and plays an important role in sensory function by providing counterpressure to the pulp of the distal finger, allowing for enhanced two-point discrimination. It is a part of the nail complex, which is also referred to as the **perionychium**. In addition to the nail, the perionychium is also comprised of the paronychium, the nail fold, the eponychium, the nail vest, the hyponychium, and the germinal and sterile matrices of the nailbed.

The **paronychium** is comprised of the skin and soft tissue lateral to the nail, including the union between the lateral nail groves and skin. It serves to protect the nail from contamination via its lateral borders. The proximal **nail fold** protects the nail at its proximal border and is covered dorsally by a stretch of skin referred to as the nail wall. The **eponychium** is an extension of the nail wall distally onto the

S. Deivasigamani
Department of Plastic and Reconstructive Surgery, Cooper University Health Systems, Camden, NJ, USA

B. Gundlach
Department of Orthopedics, Philadelphia Hand to Shoulder Center at Thomas Jefferson University Hospital, Philadelphia, PA, USA

A. Strohl (✉)
Department of Orthopedics, Philadelphia Hand to Shoulder Center at Thomas Jefferson University Hospital, Philadelphia, PA, USA

Department of Surgery - Plastic Surgery, Philadelphia Hand to Shoulder Center at Thomas Jefferson University Hospital, Philadelphia, PA, USA
e-mail: abstrohl@handcenters.com

© The Author(s), under exclusive license to Springer Nature Switzerland AG 2023
J. M. Abzug et al. (eds.), *Pediatric and Adult Hand Fractures*,
https://doi.org/10.1007/978-3-031-32072-9_19

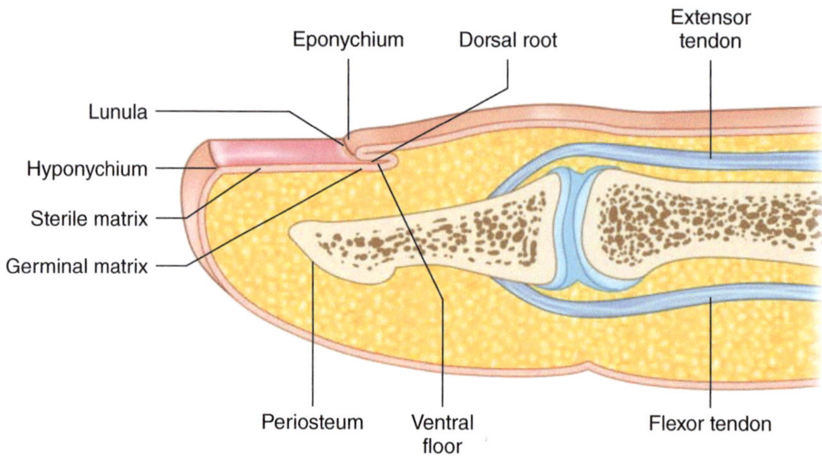

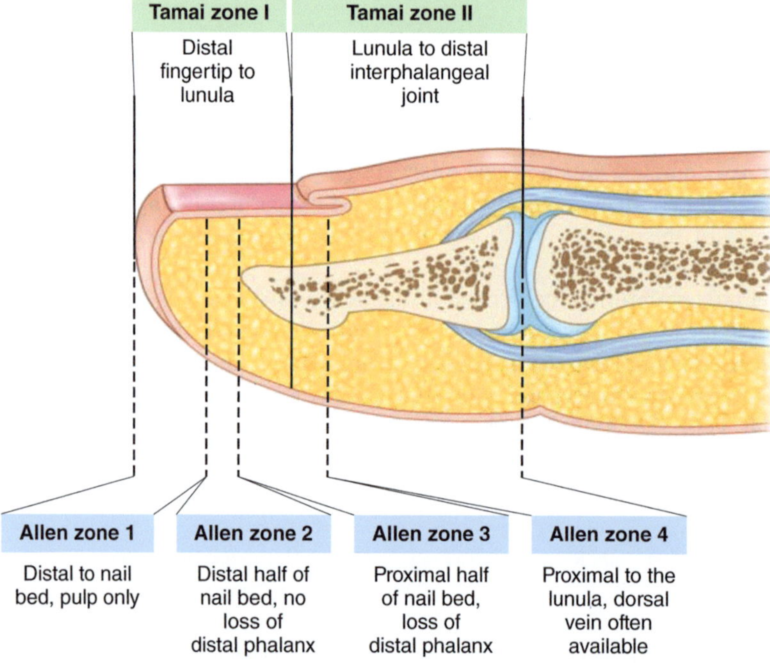

Fig. 19.1 Distal finger and nailbed anatomy. The image on the right demonstrates critical anatomical structures in the distal digit. The image on the left describes Tamai and Allen classifications for amputations through the fingertip. (Image reproduced from Green's Operative Hand Surgery Ch. 49 [1])

dorsum of the nail itself. It includes a thin epithelial layer that is adherent to the superficial aspect of the nail plate and serves to give the nail a "shiny" appearance. The **nail vest (cuticle)** is a cornified strip that attaches the eponychium to the nail. The **hyponychium** is the demarcation between the nailbed and pulp at the distal end of the nailbed. It protects the nail at its distal border both physically and an immunologically, due to its high local concentration of phagocytes.

The **nailbed** is the tissue that directly underlies and adheres to the nail. It has longitudinal grooves that correspond to the grooves of the nail plate's deep surface, which allows the nail to closely adhere to the nailbed. The nailbed consists of two histologically distinct zones: the sterile matrix and germinal matrix, which are separated by the distal border of the **lunula**, the pale semicircular area of the nailbed immediately distal to the proximal nail fold. The **germinal matrix** consists of a dorsal and volar fold that envelops the origin of the growing nail and extends distally to the distal border of the lunula. The germinal matrix is responsible for the majority of nail synthesis and is named such due to the presence of germ cells which produce the keratin and other compounds found within the nail. The **sterile matrix** extends from the distal border of the lunula to the hyponychium and adds new layers of cells to thicken the nail that has already been formed by the germinal matrix. The sterile matrix is also responsible for forming the longitudinal striations of the nail.

Distal Phalanx and Finger Pulp

The bony skeleton of the fingertip is formed by the distal phalanx (Fig. 19.2). The distal phalanx is divided into three anatomically distinct portions: the base, the shaft, and the tuft. The proximal portion of the distal phalanx, the base, articulates with the middle phalanx to form the distal interphalangeal joint (DIPJ). In each finger the flexor digitorum profundus—or in the thumb, the flexor pollicis longus—inserts on the volar base of the distal phalanx at the metaphyseal flare. Dorsally, the extensor tendons insert onto the epiphysis of their respective distal

Fig. 19.2 Bony anatomy of fingertip

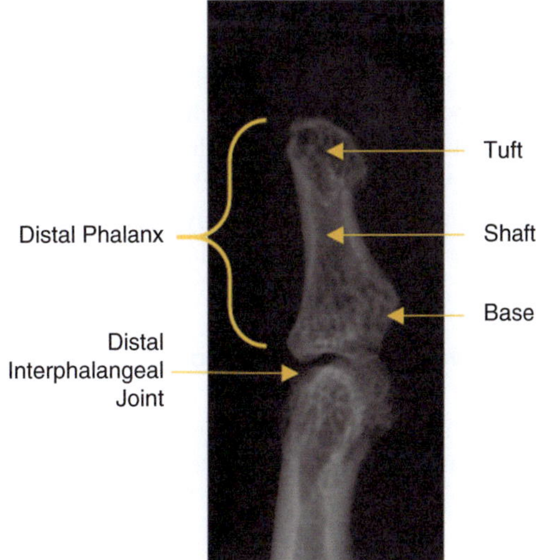

phalangeal base (Fig. 19.1). The shaft of the distal phalanx is concave on the palmar surface. The convex portion of the finger pulp overlies the concave portion of the distal phalanx and is known as the proximal pulp. The distalmost portion of the distal phalanx has a characteristic tuberosity with a proximal projection, known as the phalangeal tuft. The soft tissue overlying the phalangeal tuft on the palmar side is known as the distal pulp. The nailbed and nail overly the phalangeal tuft on the dorsal side.

Both the dorsal and proximal pulp tissue are separated by fibrous septa into discrete compartments. The dorsal and proximal pulps serve slightly different functions and have correspondingly different patterns of septation. The distal pulp is bolstered on the dorsal side by the nail, which provides counterpressure to this portion of the fingertip. The pulp is separated into wedge-shaped compartments by septa that originate in a radial pattern from the phalangeal periosteum and insert into the deep dermis. This arrangement allows for increased stability and reduced sheer in the distal pulp during pinch. The proximal pulp, conversely, is organized into several layers of spherical lobules. This conformation, in addition to the lack of a nailbed on the dorsal surface, allows for more malleability and improved grip in the proximal pulp.

Neurovascular Supply

All vessels supplying the fingertip arise from the terminal branches of the palmar digital arteries (common volar digital arteries) (Fig. 19.3). Flint [4] describes three distinct anastomotic arches over the dorsal surface of the distal phalanx that are all interconnected through several anastomotic branches. The distal arch is projected at the level of the lunula and forms a loop under the nailbed. The proximal arch courses under the proximal nail and proximal nail fold. The superficial arch overlies the base of the dorsal distal phalanx. The terminal branches of the palmar digital artery also give rise to the pulp arch, which overlies the volar surfaces of the base of the distal phalanx and supplies the pulp via longitudinal arterioles that arise from the arch. These arterioles extend over the distal tip of the digit to anastomose with the dorsal arches.

Venous drainage of the nailbed is via the dorsal venous system, wherein venules from the perionychium drain laterally and dorsally to the nailbed as well as proximal to the nail fold and then drain in a random manner over the dorsal aspect of the finger. At the level of the DIPJ, the vessel is large enough in caliber to anastomose. Lymph drainage of the perionychium shadows venous drainage and is particularly dense at the hyponychium, which helps protect the nailbed from infection.

Innervation and Sensation

The common volar digital nerves branch dorsally at the DIPJ and supply the perionychium and pulp. The pulp of the fingertip also contains many mechanoreceptors

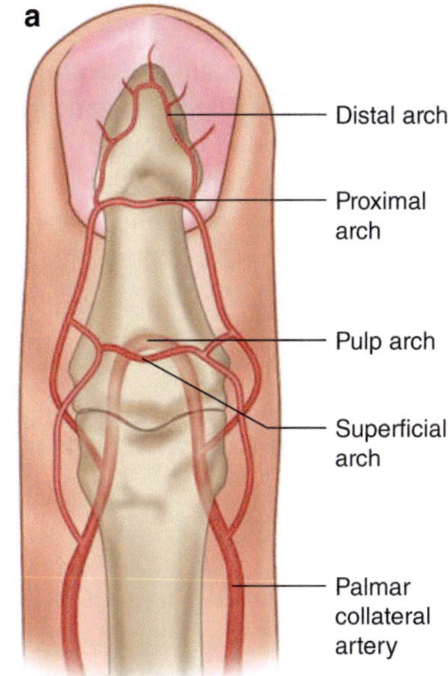

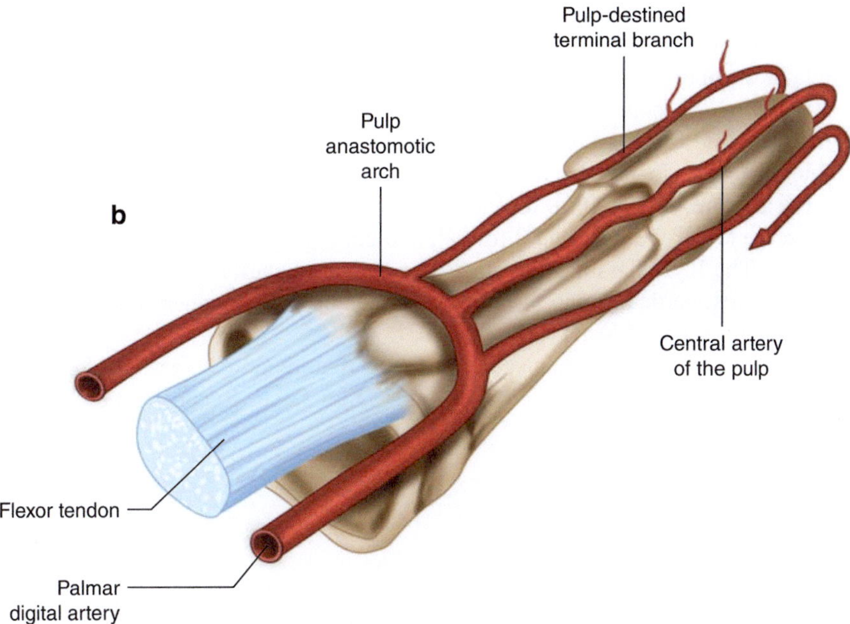

Fig. 19.3 Vascularization of fingertip. (**a**) Vascularization of the nail complex. (1) Distal arch. (2) Proximal arch. (3) Pulp arch. (4) Superficial arch. (5) Palmar collateral artery. (**b**) Pulp vascularization. (1) Pulp anastomotic arch. (2) Palmar digital artery. (3) Flexor tendon. (4) Pulp-destined terminal branch. (5) Central artery of the pulp. (Image reproduced from Emergency Hand Surgery Ch 13, Nail Trauma [2] and Ch 9, Finger and Hand Soft Tissue Defects [3])

that allow for specialized sensation. Pacinian corpuscles reside in the deep dermis and subcutaneous tissue and are important for light touch. Meissner corpuscles are in the dermal papillae and are important in detecting moving two-point discrimination, allowing for the sensation of fine touch and stroking. Merkel cells are located at the dermo-epidermal junction and respond to low-frequency vibration, allowing for detection of pressure and texture. Ruffini organs are within the dermis and respond to stretch. These sensory organelles are relevant when considering skin grafts, as full-thickness skin grafts incorporate all four organelles, whereas split-thickness skin grafts generally only incorporate Merkel cells and Ruffini organs [1–3, 5, 6].

Section II: Classification and Evaluation of Injuries

Classification

Several methods of classifying fingertip injuries have been proposed over the years. Allen describes five types of fingertip injury based on anatomical zone (Fig. 19.1) [7]. Type I injuries include only the distalmost pulp of the finger. Type II injuries involve pulp and nail loss, but no damage to the phalanx. Type III injuries involve damage to the pulp, nail, and part of the terminal distal phalanx. Type IV injuries involve damage to the pulp, nail, part of the terminal distal phalanx, as well as the lunula of the nail.

The pulp–nail–bone (PNB) classification of fingertip injury was proposed to more clearly describe the damages incurred by different structures in the fingertip (Table 19.1) [8]. In this scale, the pulp, nail, and bone each receive a separate numerical score. A score of 0 indicates no damage to the structure, while a maximum score (7 for the pulp and 8 for nail and bone) indicates complete loss of the structure. The PNB classification allows for increased clarity when describing fingertip injuries, particularly in the case of oblique lacerations when different structures may be damaged to varying degrees.

Classification of distal phalanx fractures may require more extensive description and is discussed further in section "Section IV: Soft Tissue Reconstruction" of this chapter.

Physical Exam

Physical examination of a fingertip injury should include assessment of the following factors: mechanism of injury (in particular, sharp versus crushing trauma), plane of injury (oblique versus transverse, volar versus dorsal), the level of damage (in relation to DIP joint), the degree of soft tissue damage (by assessing soft tissue stability), and whether or not there is any exposed bone. Distal phalangeal fractures often occur at the junction of the nail fold, which can obscure a subtle open fracture if not thoroughly inspected. Undiagnosed open

Table 19.1 The pulp–nail–bone classification of fingertip injuries

Pulp	
0	No injury
1	Laceration
2	Crush
3	Loss—distal transverse
4	Loss—palmar oblique partial
5	Loss—dorsal oblique
6	Loss—lateral
7	Loss—complete
Nail	
0	No injury
1	Sterile matrix laceration
2	Germinal and sterile matrix laceration
3	Crush
4	Proximal nailbed dislocation
5	Loss—distal third
6	Loss—distal two-thirds
7	Loss—lateral
8	Loss—complete
Bone	
0	No injury
1	Tuft Fracture
2	Comminuted nonarticular fracture
3	Articular fracture
4	Displaced basal fracture
5	Tip exposure
6	Loss—distal half
7	Loss—subtotal (tendon insertions intact)
8	Loss—complete

Reproduced from [8]

fractures can result in deep infection and long-lasting nailbed deformities. Similarly, large subungual hematomas can obscure the extent of a nailbed injury. Nails with painful or large subungual hematomas should be decompressed by trephination to obtain a thorough assessment of underlying nailbed injury or distal phalanx involvement. If the injury spans the nailbed, the percentage of remaining nail should be noted.

When assessing for tendon injuries, the finger should be inspected at rest. If the DIP joint at rest has a flexed posture, or there is an extensor lag, an extensor tendon injury or avulsion should be suspected. Similarly, if the fingertip's cascade is in extension relative to other fingers, and DIP joint flexion is impaired, a flexor tendon injury or avulsion should be suspected. In a flexor tendon avulsion, the retracted flexor tendon may be palpated proximally along the flexor sheath. Pain elicited on palpation of the flexor sheath can also allow for localization of the retracted tendon.

Obtaining a detailed neurovascular examination is also important to gauge the extent of injury. In the acute setting, threshold sensory testing—such as Semmes Weinstein monofilament—is more sensitive to sensory deficits. Two-point discrimination is also useful but can be difficult to fully assess in the acutely traumatized digit.

Radiographic Evaluation

When there is concern for fracture of the distal phalanx, standard, AP, lateral, and oblique radiographs should be obtained. In cases of suspected tendon avulsions, an avulsed bone fragment may be visible on either the volar or dorsal surface of the base of the distal phalanx. However, lack of a visible avulsion fragment on radiograph does not definitively rule out an avulsion injury.

MRI and ultrasound have comparatively less utility but may be helpful in identifying a retracted FDP tendon in cases of FDP tendon avulsions.

Section III: Management of Nailbed Injuries

Injury to the nailbed is very common during fingertip injury. The most commonly injured finger is the middle finger, followed by the ring, index, small, and thumb. Fractures of the distal phalanx are present in 50% of nailbed injuries, with most injuries occurring in the middle or distal third of the nailbed [9].

Nailbed injuries with underlying distal phalanx fracture are discussed further in section "Section V: Distal Phalanx Fractures" of this chapter.

Subungual Hematoma

A subungual hematoma is usually the result of a crushing injury to the fingertip which causes bleeding under the nail plate and subsequent separation of the nail from the nailbed. The pressure of the blood in this confined space can be extremely painful. A subungual hematoma may also be caused by a laceration of the nail matrix, which is easily obscured by the overlying hematoma.

Management

Not all hematomas require drainage, and a small hematoma comprising less than 25% with minimal pain can be left untreated. The hematoma will eventually be incorporated into the nail and travel distally with nail growth. Acutely painful subungual hematomas or hematomas comprising >25% of the nail should be treated with trephination. Trephination can be accomplished with a heated instrument, which can be a sterile paperclip, battery-operated cautery, 18-gauge needle, or 2 mm punch biopsy. In children, an insulin needle can be used. First, the nail should be cleaned with an alcohol swab. Then, the heated instrument can be used to carefully perforate the nail. The pooled blood from the hematoma will create a barrier protecting the nailbed from injury by the heated trephination device. Decompression of the hematoma should result in rapid relief from pain (Fig. 19.4).

In the past, subungual hematomas greater than 50% of the nail were treated with removal of the nail for nailbed inspection and repair. However, a multitude of more recent studies have shown that there is no difference in eventual nail cosmesis in patients whose subungual hematomas were treated with trephination alone or with

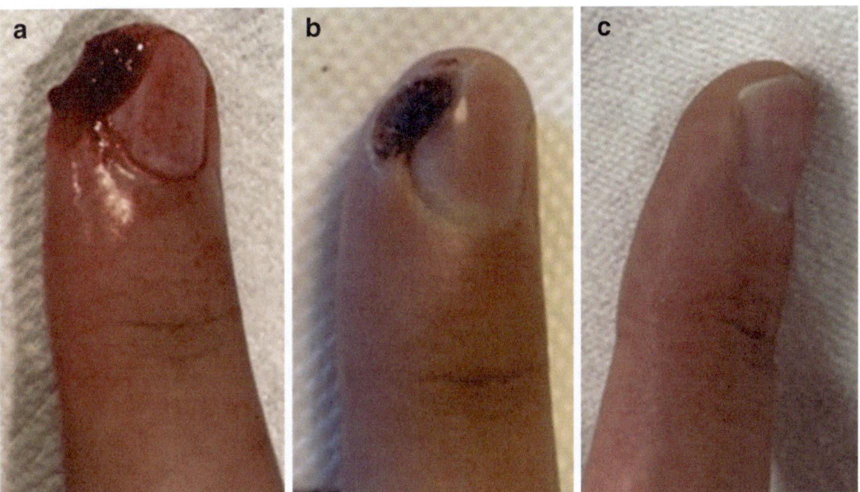

Fig. 19.4 Healing by secondary intention. (**a**) Initial soft tissue defect. (**b**) Soft tissue defect after 1 week of healing by secondary intention. (**c**) Resultant soft tissue after several weeks of healing by secondary intention

nail removal and nailbed repair [10, 11]. These findings have been reproduced in the pediatric population as well [12]. The current recommendation for management of large and painful subungual hematoma is trephination alone; however, nail removal and further exploration is recommended for fingertip trauma resulting in a punctured or lacerated nail, disruption of any nail border, or a painful subungual hematoma not relieved by trephination alone [2, 3, 5, 6].

Nail Laceration and Avulsion

Lacerations that pierce through the nail typically result from crushing forces and leave a stellate wound on the nailbed. Often, there is an associated subungual hematoma. Nail avulsion are an uncommon injury but can occur as a result of a very large subungual hematoma or very proximal nail laceration. In some cases of excessive hyperflexion of the fingertip, just the proximal nail edge can become dislocated from the nail fold.

Management of Laceration and Avulsion

A digital block should be administered prior to exploration of the nailbed and a small tourniquet—such as a dedicated finger tourniquet, Penrose drain, or the long finger of a surgical glove—should be applied around the base of the affected finger and held with a small hemostat. The nail plate can be carefully lifted from the nailbed using a small freer elevator or tenotomy scissors. It is important to not further injure the underlying matrix while elevating the nail. Beveling the instrument away from the matrix while using slow and methodically movements can prevent iatrogenic injury. The nail, once removed, should be inspected for residual tissue from the nailbed. If fragments of nailbed remain adhered to the volar surface of the avulsed nail, they should gently be released from the nail and sutured back onto the nailbed as free grafts. Grafts up to 1 cm in diameter will usually survive, even when placed on the cortex of the distal phalanx [4]; however, it is not recommended to use a nailbed graft from a neighboring finger or the great toe due to donor site morbidity as well as reports of nearly normal regeneration of the nailbed without grafts, even when the entire sterile matrix has been lost [13].

The avulsed nail can then be soaked in a povidone-iodine solution. Lacerations of the nailbed should be examined under loupe magnification and sutured using 6-0 or 7-0, absorbable sutures. Splinting the nail fold open following nail removal remains controversial, with evidence suggesting it provides no benefit and may just become a nidus for infection [14]. If one chooses to replace the nail or use a synthetic material (such as the foil from a suture package), a horizontal mattress should be placed proximally to secure the splint under the proximal nail fold, and another distally to secure it to the hyponychium.

In skeletally immature patients, a physeal fracture of the distal phalanx with an associated matrix laceration can occur, often referred to as a Seymour fracture. Due to the epiphyseal insertion of the extensor tendon, and the metaphyseal insertion of the flexor tendon, this injury results in an apex dorsal angulation through the physis. The angulation often leads to a concomitant laceration of the overlying germinal and sterile matrix. Classically, the proximal extent of the nail plate will be flipped up and exposed with disappearance of the proximal nail fold; however, these injuries can be subtle and easily missed if only relying on physical exam. Therefore radiographs—including a perfect lateral—should be obtained in all pediatric nailbed injuries to rule out a Seymour fracture. Surgical intervention with nail plate removal, fracture reduction, and matrix repair is required in all Seymour fractures. Closed reduction, matrix repair, and splinting are often enough to maintain fracture reduction; however, a retrograde pin through the distal phalanx should be placed if there is any concern for unstable fractures. Similar fracture patterns can occur in skeletally mature patients, with identical treatment recommend.

If the nail is avulsed and not available for replacement, several options exist to serve as a temporary nail, such as silicone sheeting, artificial nails, foil from a suture package, or non-adherent gauze. As with the native nail, these materials are trimmed to the shape of the nail, placed under the proximal nail fold, and secured proximally and distally with suture [2, 3, 5, 6].

Section IV: Soft Tissue Reconstruction

Fingertip injuries often result in soft tissue damage necessitating repair. Depending on the extent of the damage, the recommended repair options can range from healing by secondary intention to a local or larger regional flap. Various options and their indications are discussed here. Additionally, healing by secondary intention may allow for near-normal sensory recovery in the fingertip, whereas many described flaps for fingertip coverage cannot restore near-normal sensation.

An advancement in non-operative treatment of soft tissue fingertip injuries is the use of semi-permeable membrane dressings to create a clean, sealed barrier around the wound. A hematoma develops at the wound site and is contained within the dressing. The hematoma matures and subsequently epithelializes, providing pulp tissue that is nearly equal in thickness and sensation compared to normal digits [15, 16].

Secondary Intention

Indications
Healing by secondary intention with dressing changes is a suitable choice for tip amputations in which there is no exposed bone, particularly when the amputated portion of the fingertip is either unavailable or unusable. This is most appropriate for wounds with skin loss equal to or less than 1.5 cm.

Methods
Patients with fingertip wounds that will heal via secondary intention can perform daily dressing changes and local wound care. Semi-permeable membrane dressings should be changed weekly, and it is important to not disrupt the underlying hematoma that develops during the first few weeks. Splinting can be used to protect the healing wound from further disruption. Healing by secondary intention will occur over 4–6 weeks. Active range of motion exercises should be started within the first week to prevent joint stiffness and joint contractures (Fig. 19.4) [1–3].

Skin Grafting

Indications
Split-thickness skin grafts for coverage of exposed fingertip pulp have been found to offer no tangible advantages to healing by secondary intention. Common complaints after skin grafting include skin induration, fissuring, reduced sensation in the area of the graft, tenderness in the area of the graft, cold sensitivity, reduced two-point discrimination, and hypoesthesia. In comparison, patients whose wounds heal by secondary intention often have a good cosmetic result, preserved sensation and two-point discrimination, and complain only of cold sensitivity [1–3, 5, 17, 18].

Cap Grafting ([19], 49)

Indications
In tip amputations with no exposed bone where the amputated portion is both available and relatively devoid of contamination, it may be cleaned and

non-microsurgically reattached as a composite graft, also known as a cap graft. Cap grafting is only appropriate for Allen Zone I and Zone II sharp or blunt-cut injuries in young children. It is not appropriate in more proximal injuries in children, regardless of age, nor in adults at any Allen zone, owing to poor results [19].

Methods

After the amputated portion of the fingertip is thoroughly cleaned, it should be completely defatted and non-microsurgically repaired to the stump using absorbable sutures. Cap grafts that are reattached within 5 h of injury have been shown to have a significantly higher survival rate when compared with cap grafts reattached after 5 h [20]. Cap grafts will take several weeks to months to completely heal. In many individuals, the composite graft will develop partial or complete necrosis, but should remain in place as a biological dressing unless there is concern for underlying infection [1, 5].

Local Flaps

Volar V-Y Advancement Flap aka Atasoy

Indications

Fingertip defects that span <1 cm and are oriented in a dorsal oblique or transverse manner with exposed bone distal to the midportion of the nailbed are amenable to closure with a Volar V-Y (Atasoy) advancement flap (Fig. 19.5). In total, once can expect to obtain between 0.75 and 1 cm of length from this advancement flap. This method is not indicated for injuries where there is significant volar skin loss or in situations where there is extensive loss of skin.

Advantages

Advantages include lack of donor site defect, as well as the fact that the flap will remain sensate.

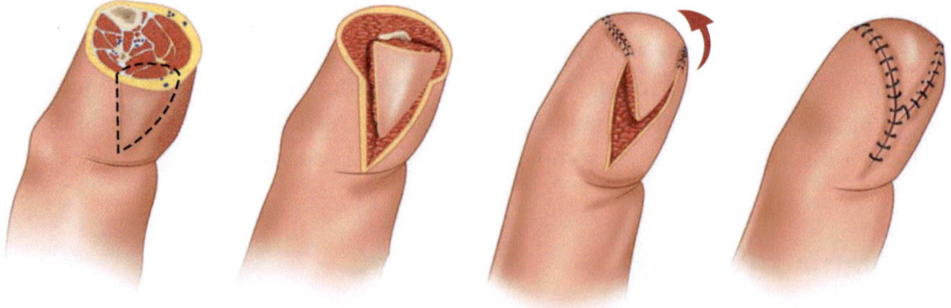

Fig. 19.5 Schematic demonstrating use of V-Y (Atasoy) advancement flap. (Reproduced from The Principles of Hand Surgery and Therapy Chapter 10: Nailbed and Fingertip Injuries [6])

Disadvantages

This flap only allows for coverage of small defects. In the case of crush injuries, damaged vasculature can render the flap unusable.

Methods

The volar digital neurovascular bundles and their terminal branches supply this flap. Digital anesthesia must first be administered and a tourniquet should be placed. This advancement flap is designed as an inverted V-shape on the volar surface of the affected distal phalanx, with the apex of the V located at the DIP joint crease and the base extending distally to the edge of the defect. The two sides of the triangle should be at least 1.5 times the length of the advancement length desired. Skin is incised through dermis until subcutaneous fat is observed, with care taken to no undermine the flap. Sharp release of any fibrous septae is then performed, and the flap is freed from the underlying distal phalanx and tendon sheath, allowing to advance distally. The flap is then carefully advanced distally, avoiding placing too much tension on the flap, which could result in tension on the vessel. Subcutaneous tissues can be carefully divided until the flap is able to cover the defect without tension. The distal end of the flap can be sutured to the nailbed and the lateral and proximal incisions are then closed in a "Y" fashion. Care should be taken not to pull the nail volarly to the suture, as this will result in a nail hook deformity. After the flap is closed, the tourniquet can be released to assess flap perfusion. Perfusion of the flap can be delayed for up to 5 min, but if perfusion remains poor beyond this, sutures should be checked for excess tension. Tight sutures should be removed until perfusion returns, and any portion of exposed subcutaneous tissue allowed to heal via secondary intention. Instead of suturing, some authors propose using an intradermal needle to transfix the flap to the distal phalanx, which might reduce the risk of a hook-nail deformity even further.

The finger can be placed in a soft dressing following repair that allows for joint motion. Sutures can be removed around 2 weeks later [1–3, 5, 6, 21].

Lateral V-Y Advancement Flap aka Kutler

Indications

The indications for the Lateral V-Y (Kutler) advancement flap are virtually identical to those of the Volar V-Y (Atasoy) advancement flap described above, but is better suited to defects approximately 0.5 cm, and no more than 1 cm, in length (Fig. 19.6).

Advantages

Advantages include lack of donor site defect and excellent preservation of flap sensation.

Disadvantages

This flap only allows for coverage of small defects. In the case of crush injuries, damaged vasculature can render the flap unusable. When compared to the Volar V-Y advancement flap, the advancement has limited mobility.

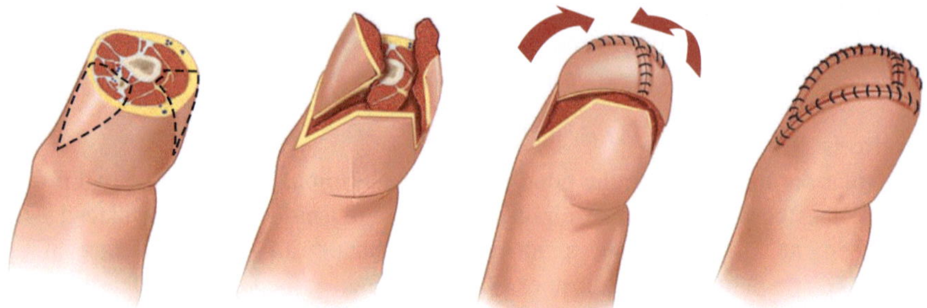

Fig. 19.6 Schematic demonstrating use of lateral V-Y (Kutler) advancement flap. (Image reproduced from The Principles of Hand Surgery and Therapy Chapter 10: Nailbed and Fingertip Injuries [6])

Methods

The branching vessels of the digital artery supply this flap. Digital anesthesia must first be administered and a tourniquet should be placed. This technique usually requires bilateral V-shaped flaps, with the apex of each V at the lateral aspects of the DIP joint. The incisions are similarly made through the dermis, and the subcutaneous tissue should be carefully mobilized from the periosteum of the distal phalanx on a deep plane by releasing the fibrous septae. The base of each triangle is advanced toward the other and sutured together, while the apex is closed in a "Y" fashion. The remaining edges of the flap can be sutured to the edges of the surrounding nailbed and skin. After the flap is closed, the tourniquet can be released to assess flap perfusion. Perfusion of the flap can be delayed for up to 5 min, but if perfusion remains poor beyond this, sutures should be checked for excess tension. Tight sutures should be removed and exposed portions of subcutaneous tissue allowed to heal via secondary intention.

The finger can be placed in a soft dressing following repair that allows for joint motion. Sutures can be removed around 2 weeks later [1–3, 5, 6].

Visor Flap

Indications

The visor flap is indicated for closure of transverse distal fingertip amputations with exposed bone.

Advantages

This flap has good cosmetic appearance and allows for preservation of existing digit length without disruption of adjacent digits or creation of scars on the palmar surface. The exposed bony portion of the stump is also well-cushioned by the flap. After this flap heals, sensation is generally adequate.

Disadvantages

The donor site requires either a split-thickness or full-thickness skin graft for closure and though sensation is adequate, it is still reduced from baseline.

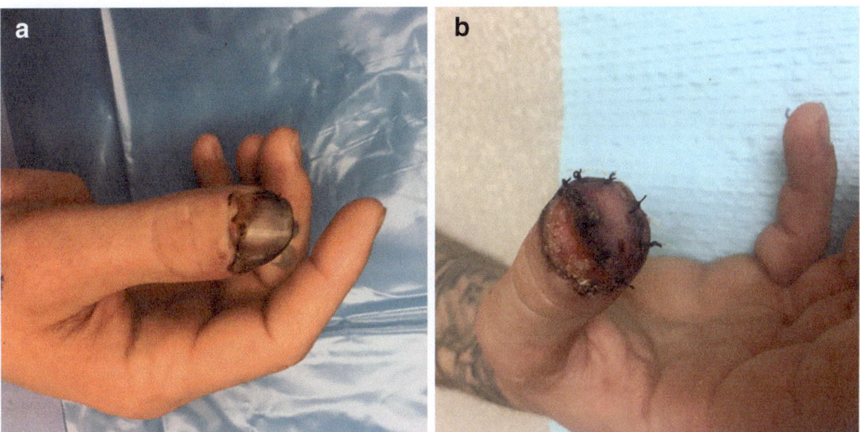

Fig. 19.7 Visor flap. (**a**) Soft tissue damage amenable to visor flap. (**b**) Visor flap after distal transposition

Methods

This is a bipedicled flap supplied by branches of the volar lateral and medial digital arteries and nerves. In this method, skin from the dorsal aspect of the finger is transposed over the distal stump like a hat, giving the flap its name. The defect is measured, and then a similarly sized rectangular flap (Fig. 19.7) is traced immediately dorsal and proximal to the defect, with the length of the flap approximating the height of the defect A proximal transverse incision is carried laterally, terminating just short of the midaxis both radially and ulnarly, and no deeper than the level of the paratenon. Two small (4–5 mm) back cuts can be made distally at either end of the incision, but these back cuts should be made through the dermis only in order to protect the nerves and vasculature. The flap is released from the underlying paratenon using blunt dissection and working through both proximal and distal wounds. The flap can then be transposed over the distal stump, with the distalmost edge of the flap advancing to the volar margin of the defect, and then secured in place with sutures. Dog ears may be left in place and will typically flatten during the healing process. The donor site should be closed with a split-thickness or full-thickness skin graft [5].

Homodigital Volar Advancement Flap aka Moberg and O'Brien Modification

Indications

This method can be used to reconstruct volar defects of the thumb, which has a lower risk of necrosis than other digits due to its shorter length, superior dorsal circulation via the princeps pollicis, and comparably mobile skin. This flap can cover defects up to 2 cm in length without need for a donor site skin graft or 3 cm with additional dissection of the flap into the palm (Fig. 19.8).

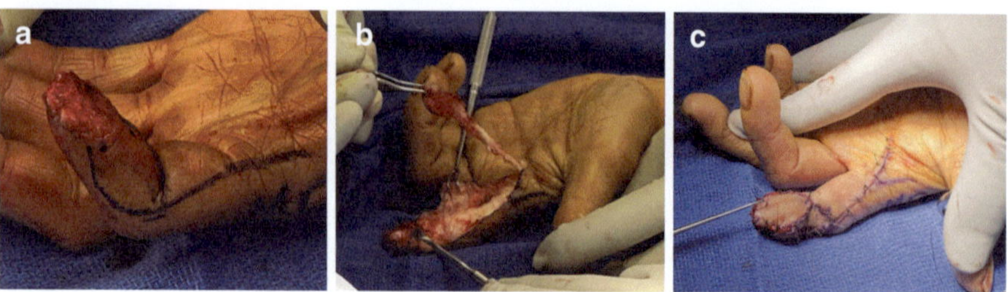

Fig. 19.8 Homodigital volar advancement flaps. (**a**) Soft tissue defect amenable to a homodigital advancement flap. (**b**) Dissection of the flap. (**c**) Inset of the flap, with digit held in flexion

Advantages

Provides near-normal sensation and allows the thumb to be covered with glabrous skin. Also allows for the length of the thumb to be maintained.

Disadvantages

There is a risk of IP joint flexion contracture, especially with large or excessively tensioned flaps. In some cases, there is also a risk for necrosis of the dorsal tip if the flap is advanced too far or if the neurovascular bundles are injured.

Methods

This is a bipedicled flap that relies on both the volar and dorsal neurovascular bundles supplying the thumb. After the dorsal tip is debrided, longitudinal incisions are made along the midaxis, ensuring the neurovascular bundles are incorporated within the flap. The flap is dissected off the underlying flexor tendon sheath, taking extreme care to preserve the neurovascular bundles. The flap should not be taken proximal to the level of the metacarpophalangeal joint; however, if additional length is needed, the flap can be designed proximally with a V-Y advancement and then islandized. The IP joint is flexed in order to achieve coverage of the defect with the flap, and the distal position of the flap can be shaped to ensure adequate coverage. Depending on the extent of damage, the distal portion of the flap may be fixed using an intradermal needle into the distal phalanx to reduce the risk of a hook-nail deformity, and the remaining edges of the flap can be sutured in place.

The O'Brien modification of this flap [22] utilizes an additional transverse incision to create a bipedicled "postage stamp" flap. The proximal transverse incision should be created at the IP crease so that the resultant donor site defect will be not only hidden, but also protected during gripping motions. The midlateral incisions allow for dissection of the neurovascular bundles bilaterally, and care should be taken to spare the adipose fat surrounding the vascular pedicle, which supports venous return. Depending on the length of the pedicle and size of the defect, coverage can be attained using flap advancement alone or flap advancement in conjunction with IP joint flexion. The flap can then be sutured into place. The donor site defect can be covered using a thick split-thickness skin graft from the hypothenar eminence, and care should be taken not to compress the pedicles with the graft [1–3, 5, 6].

Regional Flaps

For fingertip wounds that are too large for local flap coverage, a regional flap can be used. Some examples include island flaps, thenar flaps, and cross-finger flaps. Several regional flaps are two-stage procedures spaced approximately 2–4 weeks apart, and during this interim period, the fingers must remain immobilized. This period of immobilization can cause IP joint contractures and might not be appropriate for use in certain patient populations.

Thenar Flap

Indications

This method is appropriate for injuries to the index, middle, and ring fingers that are approximately 1×1.5 cm^2 in size, with exposed tendon or bone. It can be used when preservation of length is desired and other methods are not possible. This method should not be used in older patients or patients with preexisting arthritis or joint injury, as the tendency to develop PIP joint contractures is greater.

Advantages

Sensation has been reported to be higher than with skin grafts. This technique also allows for an excellent cosmetic result, including a better match in skin color and texture.

Disadvantages

There is a risk of PIP joint contractures in adults, especially if the small or ring finger is used. In all populations it is of utmost importance to follow the second phase of the surgery with early and aggressive range of motion exercises. There is also the obvious disadvantage conferred by the fact that this is a two-stage procedure, and the injured finger will be immobilized in flexion for approximately 3 weeks between the first and second stage. For these reasons, the thenar flap is used sparingly.

Methods

This flap can be as an "H" flap (Fig. 19.9), as well as a three-sided rectangular flap based along any border. To determine the flap donor site, the injured finger should be flexed toward the bulk of the thenar eminence in the position that requires the smallest amount of PIP joint flexion from the injured finger, and this point on the thenar eminence is marked with an "H" that is approximately 20% wider than the defect. Avoid placing the flap in the mid-palm region, as the latter often results in a painful donor site. The flap is incised and raised, incorporating some underlying subcutaneous fat, while taking care not to injure the underlying digital nerve of the thumb. If using an H-shaped flap, either the proximal or distal flap can be used to cover the fingertip. The flap is sutured to the fingertip, and if using an H-flap, the remaining flap is advanced within the flap defect and sutured down, closing the defect. In the rare case that the donor site cannot be closed primarily, a full-thickness skin graft may be used. A dressing is applied to support the injured finger in flexion.

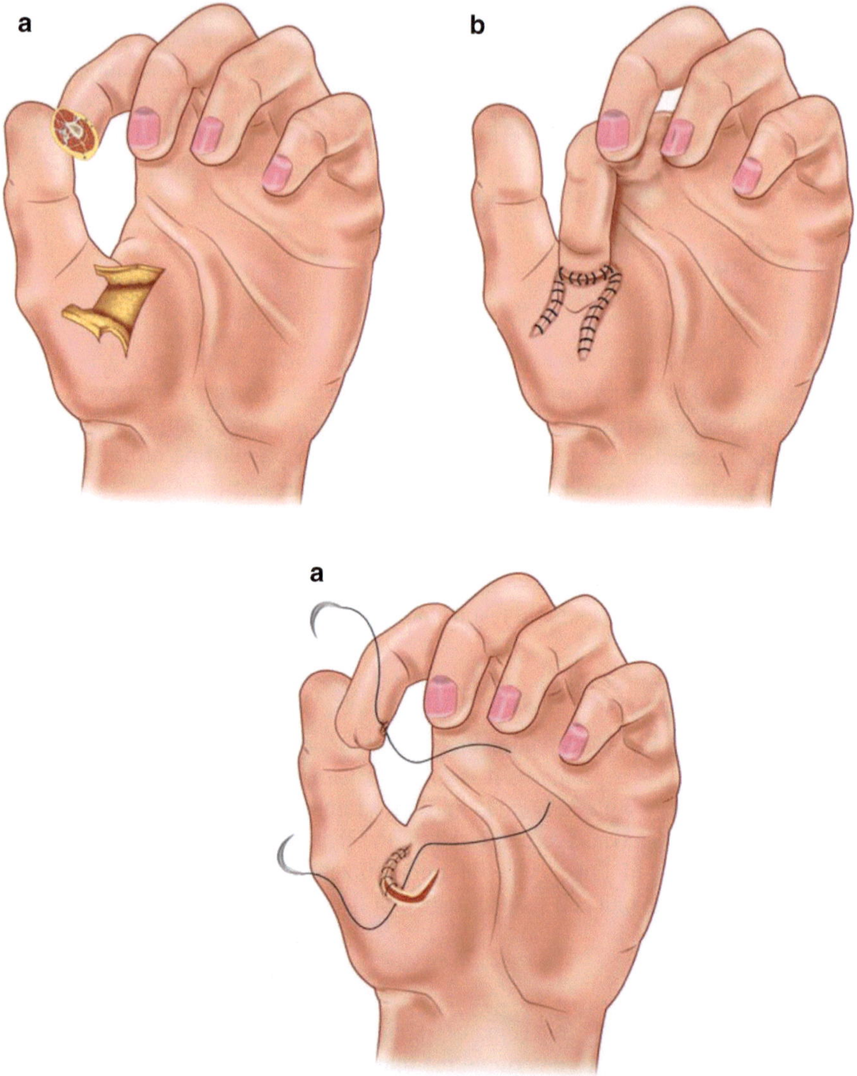

Fig. 19.9 Thenar H-flap. (**a**) Flap design. (**b**) Flap inset into thenar skin. (**c**) Flap division after 2–3 weeks. (Image reproduced from Green's Operative Hand Surgery Ch. 49 [1])

In 2–3 weeks, the second stage of the surgery is performed, in which the flap to the finger is divided at its base and sutured down to cover the remaining tip injury. The distal flap can be further advanced to cover any remaining donor site defect. Any excess skin from the pedicle can be returned to cover the donor site defect.

Postoperative rehabilitation is of utmost importance when using this method, to prevent the formation of contractures. Following the second stage of the procedure, all fingers should undergo vigorous range of motion exercises [1, 5, 6, 21].

Cross-Finger Flap

Indications
This method is appropriate for fingertip injuries 1.5×2.5 cm^2 or larger with exposed tendon or bone that require full-thickness coverage. Patients must have an uninjured adjacent digit. Similar to the thenar flap, this method is unsuitable for older patients or those who have preexisting arthritis or joint contractures (Fig. 19.10).

Advantages
When compared to the thenar flap, the cross-finger flap is larger and more versatile. Though there is still a risk for PIP joint contractures, the risk is lower than with the thenar flap.

Disadvantages
Though less than with the thenar flap, there is still a risk of PIP joint contractures in older populations. Similarly, this is a two-stage procedure, requiring the injured finger to be immobilized in flexion for approximately 3 weeks between the first and second stage. The cosmesis of this method is inferior to that of the thenar flap due to the necessity of a full-thickness skin graft over the donor site. Additionally, in

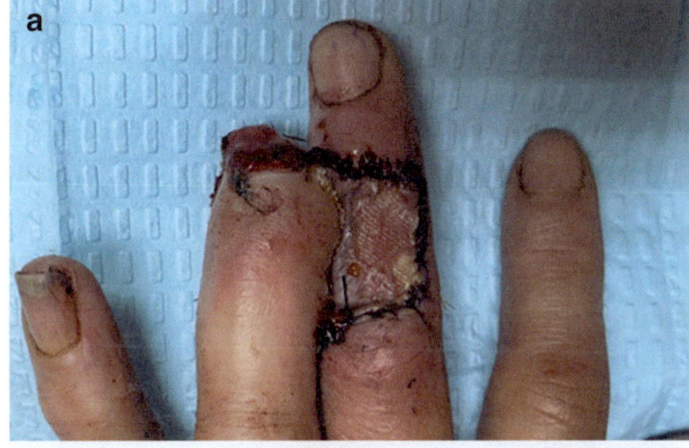
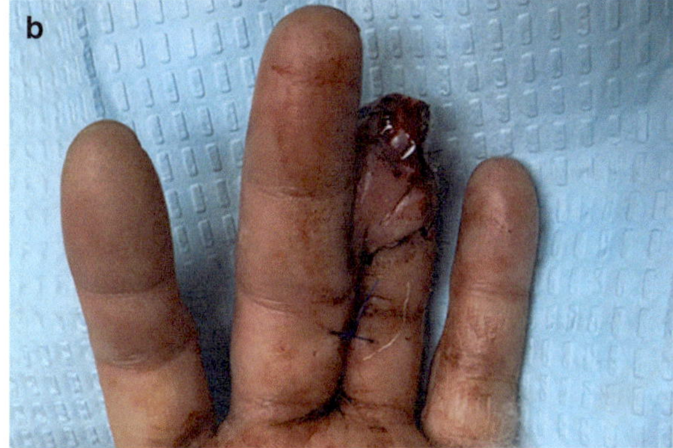

Fig. 19.10 Cross-finger flap. (**a**) Dorsal surface of cross-finger flap after inset. (**b**) Volar surface of cross-finger flap after inset

many people the dorsal finger over the middle phalanx is hair-bearing, which will continue to grow when placed onto the fingertip. For these reasons, the cross-finger flap is used as a last resort for fingertip injuries, but still sees some use in the reconstruction of more proximal digit injuries.

Methods

The recipient site is appropriately debrided and the injured finger should be positioned against the donor finger in the conformation it would be held in after the first stage of the procedure, to ensure an acceptable angle prior to beginning the procedure. The flap is then outlined on the dorsal surface of the middle phalanx of the adjacent finger as a rectangle, approximately 2 mm larger than the defect on all sides. The flap should not cross the DIP or PIP joint and should not extend volarly beyond the level of the neurovascular bundles. The side of the flap adjacent to the injured finger will serve as the hinge. An incision is made along the remaining three edges of the flap and the flap is carefully dissected off, but not penetrating through, the underlying paratenon of the extensor tendon. Subcutaneous veins can be cauterized and contained within the flap. The flap is reflected 180° on its hinge and sutured to the injured site. To cover the donor site defect, a full-thickness skin graft can be harvested from the groin, the volar wrist crease, hypothenar aspect of the hand, or antecubital fossa. The finger is wrapped in a soft dressing and either a volar or dorsal blocking splint for 2–3 weeks. Before the second stage of surgery, perfusion of the flap by the recipient digit can be assessed by placing a tourniquet around the base of the donor digit and observing for punctate bleeding within the flap. If perfusion is acceptable, the second stage of the surgery is performed to divide the flap and separate the two fingers. The skin of the pedicle can be returned to the donor site to cover the lateral defect. As with the thenar flap, the patient should undergo vigorous and early range of motion exercises after the second stage of the surgery to avoid contractures [1–3, 5, 6, 21].

Reverse Homodigital Island Flap

Indications

Fingertip injuries involving both the dorsal and volar surface, especially larger volar oblique amputations in which a lateral or volar V-Y advancement flaps are not an option. This is less reliable for coverage of defects that cross the DIP joint. This flap is also not appropriate for use in patients with a history of vasculitis, peripheral artery disease, or prior surgery on or around the volar surface of the DIP joint. This flap relies on the integrity of both digital arteries, so a digital Allen test should be performed prior to choosing this method to insure the remaining digital artery can perfuse the digit (Fig. 19.11).

Advantages

This is a one-stage procedure that does not have postoperative restrictions and can be used in older patients.

Disadvantages

This method cannot reconstruct large volumes of pulp loss.

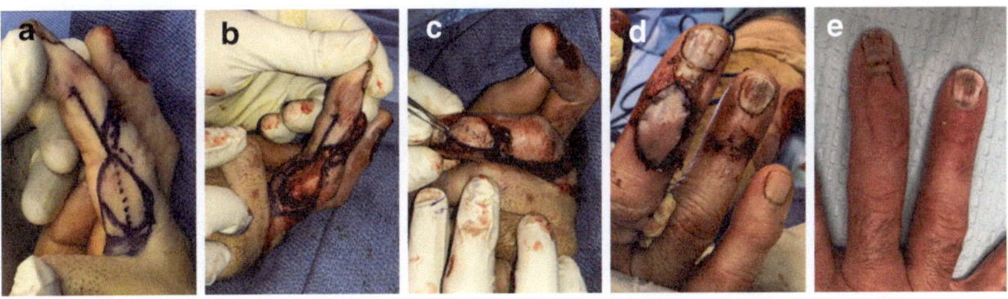

Fig. 19.11 Reverse homodigital island flap. (**a**) Design and incisions for flap. (**b**) Digit after dissection of the flap. (**c**, **d**) Digit after inset of the flap. (**e**) Digit with healed flap

Methods

This flap is perfused by the remaining digital artery via the transverse palmar digital arch just proximal to the DIP joint. The flap is first designed by tracing a template onto the donor surface at the base of the injured digit. The maximum dimensions of the flap are 3.5 cm by 2.5 cm, and the pivot point of the flap should be approximately 5 mm proximal to the DIP joint to avoid injuring the transverse arch. A midaxial incision is made proximal to the flap template to reveal the neurovascular bundle. If necessary, the flap can be adjusted to ensure that it is centered over the bundle. The borders of the flap are then incised and the volar and dorsal flaps are raised in the subdermal plane. The neurovascular bundle is carefully dissected along its course until 5 mm proximal to the DIP joint. The digital artery can be separated from the digital nerve, taking care to preserve the perivascular venules in the surrounding subcutaneous tissue; however, for a sensate flap the digital nerve should also be incorporated into the flap.

The flap and pedicle are elevated and separated from their attachments to the lateral paratenon, mobilizing the pedicle until the pivot point is reached. The flap is placed over the defect. Tunneling under the skin bridge is usually difficult in this case. Instead, an incision can be made in the skin bridge to allow the pedicle to pass through. The flap can also be innervated by connecting the cut end of the digital nerve to the contralateral digital nerve at the defect. The tourniquet can be released at this point to ensure the vascular status of the flap. If the vascular status of the flap seems compromised, the pedicle should be assessed for kinking, twisting, or compression by the skin bridge. If it is acceptable, the flap is sutured in place over the defect. The incision over the skin bridge under which the pedicle rests should be closed very loosely. The donor site can be closed primarily, or with a full-thickness skin graft if primary closure is not possible.

The hand can be splinted for 1 week following surgery, after which range of motion exercises are started. Sutures are removed at 2 weeks [1–3, 5, 6, 21].

Dorsal Metacarpal Artery aka Kite Flap

Indications

This method is appropriate in the reconstruction of thumb tip injuries where there is soft tissue and digital nerve loss with or without exposed bone (Fig. 19.12).

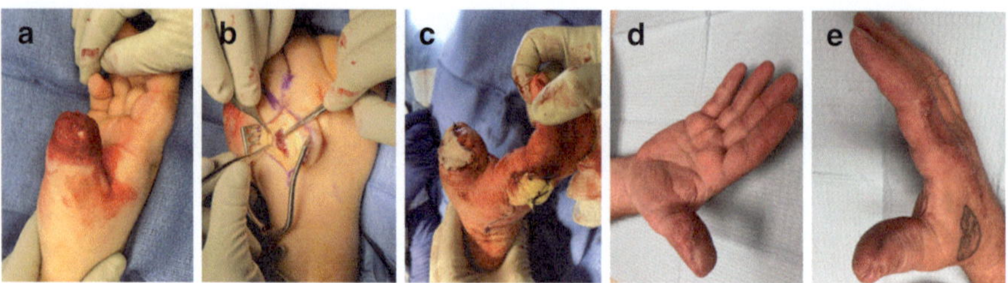

Fig. 19.12 First dorsal metacarpal artery flap. (**a**) Thumb pulp injury amenable to FDMA flap. (**b**) Design of flap. (**c**) Flap inset (**d, e**) healed FDMA flap in different patients

Advantages
This method provides reliable sensation and does not require sacrifice of the digital artery. The donor site is also more esthetically pleasing when compared to the neurovascular island flap.

Disadvantages
The secondary defect requires a skin graft for closure. Additionally, there is a risk of flap necrosis if the pedicle becomes constricted.

Methods
Because the donor site of this flap is supplied by the first dorsal metacarpal artery, a Doppler should be performed to trace the course of the artery, which will usually be located in the first dorsal interosseous fascia over the index metacarpal region (Fig. 19.12). When templating the flap over the dorsal phalanx of the proximal phalanx of the index finger, care should be taken to not allow the flap to cross the PIP joint. Incisions can be made at the borders of the flap and dissection of the pedicle can proceed proximally along the previously Doppler-traced course of the artery. Instead of exposing the pedicle, it is safer to incorporate a small strip of sagittal band and interosseous fascia with the overlying subcutaneous tissue, which also may include branches of the radial sensory nerve and subcutaneous veins. As the flap and pedicle are elevated along the plane overlying the paratenon, care must be taken not to damage the paratenon.

After the flap and pedicle are adequately elevated, a subcutaneous tunnel is bluntly dissected along the ulnar aspect of the thumb and the flap is passed through. The subcutaneous tunnel can be incised to alleviate pressure on the pedicle or to increase the area for flap inset. The flap is sutured in place and the tourniquet is released to assess vascular status. If the vascular status seems compromised, the pedicle should be assessed for twisting or kinking. The donor defect can be covered with a full-thickness skin graft.

The hand is splinted after the surgery, with a portion of the flap visible to monitor vascular status in the days following surgery. A full range of motion can begin at the time of suture removal, typically 2 weeks following surgery [1–3, 5].

Heterodigital Island Flap

Indications
This method is used in severe soft tissue injuries involving large portions of the volar surface of the thumb. In cases of irreparable damage to the digital nerve, this method can restore some sensory function (Fig. 19.13).

Advantages
It provides sensate and glabrous coverage to the tip of thumb and brings a reliable vascular supply.

Disadvantages
This method sacrifices a digital artery and can result in hypertrophic scarring around the donor site. If a large donor site is taken, the lack of pulp padding can make the site uncomfortable. In some cases, patients also report the so-called double sensitivity, where sensation is felt at both the donor and recipient site. Patients also sometimes complain of hyperesthesia, cold intolerance, and reduction in sensation over time.

Methods
Prior to beginning this procedure, a Doppler should be performed on the donor digit and the neighboring digit in the ulnar direction to ensure adequate flow from both the ulnar and radial digital artery. The donor site for this procedure is usually ulnar aspect of the middle finger (Fig. 19.13). If there is a median nerve deficit, the ulnar border of the ring finger can be used instead, although with slightly less reach than the middle finger. The thumb tip is debrided and a template of the flap is traced on the donor surface. Depending on how much tissue is needed to reconstruct the defect, the donor site can donate the entire ulnar-sided digital pulp up to the volar midline of the digit, proximally to the MCP crease, and distally within a few millimeters from the end of the finger pulp. To dissect the neurovascular pedicle within the palm, the palm is incised with Brunner incisions, which will reduce the risk of a flexion contracture. At the level of webspace, the radial digital artery to the adjacent

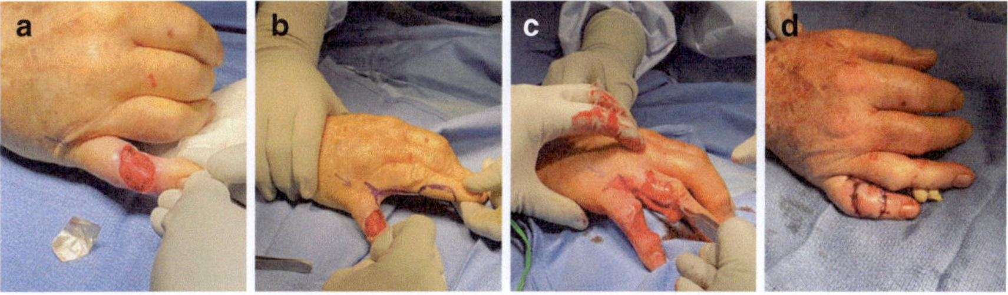

Fig. 19.13 Heterodigital island flap. (**a**) Small finger with injury amenable to heterodigital island flap. (**b**) Incisions for a ring finger donor site. (**b**) Elevation of flap. (**c**) Flap inset. (**d**) Final inset of flap over defect

finger is found and ligated, which will allow for increased reach of the flap along the common digital artery. Dissection is then continued proximally to the level of the superficial arch. When the flap and pedicle are raised, it should be dissected off the underlying flexor sheath carefully, and a perivascular cuff of tissue should be preserved, as the venous drainage is contained here.

To move the flap onto its donor site, a tunnel is created subcutaneously under the thenar skin bridge, and the flap is carefully passed through (using a Penrose drain as a guide if necessary). The flap is sutured loosely in place, and the tourniquet is released to assess vascular status. If the vascular status seems compromised, the pedicle should be assessed for twisting or kinking, as well as for compression under the thenar skin bridge. Releasing constricting bands of palmar fascia in the palm may help in this troubleshooting. After vascular status is confirmed, the donor site can be covered with a full-thickness skin graft.

The hand is splinted after the surgery, with a portion of the flap visible to monitor vascular status in the days following surgery. A full range of motion can begin at the time of suture removal, typically 2 weeks following surgery [1–3, 5, 6, 21].

Revision Amputation

Indications

Revision amputation is indicated in individuals with unsalvageable amputation injuries at any level along the finger. If length of the digit cannot be preserved due to trauma or infection, revision amputation with shortening of the phalanx can allow for immediate wound closure.

Advantages

Terminalizing a digit avoids a local or regional flap and depending on the situation can still result in a very functional digit. Amputations at or distal to the DIP joint were noted to have largely normal sensation and an average PIP joint arc of 94° [23].

Disadvantages

Terminalizing a digit can result in a poor or obvious deformity, emphasized in part by the lack of nailbed on the digit. If the nailbed is not appropriately ablated, there is a chance of forming a painful or esthetically displeasing hook-nail or nail horn deformity. Some patients experience cold intolerance. Though care is taken during the amputation to prevent symptomatic neuroma formation, neuromas are very likely to form and some can become symptomatic and painful.

Methods

Following distal bone loss, the shape and contour of the amputation stump should be shaped to resemble a tuft. This can be accomplished by rongeuring the volar and lateral condylar prominences. The digital nerves should be dissected and cut under tension so that the neuromas which will likely form do not form at the scar site. Similarly, the flexor tendon/s should be cut under traction and allowed to retract.

The nailbed should be appropriately ablated of any germinal matrix to prevent the formation of a hook-nail deformity [1–3, 6].

Other Options for Soft Tissue Coverage

In some cases, neither local nor regional flaps are amenable options for a particular patient's fingertip injury. Groin, chest, and cross-arm flaps are two-phase procedures similar to the thenar flap and can be considered in some patients, but have similar problems related to the period of immobilization.

There has been some evidence that extensive fingertip injuries with exposed bone or tendon in patients with vascular disease of poor donor tissue that are not appropriate for regional flaps can be treated with acellular dermal matrices. In this method, the wound bed is thoroughly debrided and an acellular dermal matrix is placed directly on the exposed bone or tendon and secured in place. A compressive dressing or negative-pressure device is placed on the wound for 3–4 weeks, after which a full or partial thickness skin graft is overlaid on the wound for final coverage. Several studies have found that this method leads to successful skin graft incorporation without need for intervention within 1 year [24, 25].

Current methods in microsurgery have allowed for free flaps to become an option for fingertip reconstruction. However, for the small space of a fingertip, free flaps are often complicated by bulky appearance, donor site morbidity, and unpredictable flap survival rates.

Section V: Distal Phalanx Fractures

Classification

Distal phalanx fractures can be described in a number of ways. Chen and Schneider [26] divide distal phalanx fractures into three categories: distal-tuft fractures, central-shaft fractures, and proximal-articular fractures. Tuft fractures can be either a simple transverse fracture or a comminuted fracture. Shaft fractures are usually due to crush or direct impact injuries and are usually transverse. Articular fractures are the most varied in presentation, but generally affect the volar rim, dorsal rim, or are transphyseal in the skeletally immature population.

Palmar articular fractures can be described using the Wehbé and Schneider classification system to specify the degree of DIP joint involvement (Table 19.2) [29]. This classification is useful when describing mallet fractures and determining indications for treatment.

Osteosynthesis of intraarticular distal phalangeal fractures, mallet fractures, and jersey finger injuries is beyond the scope of this chapter. In general, fixation of intraarticular fractures of the distal phalanx is indicated when the size of the fracture is large enough to destabilize the joint, leading to subluxation on lateral or PA imaging. Nonoperative treatment of stable injuries is successful in most cases. Similarly, skeletal fixation of shaft and tuft fractures is rarely indicated, due to the stability provided by the dense fibrous interconnections of the fingertip which stabilize the phalanx.

Table 19.2 Management guidelines for distal phalanx fractures

Area of injury	Type	Description	Management
Tuft	Closed fracture	Fracture with no exposed bone. Visualized on radiograph as a simple transverse fracture at the tip of the distal phalanx or a comminuted fracture	Decompress subungual hematoma for pain control and to ensure there is no obscured open fracture. Then treat the soft tissue component of injury and splint for approximately 2 weeks Rehabilitation is essential and should focus on DIP joint range of motion exercises and desensitization of healed soft tissue
			Repeat radiographs after healing often show no evidence of bony union, even if the area of injury is clinically stable and well-functioning and thus have little utility after confirming the initial diagnosis
	Comminuted open fracture	Fracture with exposed bone, with many small bone fragments connected by phalangeal periosteum or by the fibrous septations of the pulp	Substantial injuries should undergo surgical debridement of necrotic tissue and bone fragments followed by 5 days of oral antibiotics. Indications for phalangeal shortening are discussed in section "Section V: Distal Phalanx Fractures" of this chapter
			Stability and proper alignment of the injury can be achieved by placing a small 0.8 mm wire or intradermic needle through the phalanx
			Comminuted tuft fractures may progress to pseudarthrosis, which might require a second surgery to excise a bone fragment. The fingernail has a major stabilizing effect, so pseudoarthrosis may also be mitigated when the whole nail has regrown
	Longitudinal open fracture	Fracture with exposed bone. Radiographs show a longitudinal fracture of the tuft	Substantial injuries should undergo surgical debridement of necrotic tissue and bone fragments followed by 5 days of oral antibiotics
			Cerclage using 4-0 PDS can increase contact between the two fragments of the tuft and mitigate downstream risk of a split phalanx. The nailbed overlying the fracture can be closed primarily using 6-0 Monocryl and a cutaneous suture or by creating a local flap (see section "Section IV: Soft Tissue Reconstruction" for a discussion about local flap options and indications)
			Longitudinal fractures may progress to pseudoarthrosis or develop into a split phalanx, which may require a second surgery to place an intermediate bone graft into the split phalanx. The fingernail has a major stabilizing effect, so pseudoarthrosis may also be mitigated when the whole nail has regrown

Shaft	Nondisplaced closed fractures	Sufficient soft tissue stability over the site of the fracture	Nondisplaced closed fractures can be treated with protective splinting or immediate mobilization depending on the location and activity of the patient. In longitudinal injuries and distal transverse shaft fractures, daytime mobilization with nighttime dorsal splinting for 3–4 weeks is preferable as long as the patient is not performing manual labor. If the patient is performing manual labor, has substantial pain, or if the fracture is in the middle or distal third of the diaphysis, continuous dorsal splinting for 3–4 weeks is preferable Prior to splinting, any soft tissue component of the injury should be treated. After splinting, rehabilitation should focus on DIP joint range of motion
	Displaced closed fracture	Characterized by significant soft tissue injury and instability without any open bone exposure	Displaced closed fractures should be treated surgically when bone-on-bone contact is noted to be insufficient or if the dorsal cortex displacement will lead to ungual deformity Surgical fixation is achieved using divergent percutaneous wiring after manual axial compression. The wires are introduced under the distal nail edge under fluoroscopic control to about 1–2 mm. The DIP joint should not be immobilized. If the fracture is also juxtaepiphyseal, performing a temporary arthrodesis can contribute to additional stability
	Displaced open fracture	Characterized by significant soft tissue injury and instability	Open fractures should be thoroughly cleaned and irrigated before fixation is attempted, and patients should receive antibiotic therapy. Internal splinting can be done using either two Kirschner wires or 20-gauge hypodermic needles drilled across the fracture site in opposite directions. The first wire should be placed axially and the second obliquely. The nailbed is then sutured, but the nail is not usually replaced as there is a risk of infection. The internal splint can stay in place for 3–4 weeks Injuries resulting in loss of bone (due to an industrial accident, etc.) can be treated with a cement spacer kept in place with wire placed axially. After several weeks, a second surgery replaces the cement spacer with corticocancellous bone graft from the radius

(continued)

Table 19.2 (continued)

Area of injury	Type	Description	Management
Articular	Palmar (Jersey finger injuries)	Fracture of the palmar surface of the base of the distal phalanx causing avulsion of the FDP tendon. Clinical presentation is pain at or proximal to the DIP joint and loss of DIP joint flexion	Theoretically, when the FDP tendon has retracted into the palm, surgical reattachment of the FDP should occur as soon as possible, and no later than 1 week after the injury. When the FDP tendon has not retracted more proximally than the PIP joint, surgical repair can be performed as late as 4 weeks after the injury. However, in practice is often difficult to ascertain the exact location of the avulsed tendon so repair should always be done as early as possible
		Radiographically, a fracture fragment will be visualized on the palmar plate of the base of the distal phalanx. A small bony fragment attached to the avulsed tendon might be visible proximally, indicating how far the tendon has avulsed, but this is not always seen	Surgical repair is done by placing sutures in the tendon and passing it through the sheath back to the base of the distal phalanx. The tendon can be affixed to the base using suture anchors or, if the base will not support suture anchors, drill holes and nails. If the repair needs to be further reinforced, a pull-out Prolene suture can be placed through the fingernail for 6 weeks
			The hand is splinted in an intrinsic-plus position following the procedure. Rehabilitation includes passive flexion exercises and active extension to the limits of the splint within a week of repair, After 2 weeks, joint-blocking exercises for the PIP and DIP joints and tendon-gliding exercises can begin. Partial resistance is added at 6 weeks and full resistance can be started at 12 weeks
	Dorsal (bony mallet finger fractures)	Fracture of the dorsal surface of the base of the distal phalanx causing avulsion of the extensor tendon. Clinical presentation is pain at or proximal to the DIP joint and loss of DIP joint extension, with the fingertip passively held in 45° of flexion at the DIP joint	Management of bony mallet finger injuries is somewhat more controversial. Generally, a dorsal splint alone will yield satisfactory results if the injury does not involve subluxation of the DIP joint and involves less than one-third of the articular surface
			In injuries where there is joint subluxation or where greater than one-third of the articular surface is involved, wire stabilization is indicated. If closed reduction is possible, then two 0.028-in. Kirschner wires can be used to affix the fracture fragments in place. If closed reduction is not possible, open fixation with Kirschner wire, screw, or plate can be undertaken depending on the size of the avulsion fragment. After fixation, a dorsal splint should still be used
		Radiographically, a fracture fragment may be visualized on the dorsal plate of the base of the distal phalanx	In all cases, splints should remain on the finger full-time for 6–8 weeks. Splints should not traverse the PIP joint, so that early movement across that joint can be initiated. After 6–8 weeks, gentle DIP flexion exercises can begin. If the patient is involved in manual labor or extreme activity, night splinting is recommended for another 4 weeks
	Seymour's juxta-epiphyseal fracture	Transverse extraarticular fracture affecting the growth cartilage of a child's distal phalanx. This injury is generally due to hyperflexion. This is a Salter type I or II injury. Clinically, this will appear as a mallet finger with possible disruption of the nailbed by the avulsed bone	In closed fractures, a closed reduction can be used to treat the injury, followed by 4 weeks of dorsal splinting
		Radiographs will show a classic image of an angulated distal phalanx with dorsal protrusion	When the reduction cannot be performed due to nailbed disruption, the nail should first be removed. The site should be thoroughly cleaned and debrided and then fixed with a 0.8 mm axial wire. The nail matrix should be repaired using a 6-0 Monocryl and the nail can be replaced
			Complications can include premature epiphyseal arrest or pseudarthrosis. If there is painful pseudarthrosis after time has passed and the nail has regrown, a second surgery can be performed freshen the bone ends, add a bone graft, and stabilize the fracture site with a compressive screw or two Kirschner wires

Summary of management guidelines for distal phalanx fractures [26–28]

Section VI: Rehabilitation

Following initial management of the fingertip injury, wound care is focused on keeping the area protected in order to allow healing in a semi-moist environment. Non-adherent dressings are key to avoid re-injury to area and prevent significant patient discomfort with dressing changes. Non-adherent Vaseline based dressings—such as Xeroform (Covidien, Minneapolis, MN) and Adaptic gauze (Johnson & Johnson, New Brunswick, NJ)—may be utilized; however, care should be taken to avoid maceration of surrounding healthy tissues. A gauze dressing is placed over the non-adherent base layer and secured either with tape or tube gauze. Tube gauze should be applied carefully, as overzealous and tight application will lead to a tourniquet dressing. Custom thermoplastic-based cap splints can be fashioned to protect and immobilize the distal interphalangeal joint for a short course immediately following the injury. Active range of motion should be initiated within the first week to avoid stiffness. Early motion should be avoided in injuries with associated non-tuft distal phalangeal fractures, as this will require a period of immobilization to allow for fracture healing. After most local flaps, range of motion exercises can begin at 10–14 days, and in cross-finger flaps the PIP joints and donor DIP joint can be mobilized through a limited arc of motion 10–14 days after the flap is placed. After the flap is divided, the PIP joint may be immediately engaged in active range of motion exercises. Stiffness following thenar or cross-finger flaps is common, especially in the adult population, and prolonged therapy with static-progressive splinting may be necessary to achieve full extension following flap division in this patient population [6].

References

1. Kakar S. Chapter 49: Digital amputations. In: Wolfe S, Hotchkiss N, Pederson WC, Kozin SH, Cohen MS, editors. Green's operative hand surgery. 7th ed. Philadelphia, PA: Elsevier; 2017. p. 1708–52.
2. Dautel G. Chapter 13: Nail trauma. In: Merle M, Dautel G, editors. Emergency surgery of the hand. 1st ed. Amsterdam: Elsevier; 2016. p. 332–43.
3. Dautel G. Chapter 9: Finger and hand soft tissue defects. In: Merle M, Dautel G, editors. Emergency surgery of the hand. 1st ed. Amsterdam: Elsevier; 2016. p. 156–267.
4. Flint MH. Some observations on the vascular supply of the nail bed and terminal segments of the finger. Br J Plast Surg. 1955;8:186–95.
5. Mailey B, Neumeister MW. Chapter 6: The fingertip, nail plate and nail bed: anatomy, repair, and reconstruction. In: Chang J, Neligan PC, editors. Plastic surgery E-book: volume 6: hand and upper extremity. 4th ed. Philadelphia, PA: Elsevier Health Sciences; 2018. p. 122–46.
6. Schick C. Chapter 10: Nail bed and fingertip injuries. In: Principles of hand surgery and therapy. 3rd ed. Philadelphia, PA: Elsevier; 2017. p. 193–205.
7. Allen MJ. Conservative management of finger tip injuries in adults. Hand. 1980;12(3):257–65.
8. Evans DM, Bernadis C. A new classification for fingertip injuries. J Hand Surg. 2000;25(1):58–60.
9. Zook EG, Guy RJ, Russell RC. A study of nail bed injuries: causes, treatment, and prognosis. J Hand Surg [Am]. 1984;9:247–52.

10. Dean B, Becker G, Little C. The management of the acute traumatic subungual haematoma: a systematic review. Hand Surg. 2012;17:151–4.
11. Seaberg DC, Angelos WJ, Paris PM. Treatment of subungual hematomas with nail trephination: a prospective study. Am J Emerg Med. 1991;9(3):209–10.
12. Roser SE, Gellman H. Comparison of nail bed repair versus nail trephination for subungual hematomas in children. J Hand Surg [Am]. 1999;24:1166–70.
13. Ogunro O, Ogunro S. Avulsion injuries of the nail bed do not need nail bed graft. Tech Hand Up Extrem Surg. 2007;11(2):135–8.
14. O'Shaughnessy M, McCann J, O'Connor TP, Condon KC. Nail re-growth in fingertip injuries. Ir Med J. 1990;83(4):136–7.
15. Hoigné D, Hug U, Schürch M, Meoli M, Von Wartburg U. Semi-occlusive dressing for the treatment of fingertip amputations with exposed bone: quantity and quality of soft-tissue regeneration. J Hand Surg. 2014;39(5):505–9.
16. Mennen U, Wiese A. Fingertip injuries management with semiocclusive dressing. J Hand Surg. 1993;18(4):416–22.
17. Sturman MJ, Duran RJ. The late results of fingertip injuries. J Bone Joint Surg Am. 1963;45:289–98.
18. Holm A, Zachariae L. Fingertip lesions: an evaluation of conservative treatment versus free skin grafting. Acta Orthop Scand. 1974;45:382.
19. Eberlin KR, Busa K, Bae DS, et al. Composite grafting for pediatric fingertip injuries. Hand. 2015;10:28–33.
20. Moiemen NS, Elliot D. Composite graft replacement of digital tips. A study in children. J Hand Surg. 1997;22:346–52.
21. Yang G, Kamnerdnakta S, Brown M, Chung KC. Procedure 72: Flap coverage of fingertip injuries. In: Operative techniques: hand and wrist surgery. 3rd ed. Philadelphia, PA: Elsevier; 2017. p. 655–64.
22. O'Brien B. Neurovascular island pedicle flaps for terminal amputations and digital scars. Br J Plast Surg. 1968;21:258–61.
23. Wang K, Sears ED, Shauver MJ, Chung KC. A systematic review of outcomes of revision amputation treatment for fingertip amputations. Hand. 2013;8(2):139–45.
24. Taras JS, Sapienza A, Roach JB, Taras JP. Acellular dermal regeneration template for soft tissue reconstruction of the digits. J Hand Surg [Am]. 2010;35(3):415–21.
25. Weigert R, Choughri H, Casoli V. Management of severe hand wounds with Integra® dermal regeneration template. J Hand Surg. 2011;36:185.
26. Chen F, Schneider LH. Fractures of the distal phalanx. Oper Tech Orthop. 1997;7(2):107–15.
27. Merle M, Jager T. Chapter 7: Metacarpal and phalangeal fractures. In: Merle M, Dautel G, editors. Emergency surgery of the hand. 1st ed. Philadelphia, PA: Elsevier; 2016. p. 100–47.
28. Schuler MS, Roskosky M, Kinney J, Elstad Z. Chapter 2: Phalangeal fractures and interphalangeal joint injuries. In: Principles of hand surgery and therapy. 3rd ed. Philadelphia, PA: Elsevier; 2017. p. 27–55.
29. Wehbé MA, Schneider LH. Mallet fractures. J Bone Jt Surg Am. 1984;66(5):658–69.

Arthroscopy for Adult Hand Fractures

Jack G. Graham and A. Lee Osterman

Introduction

With the development of the 1.7 mm Watanabe No. 24 arthroscope in 1970, minimally invasive direct visualization of smaller joints became feasible [1]. Chen's landmark 1979 article was the first to describe arthroscopic findings of the wrist, metacarpophalangeal joints, and interphalangeal joints [2]. In the subsequent decades, small joint arthroscopy of the hand has become a valuable addition to the hand surgeon's armamentarium.

While Chen did not specifically describe arthroscopy of the thumb carpometacarpal (CMC) joint, this has arguably become greatest utility of small joint arthroscopy in the hand [2–4]. The thumb CMC joint is notoriously difficult to visualize with an open exposure, due to its saddle joint topography with recessed surfaces and complex ligamentous capsule. Direct arthroscopic visualization of the thumb CMC joint allows for accurate staging of degenerative joint disease and facilitates a variety of well-documented therapeutic interventions depending on osteoarthritis severity [4–8]. Metacarpophalangeal (MCP) joint arthroscopy can also provide diagnostic and therapeutic value. Approximately 70% of patients with rheumatoid arthritis develop inflammatory MCP joint pathology [9–11]. Arthroscopy can prove useful in staging and treating various degrees of inflammatory MCP arthropathy [12–18].

The arthroscopic approaches to the thumb CMC and MCP joints of the hand can also be used to aid in the reduction and fixation of multiple intra-articular fracture types. Classically, many of these fractures have been treated with closed reduction and percutaneous pinning. However, post-reduction fluoroscopic evaluation alone

J. G. Graham (✉)
Department of Orthopaedic Surgery, Thomas Jefferson University Hospital,
Philadelphia, PA, USA

A. L. Osterman
Philadelphia Hand to Shoulder Center, Thomas Jefferson University Hospital,
Philadelphia, PA, USA

J. M. Abzug et al. (eds.), *Pediatric and Adult Hand Fractures*,
https://doi.org/10.1007/978-3-031-32072-9_20

can underestimate residual joint incongruity and malreduction may predispose a patient to post-traumatic arthritis [19]. Direct arthroscopic visualization of fracture reduction is advantageous in judging displacement and rotational malalignment while minimizing damage to the local soft tissues when compared to traditional open techniques. In this chapter, we aim to summarize the role of arthroscopy in the management of intra-articular hand fractures and offer technical pearls gleaned from our own experience.

Intra-Articular Fractures of the Thumb Metacarpal Base

The most common thumb intra-articular fracture occurs at the volar-ulnar base and is named a Bennett fracture, after an Irish Surgeon who originally described it in 1882 [20] (Fig. 20.1). The eponymous Rolando fracture represents a comminuted, intra-articular thumb metacarpal base fracture classically described as having a "Y" or "T" fracture morphology [20] (Fig. 20.2). Contemporarily, *Green's Operative Hand Surgery* textbook refers to any comminuted articular fracture of the base of the thumb metacarpal as a Rolando fracture [21]. These injuries share a common mechanism, due to an axial force applied to the thumb while in a flexed position [22]. The volar-ulnar fragment often remains attached to the trapezium via the anterior oblique ("beak") ligament, while the thumb metacarpal shaft is typically supinated and displaced dorsally, radially, and proximally [22–24]. This deformity is caused by the combined forces of the abductor pollicis longus (APL), extensor pollicis longus (EPL), extensor pollicis brevis (EPB), and adductor pollicis [22].

Gedda classified Bennett fractures into three types [25]. Type 1 represents a large singular ulnar fragment and subluxation of the thumb metacarpal base. Type 2 is associated with an impaction fracture without subluxation of the thumb metacarpal. Type 3 represents a small ulnar avulsion fracture fragment with an

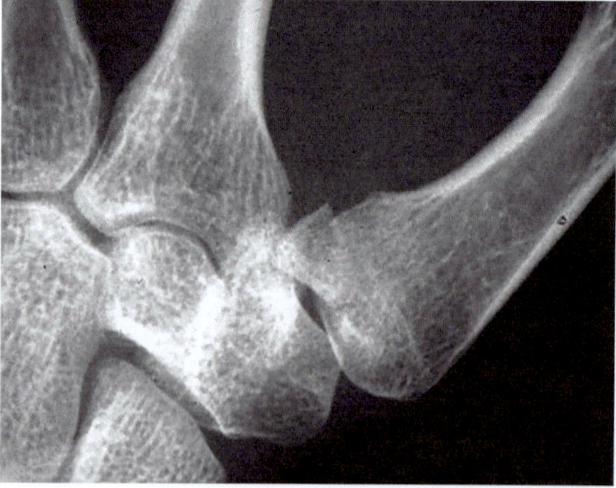

Fig. 20.1 Bennett fracture—a partial articular fracture of the thumb metacarpal volar-ulnar base noted on thumb posteroanterior radiograph

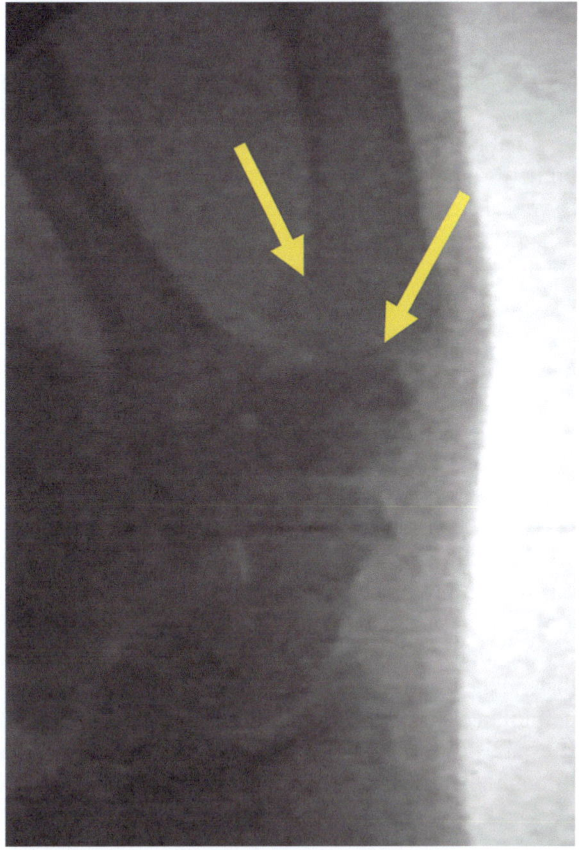

Fig. 20.2 Rolando fracture—a classic three-part intra-articular thumb metacarpal base fracture noted on thumb posteroanterior radiograph

associated metacarpal dislocation [25, 26]. Recognition of these injuries in the acute period is key. Our recommended series of radiographs for injuries involving the base of the thumb metacarpal includes a posteroanterior view of the hand, a lateral view of the thumb, and a Robert's view (true AP) of the thumb [27]. We do not routinely obtain computed tomography (CT) scans. As with any intra-articular fracture, joint congruency and an anatomic reduction is the goal. Malreduction of these fractures can lead to post-traumatic arthritis, narrowing of the first webspace, and significant functional limitations. Operative fixation is indicated in fractures with a joint step off greater than 1 mm or those with residual subluxation [22].

Arthroscopy can aid in the accurate reduction and fixation of Bennett fractures [22, 28–30]. In our experience, some Rolando fractures, such as those with a simple intra-articular split, are also amenable to arthroscopic reduction and percutaneous pinning or screw fixation. Contraindications, as detailed by Solomon and Culp, include chronic injuries, active infection, severely comminuted articular fractures, and ipsilateral upper extremity injuries precluding the use of an arthroscopy tower [22].

Technique

We use a similar technique to that described by Culp and Johnson [28]. All patients are positioned supine on the operating table or stretcher after receiving either regional or general anesthesia. A pneumatic tourniquet is applied to the proximal humerus in order to minimize potential interference with the arthroscopic traction tower. The extremity is prepared and draped in the standard manner and placed on a hand table. Currently, we use the CONMED Extremity Traction Tower for all small joint arthroscopy; however, any commercial upper extremity traction tower is acceptable.

A single sterile finger-trap is applied to the thumb and reinforced using 3M Coban Self-Adherent Wrap prior to application of 5–10 lb of traction (Fig. 20.3). The 1-R (radial to APL) and 1-U portal (ulnar to EPB) sites are marked as well as the courses of the APL and EPB tendons. After tourniquet insufflation to 250 mmHg, an 18-gauge needle is inserted into the thumb CMC joint, which is then distended using 2–3 mL of 0.9% normal saline solution A 2 mm incision is made over the 1-R portal, and after clearing subcutaneous tissue with a small hemostat, a short-barrel 1.9 mm, 30-degree inclination arthroscope is introduced into the joint. Depending on surgeon preference, additional arthroscope size options are available, including 1.5, 1.7, 2.0, 2.3, and 2.5 mm devices [13, 14, 16, 31–35].

The joint can be viewed either dry or with the injection of 5 cm^3 of saline to help distend the joint. Alternatively, a pump system set on low flow can be used. Fluid is helpful in clearing the joint of hematoma and debris. The 1-U portal (ulnar to EPB) is established first. Next, we introduce a 2.0 mm shaver into the thumb CMC joint through the thenar portal (as described by Walsh et al.) to debride fracture

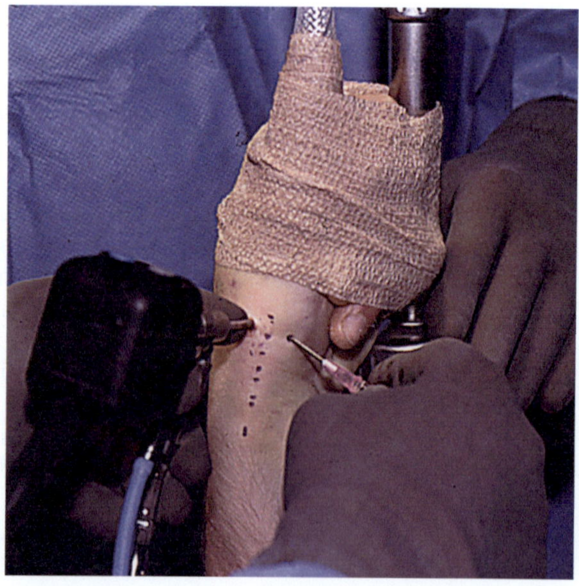

Fig. 20.3 Thumb carpometacarpal joint arthroscopy setup with 1-R and 1-U portal sites

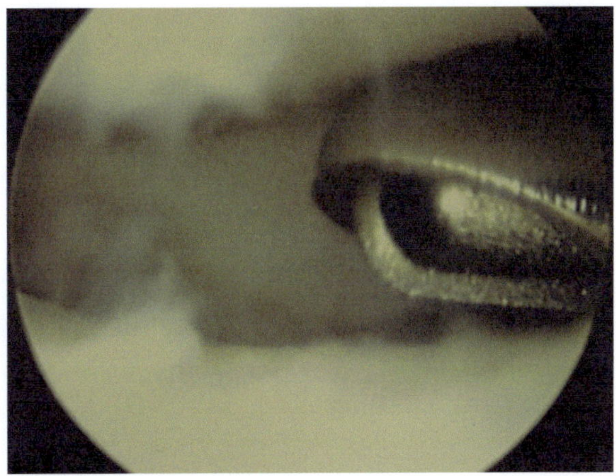

Fig. 20.4 Use of a 2.0 mm shaver through the 1-U portal allows for better visualization of thumb metacarpal base fractures; significant fracture step-off is noted

hematoma, loose cartilaginous fragments, synovium, and frayed tissue (Fig. 20.4) [36]. This allows for better joint visualization to aid in assessment of the fracture. A distinct advantage of the arthroscopic approach is the relative ease with which extrication of any interposed ligamentous or capsular tissue can be performed. These interposed tissues can often block reduction. We recommend visualization from each portal to best appreciate fracture morphology, displacement, and rotation.

A mini C-arm fluoroscopic image intensifier is brought in at a perpendicular angle to the thumb metacarpal long-axis (Fig. 20.5). A small 3-mm probe is then inserted via one of the working portals, and the fracture is carefully manipulated under direct visualization until anatomic reduction of the fragment is achieved (Fig. 20.6). A combination of reduction maneuvers is often helpful, including traction with thumb abduction and extension. Our preferred fixation method is with 0.045-in. Kirschner wires (K-wires), which are inserted percutaneously under mini C-arm guidance, while the fracture is held reduced with the probe (Fig. 20.7). These can also be used in a joystick fashion to aid in the reduction. Arthroscopically aided percutaneous screw fixation of these fractures has also been reported [29, 30]. For added stability if deemed necessary intra-operatively, K-wires can be directed across the base of the first metacarpal and into the trapezium or from the first to the second metacarpal [22]. In Bennett fractures, we recommend using two K-wires for fixation, as a single wire may not prevent loss of reduction and secondary displacement (Fig. 20.8). Additional wires can be added as needed, such as in Rolando fracture (Fig. 20.9). If placing intermetacarpal or trapeziometacarpal wires, the surgeon must be cognizant of thumb position to avoid causing an adduction deformity.

After final confirmation of anatomic reduction with the arthroscope, instruments are removed and K-wires are cut short but remain out of the skin 1–2 cm. Ideally, traction and operative time is kept to less than 1 h. The arthroscopic portal sites are closed with a single simple, interrupted 4-0 nylon suture. At the conclusion of the case, a well-padded short-arm thumb spica splint is applied to the level of the interphalangeal (IP) joint. We emphasize continuing active range of motion (ROM) of

Fig. 20.5 Mini C-arm image intensifier is aimed perpendicular to the long-axis of the thumb metacarpal to allow simultaneous arthroscopy and fluoroscopy

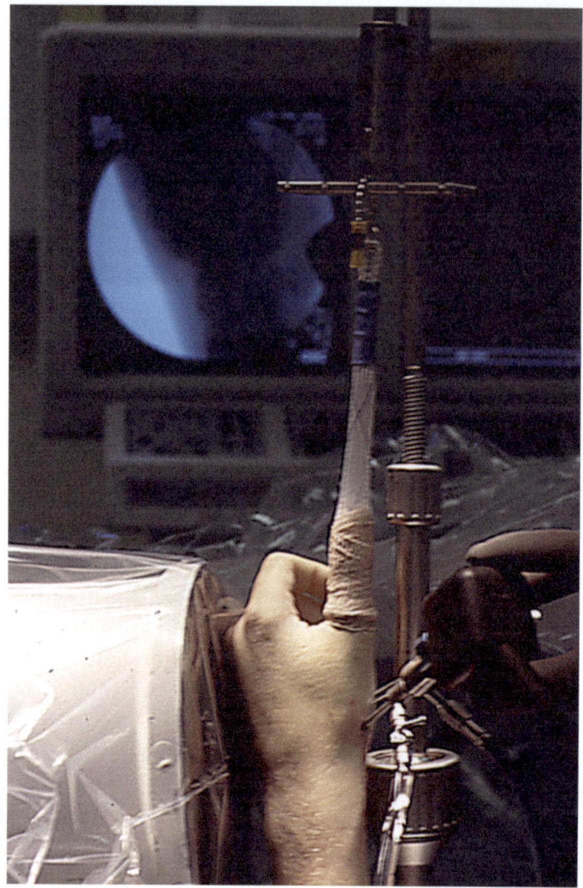

Fig. 20.6 An arthroscopic probe is used to achieve and maintain anatomic reduction of the fracture

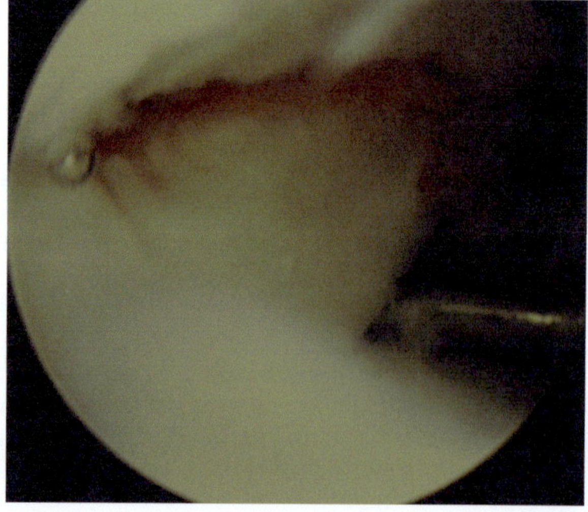

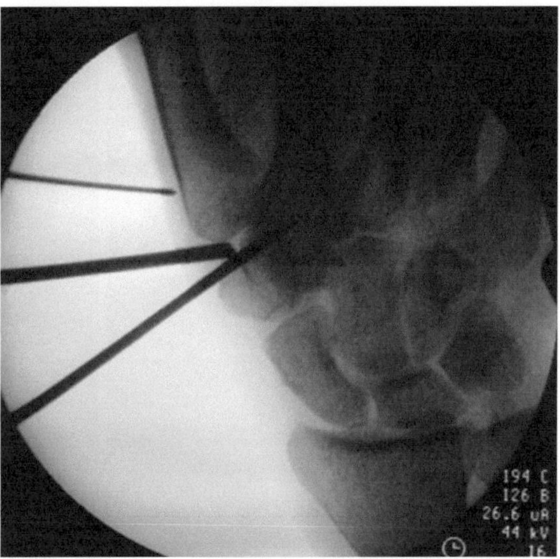

Fig. 20.7 Introduction of a K-wire fixation of an anatomically reduced Bennett fracture using fluoroscopic guidance

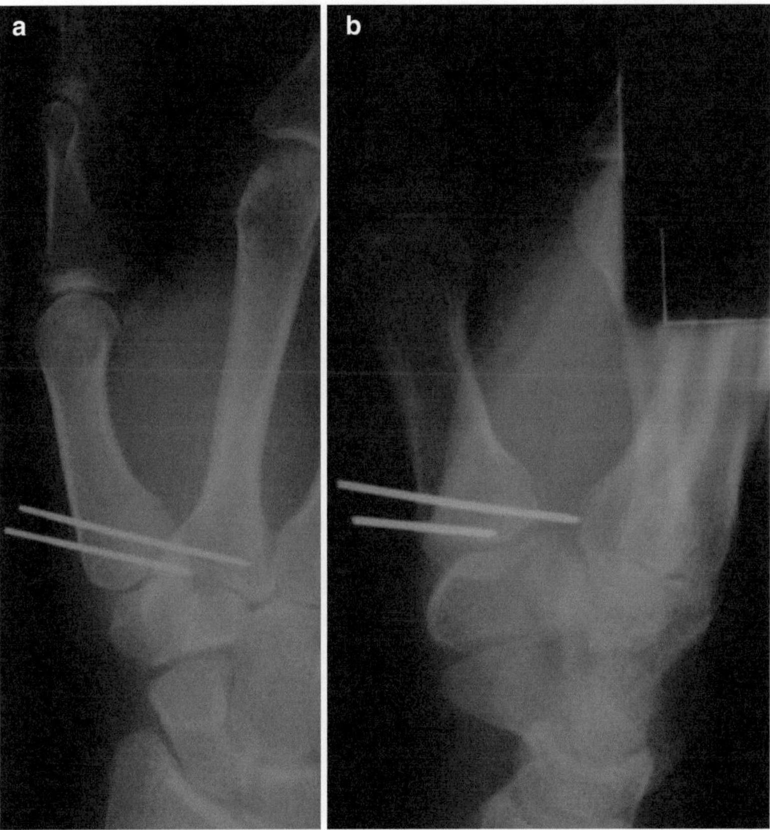

Fig. 20.8 Radiographs demonstrating final fixation of a Bennett fracture with two 0.045-in. K-wires (**a**: posteroanterior view, **b**: lateral view)

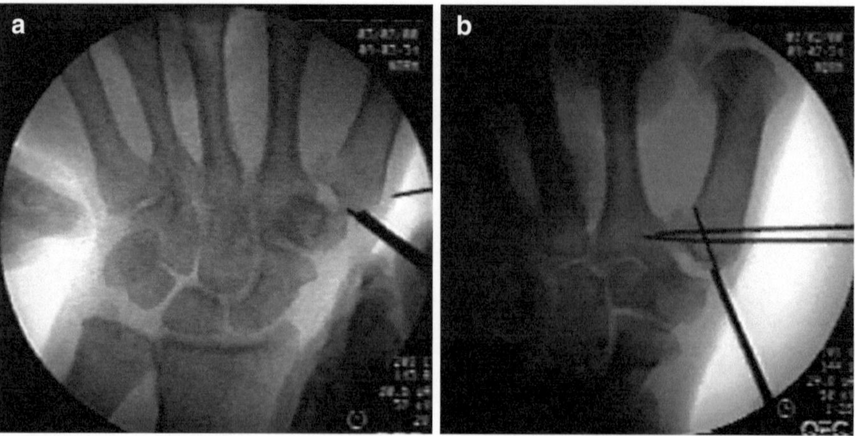

Fig. 20.9 (**a**, **b**) Introduction of multiple K-wires in an anatomically reduced Rolando fracture using fluoroscopic guidance

the uninvolved digits and the thumb IP joint immediately post-operatively. Sutures are removed within 7–14 days, and at that time the patient is transitioned to a removable, custom-molded, forearm-based thumb spica splint. K-wires are typically removed 4 weeks after surgery after adequate healing is demonstrated on follow-up radiographs. Once K-wires are removed, formal therapy is initiated targeting thumb range of motion.

Current Literature

Zemirline and colleagues performed a retrospective study of all Bennett fractures treated within their practice using arthroscopically aided percutaneous screw fixation over a 1-year period [30]. All fractures met Type I or II Gedda classification criteria and two cannulated 2.3 mm compression screws were used in each case ($n = 7$). Anatomic reduction was achieved in all cases. Their review included seven patients (mean age 29 years), although one was lost to follow-up. In the remaining six patients, with a mean follow-up of 4.5 months, dynamometer key pinch and grip strength were 73% and 85% of the contralateral side, respectively. The authors did note that arthroscopically aided anatomic reduction did not guarantee stability of the fixation. Two patients in their cohort were found to have a sub-millimeter step off at final follow-up. An additional two patients presented with secondary displacement of 1–2 mm: One patient with osteoporosis and CMC osteoarthritis and the second patient who was non-compliant with the post-operative protocol and removed his own splint.

Pomares et al. compared outcomes of arthroscopically assisted percutaneous screw fixation versus open reduction internal fixation of Bennett fractures [29]. The authors retrospectively reviewed 21 Bennett fractures with involvement of at least one-third of the joint surface. Among these, 11 patients underwent arthroscopically assisted percutaneous headless compression screw fixation and ten underwent open surgery with one to three non-cannulated, headed compression screws. The authors reported less complications in the arthroscopic group (1 of 11; 9%) than the open group (6 of 10; 60%), as well as a significantly shorter period of immobilization (3.9 weeks vs. 7.1 weeks), and less tourniquet time (42 min vs. 56 min). A single malunion was described in the open group. No significant differences were noted in QuickDASH scores, grip strength, or pinch strength. Mean follow-up (27.6 months vs. 33.3 months) and patient age (37.4 years vs. 30.2 years) were also comparable. The study was inherently limited due to its retrospective design as well as the use of different screw types between groups. These series are limited by sample size and their retrospective designs. The upside in achieving anatomic reduction of first metacarpal base fractures under direct arthroscopic visualization and in a less invasive manner makes this technique an enticing option.

In our own experience, we have seen excellent results. Fifteen fractures of the first metacarpal base (12 Bennett; 3 Rolando) were treated with the arthroscopically assisted reduction and percutaneous K-wire fixation. At most recent follow-up (mean 4.7 years), 14 of the 15 patients (93%) were asymptomatic, with mild weather-related achiness in the single remaining patient. Average pinch strength was found to be 94% that of the contralateral side and no patients required a revision surgery. Each of these patients was treated by the chapter's senior author.

Fractures Involving the Thumb Metacarpophalangeal Joint

The thumb metacarpophalangeal (MCP) joint, which represents a single compartment, is well-suited for arthroscopic intervention [12, 13, 37]. Surface anatomy landmarks are typically easy to identify, and no neurovascular structures are at risk with the common portal placement required to thoroughly evaluate the joint [37]. These factors make intra-articular fractures involving the thumb MCP joint particularly amenable to arthroscopic management.

The thumb MCP joint is a diarthrodial joint and primarily functions through flexion and extension in the sagittal plane, but it does allow for some degree of circumduction, adduction, and abduction [21]. Both static and dynamic structures provide stability to the thumb MCP joint. Dynamic stabilization is provided by the intrinsic and extrinsic tendons crossing the joint. Static stabilizers include the thumb MCP joint's bony architecture, the volar plate, joint capsule, ulnar collateral ligament (UCL), and radial collateral ligament (RCL) [38, 39].

Thumb MCP joint collateral ligament injuries are one of the most common injuries evaluated by hand surgeons [38]. Thumb UCL injuries are approximately 10 times more common than RCL injuries [40]. In UCL injuries, the most common mechanism is a sudden forceful hyperabduction (radial stress) or hyperextension stress to the thumb MCP joint [38–44]. Conversely, the RCL is most often injured due to sudden thumb MCP adduction [38, 45]. Acute UCL ruptures are often referred to as "skier's thumb," as these injuries commonly occur after a fall onto an outstretched hand while the thumb is abducted around a ski pole [46]. "Gamekeeper's thumb" refers to chronic, attritional UCL laxity, which was first described in Scottish gamekeepers who repeatedly hyperextended the necks of wounded rabbits while using the ulnar aspect of their thumb as a fulcrum [47, 48]. These terms are often confused and used interchangeably [48].

While thumb MCP UCL and RCL injuries can be purely ligamentous, associated avulsion fractures are also common. In bony UCL avulsions, the ulnar aspect of the proximal phalanx base is most often involved. Posner et al. performed a retrospective review of 500 surgical thumb MCP collateral ligament injuries. They reported 57 of 362 (16%) UCL injuries had an associated avulsion fracture, 56 (98%) of which involved the ulnar proximal phalanx base [49]. We consider arthroscopic reduction and fixation in any UCL avulsion fracture involving 20% or more of the articular surface and with 2 mm or more of displacement.

Typically, in the setting of a UCL bony avulsion fracture, the ligament itself is intact and a Stener lesion (in which the torn UCL lies superficial to the adductor aponeurosis) is not present [50–52]. However, as reported by Giele and Martin, in rare cases it is possible for minimally displaced bony avulsion and ligamentous tears to occur simultaneously [50]. These "two-level" injuries often have a non-displaced avulsion fragment as swell as a small fleck of bone in the "Stener position." Non-operative management of these rare injuries can result in chronic laxity and hand surgeons must be way of this uncommon variant [50]. In these rare cases, arthroscopic management alone should be avoided.

In 3% of RCL ruptures, Posner and colleagues noted an associated bony avulsion fracture, most often from the base of the proximal phalanx as well [49] (Fig. 20.10). Our operative indications for RCL avulsions are consistent with that of bony UCL avulsions—if the fracture involves 20% or more of the articular surface, has 2 mm of displacement, or is rotated 30 or more degrees, we opt for arthroscopic reduction and percutaneous fixation. Without early surgical intervention of grade III acute RCL tears and RCL avulsions, patients are prone to post-traumatic instability and persistent pain [53].

Technique

Our positioning, tourniquet application, and traction tower setup are the same as detailed in the *Fractures of the Thumb Metacarpal Base* section (Fig. 20.11). The extensor pollicis longus (EPL) and extensor pollicis brevis (EPB) are palpated and clearly marked. Additionally, a depression at the MCP joint line is palpated radial and ulnar to the extensor tendons and thumb MCP portals are planned and marked at these sites. As Berner described, we localize our radial and ulnar portals using 18-gauge needles which are angled slightly distal due to the convexity of the metacarpal head [12]. These are also angled approximately 45° toward the midline to allow for triangulation of the arthroscopic instruments [12]. One to two milliliters

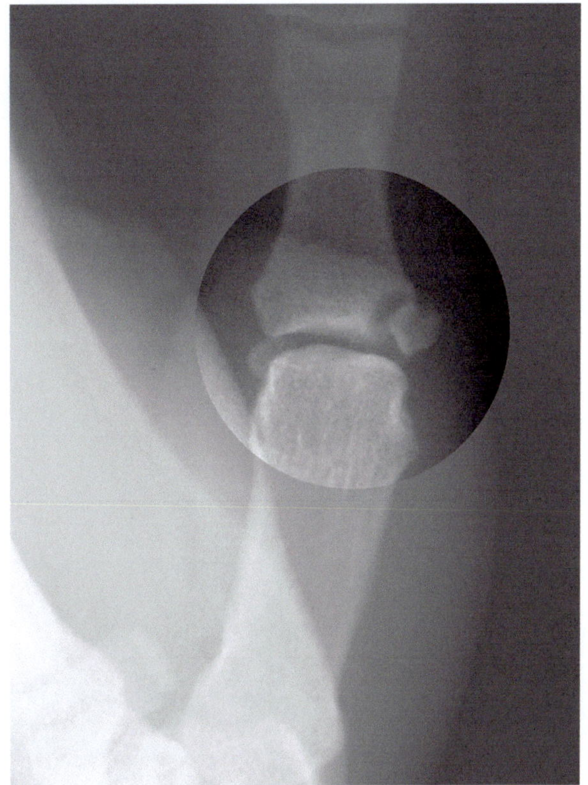

Fig. 20.10 Thumb MCP radial collateral ligament avulsion from the base of the proximal phalanx

(mL) of 0.9% normal saline solution is introduced to distend the MCP joint. Care must be taken to avoid damaging the articular cartilage of the metacarpal head [54]. Depending on the type and location of the fracture, a 1–2 mm incision is made at either the radial or ulnar thumb MCP portal site first. A small, curved hemostat should be used to carefully clear away soft tissue. Careful, atraumatic introduction of a short-barrel 1.9 mm, 30-degree arthroscope is performed. These same precautions should be taken to establish the corresponding working portal (Fig. 20.12).

Using a 2.0 mm arthroscopic shaver, hematoma, synovium, and frayed tissue is carefully cleared to allow for proper visualization of the avulsion fracture (Fig. 20.13). A 3-mm arthroscopic probe is introduced (via the radial portal in RCL avulsions and ulnar portal in UCL avulsions) and used to carefully de-rotate and anatomically reduce the avulsed fragment (Fig. 20.14). Once satisfied with our reduction, we carefully introduce a 0.035 K-wire under arthroscopic view and confirm the tip of the wire is centrally positioned on the fragment itself. A mini C-arm fluoroscopic image intensifier machine is brought in at a perpendicular angle to the thumb metacarpal long-axis.

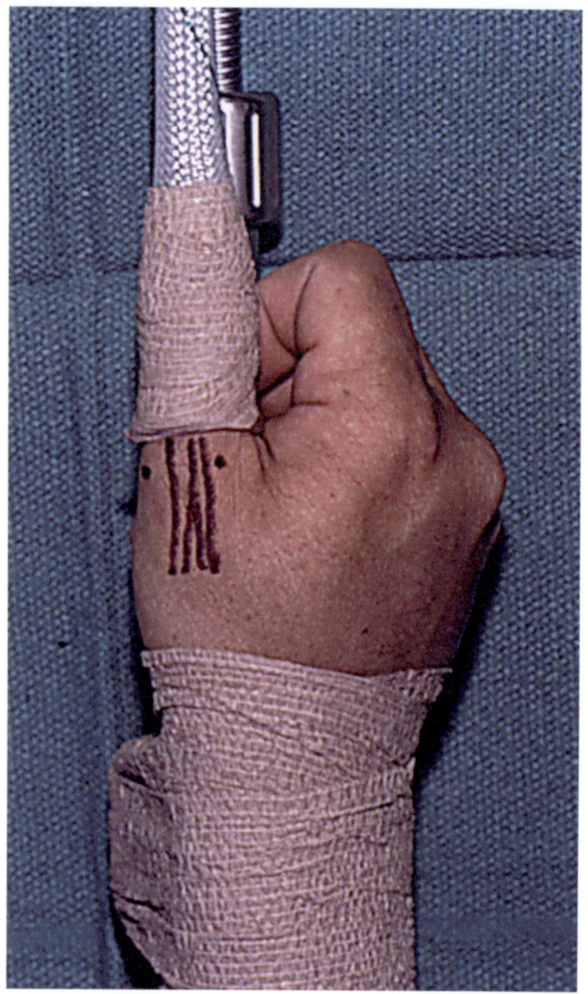

Fig. 20.11 Thumb MCP arthroscopic setup with landmarks (EPL and EPB tendons) and portal sites marked

Under fluoroscopy, the K-wire is advanced with a wire driver through the fragment, as perpendicular to the fracture line as possible. The wire should be advanced to the level of the far cortex without perforating it.

The quality of the reduction is scrutinized via direct fluoroscopic visualization and fluoroscopy. Once satisfied, we cut the K-wire with 1–2 cm of length exposed outside of the skin. An example of arthroscopically aided reduction with percutaneous pinning of an RCL avulsion fracture in one of our patients is depicted in (Fig. 20.15). The arthroscopic portal sites are closed with a single simple, interrupted 4-0 nylon suture. At the conclusion of the cases, a well-padded thumb spica splint is applied. Our post-operative protocol is the same as detailed in the thumb metacarpal base fracture section. K-wires are typically removed 4–6 weeks after surgery once adequate fracture fragment healing is demonstrated on follow-up radiographs.

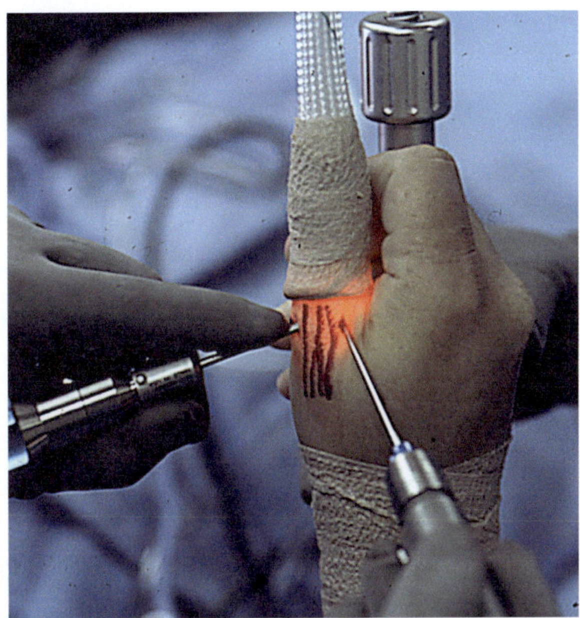

Fig. 20.12 Thumb MCP arthroscopy technique

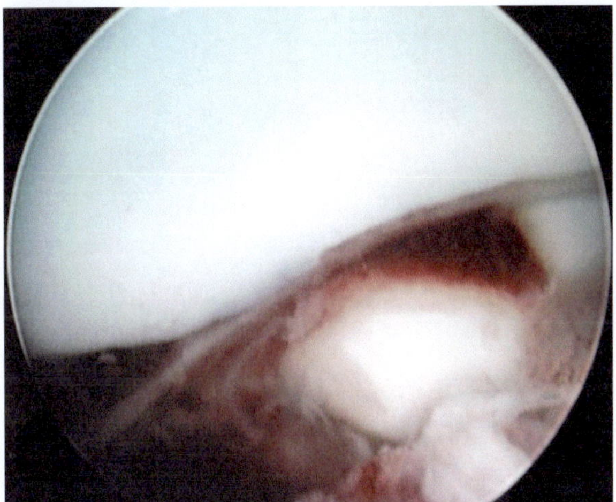

Fig. 20.13 Intra-articular displacement of an RCL avulsion fracture

Current Literature

Badia performed a retrospective study on 12 patients (mean age 18) who sustained thumb MCP UCL avulsion injuries treated with arthroscopically aided reduction and percutaneous pinning [54]. Each of the included injuries resulted from a thumb MCP joint hyperabduction mechanism and all avulsion fractures involved the ulnar proximal phalanx base. The author reported an average fracture displacement of 2.5 mm and 46° of rotation. Fixation consisted of a single 0.035-in. K-wire which

Fig. 20.14 RCL avulsion fracture reduced with arthroscopic probe

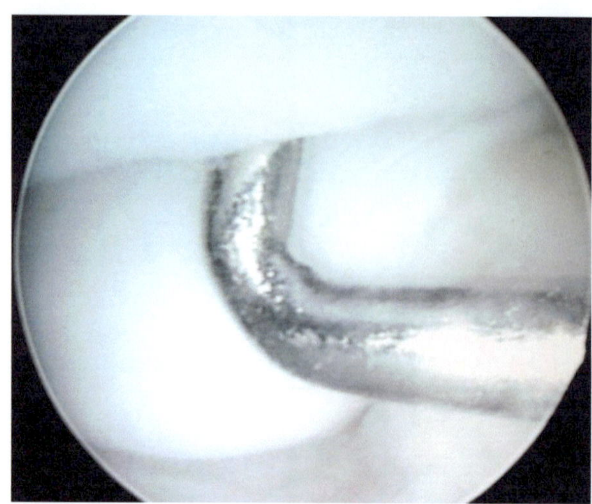

Fig. 20.15 Post-operative posteroanterior radiograph following arthroscopically aided reduction and percutaneous pinning with a single 0.0350-in. K-wire

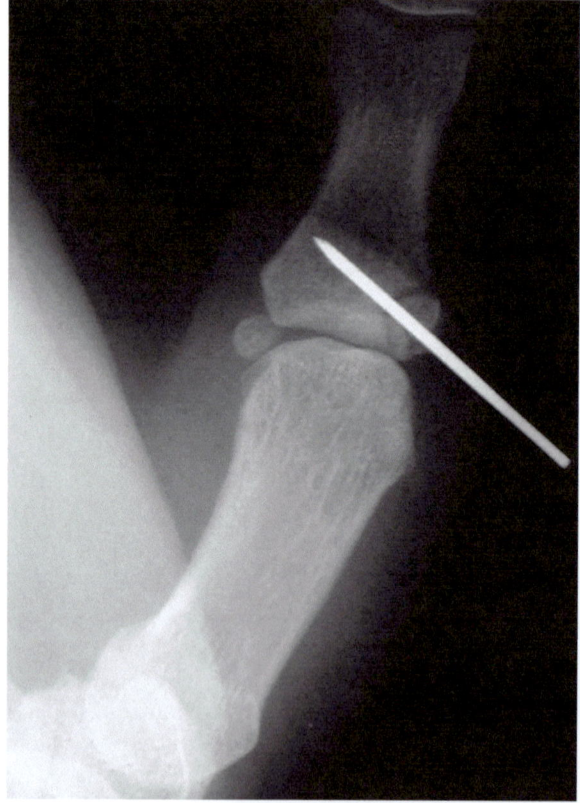

was cut underneath the skin. They reported a mean fragment healing time of 4.3 weeks post-operatively prior to pin removal. At final follow-up (34.2 months), all thumb MCP joints were stable to stress maneuvers in full extension and at 30° of MCP flexion. Mean range of motion was 0–60° of the interphalangeal (IP) joint and 0–88° at the thumb MCP. All patients returned to full activities by 3 months, and there were no reports of residual pain at final follow-up. These encouraging results closely resemble our own anecdotal experience in practice.

Intra-Articular Fractures of the Finger Metacarpophalangeal Joints

Chen first described metacarpophalangeal joint (MCP) arthroscopy in a ground-breaking 1979 article [2]. However, excluding the thumb, arthroscopy of the MCP joints in the remaining digits has been infrequently described. A small number of case series have reported results from diagnostic arthroscopy and synovectomy and/ or biopsy in rheumatoid hands [14–17, 55]. Even fewer studies have discussed arthroscopically assisted reduction and fixation of intra-articular finger MCP fractures [18, 34, 37, 56].

Intra-Articular Finger Metacarpal Head Fractures

Metacarpal head fractures represent only 4–5% of all metacarpal fractures [57]. When evaluating these injuries radiographically, standard posteroanterior, oblique, and lateral views are required. However, it can be difficult to visualize some fractures on these standard views, and evaluation of the articular surface is often improved via the Brewerton view. To obtain this projection, the dorsum of the fingers is placed flat on the X-ray imaging plate, the MCP joints are flexed to 65°, and the beam is angled 15° from ulnar to radial [58, 59].

McElfresh et al. anatomically classified 103 intra-articular metacarpal head fractures from 100 patients into the following categories: epiphyseal fractures, collateral ligamentous avulsions, osteochondral fractures, two-part fractures (sagittal vs. coronal vs. axial plane), comminuted fractures, metacarpal neck fractures with intra-articular extension, fractures with loss of bony substance (machine-associated injuries), and occult fractures leading to avascular necrosis [60]. Comminuted fractures were the most common fracture type (31%) and the index finger was most often injured digit in their series (40%) [60].

Management of intra-articular metacarpal head fractures should be made on a case-by-case basis. Due to a dearth of comparative data, the chosen operative intervention is often a result of surgeon preference and experience with certain techniques [61]. Closed, open, and arthroscopically assisted reduction and fixation are all viable options depending on fracture pattern and displacement. Authors have reported success with a variety of fixation options as well, including standard K-wires, mini-screws, headless compression screws, mini-condylar plates, and bioabsorbable pins [57, 61–68].

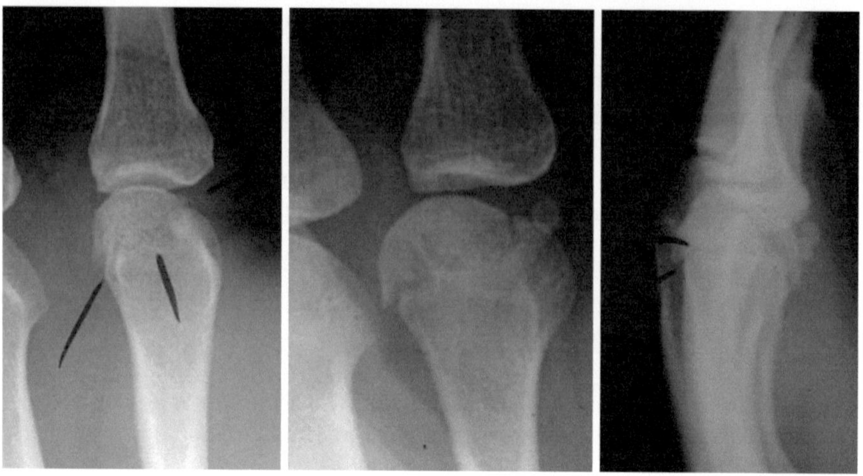

Fig. 20.16 Posteroanterior, oblique, and lateral radiographic views demonstrating a displaced, simple, oblique intra-articular metacarpal head fracture

In metacarpal head fractures with substantial bone loss secondary to saw injuries, Boulas et al. have reported good functional outcomes with osteochondral metatarsophalangeal autografting [69, 70]. Comminuted fractures, depending on severity, may not be amendable to open reduction and internal fixation at all. Alternative treatment options in these cases include arthroplasty or skeletal traction [56, 65]. In fractures well-suited for fixation, many surgeons opt for an open technique, utilizing a longitudinal dorsal approach with an extensor tendon split [57, 66].

Our indications for arthroscopically assisted reduction and percutaneous fixation of metacarpal head fractures include: fracture involvement of 20% or greater of the articular surface, fracture displacement of 1 mm or greater, and simple fracture patterns without comminution which are amendable to fixation with K-wires or screws (Fig. 20.16). We opt to intervene in these cases with the goal of minimizing post-traumatic MCP joint stiffness and functional limitations as much as possible. Computed tomography (CT) scans can be useful for surgical planning purposes (Fig. 20.17).

Technique

Our positioning, tourniquet application, and traction tower setup are the same as detailed previously in this chapter. To access the MCP joint in fingers other than the thumb, we use vertical traction through finger traps applied to the involved digit and one or more adjacent digits (Fig. 20.18). Horizontal traction has been described as an alternative technique [71].

The extensor tendon of the involved finger is palpated and clearly marked. The finger MCP joint line is palpated radial and ulnar to the extensor tendon. Portal localization is marked 1–2 mm ulnar and radial to the extensor tendon. The joint is localized from each portal site using 18-gauge needles which are angled slightly

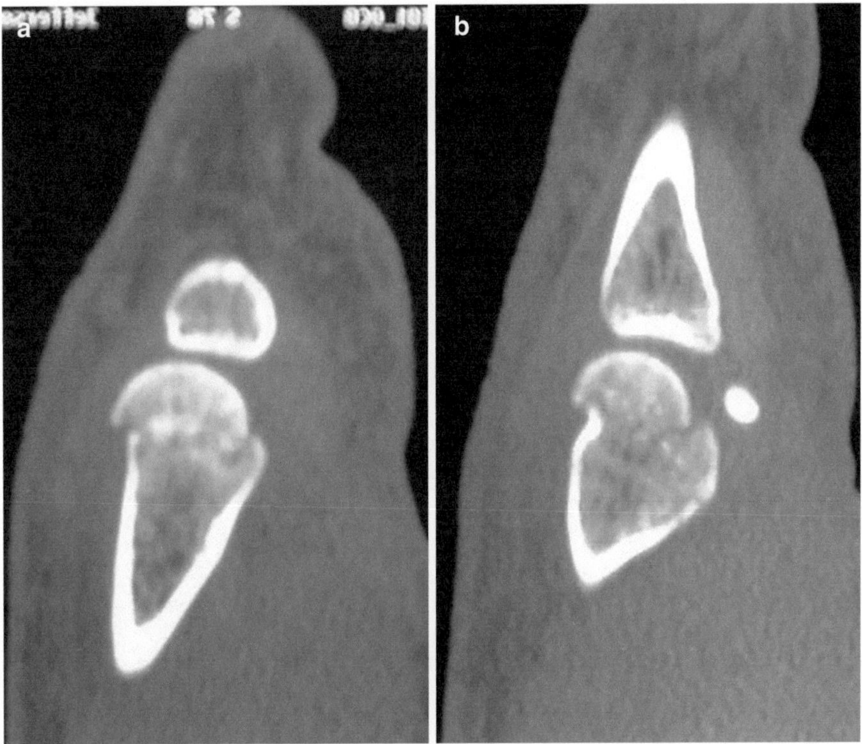

Fig. 20.17 (**a, b**) Coronal and sagittal CT views better visualizing the metacarpal head intra-articular step-off

distal and approximately 45° toward the midline as described previously. The joint is distended in a standard fashion by introducing 1–2 mL of 0.9% normal saline solution. Atraumatic introduction of the arthroscope and instruments through the viewing and working portals is performed as per our standard technique (Fig. 20.19). The 2.0 mm arthroscopic shaver is used to clear debris in the form of hematoma, synovium, and frayed tissue to best visualize the intra-articular finger MCP joint fracture and the degree of displacement (Fig. 20.20).

In metacarpal head fractures, once the fracture is well-visualized, reduction is typically achieved using the 3 mm probe (Fig. 20.21). K-wires can also be used as joysticks to manipulate the fracture fragments as needed. Gentle and precise manipulation of metacarpal head fragments is absolutely necessary to prevent additional chondral damage and mitigate the risk for subsequent avascular necrosis. The mini C-arm fluoroscopic image intensifier is utilized at a perpendicular angle to the metacarpal of the involved finger. We prefer percutaneous fixation with multiple 0.045-in. K-wires, typically in a crossing pattern (Fig. 20.22). Fluoroscopy is utilized while driving the wires across the fracture site in a retrograde fashion (Fig. 20.23). Wires are cut with 1–2 cm of length exposed outside of the skin (Fig. 20.24).

Fig. 20.18 Long finger MCP joint arthroscopic setup with landmarks (extensor tendon) and portal sites marked

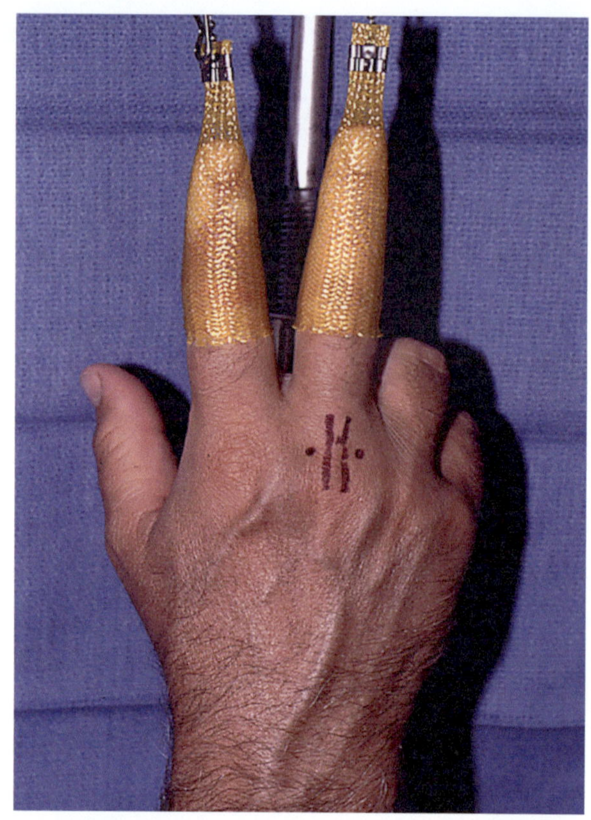

Fig. 20.19 Finger MCP arthroscopy technique

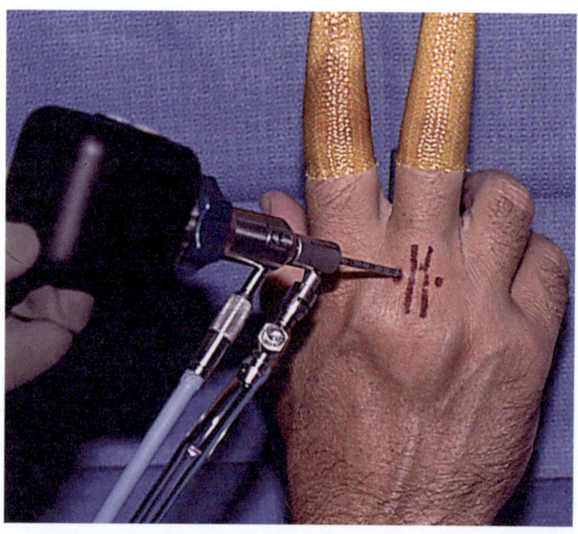

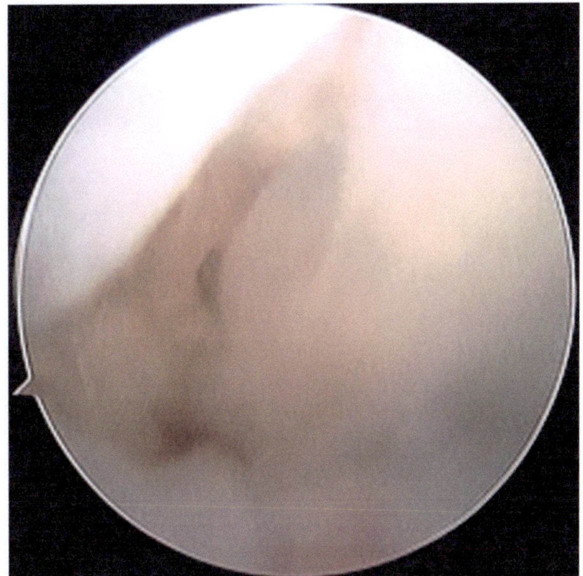

Fig. 20.20 Use of a 2.0 mm shaver allows for better visualization of the intra-articular metacarpal head fracture fractures; significant fracture step-off is noted

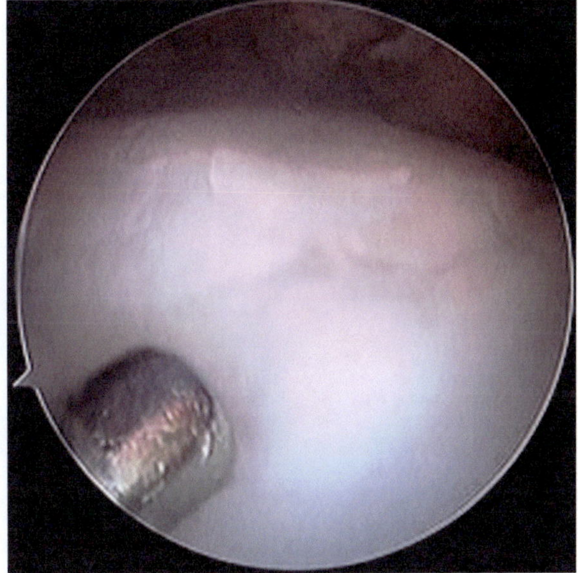

Fig. 20.21 Arthroscopically assisted reduction of intra-articular metacarpal head fracture with 3 mm probe

K-wires are typically removed 4–6 weeks after surgery once adequate fracture fragment healing is demonstrated on follow-up radiographs (Fig. 20.25). A postoperative CT scan in this case demonstrates the restoration of articular congruity (Fig. 20.26). In our experience, following arthroscopically assisted reduction and percutaneous pinning, patients have regained an average of 90% of their total active motion at final follow-up compared to the contralateral side (Fig. 20.27).

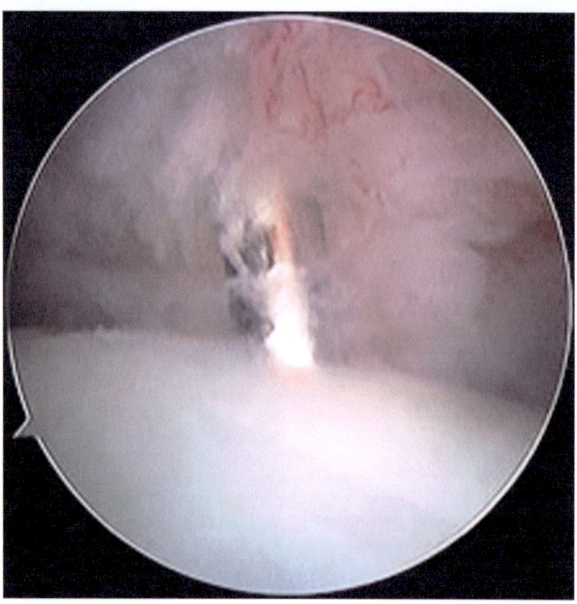

Fig. 20.22 Percutaneous 0.045-in. K-wire fixation of intra-articular metacarpal head fracture

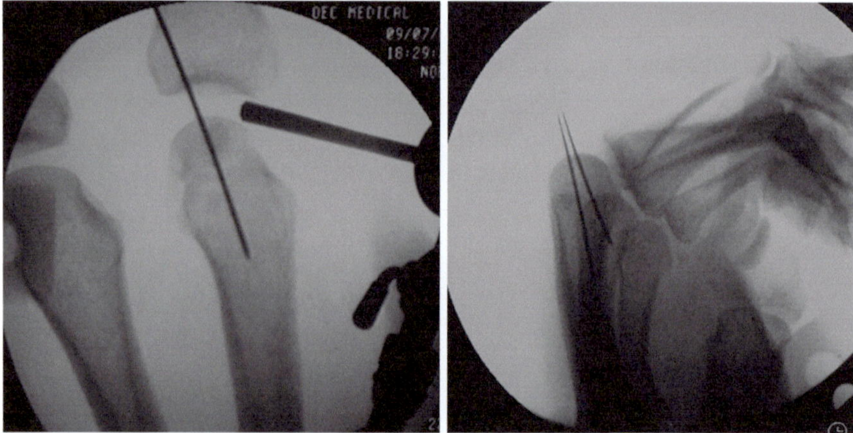

Fig. 20.23 Retrograde K-wire fixation of an anatomically reduced metacarpal head fracture using fluoroscopic guidance

Intra-Articular Finger Proximal Phalanx Base Fractures

Proximal phalanx fractures of the fingers can result from a variety of mechanisms of injury including a direct blow, fall onto an outstretched hand, and collateral ligament avulsions [21, 72]. Collateral ligament avulsions are far less common in the fingers than in the thumb [73, 74]. Intra-articular proximal phalanx base fractures

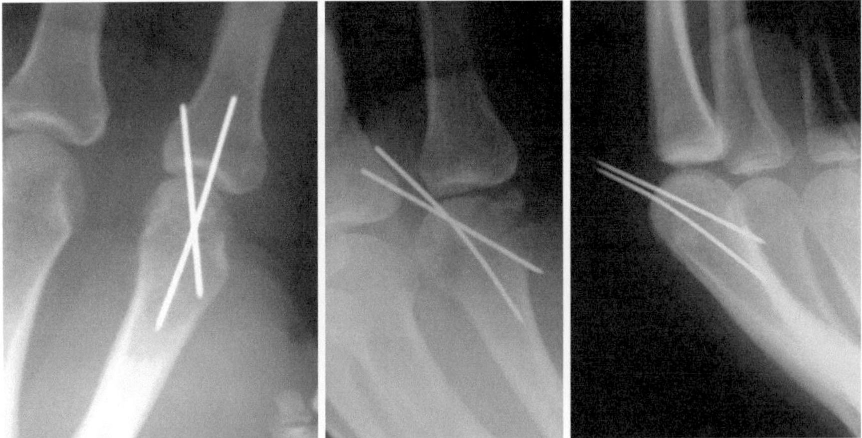

Fig. 20.24 Posteroanterior, oblique, and lateral radiographic views demonstrating the final fixation construct with two crossing 0.045-in. K-wires

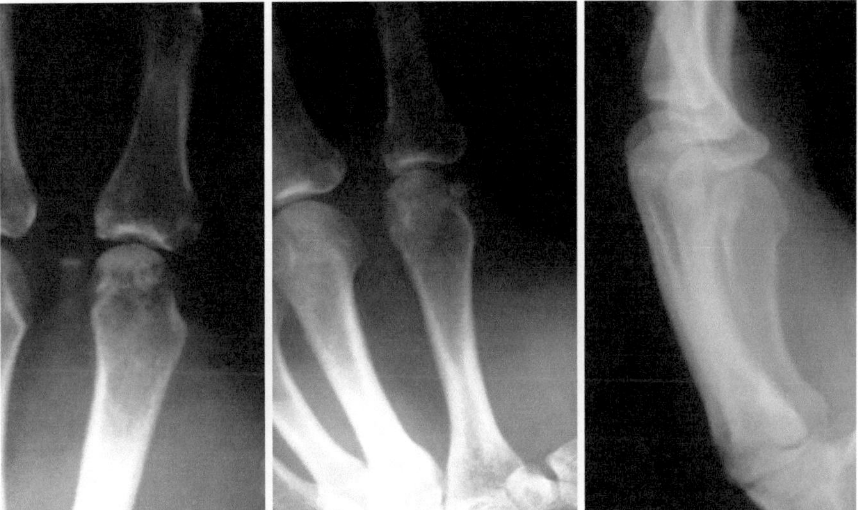

Fig. 20.25 Posteroanterior, oblique, and lateral radiographic views demonstrating healing of the metacarpal head fracture without step-off

that demonstrate any incongruity of the concave joint surface, or sourcil, meet our criteria for operative intervention in order to prevent post-traumatic arthrosis and dysfunction (Fig. 20.28). Non-displaced fractures can be managed non-operatively with vigilant follow-up and radiographic surveillance.

Classically, proximal phalanx base fractures have been treated with closed reduction and percutaneous pinning or open reduction and internal fixation. While closed

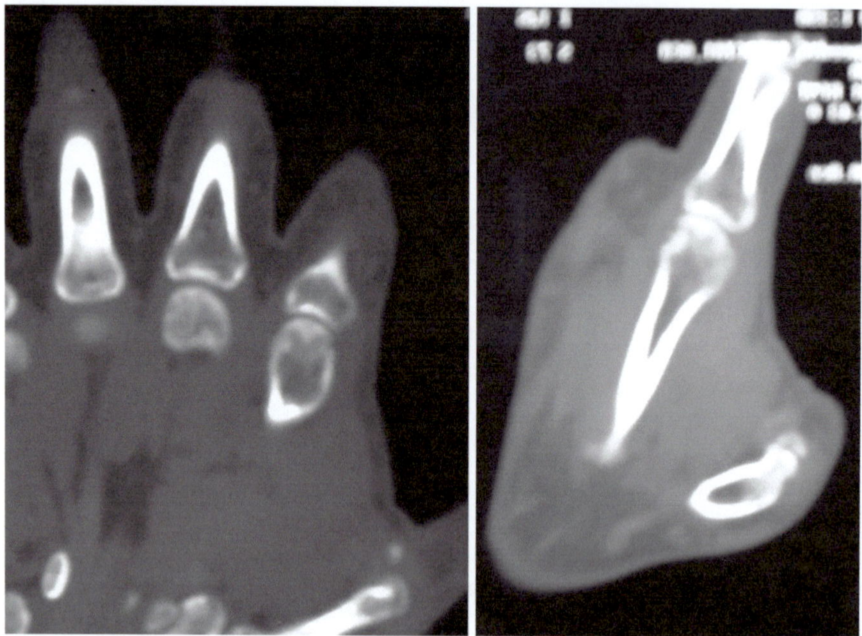

Fig. 20.26 Coronal and sagittal CT views confirming restoration of articular congruity at the MCP joint

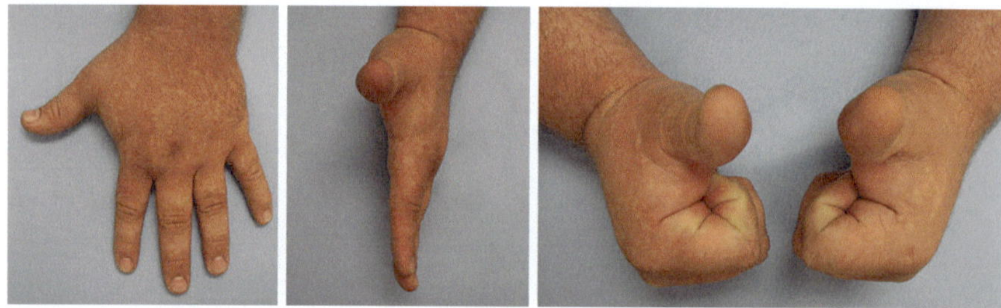

Fig. 20.27 Finger range of motion at final follow-up after metacarpal head fracture fixation

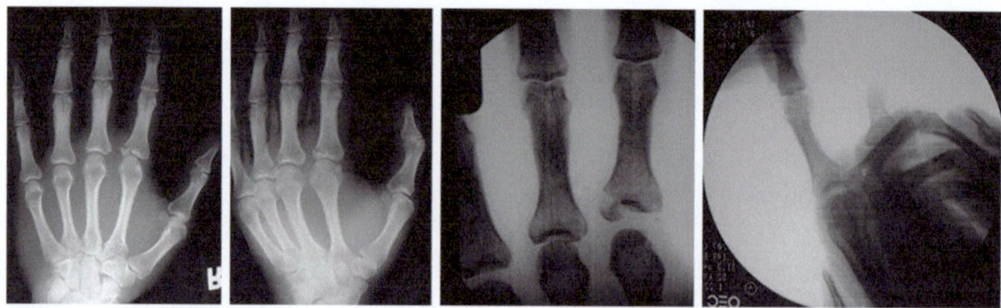

Fig. 20.28 Injury radiographs and fluoroscopy (posteroanterior, oblique, and lateral views) demonstrating a displaced, intra-articular, index finger volar-ulnar proximal phalanx base fracture

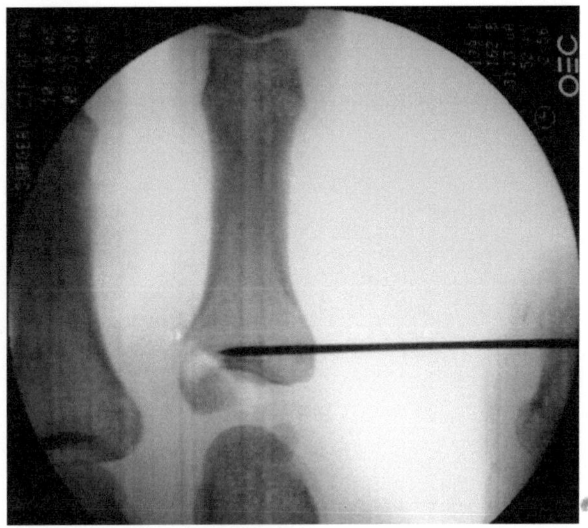

Fig. 20.29 Under fluoroscopic guidance, a K-wire entered perpendicular to the base of the proximal phalanx in a radial to ulnar direction to the level of the fracture

reduction and percutaneous pinning is less damaging to the surrounding tissues, obtaining and maintaining an anatomic reduction can be challenging. Open techniques allow for reasonable visualization of the fracture and reduction quality at the expense of significant soft tissue dissection. Dorsal and volar approaches have each been described [72, 73]. While our preferred technique has rarely been mentioned in the academic literature, we have had success with arthroscopically aided reduction and pinning of displaced, noncomminuted, intra-articular proximal phalanx base fractures.

Technique

We access the finger MCP joint arthroscopically in the exact same manner as described in the *Intra-Articular Finger Metacarpal Head Fractures* technique section. In the first case example involving a displaced, intra-articular, index finger volar-ulnar proximal phalanx base fracture, we chose to first advance a K-wire to the fracture site, from radial to ulnar under mini C-arm fluoroscopic guidance (Fig. 20.29). At the same time, the fracture was well-visualized under direct arthroscopic view (Fig. 20.30).

We first attempt to reduce these fractures using the 3 mm probe alone, but the use of K-wires as joysticks or percutaneous point-to-point reduction forceps can also be used (Fig. 20.31). Once reduction is achieved, the fracture fragment is held using one to two 0.045-in. or 0.035-in. K-wires which are advanced under fluoroscopy (Fig. 20.32). Concurrently, the arthroscope is utilized to view the articular surface of the proximal phalanx base to confirm reduction is maintained throughout this portion of the procedure (Fig. 20.33). K-wires are cut and buried below the skin (Fig. 20.34). The pins are typically removed 4–6 weeks after surgery once adequate fracture fragment healing is demonstrated on follow-up radiographs (Fig. 20.35). In the presented case, our patient regained full painless active range of motion of the

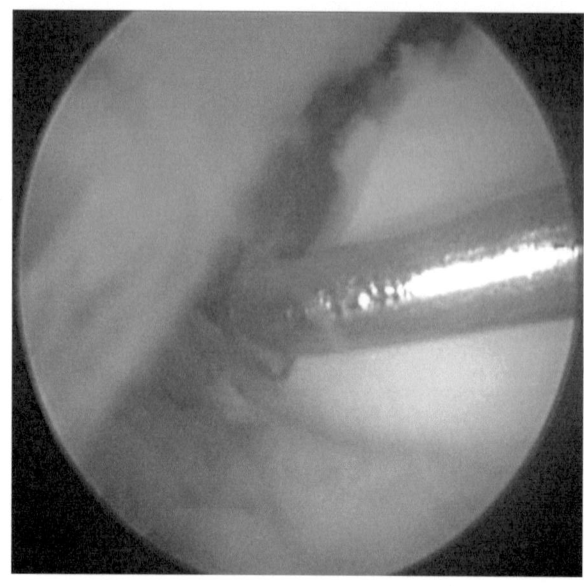

Fig. 20.30 Arthroscopic visualization of an intra-articular proximal phalanx base fracture

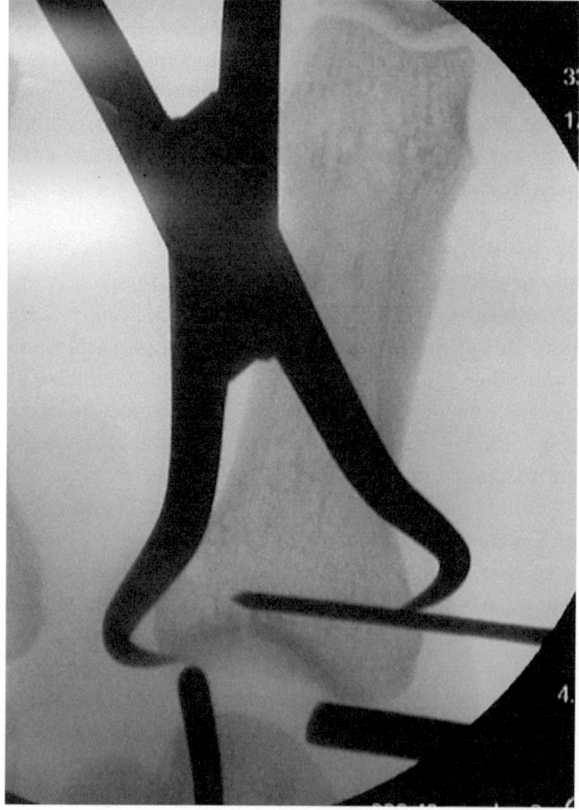

Fig. 20.31 Percutaneous reduction technique using point-to-point reduction forceps

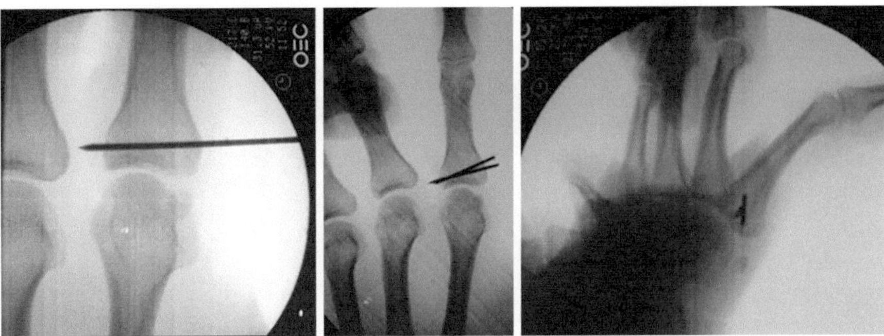

Fig. 20.32 Percutaneous pinning of fracture with final fluoroscopic images after K-wires are cut below the skin

Fig. 20.33 Arthroscopic confirmation of maintained anatomic reduction of the intra-articular proximal phalanx base fracture

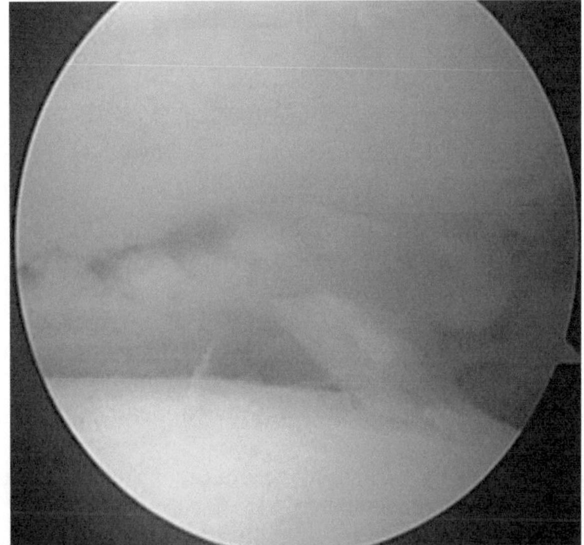

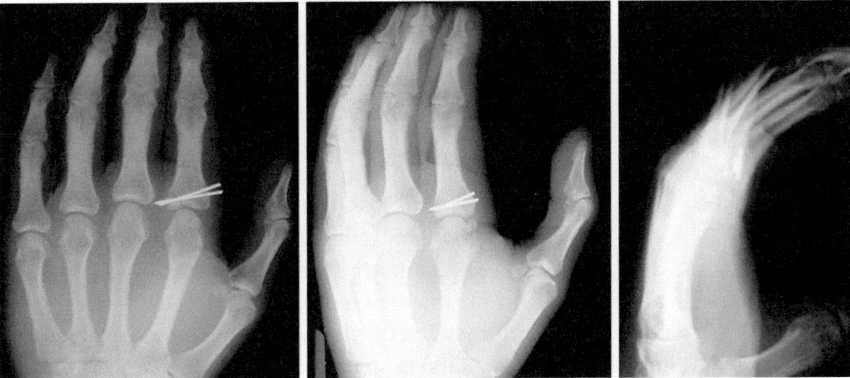

Fig. 20.34 Post-operative radiographs (posteroanterior, oblique, and lateral views) demonstrating final K-wire fixation

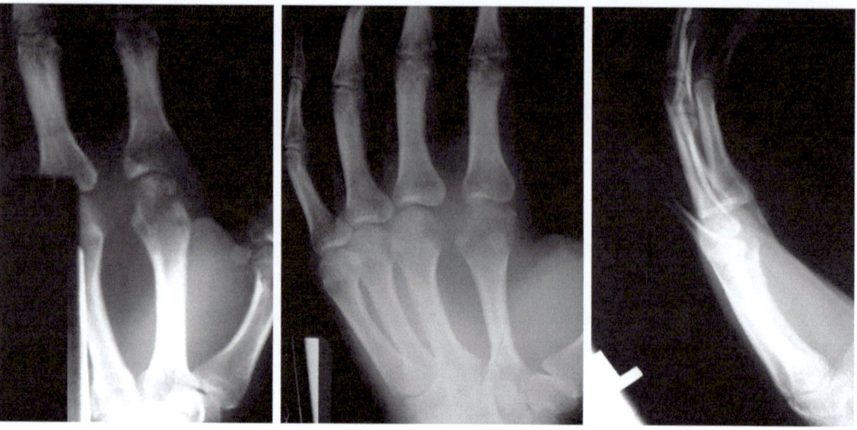

Fig. 20.35 Healed index finger intra-articular proximal phalanx base fracture—radiographs status post K-wire removal

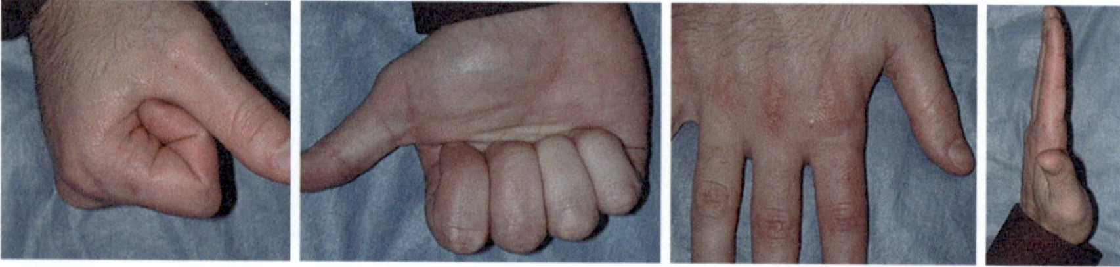

Fig. 20.36 Patient regained full active range of motion post-operatively

index finger and had an excellent cosmetic appearance after portal site healing (Fig. 20.36).

Additionally, we have found arthroscopy to be particularly helpful with impacted, die-punch proximal phalanx base fractures (Figs. 20.37 and 20.38). In this particular case, we used our standard MCP arthroscopic approach and were able to visualize the die-punch fragment (Fig. 20.39), disimpact the fragment with the arthroscopic probe (Fig. 20.40), and restore articular congruity with an anatomic reduction (Fig. 20.41). Once satisfied with the reduction, the fracture was pinned with two antegrade 0.045-in. K-wires (Fig. 20.42).

Current Literature

Few studies have reported arthroscopic reduction and fixation of metacarpal head fractures or intra-articular proximal phalanx base fractures in the second through fifth digits. In a review article revisiting their indications for metacarpophalangeal joint arthroscopy, Choi and colleagues included a case report of an intra-articular metacarpal head fracture in a skeletally mature young athlete [18]. The fracture was reduced using an arthroscopic probe and fixed with two retrograde absorbable pins. The athlete was allowed free mobilization as tolerated 2 days after surgery. Return

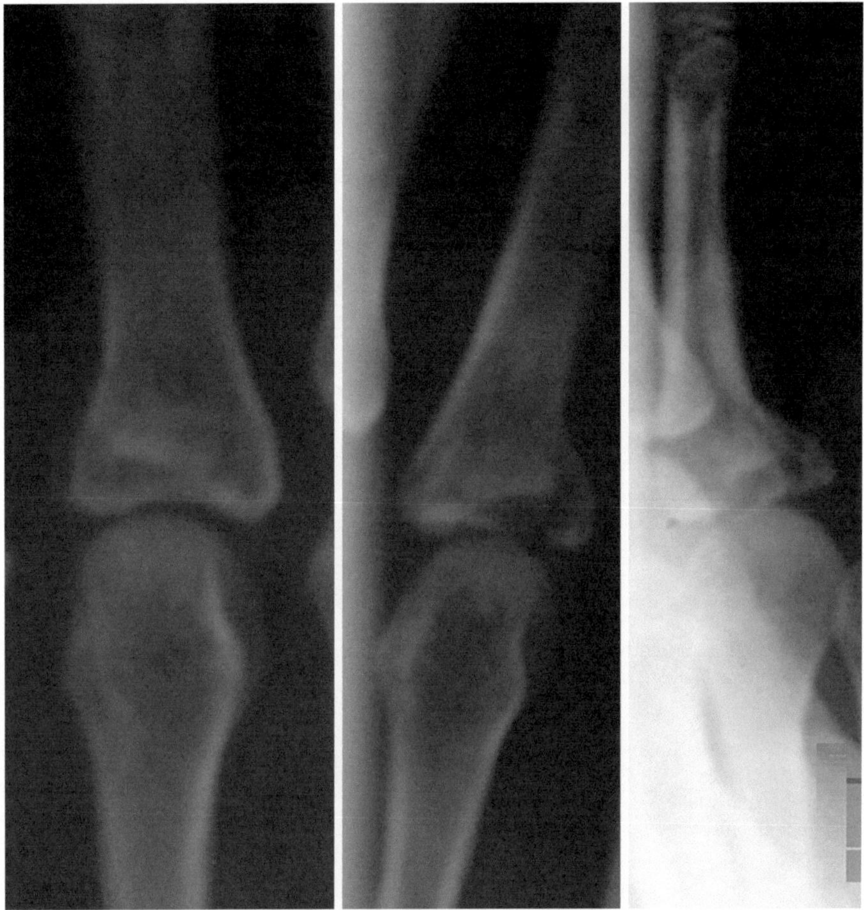

Fig. 20.37 Injury radiographs (posteroanterior, oblique, and lateral views) demonstrating a displaced, intra-articular, die-punch fracture of the ring finger proximal phalanx base

to sport time was not reported. Their final post-operative radiographs demonstrated complete fracture healing with maintained joint congruity.

Slade et al. presented findings from 14 consecutive cases of displaced, intra-articular fractures involving the MCP joint that were treated with arthroscopically aided reduction and percutaneous fixation with K-wires and/or cannulated screws [34]. Eight of these involved the non-thumb digits (two index, two long, three ring, and one small finger). At final follow-up (average 11 months), mean MCP joint range of motion was 81°. They reported an earlier return to work and a greater final ROM vs. a matched cohort; however, no statistical evaluation was provided. The authors detailed a single complication in this group, due to loss of reduction noted at 2 weeks in a comminuted, long finger proximal phalanx base pilon fracture fixed with cannulated screws after arthroscopic reduction. A revision arthroscopic

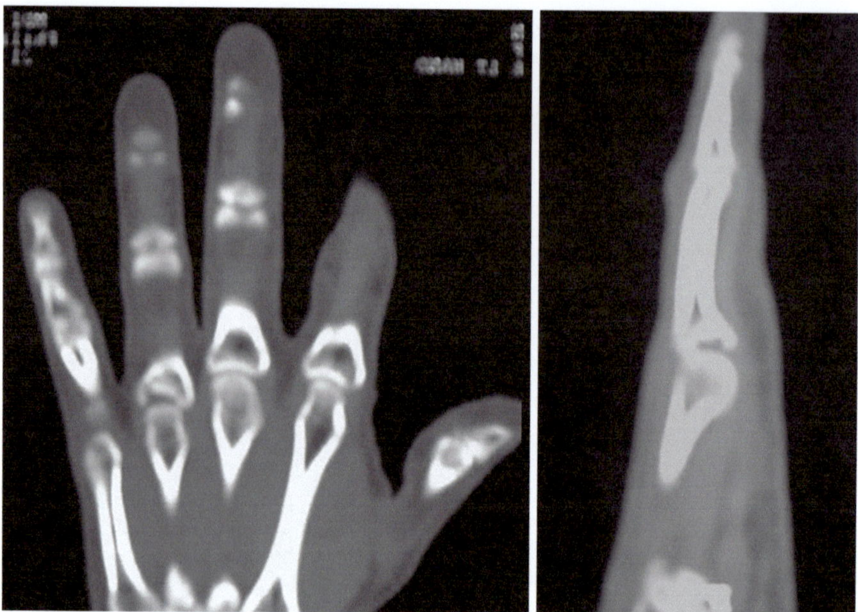

Fig. 20.38 CT scan (coronal and sagittal cuts) demonstrating a displaced, intra-articular, die-punch fracture of the ring finger proximal phalanx base

Fig. 20.39 Arthroscopic view of ring finger proximal phalanx base die-punch fracture fragment

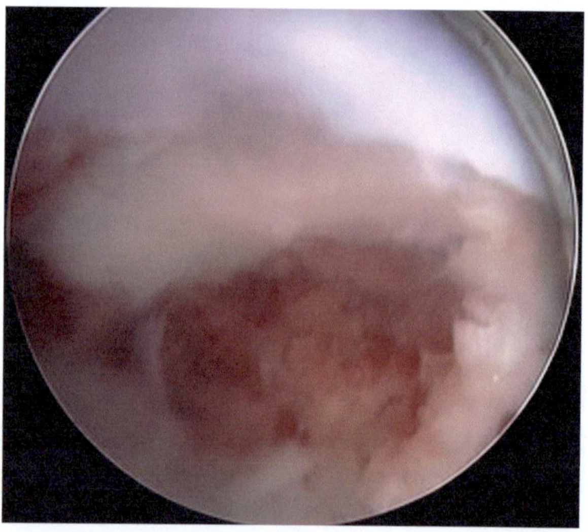

reduction and percutaneous fixation was performed, and the patient's fracture healed in anatomic position.

Erdos and colleagues described a failed attempt to percutaneously pin an intra-articular avulsion fracture involving the ulnar-volar margin of an index proximal phalanx. The fracture was reduced arthroscopically, but they reported difficulty with

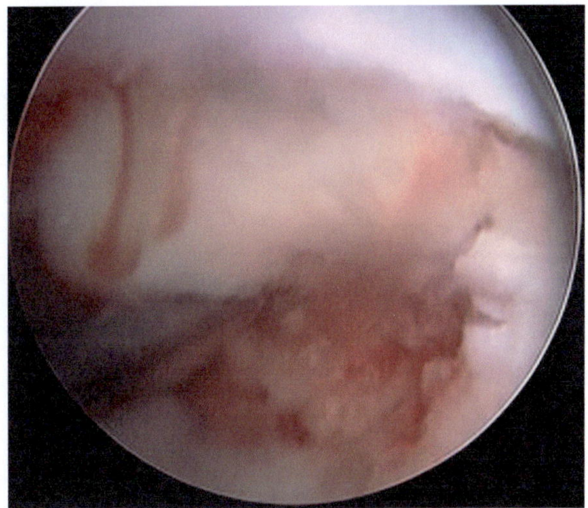

Fig. 20.40 Arthroscopic disimpaction of proximal phalanx base die-punch fracture fragment using an arthroscopic probe

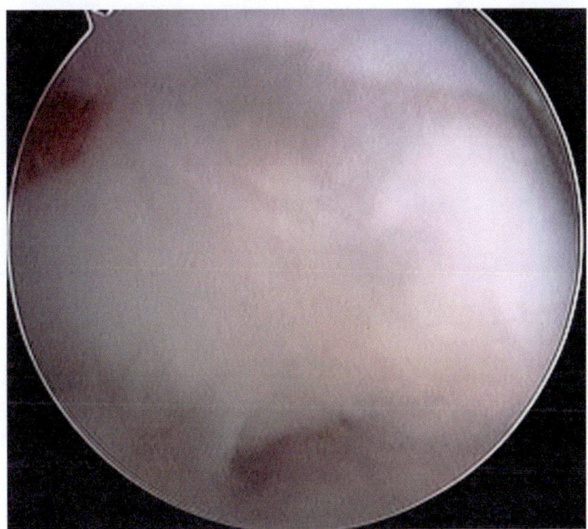

Fig. 20.41 Restoration of proximal phalanx base articular congruity

capturing and fixing the fragment while maintaining anatomic reduction. Ultimately the authors converted to an open reduction and pinning [56].

The senior author of this chapter performed a prospective study evaluating 23 consecutive patients who underwent arthroscopically assisted reduction of intra-articular fractures involving a carpometacarpal or metacarpophalangeal joint. Mean age was 42.3 years. Ten patients (43%) were male and 13 (57%) were female. Follow-up ranged from 12 to 71 months. Primary outcomes were active range of motion and maintenance of fracture reduction. Overall, patients regained 90% of their total active motion as compared to the contralateral side. There were no extensor tendon injuries. Three total complications were documented including a single

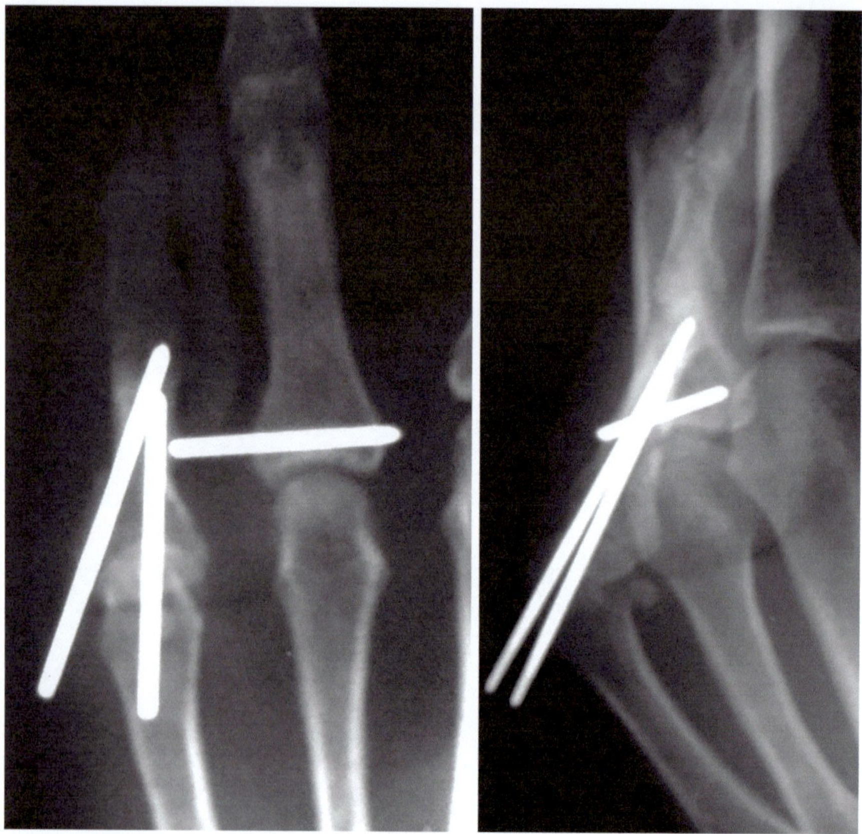

Fig. 20.42 Status post-fixation of proximal phalanx base fracture with two antegrade K-wires

pin tract infection, a case of loss of K-wire fixation, and one patient who experienced persistent digital stiffness. In our experience, overall patient satisfaction with this surgical technique is very high.

Conclusion

There are considerable advantages in the arthroscopic management of intra-articular hand fractures. Following the indications outlined in this chapter, we have had success with achieving anatomic reduction of these fractures while avoiding the significant soft tissue damage and subsequent scarring associated with the more extensive open approaches. As the role of arthroscopy continues to expand in hand surgery, we predict that arthroscopically aided reduction and fixation of hand fractures will become more prevalent over time.

References

1. Watanabe M. Present status and future of arthroscopy. Geka Chiryo. 1972;26(1):73–7. Japanese.
2. Chen YC. Arthroscopy of the wrist and finger joints. Orthop Clin North Am. 1979;10(3):723–33.
3. Badia A. Arthroscopy of the trapeziometacarpal and metacarpophalangeal joints. J Hand Surg [Am]. 2007;32(5):707–24.
4. Berger RA. A technique for arthroscopic evaluation of the first carpometacarpal joint. J Hand Surg [Am]. 1997;22(6):1077–80.
5. Badia A. Trapeziometacarpal arthroscopy: a classification and treatment algorithm. Hand Clin. 2006;22(2):153–63.
6. Menon J. Arthroscopic management of trapeziometacarpal joint arthritis of the thumb. Arthroscopy. 1996;12(5):581–7.
7. Osterman AL, Culp R, Bednar J. Arthroscopy of the thumb carpometacarpal joint. Arthroscopy. 1997;13(3):411.
8. Culp RW, Rekant MS. The role of arthroscopy in evaluating and treating trapeziometacarpal disease. Hand Clin. 2001;17(2):315–9.
9. Longo UG, Petrillo S, Denaro V. Current concepts in the management of rheumatoid hand. Int J Rheumatol. 2015;2015:648073.
10. Burke FD. The rheumatoid metacarpophalangeal joint. Hand Clin. 2011;27(1):79–86.
11. Rizzo M. Metacarpophalangeal joint arthritis. J Hand Surg [Am]. 2011;36(2):345–53.
12. Berner SH. Metacarpophalangeal arthroscopy: technique and applications. Tech Hand Up Extrem Surg. 2008;12(4):208–15.
13. Rozmaryn LM, Wei N. Metacarpophalangeal arthroscopy. Arthroscopy. 1999;15(3):333–7.
14. Sekiya I, Kobayashi M, Taneda Y, Matsui N. Arthroscopy of the proximal interphalangeal and metacarpophalangeal joints in rheumatoid hands. Arthroscopy. 2002;18(3):292–7.
15. Ostendorf B, Dann P, Wedekind F, Brauckmann U, Friemann J, Koebke J, Schulitz KP, Schneider M. Miniarthroscopy of metacarpophalangeal joints in rheumatoid arthritis. Rating of diagnostic value in synovitis staging and efficiency of synovial biopsy. J Rheumatol. 1999;26(9):1901–8.
16. Wilkes LL. Arthroscopic synovectomy in the rheumatoid metacarpophalangeal joint. J Med Assoc GA. 1987;76(9):638–9.
17. Wei N, Delauter SK, Erlichman MS, Rozmaryn LM, Beard SJ, Henry DL. Arthroscopic synovectomy of the metacarpophalangeal joint in refractory rheumatoid arthritis: a technique. Arthroscopy. 1999;15(3):265–8.
18. Choi AK, Chow EC, Ho PC, Chow YY. Metacarpophalangeal joint arthroscopy: indications revisited. Hand Clin. 2011;27(3):369–82.
19. Capo JT, Kinchelow T, Orillaza NS, Rossy W. Accuracy of fluoroscopy in closed reduction and percutaneous fixation of simulated Bennett's fracture. J Hand Surg [Am]. 2009;34(4):637–41.
20. Caldwell RA, Shorten PL, Morrell NT. Common upper extremity fracture eponyms: a look into what they really mean. J Hand Surg [Am]. 2019;44(4):331–4.
21. Wolfe SW, Pederson WC, Kozin SH, Cohen MS. Green's operative hand surgery. 8th ed. Philadelphia, PA: Elsevier; 2021.
22. Solomon J, Culp RW. Arthroscopic management of Bennett fracture. Hand Clin. 2017;33(4):787–94.
23. Ellis H. Edward Hallaran Bennett: Bennett's fracture of the base of the thumb. J Perioper Pract. 2013;23(3):59–60.
24. Bettinger PC, Berger RA. Functional ligamentous anatomy of the trapezium and trapeziometacarpal joint (gross and arthroscopic). Hand Clin. 2001;17(2):151–68.
25. Gedda KO. Studies on Bennett's fracture; anatomy, roentgenology, and therapy. Acta Chir Scand Suppl. 1954;193:1–114.

26. Guss MS, Kaye D, Rettig M. Bennett fractures a review of management. Bull Hosp Jt Dis. 2016;74(3):197–202.
27. Ladd AL. Guest editorial: The Robert's view: a historical and clinical perspective. Clin Orthop Relat Res. 2014;472(4):1097–100.
28. Culp RW, Johnson JW. Arthroscopically assisted percutaneous fixation of Bennett fractures. J Hand Surg [Am]. 2010;35(1):137–40.
29. Pomares G, Strugarek-Lecoanet C, Dap F, Dautel G. Bennett fracture: arthroscopically assisted percutaneous screw fixation versus open surgery: functional and radiological outcomes. Orthop Traumatol Surg Res. 2016;102(3):357–61.
30. Zemirline A, Lebailly F, Taleb C, Facca S, Liverneaux P. Arthroscopic assisted percutaneous screw fixation of Bennett's fracture. Hand Surg. 2014;19(2):281–6.
31. Sekiya I, Kobayashi M, Okamoto H, Iguchi H, Waguri-Nagaya Y, Goto H, Nozaki M, Tsuchiya A, Otsuka T. Arthroscopic synovectomy of the metacarpophalangeal and proximal interphalangeal joints. Tech Hand Up Extrem Surg. 2008;12(4):221–5.
32. Ryu J, Fagan R. Arthroscopic treatment of acute complete thumb metacarpophalangeal ulnar collateral ligament tears. J Hand Surg [Am]. 1995;20(6):1037–42.
33. Vaupel GL, Andrews JR. Diagnostic and operative arthroscopy of the thumb metacarpophalangeal joint. A case report. Am J Sports Med. 1985;13(2):139–41.
34. Slade JF III, Gutow AP. Arthroscopy of the metacarpophalangeal joint. Hand Clin. 1999;15(3):501–27.
35. Sekiya I, Kobayashi M, Okamoto H, Otsuka T. Progress and role of finger joint arthroscopy. Hand Clin. 2017;33(4):819–29.
36. Walsh EF, Akelman E, Fleming BC, Da Silva MF. Thumb carpometacarpal arthroscopy: a topographic, anatomic study of the thenar portal. J Hand Surg [Am]. 2005;30(2):373–9.
37. Cobb TK, Berner SH, Badia A. New frontiers in hand arthroscopy. Hand Clin. 2011;27(3):383–94.
38. Daley D, Geary M, Gaston RG. Thumb metacarpophalangeal ulnar and radial collateral ligament injuries. Clin Sports Med. 2020;39(2):443–55.
39. Tang P. Collateral ligament injuries of the thumb metacarpophalangeal joint. J Am Acad Orthop Surg. 2011;19(5):287–96.
40. Keramidas E, Miller G. Adult hand injuries on artificial ski slopes. Ann Plast Surg. 2005;55(4):357–8.
41. Coyle MP Jr. Grade III radial collateral ligament injuries of the thumb metacarpophalangeal joint: treatment by soft tissue advancement and bony reattachment. J Hand Surg [Am]. 2003;28(1):14–20.
42. Johnson JW, Culp RW. Acute ulnar collateral ligament injury in the athlete. Hand Clin. 2009;25(3):437–42.
43. Heyman P, Gelberman RH, Duncan K, Hipp JA. Injuries of the ulnar collateral ligament of the thumb metacarpophalangeal joint. Biomechanical and prospective clinical studies on the usefulness of valgus stress testing. Clin Orthop Relat Res. 1993;(292):165–71.
44. Avery DM III, Caggiano NM, Matullo KS. Ulnar collateral ligament injuries of the thumb: a comprehensive review. Orthop Clin North Am. 2015;46(2):281–92.
45. Edelstein DM, Kardashian G, Lee SK. Radial collateral ligament injuries of the thumb. J Hand Surg [Am]. 2008;33(5):760–70.
46. Gerber C, Senn E, Matter P. Skier's thumb. Surgical treatment of recent injuries to the ulnar collateral ligament of the thumb's metacarpophalangeal joint. Am J Sports Med. 1981;9(3):171–7.
47. Campbell CS. Gamekeeper's thumb. J Bone Joint Surg (Br). 1955;37(1):148–9.
48. Newland CC. Gamekeeper's thumb. Orthop Clin North Am. 1992;23(1):41–8.
49. Posner MA, Retaillaud JL, Green SM. Collateral ligament ruptures of the thumb metacarpophalangeal joint a review of 500 surgical cases. Bull Hosp Jt Dis. 2022;80(2):122–8.
50. Giele H, Martin J. The two-level ulnar collateral ligament injury of the metacarpophalangeal joint of the thumb. J Hand Surg (Br). 2003;28(1):92–3.
51. Stener B. Displacement of the ruptured ulnar collateral ligament of the metacarpo-phalangeal joint of the thumb. J Bone Joint Surg. 1962;44B(4):869–79.

52. Lark ME, Maroukis BL, Chung KC. The Stener lesion: historical perspective and evolution of diagnostic criteria. Hand. 2017;12(3):283–9.
53. Köttstorfer J, Hofbauer M, Krusche-Mandl I, Kaiser G, Erhart J, Platzer P. Avulsion fracture and complete rupture of the thumb radial collateral ligament. Arch Orthop Trauma Surg. 2013;133(4):583–8.
54. Badia A. Arthroscopic reduction and internal fixation of bony gamekeeper's thumb. Orthopedics. 2006;29(8):675–8.
55. Gáspár L, Szekanecz Z, Dezso B, Szegedi G, Csernátony Z, Szepesi K. Technique of synovial biopsy of metacarpophalangeal joints using the needle arthroscope. Knee Surg Sports Traumatol Arthrosc. 2003;11(1):50–2.
56. Erdos J, Gannon C, Baratz ME. Arthroscopy of the metacarpophalangeal joint. Oper Tech Orthop. 2007;17:133–9.
57. Diao E. Metacarpal fixation. Hand Clin. 1997;13(4):557–71.
58. Brewerton DA. A tangential radiographic projection for demonstrating involvement of metacarpal heads in rheumatoid arthritis. Br J Radiol. 1967;40(471):233–4.
59. Lane CS. Detecting occult fractures of the metacarpal head: the Brewerton view. J Hand Surg [Am]. 1977;2(2):131–3.
60. McElfresh EC, Dobyns JH. Intra-articular metacarpal head fractures. J Hand Surg [Am]. 1983;8(4):383–93.
61. Lee JK, Jo YG, Kim JW, Choi YS, Han SH. Open reduction and internal fixation for intraarticular fracture of metacarpal head. Orthopade. 2017;46(7):617–24.
62. Ford DJ, El-Hadidi S, Lunn PG, Burke FD. Fractures of the metacarpals: treatment by A. O. screw and plate fixation. J Hand Surg (Br). 1987;12(1):34–7.
63. Ouellette EA, Freeland AE. Use of the minicondylar plate in metacarpal and phalangeal fractures. Clin Orthop Relat Res. 1996;(327):38–46.
64. Sudhakar JE, Smith AM, Leslie IJ. Late treatment of a displaced intraarticular metacarpal head fracture. J Hand Surg (Br). 1997;22(5):672–3.
65. Hastings H II, Carroll C IV. Treatment of closed articular fractures of the metacarpophalangeal and proximal interphalangeal joints. Hand Clin. 1988;4(3):503–27.
66. Light TR, Bednar MS. Management of intra-articular fractures of the metacarpophalangeal joint. Hand Clin. 1994;10(2):303–14.
67. Shewring DJ, Thomas RH. Collateral ligament avulsion fractures from the heads of the metacarpals of the fingers. J Hand Surg (Br). 2006;31(5):537–41.
68. Henry MH. Fractures of the proximal phalanx and metacarpals in the hand: preferred methods of stabilization. J Am Acad Orthop Surg. 2008;16(10):586–95.
69. Boulas HJ, Herren A, Büchler U. Osteochondral metatarsophalangeal autografts for traumatic articular metacarpophalangeal defects: a preliminary report. J Hand Surg [Am]. 1993;18(6):1086–92.
70. Boulas HJ. Autograft replacement of small joint defects in the hand. Clin Orthop Relat Res. 1996;(327):63–71.
71. Hidalgo-Díaz JJ, Ichihara S, Taleb C, Gouzou S, Facca S, Naroura I, Bodin F, Liverneaux P. Metacarpophalangeal joint arthroscopy in the fingers other than the thumb: retrospective comparison of horizontal versus vertical traction. Chir Main. 2015;34(3):105–8.
72. Eberlin KR, Babushkina A, Neira JR, Mudgal CS. Outcomes of closed reduction and periarticular pinning of base and shaft fractures of the proximal phalanx. J Hand Surg [Am]. 2014;39(8):1524–8.
73. Kuhn KM, Dao KD, Shin AY. Volar A1 pulley approach for fixation of avulsion fractures of the base of the proximal phalanx. J Hand Surg [Am]. 2001;26(4):762–71.
74. Sakuma M, Nakamura R, Inoue G, Horii E. Avulsion fracture of the metacarpophalangeal joint of the finger. J Hand Surg (Br). 1997;22(5):667–71.

WALANT for Adult Hand Fractures

21

Donald H. Lalonde

What Is WALANT?

WALANT stands for Wide Awake Local Anesthesia No Tourniquet. It is pure local anesthesia with 1% lidocaine and 1:100,000 epinephrine. This is an alternative to tourniquet surgery with sedation and nerve blocks or general anesthesia. It is tumescent local anesthesia. This means enough visible and palpable local anesthesia so that you can see it and feel it at least 2 cm beyond anywhere you will cut, insert a K wire, or manipulate a fracture. This is like an extravascular Bier Block, but only where you need it.

Why Use WALANT for Hand and Finger Fractures?

1. Pure local anesthesia is safer than sedation in hand surgery, especially in ASA three or four patients with multiple medical comorbidities. The safest sedation is no sedation.
2. WALANT makes the surgery less expensive by eliminating sedation and main operating room sterility [1, 3] and therefore more available to patients with limited means [4].
3. When fingers are crooked because of fractures, the patient can be the best judge of whether his finger is straightened when he flexes and extends it during the surgery after reduction. He has been looking at the finger for years and knows better than the surgeon if it is straight or not.
4. The surgeon has an hour of uninterrupted time to educate the unsedated patient during the surgery to decrease the risk of many post-operative complications.

D. H. Lalonde (✉)
Division of Plastic Surgery, Dalhousie University, Saint John, NB, Canada
e-mail: dlalonde@drlalonde.ca

© The Author(s), under exclusive license to Springer Nature Switzerland AG 2023
J. M. Abzug et al. (eds.), *Pediatric and Adult Hand Fractures*,
https://doi.org/10.1007/978-3-031-32072-9_21

5. The surgeon can assess the intraoperative stability of fracture fixation as the patient takes the fingers through a full range of motion under fluoroscopy after reduction. Adjustments in K wire number or placement can be made if necessary. The surgeon can then be confident to start pain guided early protected movement at 3–5 days after K wiring, just like after flexor tendon repair.

6. WALANT can make K wiring of hand fractures much more convenient for patients who can have this performed in minor procedure rooms during daytime hours instead of in the main operating room which may end up being during evening or night hours [3, 1, 5]. They spend much less time at the hospital because they have no recovery from sedation.

7. It eliminates the costs, solid waste, fasting, intravenous insertion, nausea, and vomiting associated with sedation and unnecessary main operting room sterility.

How to Inject the Local Anesthesia for WALANT Hand Fracture Reduction

Local anesthesia injection should barely hurt at all if you follow simple rules to minimize injection pain [6, 7].

- Use 27 or 30 gauge needles instead of 25 gauge
- Don't blast local in quickly! Slow down!
- Buffer acidic local with bicarbonate in a 10:1 ratio
- Insert needle perpendicular to skin
- Don't inject in the dermis
- Stabilize the syringe with both hands to avoid needle pain until needle entry site is numb
- Use sensory noise for needle insertion
- Blow in more than 2 mL before moving the needle at all
- Don't advance sharp needle tips anywhere that is not numb
- Only reinsert needles in completely numbed skin
- Always inject too much volume instead of not enough (except in fingers)
- Ask for patient pain feedback every time so you can count the number of times they feel pain and score yourself
- Always inject from proximal to distal
- Never inject into the tendon sheath. It hurts more and is not necessary.

Other Suggestions to Eliminate Problems with WALANT Local Anesthesia Injection

- As long as you respect the limit of 7 mg/kg of lidocaine with epinephrine, it is always better to inject too much local anesthesia as opposed to not enough. No one ever complained about being too numb, and you want zero pain during the surgery. However, you do not need more than 2 mL on either the volar or dorsal aspect of each of the proximal and middle phalanges, or more than 0.5 mL on the volar or dorsal aspect of the distal phalanx.

- Inject the anesthetic solution a minimum of 30 min before surgery to allow the epinephrine to take optimal effect and provide an adequately dry working field [8].
- Inject patients in a waiting area before they come into the procedure room to give the local anesthetic time to work.
- We inject supine patients lying down on stretchers to decrease the risk of their fainting, and we always warn them about the possible epinephrine rush to avoid concerns and the false assumption that this is an allergic response [9].
- Remember that if you do not have epinephrine in a middle phalanx but you have lidocaine with epinephrine blocking the nerve proximally, the lidocaine will cause increased bleeding in the middle phalanx because of the sympathetic blockade. You should have epinephrine wherever you are going to cut when you do not use a tourniquet.
- If you are only using K wires for a percutaneous reduction and not cutting through the skin, it is still worth having epinephrine in the soft tissue around the bone you are K wiring, even if that tissue is numb from proximal blocks. Epinephrine will provide less internal bleeding in the periosteal tissue, which means less callus and less scar for the patient to work through later.

Where to Inject the Local Anesthetic for Finger Fracture Reduction

1. Inject 5–10 mL of 1% lidocaine with 1:100,000 epinephrine (buffered with 0.5–1.0 mL of 8.4% sodium bicarbonate) between both common digital nerves in the subcutaneous fat of the distal palm. Do not inject in the flexor tendon sheath as that causes a lot of unnecessary pain (see Fig. 21.1).
2. While the palm is numbing, perform the first dorsal injection. Once again, inject 5–10 mL on the dorsal hand just proximal to the MP joint over the metacarpal in the subcutaneous fat.
3. Next, inject 2 mL in the subcutaneous fat between both digital nerves on the volar side of the mid-proximal phalanx.

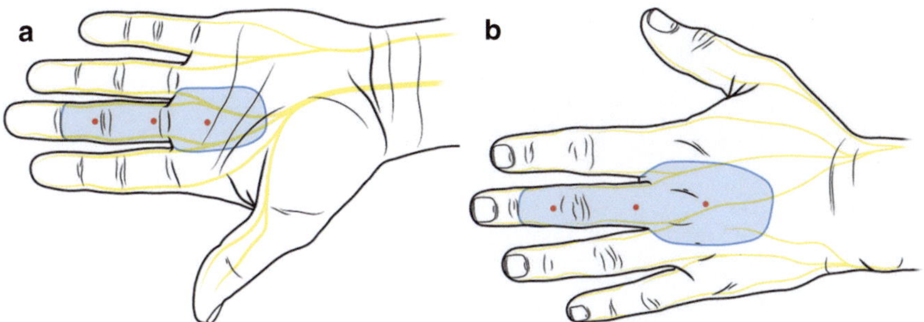

Fig. 21.1 Where to inject local anesthesia for finger fracture reduction. The red dots are the injection points between the digital nerves in the subcutaneous fat. (Reproduced with permission [10])

4. Then inject 2 mL in the subcutaneous fat over the mid-dorsal proximal phalanx.
5. You can repeat the 2 mL volar and the 2 mL dorsal in the middle of the middle phalanx if you will be operating at the middle phalanx level.
6. Although you can inject 0.5 mL in the distal phalanx volarly or dorsally, this is usually not required. For distal phalanx fractures, the author sometimes uses a finger tourniquet if better visibility is required after blocking the finger with local anesthesia. For a finger tourniquet, he prefers cutting out of the distal fingertip of a sterile glove worn by the patient, and then the finger of the glove rolled proximally.

Where to Inject the Local Anesthetic for Metacarpal Fracture Reduction

1. For hand metacarpals, inject at least 20 mL of local anesthesia from proximal to distal as shown in Fig. 21.2. The entire metacarpal periosteum affected by K wires, screw, or fracture manipulation should be bathed with lidocaine with epinephrine.
2. The volar aspect of the metacarpals need to be bathed in local anesthesia. This can be done via needles inserted on the dorsal side of the hand as shown in Fig. 21.2. Start by injecting proximally (21.2a), followed by middle (21.2b) and then distal (21.2c) injection.

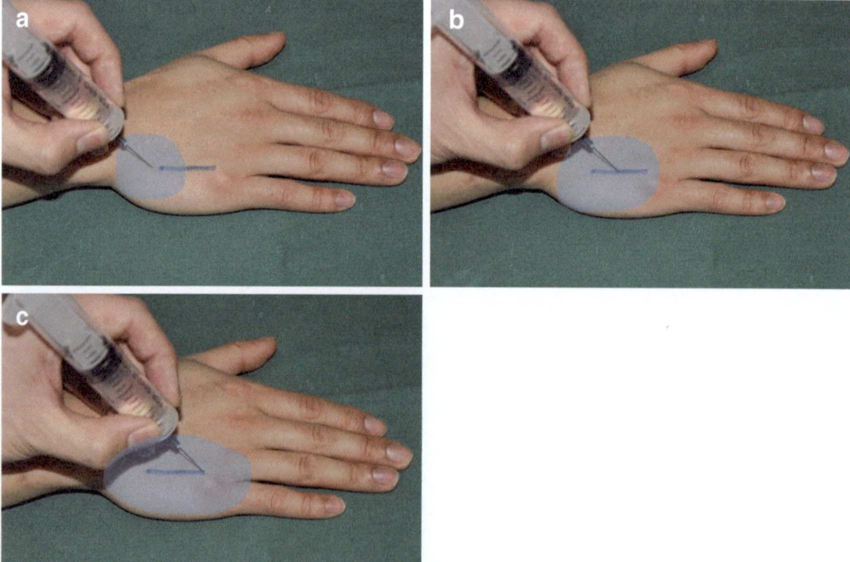

Fig. 21.2 Where to inject tumescent local anesthesia for operative reduction of metacarpal fracture. (Reproduced with permission [11])

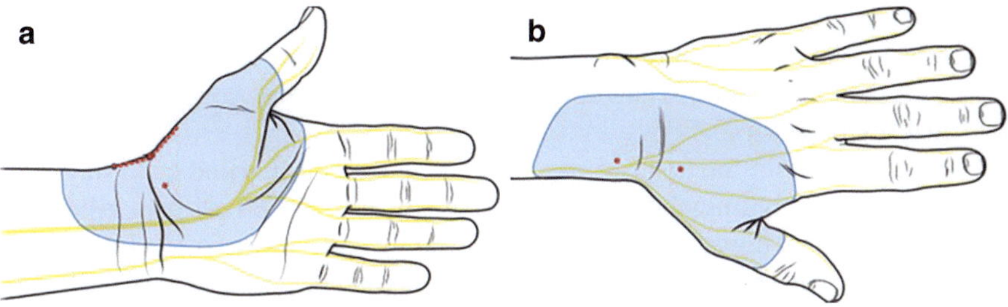

Fig. 21.3 Where to inject tumescent local anesthesia for operative reduction of Bennet fracture (base of thumb metacarpal). This is like the local anesthesia for trapeziectomy. (Reproduced with permission [12])

3. If the adjacent bones are to be involved, they also should be bathed circumferentially with local anesthesia.
4. For Bennet's fracture dislocations, it is useful to numb the whole radial side of the hand as in Fig. 21.3 which is the same approach as for WALANT trapeziectomy.
5. Manipulation of the fractured part should be totally pain free before starting the surgery.

Wrist and Distal Radius Fracture Reduction

All wrist and distal radius fractures are also amenable to WALANT surgery [13, 14].

Patients Need to See Their Finger Move During Surgery

Patients need to look at their fingers or thumb to help them move the digit after you reduce the fracture, since they cannot feel the numbed digit move. If you are using main operating room sterility, take down drapes so they can see the finger if you are asking them to move it. Although most patients do not mind looking at the wound, you can cover it with a towel as they flex and extend the tip of the finger or thumb.

Intraoperative Unsedated Patient Education During WALANT Hand Fracture Reduction

Patient education is one of the most important keys to improving the results of hand fracture management. I love to explain to patients that the biggest problem with finger fractures is stiffness. During the surgery, I tell them that they can avoid this by following some simple rules.

1. Follow pain guided healing. I tell them that if they follow the rules, all they will need for pain is ibuprofen (800 mg) to which they can add acetaminophen (1000 mg) if they need more relief for the first 2–3 days after fracture surgery.

However, they need to be a "one armed man" with the operated hand higher than the heart and quiet at all times because they do not know what hurts when they are on pain medication. They do not need narcotics if they keep their hand elevated and quiet for 3–5 days.

2. I tell them that for the first 3–5 days after surgery, their K wired hand stays elevated and mostly immobilized. This allows them to get off all pain killers, so they know what hurts. This also lets the swelling come down. It lets bleeding in the fracture site stop to avoid adding more callus and scar which lead to stiffness. Totally avoiding pain killers and pain guided movement will also prevent skin infection around K wire sites and loss of fracture reduction when they start moving their hand with the hand therapist at 3–5 days with early protected pain guided movement [15].

3. I explain to them the importance of early protected movement with the therapist, so their fingers do not get stiff. Starting at 3–5 days after surgery, they will not be using their fingers, just keeping them moving a little so they do not get stuck in scar.

4. We take advantage of the uninterrupted operating time to discuss return to work and activities, as well as realistic outcomes of their fracture problem.

References

1. Gillis JA, Williams JG. Cost analysis of percutaneous fixation of hand fractures in the main operating room versus the ambulatory setting. J Plast Reconstr Aesthet Surg. 2017;70(8):1044–50.
2. Gillis JA, Lalonde J, Alagar D, Azzi A, Lalonde DH. K-wire Fixation of Closed Hand Fractures Outside the Main Operating Room Does Not Increase Infections. Plast Reconstr Surg Glob Open. 2022 Nov 21;10(11):e4679. https://doi.org/10.1097/GOX.0000000000004679. PMID: 36438460; PMCID: PMC9682614.
3. Yu J, Ji TA, Craig M, McKee D, Lalonde DH. Evidence-based sterility: the evolving role of field sterility in skin and minor hand surgery. Plast Reconstr Surg Glob Open. 2019;7(11):e2481.
4. Steve AK, Schrag CH, Kuo A, Harrop AR. Metacarpal fracture fixation in a minor surgery setting versus main operating room: a cost-minimization analysis. Plast Reconstr Surg Glob Open. 2019;7(7):e2298.
5. Garon MT, Massey P, Chen A, Carroll T, Nelson BG, Hollister AM. Cost and complications of percutaneous fixation of hand fractures in a procedure room versus the operating room. Hand. 2018;13(4):428–34.
6. Lalonde DH. How to inject local anesthesia with minimal pain. In: Lalonde DH, editor. Wide awake hand surgery. New York, NY: Thieme; 2016. p. 37–48.
7. YouTube. Lecture on how to inject local anesthesia with minimal pain for hand fractures. n.d.. https://youtu.be/IcSizvzD6LM. Accessed 26 Jun 2021.
8. McKee DE, Lalonde DH, Thoma A, et al. Optimal time delay between epinephrine injection and incision to minimize bleeding. Plast Reconstr Surg. 2013;131:811–4.
9. Greene B, Lalonde D, Seal S. Incidence of the "adrenaline rush" and vasovagal response with local anesthetic injection. Plast Reconstruct Surg Glob Open. 2021;9(6):e3659.
10. Lalonde DH. Finger fractures. In: Lalonde DH, editor. Wide awake hand surgery. New York, NY: Thieme; 2016. p. 237–42.
11. Xing SG, Tang JB, Lalonde DH. Metacarpal fractures. In: Lalonde DH, editor. Wide awake hand surgery. New York, NY: Thieme; 2016. p. 243–6.

12. Lalonde DH, Amadio PC, Cook G. Trapeziectomy with or without ligament reconstruction. In: Lalonde DH, editor. Wide awake hand surgery. New York, NY: Thieme; 2016. p. 165–9.
13. Kurtzman JS, Etcheson JI, Koehler SM. Wide-awake local anesthesia with no tourniquet: an updated review. Plast Reconstr Surg Glob Open. 2021;9(3):e3507.
14. Abd Hamid MH, Abdullah S, Ahmad AA, Narin Singh PSG, Soh EZF, Liu CY, Sapuan J. A randomized controlled trial comparing wide-awake local anesthesia with no tourniquet (WALANT) to general anesthesia in plating of distal radius fractures with pain and anxiety level perception. Cureus. 2021;13(1):e12876.
15. Gregory S, Lalonde DH, Fung Leung LT. Minimally invasive finger fracture management: wide-awake closed reduction, K-wire fixation, and early protected movement. Hand Clin. 2014;30(1):7–15.

Rehabilitation and Orthoses for Adult Hand Fractures

22

Stacy Rumfelt, Teresa Mintz, and Ashley Brooks

Introduction

Hand fractures constitute approximately 10% of all musculoskeletal fractures, with the distal phalanx being the most common hand fracture [1]. These injuries can be catastrophic to a person's functional independence, work, engagement, family roles, and mental health [2]. Skilled management is critical to return to these functions and includes careful consideration of bony and soft tissue structure healing, anatomy, and surgical procedures. Hand therapy combines the philosophy and techniques of occupational and physical therapy and is defined as the "art and science of rehabilitation of the upper limb" [3]. Hand therapists are highly trained professionals who evaluate and treat upper extremity injuries in both conservative and surgical cases in order to restore movement and function. Patients who receive hand therapy have improved outcomes in motion and function [4, 5]. The information stated in this chapter is representative of the most current evidence available and the professional opinions of experienced clinicians. The authors of this chapter are occupational therapists (OTs), and therefore narration, evaluation, and intervention techniques will be described from this professional perspective. This chapter will describe the hand therapy process and how to use it to provide evidence-based protocols for phalanx and metacarpal fractures.

Hand therapy's lineage dates back to WWI, with the beginning of the broader discipline of occupational therapy (OT). Volunteers were recruited across the USA

S. Rumfelt (✉)
Occupational/Hand Therapy Department, OrthoCarolina, Gastonia, NC, USA
e-mail: Stacy.Rumfelt@orthocarolina.com

T. Mintz
Occupational/Hand Therapy Department, OrthoCarolina, Rock Hill, SC, USA
e-mail: Teresa.Mintz@orthocarolina.com

A. Brooks
Atlanta, GA, USA

J. M. Abzug et al. (eds.), *Pediatric and Adult Hand Fractures*,
https://doi.org/10.1007/978-3-031-32072-9_22

to train as practitioners of this nascent field and lead soldiers in functional tasks to facilitate return of function [6]. During WWII, there was an unprecedentedly high number of upper extremity injuries sustained by soldiers during combat. Dr. Sterling Bunnell, the "founding father" of hand surgery, was appointed as a consultant to the Secretary of War by the U.S. Surgeon General and established hand treatment centers for the U.S. Army [6]. Dr. Bunnell heralded OT as a critical component of recovery for these soldiers and expressed appreciation for their dedication to restoring the special function of the hand [6]. It was not until the Vietnam War, when surgery specialties—and subsequently hand surgery—would emerge as areas of specialized practice. Highly specialized hand surgeries for tendon and bone repairs were developed during this time and required the concomitant specialization of therapists to guide the recovery of these patients [6]. The phrase "hand therapy," however, would not be coined until 1977 when the national organization, American Society of Hand Therapists was formed [7]. Today the practice consists of just over 7000 certified hand therapists (CHT's), who are licensed as OTs and PTs, who provide skilled care internationally [8].

Evaluation

From the beginning, communication of information is a critical component of a patient's care. The most efficient care should consist of a triad of communication between the surgeon/physician, the therapist, and the patient. Surgeons should communicate to the treating therapist the fracture type, location, method, and quality of stabilization, as well as any complications or precautions [9]. Providing a surgical report, radiographic findings, and discussion of any additional details about the patient can be instrumental in the treatment planning by the therapist. Conveying this information early on enables a therapist to determine the course of treatment according to expected healing timelines and stability of structures while also navigating any complications or comorbidities [9]. For example, early conveyance of information concerning a strong stabilization of a metacarpal shaft fracture will enable the therapist to confidently pursue a more aggressive approach in treatment, but if this information is not relayed early on a therapist will typically default to the most conservative management. Likewise, it is the responsibility of the therapist to relay pertinent information to the surgeon concerning progress or lack thereof during treatment [10]. The final component is effectively educating the patient to take proper care of their injury and entrusting that they will relay accurate information to the professionals concerning new or changing symptoms that may affect their outcome. Deficiency in this fluid interprofessional and interpersonal communication may cause a permanent loss of motion and function for the patient.

After the patient is referred to therapy, initiation of treatment starts with a thorough evaluation performed by the therapist consisting of medical history intake, an occupational profile, objective measurements, assessment, and treatment planning. An occupational profile is defined as "a summary of a client's (person's, group's, or population's) occupational history and experiences, patterns of daily living, interests, values, needs, and relevant contexts" [11]. Objective measurements of edema, range of motion, pain, sensation, and strength are also assessed as appropriate. These client factors (body functions and body structures) are evaluated and then assessed for deficiencies and differences as compared to the non-injured side or from pre-injury recall. This information is used to set functional and clinical goals for the patient/s and guides the intervention/s used to create meaningful and effective treatments in order to restore function.

Client Factors

Edema

Edema typically occurs immediately at the time of injury, in this instance, fracture. It is a physiologic response to injury and is the result of the inflammatory process which consists of a variety of cellular mediators streaming to the area of trauma in order to begin the healing process. These mediators consist of cytokines, growth factors, and prostaglandins, which help to stop bleeding. Although inflammation and the resultant edema are normal and natural responses to injury, they can cause a multitude of complications during the immobilization period following fracture in both operative and nonoperative cases. Interstitial fluid accumulates in the extracellular spaces and can lead to restriction in range of motion. This added fluid causes pressure within the joint capsule often providing feedback to the nervous system in the form of pain signals [12]. Pain signals are a protective response to injury and as such patients often self-limit motion leading to capsular stiffness and additional fluid accumulation. Fibrin deposits cause permanent physiologic changes in capsular composition leading to fibrosis and ongoing stiffness [12, 13]. It is imperative that edema be addressed early in the therapy process and plan of care when treating fractures to avoid loss of motion and function [13]. If not, its presence can complicate the restorative phase of fracture management and require additional interventions outside of edema management to resolve the joint stiffness.

Common edema management strategies in the acute/immobilization period first and foremost include patient education. Arming the patient with information regarding the healing process is critical to their understanding of what they are experiencing and why. Knowledge is a key component for recovery and increases adherence to home programs that in this case will consist of edema management. Without proper instruction the patient may forgo simple strategies such as rest, elevation, and muscle pumping, thus leading to further accumulation of fluid in the hand or digit/s. Manual edema mobilization techniques are a unique set of manual therapy strokes combined with pump point stimulation and exercise that can be performed by the therapist and implemented at home by the patient several times daily. Used in conjunction with other edema management interventions, these techniques could prove beneficial in the reduction of swelling [14–16]. Compressive wrapping can be instituted early on in the protective phase for the operative and nonoperative patient. The operative patient may have surgical incisions, pins, or wounds that are healing, and compression wrapping with conforming gauze can prove beneficial in the wound healing process if circulation is not compromised. Minimizing edema promotes wound contraction and lessens the risk of infection as the lymphatic system can communicate at the level of the injury [12, 13]. Depending on the location of fracture, use of tubigrip stockinette can add an additional amount of compression. One must monitor patient tolerance to this type of compression as it is not necessarily a true gradient pressure. Modalities such as high volt electrical current (HVPC), H-wave, cryotherapy, and game ready systems can also be implemented both in the protective and restorative phases of rehabilitation [12].

During the subacute or restorative phases of healing, edema can turn from a watery transudate to that of brawny or fibrotic exudate [13]. Physiologically, the longer that the edema resides in the extracellular spaces the more the protein rich interstitial fluid thickens. Macrophages are sent to the area to begin proteolysis, but when the macrophages congest the area fibrosis and ligamentosis develop, which require more aggressive interventions to effect edema reduction [12, 13, 15]. The scaffolding or bonds of this gel-like fluid forms scar tissue and can lead to irreversible loss of motion if not addressed in a timely fashion [12]. Interventions in this phase may include pulsed ultrasound [17] and fibrosis techniques to manually break through the protein rich edema that allow for drainage of fluids [18]. Over the counter or custom compression gloves can be worn during the day as an external support for the skin so as to prevent accumulation of fluid as the patient goes about their daily routines, and Kinesio Taping for edema can facilitate lymphatic drainage from distal to proximal [19]. In conclusion, it is of utmost importance that the therapist identifies edema during the evaluation, educates the patient, and intervenes appropriately in order to prevent adverse and long standing consequences that may interfere with patient roles, routines, and daily activities [12, 13, 19, 20].

Clinical Considerations
- Avoid compression if there is arterial involvement so as to avoid compromise of circulation.
- Avoid heat during the acute phase of swelling so as to avoid further accumulation of fluids distally.
- Refrain from use of cryotherapy with concomitant diagnosis such as nerve repairs or replantations and with those patients who have sensory loss.
- Utilize light hands-on edema mobilization techniques to facilitate lymphatic drainage. Avoid retrograde massage, string wrapping, and ace wraps that compress the superficial lymphatics [18, 19].
- Minimize use of lymphatic drainage with those patients who have comorbidities such as untreated cancer, deep vein thrombosis, pulmonary embolism, untreated infection, chronic heart failure, or renal failure [18, 19].
- Chip bags are an effective means of affecting brawny edema over the dorsal hand in the subacute phase of injury [18].
- Avoid Kinesio Taping on fragile or new skin.
- Do not use HVPC on those clients who have a history of seizure or cardiac conditions including pacemakers [17].

Range of Motion

Restoration of range of motion (ROM) after a hand fracture is vital to regaining functional use of the hand. Early ROM can assist with edema, facilitate smooth tendon gliding, minimize scar adhesions, and minimize risk of joint contractures. Once a fracture is stabilized, either by way of open or closed reduction, initiation of motion will be dependent on the stage of fracture healing.

The goal of hand therapy is to safely introduce ROM while maintaining fracture stability. The therapist must understand fracture type, various forms of fixation, and stages of fracture healing to safely introduce ROM. Ideally, the hand therapist has access to radiology reports and operative reports to understand the management of the fracture. If this information is unavailable, it is imperative that the hand therapist be provided with the fracture date and method of fixation [21, 22].

There are two ways that a fractured bone can heal: primary and secondary bone healing. Primary bone healing occurs when the fractured ends are compressed or closely approximated to eliminate any interfragmentary gap and stabilized to eliminate any movement. This level of rigid fixation is usually obtained surgically with plating or screws. Because there is no motion that occurs at the fracture site, new bone is generated directly across the fracture fragments without the formation of a callus. Secondary healing occurs when there is a small amount of motion at the fracture site. This motion causes a formation of a callus, which through the three stages of healing is eventually remodeled into bone. Secondary healing is usually seen with cast immobilization, K-wire, or intramedullary pins [23–25].

There are three overlapping stages of bone healing that occur with secondary healing: inflammation, repair, and remodeling. The inflammatory phase begins immediately after bone injury with the formation of a local hematoma or fibrin clot. This provides the initial structural stability and framework for producing new bone. This phase usually peaks at 48 h and can last up to 1 week. During the inflammatory stage of healing, an initial period of immobilization may be indicated to protect healing tissues.

The repair stage of healing begins within the first 2 weeks and replaces the hematoma with a soft callus. This soft callus acts as a temporary bridge to stabilize the fracture; however, this soft callus can easily bend and deform if not adequately supported. It is during this time that ROM is delayed or restricted until a clinical union can be present at about week 3. Active range of motion (AROM) can usually be initiated between weeks 4 and 6 as the callus can be considered "clinically stiff" but is not strong enough to bear a functional load. The soft callus will continue to organize and remodel into a hard callus over the next several weeks. The development of a hard callus provides more structure and strength to the bone [21, 23], therefore, is not until 6–8 weeks that passive range of motion (PROM) or use of a dynamic orthosis can be initiated to prevent soft tissue contractures. Early strengthening with light resistance can usually be initiated after 8 weeks, but unrestricted use, heavy work, or return to sports is usually restricted until after 10–12 weeks when the hard callus begins to transition to lamellar bone during the remodeling phase of healing. This phase can last for months to years. During the remodeling phase, bone responds to loading characteristics according to Wolff's law in which activity, external forces, functional demands, and growth facilitate the remodeling process.

There are three types of ROM: active (AROM), active assisted (AAROM), and passive ROM (PROM). Each may be used depending on the stage of fracture healing, type of fixation, and stability of the fracture.

AROM/AAROM

Active range of motion (AROM) is patient-controlled and is the voluntary activation of muscle contraction on the joint. Active assistive range of motion (AAROM) requires active muscle recruitment and is assisted by a low load external force, either from the patient, therapist, or use of leverage to assist with movement. Physiological benefits of AROM and A/AROM exercises include: facilitation of differential tendon gliding, promotion of strength and endurance, improvement of lymphatic drainage, and minimization of scar adhesions.

AROM should be initiated as quickly as possible depending on the nature of fixation and fracture stability to prevent adhesions and soft tissue contractures. With primary fixation, this may be as early as 1 week and with secondary healing, usually around 3–4 weeks.

Tendon gliding exercises (Fig. 22.1) are paramount to prevent adhesions and are a safe way to initiate AROM. The amount of differential gliding between the flexor digitorum profundus (FDP) and flexor digitorum superficialis (FDS) varies with each position.

- Tabletop (intrinsic plus) to facilitate extensor hood glide to attain PIP extension
- Hook fist provides maximal differential glide of FDS and FDP as well as extensor gliding of EDC to minimize adhesions with metacarpal fractures.
- Full composite fist for maximal gliding of the FDP
- Flat fist for maximal gliding of FDS

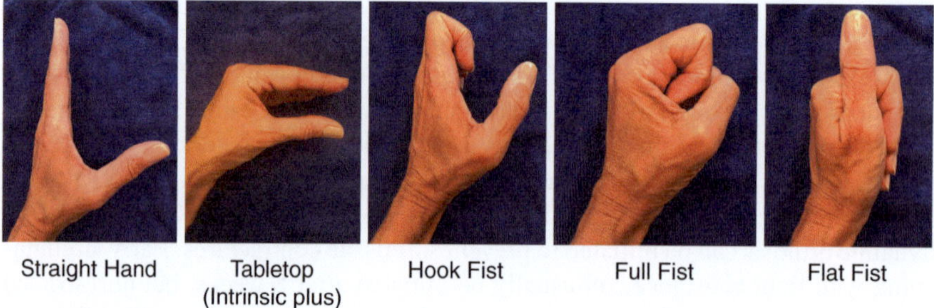

Fig. 22.1 Tendon gliding

Often when asking a patient to perform tendon gliding exercises, joints that are not hindered move the most and the stiffest joints move the least. Best outcomes may not be attained unless mechanical leverage is provided. Stabilizing or blocking movement from mobile joints and directing mechanical forces to the stiffer joints is considered A/AAROM exercises.

A/AAROM exercises may include:

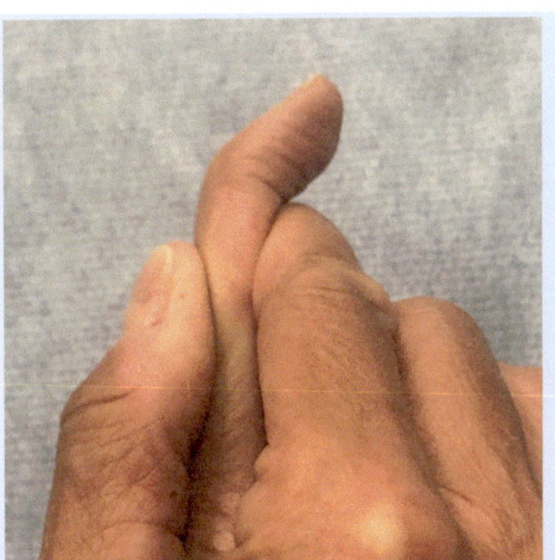

FDP tendon gliding: Blocking PIP in extension and active DIP flexion.

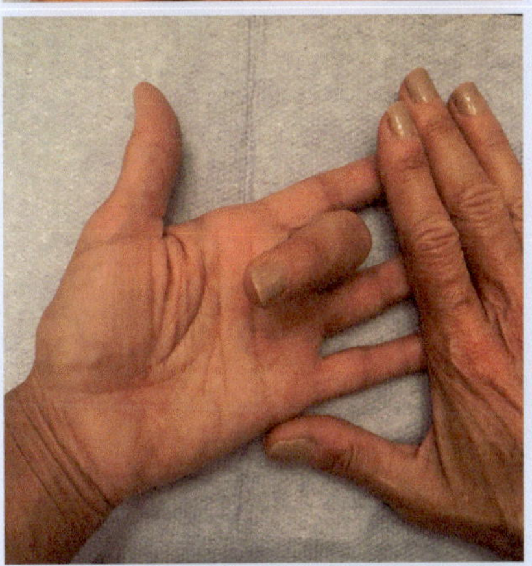

FDS tendon glides: Requires inhibition of the FDP tendon which also contributes to PIP joint flexion. This is achieved by manually restricting DIP motion in the unaffected digits with attempted PIP flexion in the involved digit.

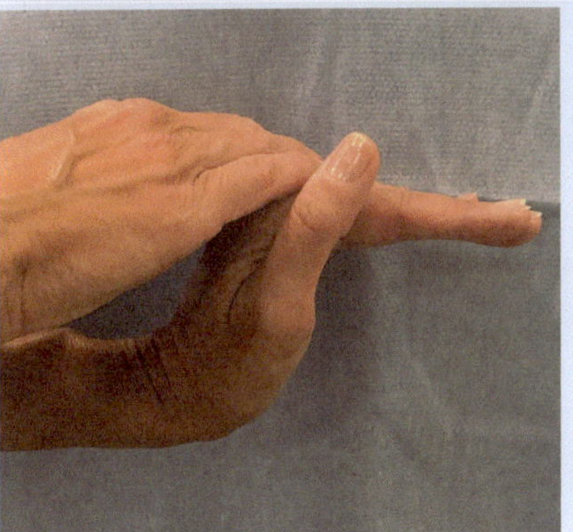

Reverse blocking: MP joints are held or blocked into flexion (intrinsic plus) and active IP extension is performed to help facilitate terminal IP extension from the lumbricals and interossei.

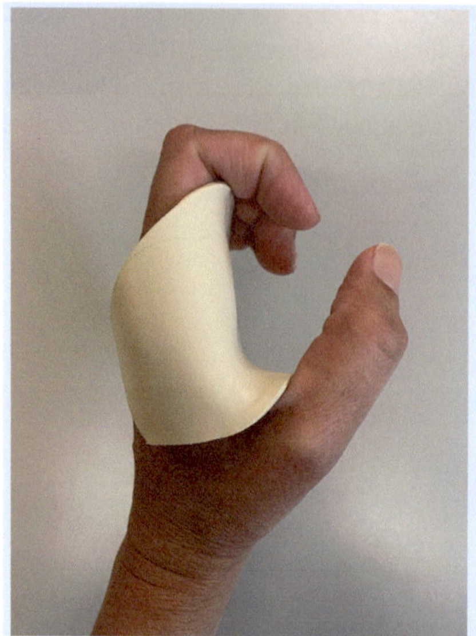

Blocked active hook exercise: To assist with maximal differential excursion of FDP and FDS and for intrinsic stretching. The hand therapist may fabricate a static MP blocking exercise orthotic.

Other important exercises can include:

- Six pack exercises [tendon glides (Fig. 22.1) plus digital ABD/ADD, thumb opposition]

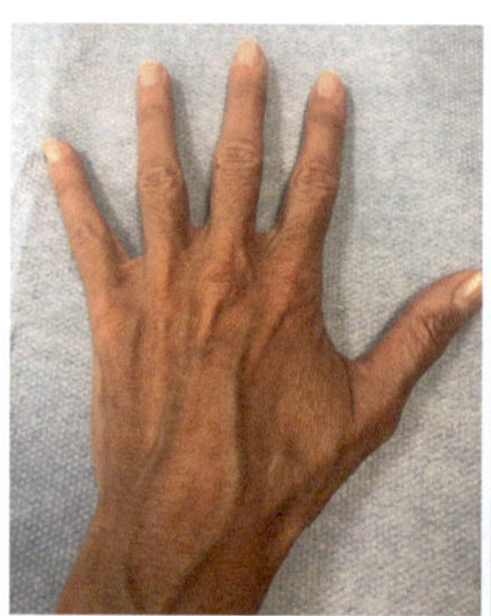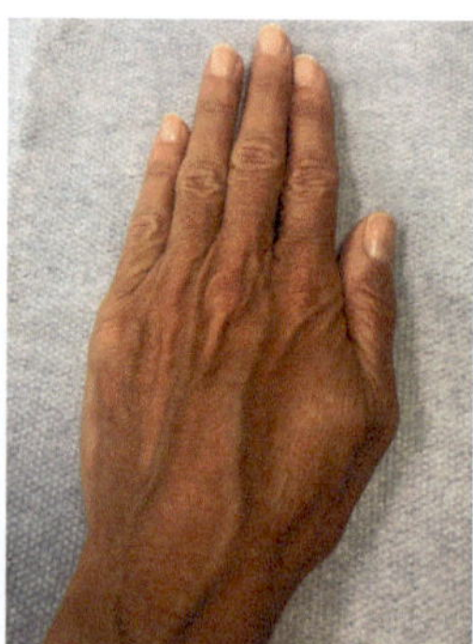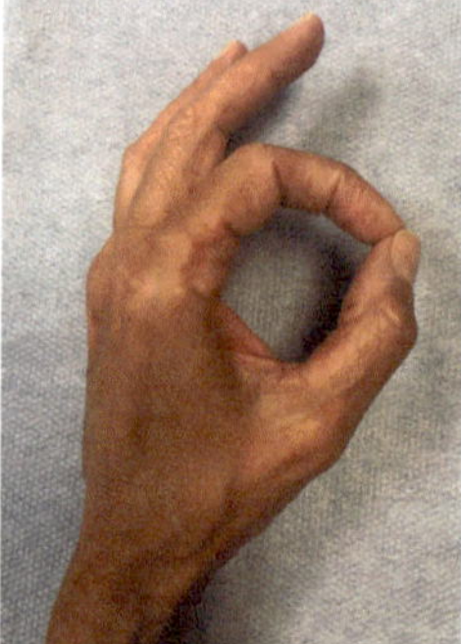

- Finger lifts from tabletop
- Place and hold

Best outcomes for ROM and establishing neuromuscular re-education or cortical involvement are achieved when the patient is able to reinforce movement with a functional activity. If cleared to perform AROM or AA/ROM the patient should begin performing light activities such as manipulation of unweighted dexterity balls, towel scrunches for finger flexion and extension, picking up cotton balls, and rice transfer for promotion of light grasp.

PROM

Passive range of motion (PROM) is the use of external force, either by the patient, therapist, or device to maximal tissue tolerance and/or resistance. Passive motion often is not initiated until the remodeling stage of healing has started, approximately 6–8 weeks after the fracture [26]. PROM helps to stretch tight joint capsules, tight muscles and minimizes the risk of joint contractures. The hand therapist may use mobilization techniques, static progressive orthosis, or dynamic orthosis to maximize PROM.

Many factors can contribute to loss of full ROM. Prolonged immobilization can occur for many reasons such as delayed healing, persistent edema, and muscle guarding or movement avoidance from the patient. This will limit the joint's ability to move in its full arc of motion. When the new collagen is laid down in a shortened position due to lack of full motion, restrictions with ROM become more fixed as remodeling continues to develop, and a joint contracture or stiffness can develop.

Passive ROM and joint mobilization are examples of the use of high load across the joint over a brief period of time. The hand therapist or patient applies a steady force up to maximal tissue tolerance or resistance. It is important to avoid aggressive high load force causing significant pain as this can cause tissue injury. The use of static progressive and dynamic orthoses use the concept of low load prolonged stress (LLPS) which applies low stress over a longer period of time (see section "Orthosis/Splinting") [27].

Pain

One of the major risk factors impeding recovery is pain. Pain intensity scores during the acute post-injury phase can determine the patient's outcomes and reduce any long-term disability. Therefore, it is important to implement pain management strategies early in the rehabilitation program to improve functional outcomes and prevent maladaptive pain responses [28–30]. Acute pain can result from the inflammatory response triggered by trauma to tissues, which includes the release of antibodies and proteins and increased blood flow to the damaged areas. The common signs of inflammation are redness, heat, swelling, and pain. The inflammatory stage, which usually lasts for about 7 days, is the first stage in fracture healing and must occur for proper bone healing to occur [31]. Nociceptors alert us to certain high thresholds of stimuli that can potentially injure tissues, such as temperatures, mechanical forces, and inflammatory mediators [32, 33]. The nociceptive pathways send danger signals, not pain signals, to the spinal cord and then on to the brain [32, 33]. During the acute inflammatory pain stage, it is important to educate the patient on the purpose and role that inflammation has in the healing process; that it is indicative of a healthy immune response and is necessary for proper bone healing [31].

The association between pain intensity and severity of tissue damage varies greatly among patients, and local tissue pathology is neither necessary nor needs to be appreciated to experience pain [34]. Pain involves a complex relationship between the biological processes that interact within psychosocial contexts [35]. "According to recent evidence-based pain control theories, the neuromatrix paradigm codes pain characteristics according to cognitive, emotional, and sensorial dimensions. Understanding the underlying mechanisms of the paradigm offers specific rehabilitation strategies that address cognitive, emotional, and sensory aspects of pain" [30]. Pain experienced by patients can be influenced by several psychosocial factors such as the tendency to catastrophize, depression, stress, belief systems about pain, and fear of movement [36].

In the acute inflammatory phase of healing, the doctor may prescribe medication to alleviate pain. The literature on the use of NSAIDS for pain and the effects on possibly delaying fracture healing are conflicting [37, 38]. Studies have shown that opiates are not associated with improved patient outcomes and are associated with high risk of abuse and are generally not prescribed [38].

As we know, pain is a complex intertwining of physical, physiological, and emotional factors. It is important to address pain early and throughout the rehabilitative course to prevent maladaptive pain responses. Hand therapists can use a variety of physical agent modalities to help alleviate pain associated with changes in tissue pathology. The use of cryotherapy, electrical stimulation modalities, such as TENS, IFC, or high volt, can also be used for acute pain [36]. As the fracture and soft tissues heal, exercises and movement have been shown to help with decreasing pain, although educating patients on proper exercise techniques is required [39]. Patients recovering from a hand fracture may develop maladaptive nociception (defined as disabling misconception regarding pain) with over guarding or protectiveness, which has been associated with posttraumatic stiffness and delayed recovery [40]. It is important for the patient to understand the benefits of early motion, exercise, and light functional use for best outcomes. It is also important that patients understand it is not beneficial to exercise to cause pain, or to work through pain and that patients do not exercise with the outdated philosophy of "no pain, no gain."

Hand therapists are equipped with training and knowledge to educate and counsel patients about their pain perception, teaching strategies to self-manage pain along the patient's course of recovery. Strategies to help patients cope with pain are evolving with the growing understanding of the complexities of pain. The use of graded motor imagery, mirror therapy, deep breathing, and desensitization are effective tools [41].

Strength

Regardless of the method of fixation, either by primary or secondary healing, strengthening programs should not be initiated until the remodeling phase has begun at around 6–8 weeks and the patient has been cleared by the surgeon [21, 23, 42]. Progressive strengthening or resistive exercises are incorporated into therapy to help to build strength, improve joint ROM, promote soft tissue and tendon excursion. Strength should be monitored for trending improvement with a dynamometer. The use of putty, rubber band resistance, and various functional activities can be used to improve strength, thereby improving different functional grasps and pinches [26]. Neuromuscular electrical stimulation (NMES) can be used for motor recruitment for atrophied and weak muscles due to prolonged immobilization.

Pin Site Care

Percutaneous pinning is commonplace for those fractures that are unstable, whereas mini-external fixators are utilized for comminuted and intra-articular fractures of the hand. Both consist of pins or wires that traverse through the skin, fascia, and bone in order to provide stability and reduction or stabilization of the fracture. When pins or wires are used for fracture management, there are a variety of factors that can increase the likelihood of infection which may eventually lead to loosening of the hardware, compromise of fracture reduction and increased likelihood of osteomyelitis [43, 44]. It is imperative as therapists that we provide the patient with adequate education regarding pin site care and recognizing signs of infection in order to minimize this likelihood. Common factors that predispose patients to pin site infections include bacteria that exist naturally on the skin, swelling that reduces the lymphatic system's ability to provide immunity on the skin's surface, comorbidities (i.e., diabetes, rheumatoid arthritis, circulatory issues, smoking), and use of steroids which compromises the body's ability to heal [43]. At this time, there is no consensus on pin site care in the literature due to the heterogeneity of studies. Current strategies to prevent infection include preoperative prophylactic antibiotics, attention to pin insertion in order to minimize trauma to the soft tissue, use of coated pins, limiting motion of tissues around the pins, and finally pin site care itself [43–45]. Current literature cites a variety of cleaning solutions used in pin care which may include normal saline, half strength hydrogen peroxide, chlorhexidine gluconate solution 4.0%, soap with water, 70% isopropyl alcohol, or no cleaning at all; however, at this time, there is not a consensus on which is superior. Chlorhexadine has preliminary evidence that it may be useful for decreasing pin site colonization, antibiotic use, and pain; however, more research is needed [43, 46]. Frequency of pin site care is also up for debate. Ranges vary in current studies from:

- daily for the first 3 days
- use of an occlusive dressing around the pins changed every 5–7 days
- use of gauze if exudate or no use if no exudate
- Chlorhexadine dressing for the first 7 days followed by twice daily cleaning with chlorhexadine for the duration of fixation
- daily or weekly cleaning with 0.9% saline

Showers can take place once the pin sites have healed. Patients are also permitted to swim in a chlorinated pool but should take extreme care not to bathe in tub water or swim in lake or ocean water [43, 44, 46]. In conclusion, it is critical that the hand therapist uses good clinical reasoning while communicating with their referring physicians until the literature substantiates a gold standard in pin site care.

Adherence

Adherence or compliance is an aspect of the therapeutic process that is garnering more interest as current research has shown a direct relationship between adherence and outcomes [47–50]. Adherence in hand therapy can be defined as keeping appointments, following through with prescribed home programs, taking the practitioner's advice and using correct form [47, 50]. Taking time to provide the patient with education on the importance of complying in these areas is critical and can directly and profoundly affect their overall success in therapy. Research has identified several key factors that can impact the patient's ability to adhere to the various aspects of their therapy experience. These factors include locus of control, self-efficacy, pain, threat and beliefs, physical activity level, psychological symptoms, perceived barriers, social support, and time [48, 50]. When patients fail to adhere or comply with their home exercise programs (HEP) the cost of care increases not only from a financial standpoint but from a time investment as well. Additional therapy visits may be required to achieve desired outcomes. Therapist burden including energy, time, and more aggressive interventions may have to be implemented to restore function in the upper extremity injured patient. Finally, costs to the patient or insurance may come in the form of additional surgical procedures needing to be performed to restore AROM [50].

In order to maximize outcomes, it is imperative that the hand therapist crafts an evidence-based, individualized program that is not only feasible for the patient to complete but also supported by family or an accountability partner. This has shown to be an effective strategy to improve adherence [50]. Other strategies to positively influence adherence and reduce barriers include: written diaries or use of self-reporting tools; however, these are subjective accounts and often are not accurate as patients tend to overestimate their participation in their HEP. Use of patient/therapist contracts and written instructions has also been found to have positive effects on adherence [47]. Coaching through the use of videoconferencing, instant or text messaging, and email can provide additional feedback and supervision that patients may require once they leave the clinic setting in order to ensure proper form and frequency. Accessibility of the HEP is also a consideration when contemplating the use of technology versus paper handouts. Maximizing convenience and accessibility of the HEP can play a key role in the program's success [49]. Patient education, behavior modification, self-monitoring, and use of new technologies in the form of apps may also increase consistency and adherence [50].

Currently, there is no gold standard for measuring adherence outside of the self-report which is often biased and self-serving. Patients tend to over report the frequency and number of repetitions completed when keeping an exercise diary [50]. In order to lessen this bias, therapists have begun to utilize technology in the form of various home exercise apps to record compliance. Novel research is being conducted in this area as the majority of clients own a smartphone and improvements in outcomes in other medical specialty areas studied have documented results as statistically significant [49].

In the absence of technology, in-clinic strategies may be utilized and include limiting prescribed HEP to the fewest exercises possible to make gains. Research conducted in this area reveals that a maximum of four exercises is optimal for HEP adherence. Therapists should consider relying on the most effective and efficient exercises to obtain outcomes or rotating a low number of exercises throughout the course of treatment to maximize both outcome and adherence [48].

> **Clinical Considerations**
> - Assign no more than four exercises at any one time to increase adherence to HEP.
> - Consider using technology (home exercise apps, texting, videoconferencing, or email) to improve guidance and feedback regarding form and frequency,

Protocols

Now that we have discussed the various elements of evaluation and treatment for hand therapy, we will apply these concepts with available current evidence to provide protocols for these common hand fractures (Tables 22.1, 22.2, 22.3, 22.4, 22.5, and 22.6). These are based on assumed normal tissue healing timelines without complication. Please defer to your referring physician's preference, radiographic evidence, and clinical judgment.

Table 22.1 Rehab of stable metacarpal fractures second to fifth

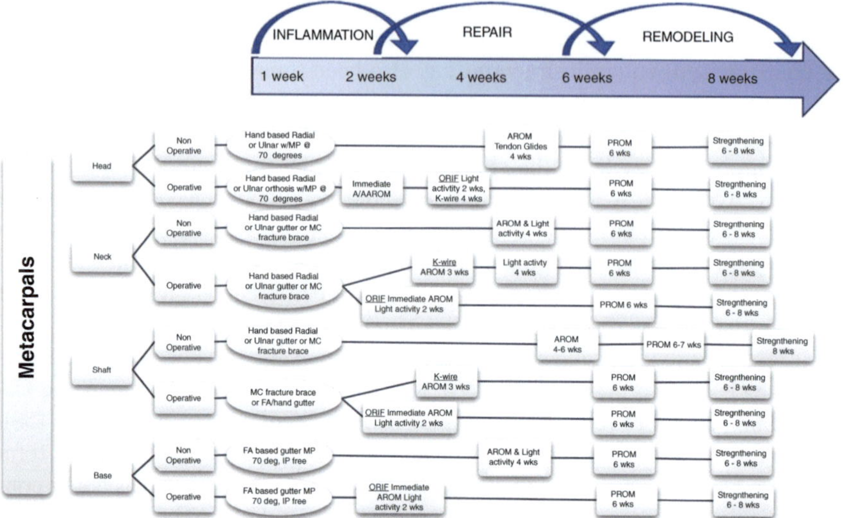

References [21, 51–56]

Table 22.2 Rehab of stable proximal phalanx fractures

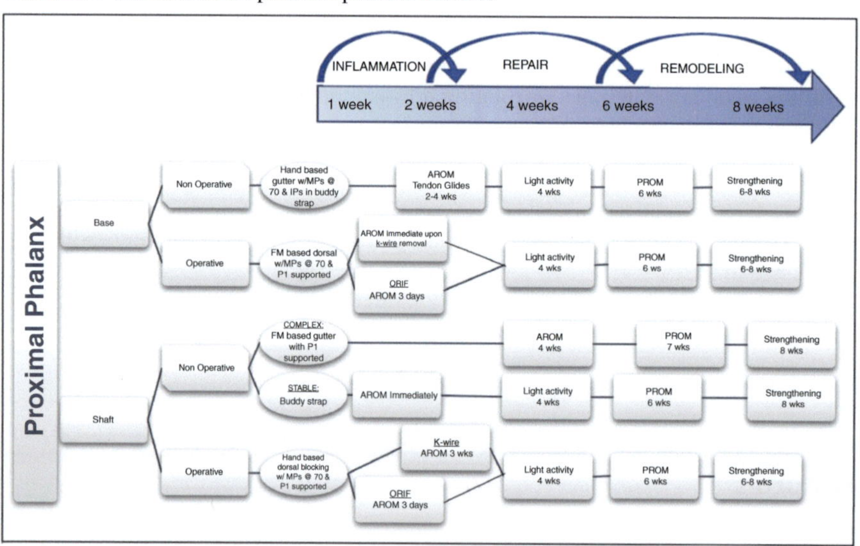

References [21, 42, 53, 55, 57]

Table 22.3 Rehab of stable middle phalanx fractures

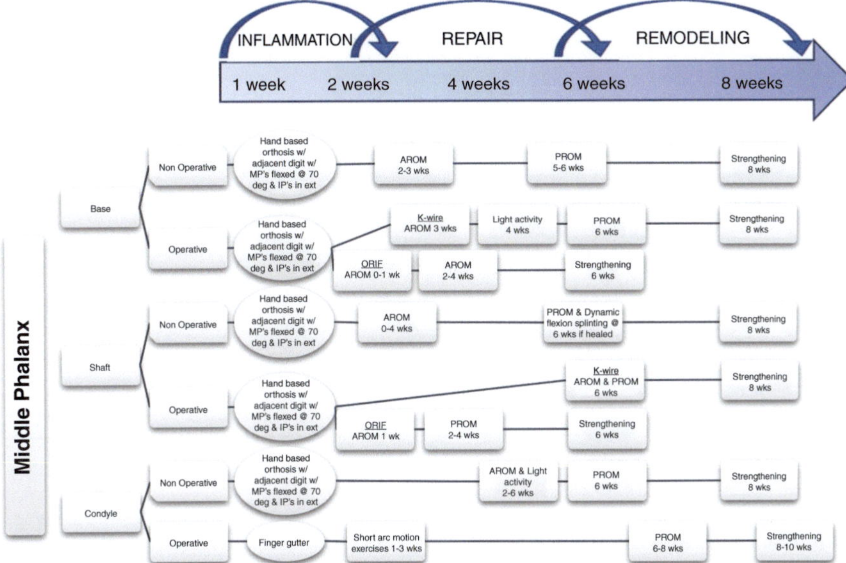

References [21, 52, 53, 55, 58]

Table 22.4 Rehab of PIP dislocations and pilon fractures

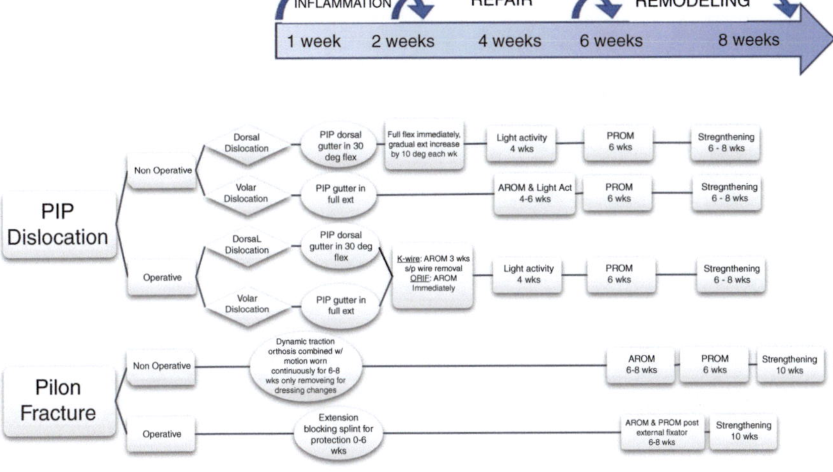

References [21, 52, 55]

Table 22.5 Rehab of distal phalanx fractures

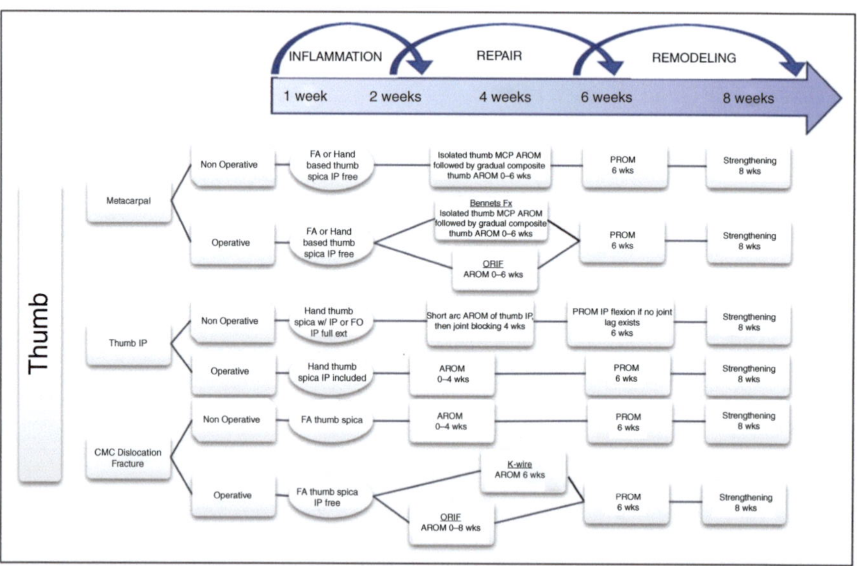

References [21, 52, 53, 55, 58]

Table 22.6 Rehab of stable thumb fractures

References [51, 52, 59, 60]

Orthosis/Splinting

Orthosis as defined by ASHT is "used to describe a single device. A rigid or semi-rigid device that supports a weak or deformed body member or restricts or eliminates motion in a diseased or injured part of the body" [61]. An effective orthosis should enhance the rehabilitation and functional recovery from a hand fracture. A well fit orthosis should prevent joint contractures, regain range of motion, improve functional outcomes, all while protecting the healing structures. However, an improper fit can result in skin breakdown, pain, deformities, non-compliance, and dysfunction. Historically, this process was referred to as splinting; however, the professional nomenclature changed in 2008 in order to better encompass the complex nature involved with this intervention [62]. For the sake of accurate interprofessional communication, integrated use of the phrase "orthosis" is strongly encouraged and will be used during discussion in this chapter. Orthosis fabrication and fitting requires a therapist to have an in-depth understanding of upper extremity anatomy, pathology, and kinesiology all while executing expert clinical reasoning and creative problem solving. Rehabilitation goals related to orthoses should support musculoskeletal healing as well as occupational performance [63]. A hand therapist can be an excellent resource to help guide the decision-making process that will promote musculo-skeletal healing in addition to improving patient adherence and satisfaction while meeting therapeutic goals. In this section we will discuss the types of orthoses available, general considerations for optimal fabrication and fit, and strategies for working alongside the therapist to choose an orthosis and ensure excellent results.

There are four primary categories of orthosis to consider depending on the therapeutic goal: static, serial static, dynamic, or static progressive. All of these types can be custom fabricated, and most are also available as a prefabricated option that can then be professionally custom fit in the clinic. In addition to the patient's injury or condition, lifestyle, cognition, home environment, and financial burden are also considered with orthosis design and selection. Below we will define and speak to each one of these options, see Table 22.7 for additional examples.

- **Static Orthosis**—A rigid support, used for protection, stabilization, or comfort. Typically used immediately following an injury [62]. *Example: A hand based ulnar gutter orthosis.*
- Unlike in the lower extremity, the hand has muscles that cross multiple joints. Therefore, static blocking and exercise orthoses can be used to transfer force and motion from blocked to available joints in order to promote ROM [64]. *Example: MP extension blocks orthosis for intrinsic tightness and a Yoke orthosis, also known as relative motion orthosis for PIP Extension.*
- **Serial Static Orthosis**—A rigid support that is applied to promote joint ROM at the tissue length's end range in order to promote tissue elongation. This orthosis is modified as the tissue changes in order to make additional gains in passive motion [62]. This orthosis is typically used for chronic joint contractures and should be worn for the majority of the day and night in order to promote lasting changes. This can be used for a PIP flexion contracture to promote passive extension. *Example: Circumferential finger orthosis remodeled weekly.*

Table 22.7 Orthosis pics and table

Orthosis type	Purpose	Examples
Hand based ulnar gutter orthosis	• Third, fourth, and fifth metacarpal fractures • Proximal phalanx fractures	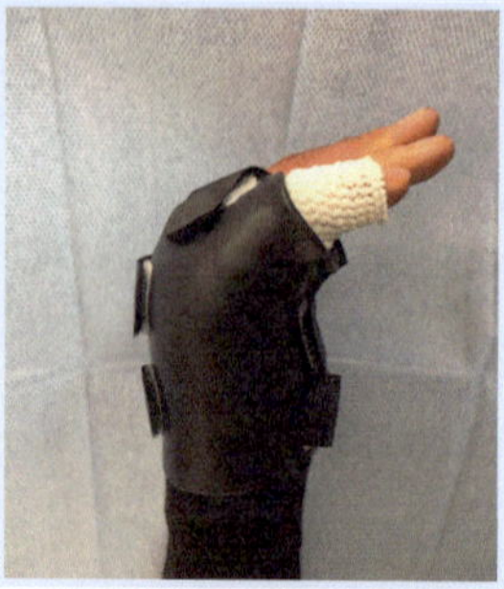
Hand based thumb spica orthosis	• First metacarpal fractures	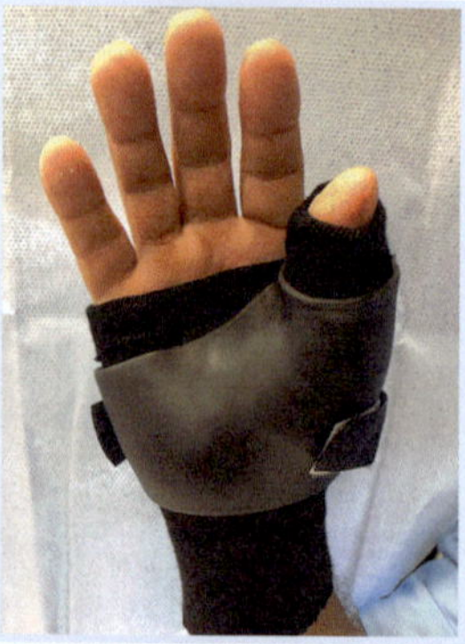
Hand based radial gutter orthosis	• Management of proximal phalangeal fractures	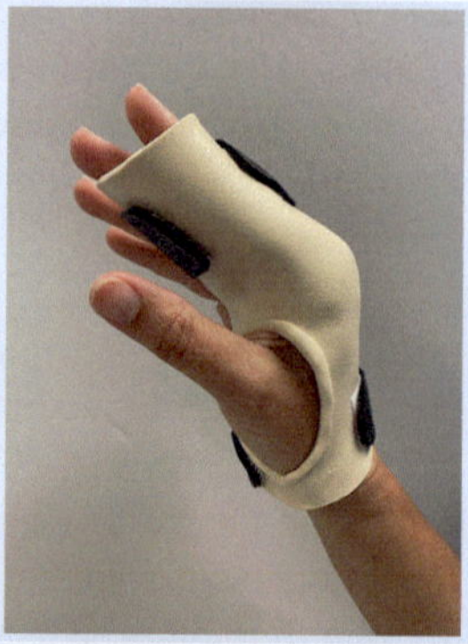
Forearm-based radial gutter orthosis	• Second and third metacarpal fractures • Second and third phalangeal fractures	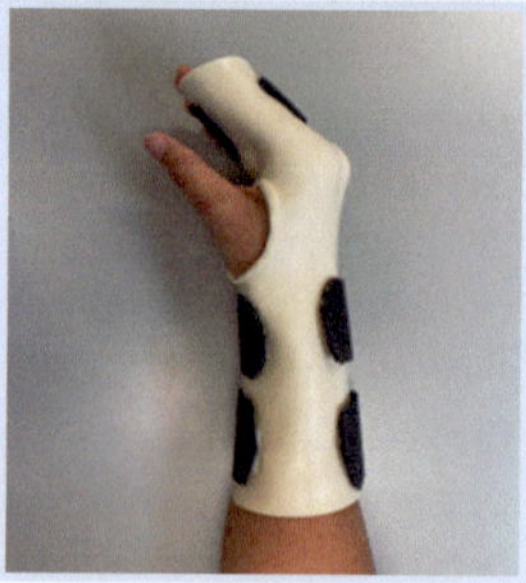

Table 22.7 (continued)

Orthosis type	Purpose	Examples
Functional fracture orthosis with 3 point stabilization	• Used to manage metacarpal fractures that are stable in order to allow for normal active motion of the uninvolved joints	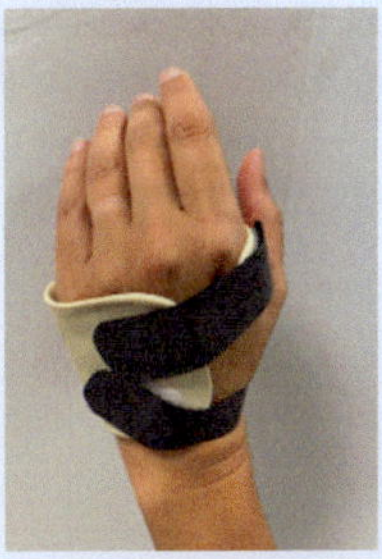 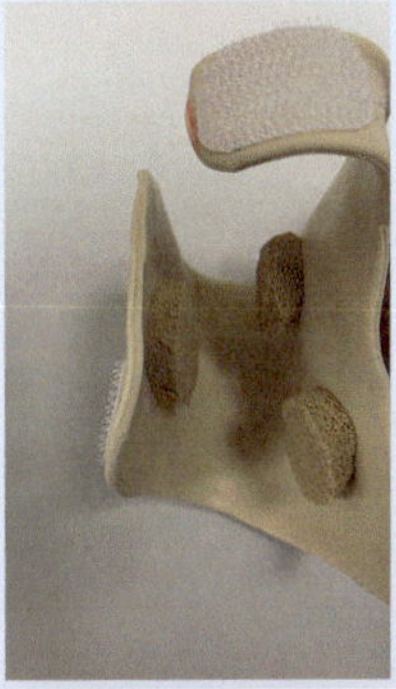
Mallet orthosis	• Bony avulsion fracture of the tip distal to the DIP joint	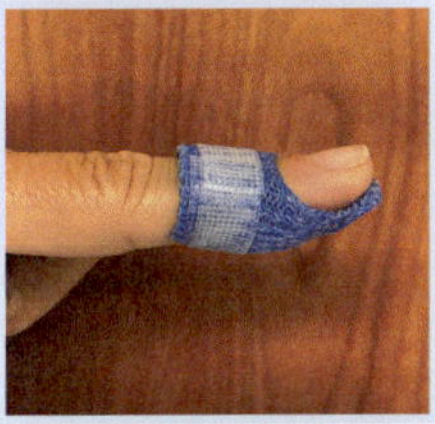 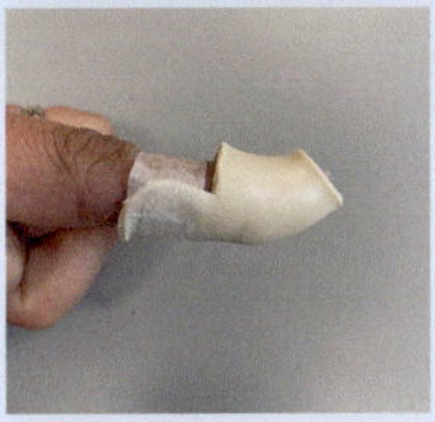
Dorsal gutter orthosis	• Middle phalanx volar avulsion with possibility of dorsal subluxation • PIPJ dorsal dislocations	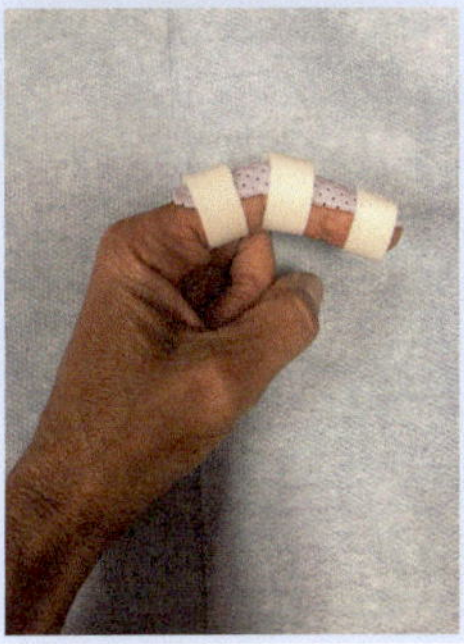

(continued)

Table 22.7 (continued)

Orthosis type	Purpose	Examples
Static progressive finger flexion orthosis	• Management and progressive mobilization of the stiff hand once the fracture is deemed healed	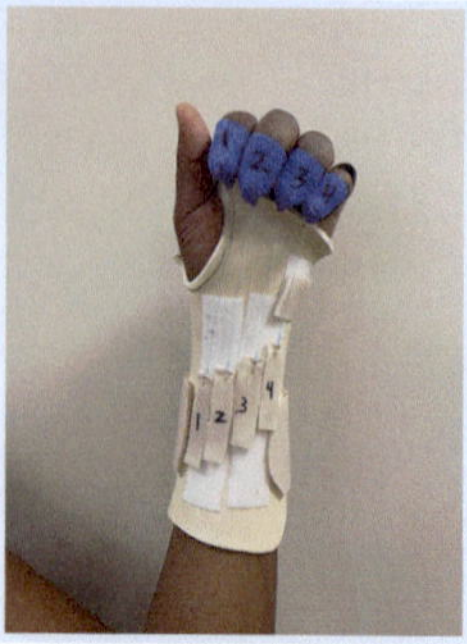
Blocking orthosis	• Used to isolate motion at the IP's during AROM depending on length of orthosis used • Addresses intrinsic stiffness	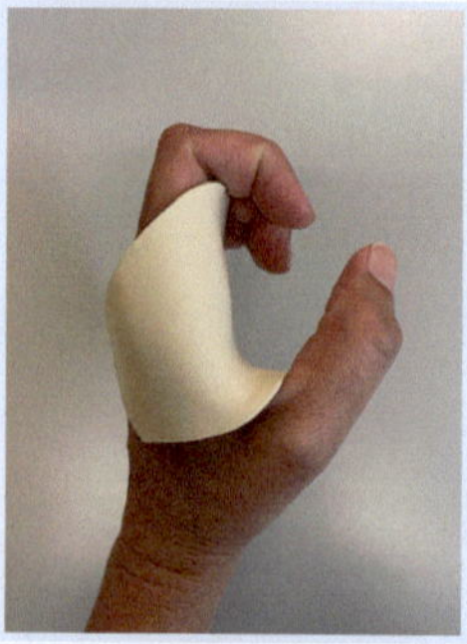
Relative motion orthosis	• Used to manage lack of PIP extension/contracture by facilitating length of the extensor hood and lumbricals while relaxing the FDP	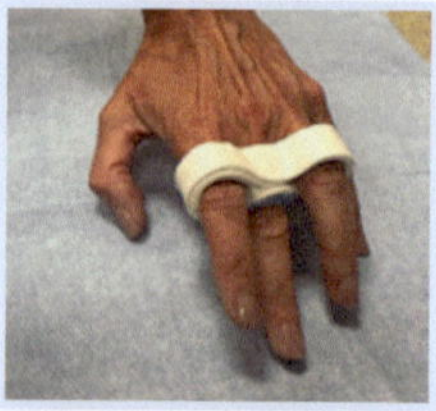
aka: Reverse Yoke		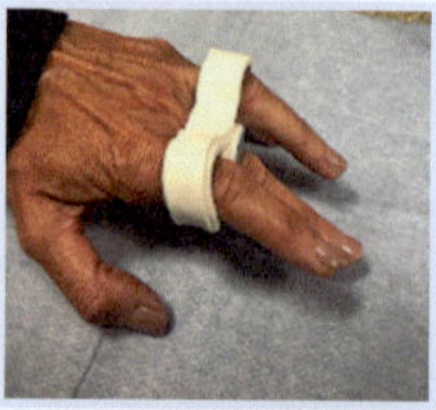
Serial orthosis	• Used to progressively lengthen tissues over time when contracture is present • Typically, remodeled weekly	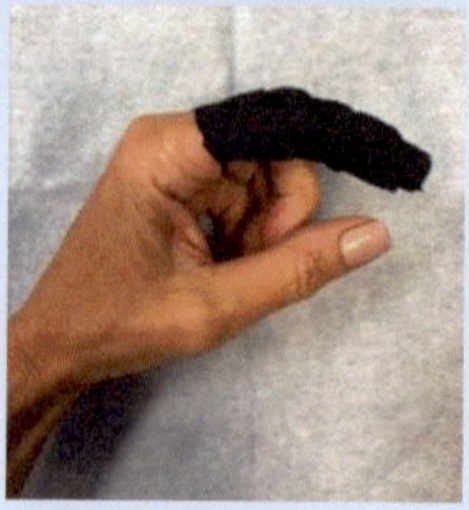

References [21, 27, 51, 55, 59, 62–67]

- **Dynamic Orthosis**—Typically a static orthosis with elastic (dynamic) components that apply increasing pressure and angles of force to stiff joints in order to increase length of tissue with a low load prolonged stretch can also be used to allow active assist motion or resistive exercise against the elastic components [62]. *Example: LMB orthosis for PIP extension.*
- **Static Progressive Orthosis**—Use of static components such as turnbuckles and strings in order to apply consistent pressure and angles of force to stiff joints in order to increase the length of tissue with a low load prolonged stretch [62]. *Example: Static progressive finger flexion orthosis.*

As the patient progresses through their rehabilitation, they may benefit from one or several orthoses in order to meet their rehabilitation goals. Both tissue healing and quality of collagen fibers help to determine which orthosis may be most appropriate at a given time during the process [65]. A static orthosis may be most appropriate post-op to support the healing structure, prevent contracture, and reduce pain [64], while a dynamic or static progressive orthosis is more beneficial to gain range of motion in the latter fibroblastic and remodeling phases when stiffness is more prevalent and collagen fibers are more dense [27]. Too much tissue stress, and it may re-trigger an inflammatory response, which will in turn create more fibrotic tissue [27]. A hand therapist will be able to help determine what type of orthosis may be beneficial during each stage of rehabilitation and educate the patient on donning and doffing as well as appropriate wear schedules in order to maximize potential gains.

L-codes are billing codes used by CMS; their descriptors are simple and useful for determining the general shape of an orthosis both for fabrication referrals and for determining appropriate billing [61]. The first letter of each body part being supported followed by an "O" for orthosis is a universal way to describe orthoses [62]. For example, FO would refer to a non-articulating finger orthosis, and WHO refers to an articulating wrist, hand, orthosis. This conveys to the therapist if a hand or forearm-based orthosis is being requested by the physician. As a rule, it is generally expected that the structures immediately above and below a fracture site will be immobilized. However, if a physician is confident in a repair or the fracture is non-displaced and stable, then a less restrictive orthosis may be considered as appropriate. For example, a nondisplaced metacarpal midshaft fracture may be treated with a simple non-articulating cuff orthosis or an HO (hand orthosis). This technique provides 3 point pressure anterior and posterior to the fracture over the length of the metacarpals and relies on the stabilizing capacity of the intrinsic muscles in lieu of a more restrictive orthosis (see Table 22.7) [51]. Below are some additional considerations for the patient's orthosis.

- **Immobilization**—The orthosis should only support the necessary structures for fracture healing and never immobilize unnecessarily. This allows for proximal and distal gliding of structures and generally improves compliance with patient wear of orthosis. During fabrication, the skin creases of non-immobilized joints should be fully visible in order to ensure movement at these joints [21].

- **Position of Hand and Wrist**—Following a fracture, the metacarpophalangeal joints should be placed in a flexed position of 70–90° in order to prevent shortening of the collateral ligaments and extension contracture or also known as safe position. The interphalangeal joints should be placed at 0° to prevent flexion contracture of the PIPs unless there is injury to the volar plate. The wrist may be placed in a comfortable 20° of extension to place in a position of function and prevent compression of structures at this level [21].
- **Strap Application**—These should enhance the intended purpose of the orthosis while respecting the delicate underlying anatomical structures, especially arteries, veins, and nerves [64]. Straps should be wide to distribute pressure and are typically applied over joints and may also have additional straps proximal and distal to prevent unnecessary motion and migration of the orthosis.
- **Pressure Points and Edema**—The extremity will change form throughout the healing process, and therefore the orthosis will need to be modified accordingly. Bony prominences are especially susceptible to pressure sores and can lead to skin breakdown if left unattended. An exceptionally edematous hand is at risk for poor lymphatic drainage with improper application of tight thin strapping, forming a sort of tourniquet effect [64]. The strap application and positioning of orthosis should be monitored at follow-up appointments by both physicians and therapists.

When referring a patient to a hand therapist, clear interprofessional communication is key for ensuring optimal outcomes. At a minimum, referrals should include a detailed description of the injured body part and extent of injury, any surgery performed and date, precautions, and the specific requested orthosis [59]. In complex cases, it may be beneficial to directly call the therapist to discuss details of the patient's case. If direct communication is not an option, then a completed surgical report will provide critical information for the therapist to consider during evaluation and orthosis fabrication. Factors such as open wounds or external wires can be accommodated during orthosis fabrication with creative solutions, e.g., blowing out the material with a hot gun or creating bridges with extra material. Additional information that is beneficial for patient care includes relaying the exact location of the fracture, the surgeon's confidence in stabilization, and any additional structures injured. Upon evaluation, if the therapist believes there is an orthosis that will be more suitable, then they should reach out to the referring physician to discuss an alternative option and adjust the plan of care accordingly. As stated, prior, when a therapist does not have all the information needed to make informed clinical decisions, then they will typically default to the most conservative treatment and orthosis fabrication approach. This can compromise the care and progress of the patient's rehabilitation, especially if unnecessary joints are immobilized. A good working interprofessional relationship and communication is key to ensuring an appropriate orthosis choice, fabrication, fit, wear, and care for a patient's successful outcome.

> **Clinical Considerations**
> - The decision to include the IPs with metacarpal and proximal phalanx fractures is dependent on fracture stability, patient factors, and surgeon's preference. However, unaffected joints should be left free when possible to avoid secondary contractures.
> - Thermoplastic material comes in a wide variety of options in order to suit your patient's needs, including thickness, perforation, memory, as well as color.

References

1. Sebastin S, Chung K, Ono S. Overview of finger, hand, and wrist fractures. UpToDate. https://www.uptodate.com/contents/overview-of-finger-hand-and-wrist-fractures. Accessed 27 Jul 2021.
2. Beleckas CM, Wright M, Prather H, Chamberlain A, Guattery J, Calfee RP. Relative prevalence of anxiety and depression in patients with upper extremity conditions. J Hand Surg [Am]. 2018;43(6):571.e1–8.
3. Asht.org. What we do. 2016. https://www.asht.org/about/what-we-do. Accessed 4 Aug 2021.
4. Weinstock-Zlotnick G, Mehta SP. A systematic review of the benefits of occupation-based intervention for patients with upper extremity musculoskeletal disorders. J Hand Ther. 2019;32(2):141–52.
5. Case-Smith J. Outcomes in hand rehabilitation using occupational therapy services. Am J Occup Ther. 2003;57(5):499–506.
6. Yakobina SC, Yakobina SR, Harrison-Weaver S. War, what is it good for? Historical contribution of the military and war to occupational therapy and hand therapy. J Hand Ther. 2008;21(2):106–13.
7. Pendergast Lauckhart K, Kasch M. The spirit of our creators. ASHT Times. 2002;9(1):3.
8. Htcc.org. Hand therapy certification commission - who is a CHT. https://www.htcc.org/consumer-information/the-cht-credential/who-is-a-cht. Accessed 4 Aug 2021.
9. Bano KY, Kahlon RS. Radial head fractures—advanced techniques in surgical management and rehabilitation. J Hand Ther. 2006;19(2):114–36.
10. Valdes K, Szekeres M, MacDermid JC. Hand therapists report perceived differences in patient referrals from hand surgeons vs other referral sources: a survey study. J Hand Ther. 2017;30(3):314–9.
11. American Occupational Therapy Association. Occupational therapy practice framework: domain and process—fourth edition. Am J Occup Ther. 2020;74(Suppl 2):7412410010.
12. Rodrick J. Treatment of post-surgical edema in the orthopedic patient—a case report. 2014
13. Sorenson MK. The edematous hand. Phys Ther. 1989;69(12):1059–64.
14. Howard SB, Krishnagiri S. The use of manual edema mobilization for the reduction of persistent edema in the upper limb. J Hand Ther. 2001;14(4):291–301.
15. Miller LK, Jerosch-Herold C, Shepstone L. Effectiveness of edema management techniques for subacute hand edema: a systematic review. J Hand Ther. 2017;30(4):432–46.
16. Artzberger S. Hand manual edema mobilization: overview of a new concept in hand edema reduction. E-Doc SAJHT. 2003;1:1.
17. Bracciano AG. Physical agent modalities. Thorofare, NJ: SLACK; 2008.
18. Zuther JE, Norton S. Lymphedema management: the comprehensive guide for practitioners. New York, NY: Thieme; 2013.
19. Villeco JP. Edema: a silent but important factor. J Hand Ther. 2012;25(2):153–62.
20. Shier B. The impact of lymphedema on occupational performance, an opportunity for occupational therapy. 2013.

21. Hardy MA. Principles of metacarpal and phalangeal fracture management: a review of rehabilitation concepts. J Orthop Sports Phys Ther. 2004;34(12):781–99.

22. Krop PN. Fractures: general principles of surgical management. In: Mackin EJ, Callahan AD, Skirven TM, Schneider LH, Osterman AL, editors. Rehabilitation of the hand and upper extremity. St. Louis, MO: Mosby; 2002. p. 371–9.

23. LaStayo PC, Winters KM, Hardy M. Fracture healing: bone healing, fracture management, and current concepts related to the hand. J Hand Ther. 2003;16(2):81–93.

24. Ghiasi MS, Chen J, Vaziri A, Rodriguez EK, Nazarian A. Bone fracture healing in mechano-biological modeling: a review of principles and methods. Bone Rep. 2017;6:87–100.

25. Loi F, Córdova LA, Pajarinen J, Lin TH, Yao Z, Goodman SB. Inflammation, fracture and bone repair. Bone. 2016;86:119–30.

26. Hays PL, Rozental TD. Rehabilitative strategies following hand fractures. Hand Clin. 2013;29(4):585–600.

27. Glasgow C, Tooth LR, Fleming J. Mobilizing the stiff hand: combining theory and evidence to improve clinical outcomes. J Hand Ther. 2010;23(4):392–401.

28. MacDermid JC, Roth JH, Richards RS. Pain and disability reported in the year following a distal radius fracture: a cohort study. BMC Musculoskelet Disord. 2003;4(1):1–3.

29. Dekkers MK, Søballe K. Activities and impairments in the early stage of rehabilitation after Colles' fracture. Disabil Rehabil. 2004;26(11):662–8.

30. Dilek B, Ayhan C, Yagci G, Yakut Y. Effectiveness of the graded motor imagery to improve hand function in patients with distal radius fracture: a randomized controlled trial. J Hand Ther. 2018;31(1):2–9.

31. Maruyama M, Rhee C, Utsunomiya T, Zhang N, Ueno M, Yao Z, Goodman SB. Modulation of the inflammatory response and bone healing. Front Endocrinol. 2020;11:386.

32. Bongiorno L. Explain pain. 2020. https://www.noigroup.com/.

33. Dubin AE, Patapoutian A. Nociceptors: the sensors of the pain pathway. J Clin Invest. 2010;120(11):3760–72.

34. Fedorczyk JM, Barbe MF. Pain management: principles of therapists' intervention. In: Mackin EJ, Callahan AD, Skirven TM, Schneider LH, Osterman AL, editors. Rehabilitation of the hand and upper extremity. St. Louis, MO: Mosby; 2002. p. 1725–41.

35. Hamasaki T, Pelletier R, Bourbonnais D, Harris P, Choinière M. Pain-related psychological issues in hand therapy. J Hand Ther. 2018;31(2):215–26.

36. Koman LA, Smith BP, Smith TL. Reflex sympathetic dystrophy (complex regional pain syndromes-types 1 and 2). In: Mackin EJ, Callahan AD, Skirven TM, Schneider LH, Osterman AL, editors. Rehabilitation of the hand and upper extremity. St. Louis, MO: Mosby; 2002. p. 1707–23.

37. Mitchell SA, Majuta LA, Mantyh PW. New insights in understanding and treating bone fracture pain. Curre Osteopor Rep. 2018;16(4):325–32.

38. Hsu JR, Mir H, Wally MK, Seymour RB. Clinical practice guidelines for pain management in acute musculoskeletal injury. J Orthop Trauma. 2019;33(5):e158.

39. Merkle SL, Sluka KA, Frey-Law LA. The interaction between pain and movement. J Hand Ther. 2020;33(1):60–6.

40. Roh YH, Noh JH, Oh JH, Gong HS, Baek GH. Retraction notice. To what degree do pain-coping strategies affect joint stiffness and functional outcomes in patients with hand fractures? Clin Orthop Relat Res. 2020;478(11):2687.

41. Cochrane SK, Calfee RP, Stonner MM, Dale AM. The relationship between depression, anxiety, and pain interference with therapy referral and utilization among patients with hand conditions. J Hand Ther. 2022;35:24.

42. Freeland AE, Hardy MA, Singletary S. Rehabilitation for proximal phalangeal fractures. J Hand Ther. 2003;16(2):129–42.

43. Kazmers NH, Fragomen AT, Rozbruch SR. Prevention of pin site infection in external fixation: a review of the literature. Strat Trauma Limb Reconstr. 2016;11(2):75–85.

44. Ferreira N, Marais LC. Prevention and management of external fixator pin track sepsis. Strat Trauma Limb Reconstr. 2012;7(2):67–72.

45. Solari M, Kapur B, Benjamin-Laing H, Klass BR, Cheung G, Brown DJ. Reducing the incidence of pin site infection in hand surgery with the use of a protocol from Ilizarov. J Hand Surg. 2021;46:482.

46. Smith MA, Dahlen NR, Bruemmer A, Davis S, Heishman C. Clinical practice guideline surgical site infection prevention. Orthop Nurs. 2013;32(5):242–8.

47. Lyngcoln A, Taylor N, Pizzari T, Baskus K. The relationship between adherence to hand therapy and short-term outcome after distal radius fracture. J Hand Ther. 2005;18(1):2–8.

48. Bachmann C, Oesch P, Bachmann S. Recommendations for improving adherence to home-based exercise: a systematic review. Physikalische Medizin, Rehabilitationsmedizin, Kurortmedizin. 2018;28(1):20–31.

49. Lambert TE, Harvey LA, Avdalis C, Chen LW, Jeyalingam S, Pratt CA, Tatum HJ, Bowden JL, Lucas BR. An app with remote support achieves better adherence to home exercise programs than paper handouts in people with musculoskeletal conditions: a randomised trial. J Physiother. 2017;63(3):161–7.

50. Argent R, Daly A, Caulfield B. Patient involvement with home-based exercise programs: can connected health interventions influence adherence? JMIR mHealth uHealth. 2018;6(3):e47.

51. Toemen A, Midgley R. Hand therapy management of metacarpal fractures: an evidence-based patient pathway. Hand Ther. 2010;15(4):87–93.

52. Haughton DN, Jordan D, Malahias M, Hindocha S, Khan W. Suppl 1: principles of hand fracture management. Open Orthopaed J. 2012;6:43.

53. Oetgen ME, Dodds SD. Non-operative treatment of common finger injuries. Curr Rev Musculoskel Med. 2008;1(2):97–102.

54. Diaz-Garcia R, Waljee JF. Current management of metacarpal fractures. Hand Clin. 2013;29(4):507–18.

55. Cooper C, Wietlisbach CM. Fundamentals of hand therapy. St. Louis, MO: Mosby; 2014.

56. Keller MM, Barnes R, Brandt C, Hepworth LM. Hand rehabilitation programmes for second to fifth metacarpal fractures: a systematic literature review. S Afr J Physiother. 2021;77(1):1536.

57. Rajesh G, Ip WY, Chow SP, Fung BK. Dynamic treatment for proximal phalangeal fracture of the hand. J Orthop Surg. 2007;15(2):211–5.

58. Cannon NM. Rehabilitation approaches for distal and middle phalanx fractures of the hand. J Hand Ther. 2003;16(2):105–16.

59. Gallagher KG, Blackmore S, Corbin S, Feldscher S. Intra articular hand fractures and joint injuries: Part 2 - Therapy management. In: Rehabilitation of the hand and upper extremity. 7th ed. Philadelphia, PA: Elsevier; 2021. p. 322–44.

60. McNemar TB, Howell JW, Chang E. Management of metacarpal fractures. J Hand Ther. 2003;16(2):143–51.

61. Asht.org. Coding. 2016. https://www.asht.org/practice/durable-medical-equipment-dme/orthotics/coding. Accessed 4 Aug 2021.

62. Jacobs MLA, Austin NM. Orthotic intervention for the hand and upper extremity; Fabrication process manual for Orthotic intervention for the hand and upper extremity. Philadelphia, PA: Lippincott Williams & Wilkins; 2021.

63. McKee P, Rivard A. Foundations of orthotic intervention. In: Rehabilitation of the hand and upper extremity. 6th ed. Philadelphia, PA: Elsevier; 2011. p. 1565–81.

64. Colditz J. Therapist's management of the stiff hand. In: Rehabilitation of the hand and upper extremity. 6th ed. Philadelphia, PA: Elsevier; 2011. p. 894–921.

65. Flowers KR. A proposed decision hierarchy for splinting the stiff joint, with an emphasis on force application parameters. J Hand Ther. 2002;15(2):158–62.

66. Chinchalkar SJ, Pipicelli JG. Addressing extensor digitorum communis adherence after metacarpal fracture with the use of a circumferential fracture brace. J Hand Ther. 2009;22(4):377–81.

67. Feehan LM. Therapy management of extraarticular hand fractures. In: Rehabilitation of the hand and upper extremity. 7th ed. Philadelphia, PA: Elsevier; 2021. p. 295–309.

Index